# Tumor Board Review

# Tumor Board Review

## Guideline and Case Reviews in Oncology

### SECOND EDITION

*Editors*

**Robert F. Todd III, MD, PhD**
Margaret M. Alkek Distinguished Chair of Medicine
Baylor College of Medicine
Houston, Texas

**Kathleen A. Cooney, MD**
Frances and Victor Ginsberg Professor of Hematology/Oncology
Chief, Division of Hematology/Oncology
Professor of Internal Medicine and Urology
University of Michigan Medical School;
Deputy Director, Cancer Clinical Services
University of Michigan Comprehensive Cancer Center
Ann Arbor, Michigan

**Teresa G. Hayes, MD, PhD**
Associate Professor of Medicine
Director, Hematology/Oncology Fellowship Program
Baylor College of Medicine
Houston, Texas

**Martha Pritchett Mims, MD, PhD**
Dan L. Duncan Professor
Chief, Section of Hematology/Oncology
Associate Director for Clinical Research
Dan L. Duncan Cancer Center
Baylor College of Medicine
Houston, Texas

**Francis P. Worden, MD**
Professor of Internal Medicine
Director, Hematology/Oncology Fellowship Program
University of Michigan Medical School
Ann Arbor, Michigan

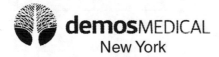
**demos**MEDICAL
New York

Visit our website at www.demosmedical.com

ISBN: 978-1-62070-060-0
E-book ISBN: 978-1-61705-223-1

Acquisitions Editor: Rich Winters
Compositor: Newgen Knowledge Works

Medicine is an ever-changing science. Research and clinical experience are continually expanding our knowledge, in particular our understanding of proper treatment and drug therapy. The authors, editors, and publisher have made every effort to ensure that all information in this book is in accordance with the state of knowledge at the time of production of the book. Nevertheless, the authors, editors, and publisher are not responsible for errors or omissions or for any consequences from application of the information in this book and make no warranty, expressed or implied, with respect to the contents of the publication. Every reader should examine carefully the package inserts accompanying each drug and should carefully check whether the dosage schedules mentioned therein or the contraindications stated by the manufacturer differ from the statements made in this book. Such examination is particularly important with drugs that are either rarely used or have been newly released on the market.

Library of Congress Cataloging-in-Publication Data
Tumor board review: guideline and case reviews in oncology / editors, Robert F. Todd, III, Kathleen A. Cooney, Teresa G. Hayes, Martha Pritchett Mims, Francis P. Worden. — Second edition.
    p. ; cm.
  Includes bibliographical references and index.
  ISBN 978-1-62070-060-0 — ISBN 978-1-61705-223-1 (e-book)
  I. Todd, Robert F., III, editor. II. Cooney, Kathleen A., editor. III. Hayes, Teresa G., editor. IV. Mims, Martha Pritchett, editor. V. Worden, Francis P., editor.
  [DNLM: 1. Neoplasms—Case Reports. 2. Neoplasms—Practice Guideline. 3. Evidence-Based Medicine—Case Reports. 4. Evidence-Based Medicine—Practice Guideline. QZ 200]

RC254
616.99′4—dc23                                                                                          2014040453

Special discounts on bulk quantities of Demos Medical Publishing books are available to corporations, professional associations, pharmaceutical companies, health care organizations, and other qualifying groups. For details, please contact:

Special Sales Department
Demos Medical Publishing
11 West 42nd Street, 15th Floor
New York, NY 10036
Phone: 800–532-8663 or 212–683-0072
Fax: 212-941-7842
E-mail: specialsales@demosmedical.com

Printed in the United States of America by Bradford & Bigelow.
14 15 16 17 / 5 4 3 2 1

# Contents

# Contributors

Matthew L. Anderson, MD, PhD
Assistant Professor of Obstetrics and Gynecology
Director of Clinical Research (Gynecology)
Baylor College of Medicine
Houston, Texas

Dana E. Angelini, MD
Fellow, Division of Hematology/Oncology
Department of Internal Medicine
University of Michigan Medical School
Ann Arbor, Michigan

Ahmed Awais, MD
Staff Physician
Callahan Cancer Center
North Platte, Nebraska

Diego J. Bedoya, MD
Clearview Cancer Institute
Hunstville, Alabama

Kavitha Beedupalli, MD
Fellow, Section of Hematology/Oncology
Department of Medicine
Baylor College of Medicine
Houston, Texas

Dale Bixby, MD, PhD
Assistant Professor of Internal Medicine
Division of Hematology/Oncology
University of Michigan Medical School
Ann Arbor, Michigan

Mariela Blum, MD
Assistant Professor
Department of Gastrointestinal Medical Oncology
Division of Cancer Medicine
University of Texas MD Anderson Cancer Center
Houston, Texas

Catherine M. Bollard, MD, FRACP, FRCPA
Professor of Pediatrics and Microbiology, Immunology
    and Tropical Medicine
Department of Pediatrics
The George Washington University;
Department of Blood and Marrow Transplantation
Children's National Health System
Washington, DC

Ronald J. Buckanovich, MD, PhD
Associate Professor of Internal Medicine
Division of Hematology/Oncology
Assistant Professor of Obstetrics and Gynecology
University of Michigan Medical School
Ann Arbor, Michigan

Shamail Butt, MD
Fellow, Section of Hematology/Oncology
Department of Medicine
Baylor College of Medicine
Houston, Texas

Michelina M. Cairo, MD
Texas Oncology
Houston, Texas

Elizabeth Yu Chiao, MD, MPH
Associate Professor of Medicine
Section of Infectious Disease
Baylor College of Medicine
Houston, Texas

Rashmi Chugh, MD
Associate Professor of Internal Medicine
Division of Hematology/Oncology
University of Michigan Medical School
Ann Arbor, Michigan

Erin F. Cobain, MD
Fellow, Division of Hematology/Oncology
Department of Internal Medicine
University of Michigan Medical School
Ann Arbor, Michigan

Lan Coffman, MD, PhD
Fellow, Division of Hematology/Oncology
Department of Internal Medicine
University of Michigan Medical School
Ann Arbor, Michigan

Kathleen A. Cooney, MD
Frances and Victor Ginsberg Professor of Hematology/Oncology
Chief, Division of Hematology/Oncology
Professor of Internal Medicine and Urology
University of Michigan Medical School;
Deputy Director, Cancer Clinical Services
University of Michigan Comprehensive Cancer Center
Ann Arbor, Michigan

Gerald S. Cyprus, MD
Professor of Medicine
Section of Hematology/Oncology
Baylor College of Medicine
Houston, Texas

Daniel Da Graca, MD
Kaiser Permanente
Hillsboro, Oregon

Elizabeth J. Davis, MD
Fellow, Division of Hematology/Oncology
Department of Internal Medicine
University of Michigan Medical School
Ann Arbor, Michigan

Sumana Devata, MD
Fellow, Division of Hematology/Oncology
Department of Internal Medicine
University of Michigan Medical School
Ann Arbor, Michigan

Concepcion R. Diaz-Arrastia, MD
Associate Professor of Obstetrics and Gynecology
Chief, Division of Gynecologic Oncology
Baylor College of Medicine
Houston, Texas

Irina Y. Dobrosotskaya, MD, PhD
Division of Hematology/Oncology
Henry Ford Hospital
Detroit, Michigan

Ahmed A. Eid, MD
Assistant Professor, Oncology
University of Texas MD Anderson Cancer Center
Houston, Texas

Ray Esper, MD, PhD
Fellow, Division of Hematology/Oncology
Department of Internal Medicine
University of Michigan Medical School
Ann Arbor, Michigan

Shan Guo, MD
Assistant Professor
Division of Oncology
University of Texas Health Science Center Medical School
Houston, Texas

Megan Rist Haymart, MD
Assistant Professor of Internal Medicine
Division of Endocrinology
University of Michigan Medical School
Ann Arbor, Michigan

Jesus H. Hermosillo-Rodriguez, MD
Fellow, Section of Hematology/Oncology
Department of Medicine
Baylor College of Medicine
Houston, Texas

Leonel F. Hernandez-Aya, MD
Fellow, Division of Hematology/Oncology
Department of Internal Medicine
University of Michigan Medical School
Ann Arbor, Michigan

Maha H. Hussain, MD, FACP, FASCO
Cis Maisel Professor of Oncology
Division of Hematology/Oncology
Professor of Internal Medicine and Urology
University of Michigan Medical School;
Associate Director for Clinical Research
University of Michigan Comprehensive Cancer Center
Ann Arbor, Michigan

Kunal C. Kadakia, MD
Fellow, Division of Hematology/Oncology
Department of Internal Medicine
University of Michigan Medical School
Ann Arbor, Michigan

Gregory P. Kalemkerian, MD
Professor of Internal Medicine
Division of Hematology/Oncology
University of Michigan Medical School
Ann Arbor, Michigan

Jasmine Kamboj, MBBS
Fellow, Section of Hematology/Oncology
Department of Medicine
Baylor College of Medicine
Houston, Texas

Ghana Kang, MD
Fellow, Section of Hematology and Oncology
Department of Medicine
Baylor College of Medicine
Houston, Texas

Rami N. Khoriaty, MD
Clinical Lecturer of Internal Medicine
Division of Hematology/Oncology
University of Michigan Medical School
Ann Arbor, Michigan

Jenny J. Kim, MD
Assistant Professor of Oncology
Johns Hopkins Sidney Kimmel Comprehensive Cancer Center
Baltimore, Maryland

Priya Gomathi Kumaravelu, MD
Fellow, Section of Hematology/Oncology
Department of Medicine
Baylor College of Medicine
Houston, Texas

Christopher D. Lao, MD, MPH
Associate Professor of Internal Medicine
Division of Hematology/Oncology
University of Michigan Medical School
Ann Arbor, Michigan

Daniel Lebovic, MD
Assistant Professor of Internal Medicine
Division of Hematology/Oncology
University of Michigan Medical School
Ann Arbor, Michigan

Dongxin Liu, MD
Houston Cancer Institute
Houston, Texas

Premal Lulla, MD, MBBS
Chief Fellow, Section of Hematology/Oncology
Department of Medicine
Baylor College of Medicine
Houston, Texas

Garrett R. Lynch, MD
Professor of Medicine
Section of Hematology/Oncology
Baylor College of Medicine
Houston, Texas

John Magenau, MD
Assistant Professor of Internal Medicine
Division of Hematology/Oncology
University of Michigan Medical School
Ann Arbor, Michigan

Sami N. Malek, MD
Associate Professor of Internal Medicine
Division of Hematology/Oncology
University of Michigan Medical School
Ann Arbor, Michigan

Binu Malhotra, MD
Medical Oncologist/Hematologist
Covenant Cancer Care Center
Saginaw, Michigan

Atisha P. Manhas, MD
Texas Oncology
Methodist Dallas Cancer Center
Dallas, Texas

Abhishek Marballi, MD
Fellow, Section of Hematology/Oncology
Department of Medicine
Baylor College of Medicine
Houston, Texas

Andrei Marconescu, MD
Fellow, Section of Hematology/Oncology
Department of Medicine
Baylor College of Medicine
Houston, Texas

Kevin McDonnell, MD, PhD
Clinical Instructor of Medicine
University of Southern California
Los Angeles, California

Karen McLean, MD
Assistant Professor of Obstetrics and Gynecology
University of Michigan Medical School
Ann Arbor, Michigan

Courtney N. Miller-Chism, MD
Assistant Professor of Medicine
Section of Hematology/Oncology
Baylor College of Medicine
Houston, Texas

Martha Pritchett Mims, MD, PhD
Dan L. Duncan Professor
Chief, Section of Hematology/Oncology
Associate Director for Clinical Research
Dan L. Duncan Cancer Center
Baylor College of Medicine
Houston, Texas

Colin J. Mooney, MD
Staff Physician
Kramer Cancer Center
West Bend, Wisconsin

Benjamin L. Musher, MD
Assistant Professor of Medicine
Section of Hematology/Oncology
Baylor College of Medicine
Houston, Texas

Kiran Naqvi, MD
Fellow, Section of Hematology/Oncology
Department of Medicine
Baylor College of Medicine
Houston, Texas

Pamela New, MD
Associate Professor of Clinical Neurosurgery
Department of Neurosurgery/Neuro-Oncology
The Methodist Hospital Research Institute/Weil Cornell
   Medical Center
Houston, Texas

Polly A. Niravath, MD
Assistant Professor of Medicine
Lester and Sue Smith Breast Center
Baylor College of Medicine
Houston, Texas

Alexander T. Pearson, MD, PhD
Fellow, Division of Hematology/Oncology
Department of Internal Medicine
University of Michigan Medical School
Ann Arbor, Michigan

**Vedran Radojcic, MD**
Fellow, Division of Hematology/Oncology
Department of Internal Medicine
University of Michigan Medical School
Ann Arbor, Michigan

**Yuval Raizen, MD**
Private Practice Oncology
Oncology Consultants
Houston, Texas

**Nithya Ramnath, MBBS**
Associate Professor of Internal Medicine
Division of Hematology/Oncology
University of Michigan Medical School;
Associate Section Chief, Medical Oncology
Department of Internal Medicine
Ann Arbor Veterans Administration Health System
Ann Arbor, Michigan

**Carlos A. Ramos, MD**
Assistant Professor of Medicine
Section of Hematology/Oncology
Center for Cell and Gene Therapy
Baylor College of Medicine
Houston, Texas

**Bruce G. Redman, DO**
Professor of Internal Medicine
Division of Hematology/Oncology
University of Michigan Medical School
Ann Arbor, Michigan

**Mothaffar F. Rimawi, MD**
Associate Professor of Medicine
Clinical Director, Lester and Sue Smith Breast Center
Baylor College of Medicine
Houston, Texas

**Gustavo Rivero, MD**
Assistant Professor of Medicine
Section of Hematology/Oncology
Baylor College of Medicine
Houston, Texas

**Igor I. Rybkin, MD, PhD**
Senior Staff Oncologist
Josephine Ford Cancer Institute
Henry Ford Health System
Detroit, Michigan

**Assuntina G. Sacco, MD**
Assistant Professor of Medicine
Section of Hematology/Oncology
University of California, San Diego Moores Cancer Center
La Jolla, California

**Yvonne Sada, MD, MPH**
Assistant Professor of Medicine
Section of Hematology/Oncology
Baylor College of Medicine
Houston, Texas

**Benjamin Y. Scheier, MD**
Fellow, Division of Hematology/Oncology
Department of Internal Medicine
University of Michigan Medical School
Ann Arbor, Michigan

**Scott M. Schuetze, MD, PhD**
Professor of Internal Medicine
Divison of Hematology/Oncology
University of Michigan Medical School
Ann Arbor, Michigan

**Erlene K. Seymour, MD**
Fellow, Division of Hematology/Oncology
Department of Internal Medicine
University of Michigan Medical School
Ann Arbor, Michigan

**Ann W. Silk, MD**
Assistant Professor of Internal Medicine
Rutgers Cancer Institute of New Jersey
New Brunswick, New Jersey

**David C. Smith, MD**
Professor of Internal Medicine and Urology
Associate Chief, Division of Hematology/Oncology
University of Michigan Medical School
Ann Arbor, Michigan

**Moshe Talpaz, MD**
Alexander J. Trotman Professor of Leukemia Research
Division of Hematology/Oncology
Professor of Internal Medicine
University of Michigan Medical School;
Associate Director, Translational Research
University of Michigan Comprehensive Cancer Center
Ann Arbor, Michigan

**Muhammad A. Tarakji, MD**
Physician
Department of Hematology/Oncology
Presbyterian Cancer Center
Albuquerque, New Mexico

**Miho Teruya, MD, MPH**
Fellow, Section of Hematology/Oncology
Department of Medicine
Baylor College of Medicine
Houston, Texas

**Celestine S. Tung, MD**
Assistant Professor of Obstetrics and Gynecology
Division of Gynecologic Oncology
Baylor College of Medicine
Houston, Texas

**Mark M. Udden, MD**
Professor of Medicine
Section of Hematology/Oncology
Baylor College of Medicine
Houston, Texas

**Susan G. Urba, MD**
Professor of Internal Medicine
Division of Hematology/Oncology
University of Michigan Medical School
Ann Arbor, Michigan

**Janet Wang, MD**
Palo Alto Medical Foundation
Santa Cruz, California

**Yue C. Wang, MD**
Fellow, Section of Hematology/Oncology
Department of Medicine
Baylor College of Medicine
Houston, Texas

**Alissa A. Weber, MD**
Hematologist/Oncologist
Dean Health System
Madison, Wisconsin

**Josh Wilfong, DO**
Fellow, Division of Hematology/Oncology
Department of Internal Medicine
University of Michigan Medical School
Ann Arbor, Michigan

**Marian Yvette Williams-Brown, MD, MMS, FACOG**
Assistant Professor of Obstetrics and Gynecology
Division of Gynecologic Oncology
Baylor College of Medicine
Houston, Texas

**Francis P. Worden, MD**
Professor of Internal Medicine
Director, Hematology/Oncology Fellowship Program
University of Michigan Medical School
Ann Arbor, Michigan

**Sarvari Yellapragada, MD**
Assistant Professor of Medicine
Section of Hematology/Oncology
Baylor College of Medicine
Houston, Texas

**Aihua Edward Yen, MD**
Assistant Professor of Medicine
Section of Hematology/Oncology
Baylor College of Medicine
Houston, Texas

**Musa Yilmaz, MD**
Fellow, Section of Hematology/Oncology
Department of Medicine
Baylor College of Medicine
Houston, Texas

**Ruiling Xu Yuan, MD**
Fellow, Section of Hematology/Oncology
Department of Medicine
Baylor College of Medicine
Houston, Texas

**Mark M. Zalupski, MD**
Professor of Internal Medicine
Division of Hematology/Oncology
University of Michigan Medical School
Ann Arbor, Michigan

**Jingsong Zhang, MD, PhD**
Assistant Member
Department of Genitourinary Oncology
Department of Cancer Imaging and Metabolism
Chemical Biology and Molecular Medicine Program
Moffitt Cancer Center
Tampa, Florida

**Jun Zhang, MD**
Assistant Professor of Medicine
Section of Hematology/Oncology
Baylor College of Medicine
Houston, Texas

**Paul Zhang, MD, PhD**
Attending Physician
Integrative Cancer Treatment Center
Houston Medical Center
Houston, Texas

# Preface to the Second Edition

Thankfully, medical oncology is a rapidly evolving field, and significant progress has been made in the diagnosis and management of several forms of cancer in the 3 years since the publication of the first edition. In the second edition of *Tumor Board Review: Guideline and Case Reviews in Oncology*, we have maintained the same case-based format introduced in the first edition, but have updated the "Evidence-Based Case Discussion" of each case to include the most recent advances in diagnosis and treatment that have emerged from recently published clinical trials. Most prominent among the diagnostic advances is the further identification of genetic mutations that point to selective anticancer drug sensitivity (e.g., Braf mutations in melanoma). Similarly, the results of several phase III clinical trials have demonstrated the efficacy of a growing number of "targeted agents" in the treatment of several solid tumors and hematological malignancies. Accordingly, the content of the second edition represents our best effort to incorporate and highlight the latest, clinically relevant knowledge in our field.

The second edition continues to represent a joint effort between oncology faculty and subspecialty fellows based at the Baylor College of Medicine (Houston, Texas) and the University of Michigan Medical School (Ann Arbor, Michigan). Both institutions are the homes of NCI-designated Cancer Centers: the Dan L. Duncan Cancer Center and the University of Michigan Comprehensive Cancer Center, and contributors to the second edition were selected based on their interest and expertise in the relevant cancers. The editors gratefully acknowledge the contributions of our trainee and faculty authors, as well as the support staff who assisted in the preparation of each chapter. We also thank the editorial staff of Demos Medical Publishing, particularly Richard Winters, executive editor (who originated the tumor board concept), and Joseph Stubenrauch, managing editor.

*Robert F. Todd III, MD, PhD*
*Kathleen A. Cooney, MD*
*Teresa G. Hayes, MD, PhD*
*Martha Pritchett Mims, MD, PhD*
*Francis P. Worden, MD*

# Preface to the First Edition

As physicians, we generally practice medicine on one patient at a time, focusing our knowledge base on the specific problems of each individual. As trainees, we are urged to learn as much as we can from each patient who provides a case-specific context for applying the broader body of information derived from textbooks, lectures, and other didactic materials. In the academic practice of oncology, we encourage our trainees to attend tumor boards, which, by applying the knowledge and expertise of relevant oncology specialists to the problems of individual patients, serve as a wonderful venue for learning the practice of oncology. The tumor board as a venue for learning was the concept we applied to the design of *Tumor Board Review: Guideline and Case Reviews in Oncology*. Each of the 32 chapters follows a uniform format: a concise summary of the epidemiology, risk factors, natural history, and pathology of each major organ-specific tumor type; an abbreviated display of the relevant staging (generally based on the *American Joint Commission on Cancer [AJCC] Staging Manual, 7th edition*); and several "tumor board-style" illustrative patient case summaries (representative of major stage categories of each tumor), each followed by an evidence-based case discussion that reviews the current guidelines and rationale for the diagnostic and therapeutic steps taken. Clearly, it was our intention to make the case summaries and accompanying evidence-based discussion (the latter including helpful management algorithms) the dominant focal point of the book. The authors of each chapter have endeavored to provide the most up-to-date evidence on which treatment decisions are based, including the latest advances in targeted cancer therapy.

We are hopeful that several categories of readers will find *Tumor Board Review* particularly useful, including oncology subspecialty trainees and practitioners who are preparing for subspecialty certification or recertification, respectively; trainees at all levels (e.g., medical students, residents, and subspecialty fellows) who are seeking a readable, case-based review of the relevant oncology literature; and oncologists in practice who are looking for a concise opportunity to refresh their knowledge across the broad field of medical oncology.

The development of *Tumor Board Review* was made possible by the combined efforts of selected subspecialty fellows and expert faculty of two academic institutions, the Baylor College of Medicine (Houston, Texas) and the University of Michigan Medical School (Ann Arbor, Michigan). The editors gratefully acknowledge the dedicated participation of our trainee and faculty authors, and the support staff of both academic centers, the latter including the invaluable editorial support of Ms. Leneva Moore at Baylor. The successful completion of this project was made possible by the editorial and publishing staff of Demos Medical Publishing, especially Richard Winters, executive editor (who originated the tumor board concept), and Dana Bigelow, production editor.

*Robert F. Todd III, MD, PhD*
*Kathleen A. Cooney, MD*
*Teresa G. Hayes, MD, PhD*
*Martha Pritchett Mims, MD, PhD*
*Francis P. Worden, MD*

# 1

# Head and Neck Cancer

ASSUNTINA G. SACCO, IRINA Y. DOBROSOTSKAYA, AND FRANCIS P. WORDEN

## EPIDEMIOLOGY, RISK FACTORS, NATURAL HISTORY, AND PATHOLOGY

Squamous cell carcinoma of the head and neck (SCCHN) accounts for about 3% of new cancers diagnosed in the United States each year, with roughly 3-fold higher incidence in men compared to women. The American Cancer Society estimated that about 55,000 Americans were diagnosed with SCCHN in 2014, and approximately 12,000 patients died of this disease in that year.

SCCHN is related to several environmental and lifestyle risk factors. Of these, tobacco exposure and alcohol consumption are the 2 main causes, and when combined, they increase the risk by about 100-fold compared to nonusers. Epstein-Barr virus (EBV) is present in a significant proportion of nasopharyngeal cancers, while carcinogenic strains of human papillomavirus (HPV) have been recognized as a major contributor to carcinogenesis, especially within the oropharynx (about 70% of squamous cell cancer [SCC] of tonsils and base of tongue). HPV-related cancers of the head and neck are more prevalent in younger patients (aged 40–60 years), whereas traditional smoking- and alcohol-related SCCHN is diagnosed more frequently in patients older than 60 years. HPV-associated oropharynx cancers tend to have a better prognosis for reasons that are not completely understood. This may reflect a difference in tumor biology or simply more favorable host factors such as younger age and fewer comorbidities (and therefore better tolerance of treatments).

Significant advances in the treatment of SCCHN have been possible due to progressive improvement in surgical techniques, radiation modalities, and chemotherapeutic regimens. The multimodality approach allows cure even in locally advanced, unresectable cancers. Furthermore, organ preservation is achievable in a considerable number of these patients. This is due to the good results that can be achieved with definitive chemoradiation in patients with locally advanced tumors. Patients with early-stage disease (stage I or II) without high-risk features are treated with a single-modality approach, either surgery or radiation, depending on which technique allows for better function preservation. Positive margins necessitate re-excision or radiation treatment in most cases. Adverse features such as extracapsular extension, vascular embolism, and perineural invasion should prompt consideration for adjuvant therapy.

Patients with locally advanced, curable disease are treated with surgery followed by radiation with or without chemotherapy, or with definitive chemoradiation. The latter is used for inoperable tumors or for organ-preservation purposes. Adjuvant chemoradiation is preferred over adjuvant radiation alone in patients with >2 positive lymph nodes (LNs), positive surgical margins, or nodal disease with extracapsular extension.

Induction chemotherapy followed by definitive locoregional treatment may be considered in a subset of patients with advanced nodal disease. Patients with metastatic or incurable, recurrent disease may benefit from palliative chemotherapy, depending on their functional status.

Because of the great heterogeneity among SCCHNs, treatment is based on the primary site of origin (see Table 1.1). For example, oral cavity tumors are treated primarily with surgery because advances in reconstruction using microvascular techniques have led to improved functional outcomes. Locally advanced oropharynx and nasopharynx SCC, on the other hand, are invariably treated with combined chemoradiation, and locally advanced larynx and hypopharynx cancers can be treated either with organ preservation approaches or total laryngectomy followed by radiation with or without chemotherapy.

**Table 1.1** Primary Sites of Origin for SCCHN

| Area | Components |
|---|---|
| Oral cavity | Lips, alveolar ridge, hard palate, buccal mucosa, anterior 2/3 tongue, floor of mouth, retromolar trigone |
| Oropharynx | Palatine tonsils, posterior 1/3 tongue, vallecula, lingual tonsil, midportion of posterior pharyngeal wall, inferior surface of soft palate, uvula |
| Nasal cavity | Nasal septum; mucosa of floor of nasal cavity; superior, middle, and inferior turbinates |
| Nasopharynx | Superior surface of soft palate, upper portion of posterior pharyngeal wall above the level of uvula |
| Hypopharynx | Postcricoid area, pyriform sinuses |
| Larynx | *Supraglottis*: Supra and infrahyoid epiglottis, aryepiglottic folds, arytenoids, false cords<br>*Glottis*: True vocal cords, anterior and posterior commissures, region 1 cm below plane of true cords<br>*Subglottis*: Region from 1 cm below true cords to the cervical trachea |

SCCHN, squamous cell cancer of the head and neck.

## STAGING

### Overview of Staging

The most useful classification subdivides SCCHN into early-stage (I–II), advanced but potentially curable (stage III–IVB), and incurable (stage IVC) disease, because the treatment differs significantly among these groups. Early-stage disease generally indicates primary tumor not >4 cm in size with no LN involvement. The exception is nasal cavity and ethmoid sinus (stage I or II allows invasion of some regional bony structures) and nasopharynx (stage II allows LN involvement). Advanced but potentially curable disease implies extensive local involvement and/or progressively more bulky LN disease. Incurable disease implies the presence of distant metastases.

### Site-Specific Staging for SCCHN

Table 1.2 provides staging of head and neck cancers (HNCs; derived from *National Comprehensive Cancer Network (NCCN) Clinical Practice Guidelines for Treatment of Head and Neck Cancers*, v.2.2014) (1).

**Table 1.2** Site-Specific Staging of Head and Neck Cancer

**Oral Cavity**

| | |
|---|---|
| Stage I | Tumor ≤2 cm, no LN involvement |
| Stage II | Tumor >2 cm but ≤4 cm, no LN involvement |
| Stage III | Tumor >4 cm with or without a single, ipsilateral LN ≤3 cm<br>*or*<br>A smaller tumor with involvement of a single, ipsilateral LN ≤3 cm |
| Stage IVA | Tumor may invade skin of face, cortical bone of the face but not the skull, may invade extrinsic tongue muscles, maxillary sinus, with or without LN involvement ≤6 cm<br>*or*<br>A smaller tumor with LN involvement ≥3 cm but ≤6 cm |
| Stage IVB | Tumor invades very deep such as masticator space, pterygoid plates, base of skull, encases carotid artery, with or without LN involvement (any size)<br>*or*<br>A smaller tumor with LN involvement >6 cm |
| Stage IVC | Distant metastases are present, irrespective of tumor size or LN involvement |

**Oropharynx**

| | |
|---|---|
| Stage I | Tumor ≤2 cm, no LN involvement |
| Stage II | Tumor >2 cm but ≤4 cm, no LN involvement |
| Stage III | Tumor >4 cm or involves lingual surface of epiglottis with or without a single, ipsilateral LN ≤3 cm<br>*or*<br>A smaller tumor with involvement of a single, ipsilateral LN ≤3 cm |
| Stage IVA | Tumor may invade larynx, hard palate, mandible, medial pterygoid space or extrinsic tongue muscles, with or without LN involvement ≤6 cm<br>*or*<br>A smaller tumor with LN involvement ≥3 cm but ≤6 cm |
| Stage IVB | Tumor may invade base of skull, pterygoid plates, lateral pterygoid muscle, extend to lateral nasopharynx or encase carotid arteries, with or without LN involvement (any size)<br>*or*<br>A smaller tumor with LN involvement >6 cm |
| Stage IVC | Distant metastases are present, irrespective of tumor size or LN involvement |

*(continued)*

**Table 1.2** Site-Specific Staging of Head and Neck Cancer (*continued*)

**Nasopharynx**

| | |
|---|---|
| Stage I | Tumor is limited to nasopharynx, nasal cavity, or oropharynx, no LN involvement |
| Stage II | Tumor may involve parapharyngeal space or be less extensive, unilateral involvement of cervical LN, or uni- or bilateral involvement of retropharyngeal LNs ≤6 cm |
| Stage III | Tumor extends into base of skull or paranasal sinuses and/or there is bilateral involvement of cervical or retropharyngeal LNs ≤6 cm |
| Stage IVA | Tumor may involve intracranial structures, cranial nerves, orbit, infratemporal fossa, masticator space, or hypopharynx and there may be bilateral involvement of cervical or retropharyngeal LNs ≤6 cm |
| Stage IVB | Any tumor size as above with LN >6 cm or involvement of LNs in supraclavicular fossa |
| Stage IVC | Distant metastases are present, irrespective of tumor size or LN involvement |

**Hypopharynx**

| | |
|---|---|
| Stage I | Tumor ≤2 cm and is limited to 1 subsite in hypopharynx, no LN involvement |
| Stage II | Tumor >2 cm but ≤4 cm and may extend to >1 subsite of hypopharynx, no LN involvement |
| Stage III | Tumor >4 cm or involves esophagus or causes fixation of hemilarynx with or without a single, ipsilateral LN ≤3 cm<br>*or*<br>A smaller tumor with involvement of a single, ipsilateral LN ≤3 cm |
| Stage IVA | Tumor invades thyroid/cricoid cartilage, hyoid bone, thyroid gland, esophagus or central compartment, with or without LN involvement ≤6 cm<br>*or*<br>A smaller tumor with LN involvement ≥3 cm but ≤6 cm |
| Stage IVB | Tumor may invade prevertebral fascia, encase carotid artery, involve mediastinal structures, with or without LN involvement (any size)<br>*or*<br>A smaller tumor with LN involvement >6 cm |
| Stage IVC | Distant metastases are present, irrespective of tumor size or LN involvement |

**Larynx**

| | |
|---|---|
| Stage I | Tumor is confined to 1 larynx site, normal vocal cord mobility, no LN involvement |
| Stage II | Tumor extends to include other larynx site, and/or with impaired vocal cord mobility, no LN involvement |
| Stage III | Tumor is limited to larynx with vocal cord fixation and/or invades any of the following: postcricoid area, pre-epiglottic tissues, paraglottic space, and/or minor thyroid cartilage erosion (inner cortex), with or without a single, ipsilateral LN ≤3 cm<br>*or*<br>A smaller tumor with involvement of a single, ipsilateral LN ≤3 cm |
| Stage IVA | Tumor invades cricoid or thyroid cartilage and/or invades extralaryngeal tissues (trachea, soft tissues of neck, deep extrinsic muscles of the tongue, strap muscles, thyroid, or esophagus), with or without LN involvement ≤6 cm<br>*or*<br>A smaller tumor with LN involvement ≥3 cm but ≤6 cm |
| Stage IVB | Tumor invades prevertebral space, encases the carotid artery, or invades mediastinal structures, with or without LN involvement (any size)<br>*or*<br>A smaller tumor with LN involvement >6 cm |
| Stage IVC | Distant metastases are present, irrespective of tumor size or LN involvement |

LN, lymph node.

## CASE SUMMARIES

### Locoregionally Advanced Disease

J.S. is a 56-year-old male who initially presented to his primary care physician 3 months after noticing a small, pea-sized right neck mass that subsequently started to grow. Treatment with antibiotics and steroids brought initial, short-lived relief, but then the neck mass further increased in size. He underwent fine-needle aspiration of his neck mass, which revealed undifferentiated SCC. A CT scan of his neck demonstrated multiple enlarged, necrotic LNs in the right cervical chain. J.S. deferred further medical and surgical management and pursued alternative treatment with herbal medications. His neck mass remained stable until 5 months after his initial presentation when it increased in size. He sought medical care after developing dysarthria, difficulty chewing, and a sensation of airway narrowing. J.S. had no other medical problem and did not take any medications. He had a 60-pack-year smoking history and a history of excessive alcohol consumption. His family history was noncontributory.

On physical examination, there was a palpable 8-cm firm, fixed conglomerate of LNs at levels I through V in his right neck, which were adherent to the sternocleidomastoid muscle. The remainder of his physical examination was unremarkable.

On fiberoptic examination, the right tonsil was enlarged, and there was a 4.5-cm area of fullness in the right glossotonsillar sulcus, tonsillar fossa, and the tongue base. This was biopsied and revealed an invasive, poorly differentiated non-keratinizing SCC. A full-body PET/CT and contrast CT scan of his neck revealed a 4-cm, $^{18}$F-fludeoxyglucose (FDG)-avid mass emanating from the right glossotonsillar sulcus that invaded tongue muscles and encased the right carotid artery. Multiple, enlarged, FDG-avid right neck LNs forming a 7-cm conglomerate mass were also noted. There was no evidence of distant disease.

## Evidence-Based Case Discussion

### Combined Chemoradiation

The aforementioned patient has T4b, N3, and M0 (stage IVB) SCC of the right tonsil. Given the nature of its carotid involvement, the tumor is unresectable, but still may be curable in 10–15% of patients. The current standard of care for such a tumor is definitive, concurrent chemoradiation, which employs a platinum-containing regimen. There is stronger evidence supporting the use of cisplatin versus carboplatin, and cisplatin (100 mg/m²) every 21 days with radiation, which is generally recommended. A carboplatin-based combination regimen (such as carboplatin–paclitaxel or carboplatin–FU) may be considered if toxicities of cisplatin are prohibitive. Cisplatin is more likely than carboplatin to cause neuropathy, hearing loss, and renal failure, whereas carboplatin has a higher risk of cytopenias, especially thrombocytopenia. Cisplatin is also more emetogenic when given in high doses (>80 mg/m²). Unlike cisplatin, carboplatin is generally used in combination with other drugs in the setting of concurrent chemoradiation. The most efficacious combinations include carboplatin with 5-FU or carboplatin with a taxane. In patients who are not candidates for platinum-based therapies (i.e., poor renal function or severe sensory neuropathy), cetuximab alone may be given as a radiosensitizing agent, although the efficacy of this targeted agent has not been compared directly to that of cisplatin with radiation. Recently, there has been a renewed interest in the addition of induction chemotherapy prior to definitive chemoradiation in an effort to improve survival outcomes.

### Induction Chemotherapy

The interest in induction chemotherapy for locally advanced HNC has undergone a revival. The rationale for its use is related to the possibility for better delivery of chemotherapy to the tumor tissue not yet affected by radiation and improved distant control. Historically, the treatment of such locally advanced SCCHN used to be confined to surgery and radiation therapy. Local control was difficult, and the pattern of recurrence was more frequently local than systemic. Furthermore, the site-specific differences in prognosis and treatment were not clear. More recently, better radiation techniques and surgical approaches improved local control and survival in such patients. However, there is still room for improvement in both local and distant disease control.

The earlier trials performed before the 1990s included mostly laryngeal cancer patients and showed that induction chemotherapy, when added to local control measures (either surgery or radiation), did not adversely affect survival and allowed superior organ preservation outcomes by reducing the need for extensive surgery (e.g., Veterans Affairs Laryngeal Cancer Study Group (2) study published in 1991). Similar results were seen in the RTOG 91–11 trial published in 2003. Of note, radiation therapy was not given concurrently with chemotherapy; this concept was introduced later. The earliest meta-analysis of the role of chemotherapy in HNC by the Meta-analysis of Chemotherapy in Head and Neck Cancer (MACH-NC) group evaluated 63 trials, including 10,741 previously untreated patients with various head and neck SCC locations treated between 1965 and 1993 (3). It showed improved survival with the addition of chemotherapy to local treatment (surgery or radiation or both) with absolute benefit of 4% at 2 and 5 years. The analysis of timing of chemotherapy showed that overall survival (OS) was better with concomitant, but not neoadjuvant or adjuvant chemotherapy versus local therapy alone. Subgroup analysis showed better survival with chemotherapy in patients younger than 61 years, males, Eastern Cooperative Oncology Group performance status (ECOG PS) 0 or 1, stage IV disease, with tumors of oral cavity, and marginally of hypopharynx. This contributed to the subsequent shift in treatment paradigm from radiation to chemoradiation, both as a definitive treatment in inoperable patients and part of adjuvant treatment after surgery. The overall analysis of induction chemotherapy did not show a survival benefit, except for platinum and 5-fluorouracil (5-FU)-based regimens (hazard ratio [HR] = 0.88, 0.79–0.97). An update to the aforementioned meta-analysis by the MACH-NC group was recently published (4). It analyzed an additional 24 new trials, to bring the total number of trials to 87 and number of patients to 16,485. It included analysis of 31 induction chemotherapy trials including 5311 patients. There was no survival advantage to induction chemotherapy (HR of death = 0.96, 0.9–1.02, P = .18), although the FU–platinum-based therapies once again proved to be better than other analyzed regimens (HR of death = 0.9, 0.82–0.99), and there was significant benefit for prevention of distant metastases (HR = 0.73, 0.61–0.88, P = .001). Subsequent phase III studies of advanced curable disease showed better survival with neoadjuvant cisplatin and 5-FU as well as improved locoregional control compared to local therapy alone (5–7). In a study by Paccagnella et al. (8), the induction chemotherapy group ($n$ = 118) received 4 cycles of cisplatin plus 5-FU followed by locoregional treatment: surgery followed by radiation in operable patients or radiation alone in inoperable patients. The comparison group ($n$ = 119) received locoregional treatment alone. There was a significantly lower rate of distant metastases in the induction chemo group for both operable and inoperable patients. However, the OS benefit from induction chemotherapy was limited to inoperable patients (at 3 years, OS was 24% vs. 10%, $P$ = .04). In this study, the majority of patients had oropharyngeal cancer (54–59%); they were younger than 70 years, most had stage IVA or B disease (63–64%), and most patients were inoperable (71–73%). A later update by Zorat et al. (9) confirmed these findings: The OS benefit was limited to inoperable patients (10-year survival = 16% vs. 6%, $P$ = .04). In a similar phase III study by Domenge et al. (10), only younger patients (aged 69 years or younger) with curable oropharyngeal disease were included. The chemotherapy group ($n$ = 157) received a similar induction chemotherapy with cisplatin and 5-FU, followed by surgery and/or radiation therapy. The nonchemotherapy group ($n$ = 161) received only locoregional treatment. This study demonstrated an OS benefit, which was conferred by neoadjuvant chemotherapy in both resectable and unresectable patients (median survival = 5.1 years vs. 3.3 years, $P$ = .03).

## TPF-Induction Chemotherapy

In an effort to capitalize on the potential survival benefit of induction chemotherapy, taxanes have been added to platinum and 5-FU. The combination of docetaxel, cisplatin, and 5-fluorouracil (TPF) has recently emerged as the standard induction chemotherapy regimen if induction chemotherapy is to be considered. TPF was shown to improve OS when compared to treatment with neoadjuvant cisplatin and 5-FU followed by radiation (5,11). These findings set the stage for the investigation of induction chemotherapy followed by chemoradiation in locally advanced SCCHN. Posner et al. demonstrated an improvement in OS and progression-free survival (PFS) when TPF was compared to cisplatin/5-fluorouracil (PF) as induction chemotherapy followed by treatment with weekly carboplatin combined with radiation (6).

Subsequent randomized trials were performed to directly compare TPF induction followed by concurrent chemoradiation to definitive chemoradiation alone. A Spanish randomized phase III trial comparing 3 treatment arms (definitive chemoradiation vs. induction with PF followed by chemoradiation vs. induction with TPF followed by chemoradiation) included 439 patients with locally advanced, nonmetastatic stage III/IV SCCHN (12). While there were concerns related to study methodology, an intention-to-treat analysis demonstrated no advantage of an induction approach over concurrent chemoradiation with respect to locoregional control, time-to-treatment failure, PFS, and OS.

The Docetaxel Based Chemoradiotherapy Plus or Minus Induction Chemotherapy to Decrease Events in Head and Neck Cancer (DeCIDE) study was a phase III, multinational trial of 280 patients randomized to receive either definitive chemoradiation alone or 2 cycles of induction with TPF followed by the same chemoradiation as the control arm (13). Patients with previously untreated SCCHN with N2/N3 disease and no distant metastases were included. Fifty-eight percent of patients had oropharyngeal primaries and 88% had N2 disease. Poor accrual led to modification of the sample size and statistical plan; however, the 280 subjects accrued were still able to provide 80% power to detect an HR of 0.5 for OS ($\alpha$ = 0.05). The primary end point was OS. Results presented at the American Society of Clinical Oncology (ASCO) 2012 meeting showed no statistically significant difference between the 2 arms for OS (HR = 0.91, confidence interval [CI] [0.59–1.41], $P$ = .68). While the rate of distant recurrence (with preserved locoregional control) was improved in the induction arm ($P$ = .043), there were no significant differences in recurrence-free or distant failure-free survival. Both treatment arms were able to successfully deliver the prescribed chemotherapy and radiation; however, the induction arm was associated with increased toxicity. Specifically, grade 3–4 neutropenia rates during subsequent chemoradiation were significantly higher in the induction arm ($P$ = .02). More concerning was the observation that induction led to an increased rate of early treatment-related deaths (4 deaths during induction [3.5%] and 9 deaths [10%] during subsequent chemoradiation) as compared to 4 deaths (3.8%) in the chemoradiation-alone arm, undoubtedly contributing to the study outcomes.

The PARADIGM study was a phase III, multi-institutional trial of 145 patients randomized to receive either TPF induction followed by chemoradiation versus chemoradiation alone (14). The induction arm received 3 cycles of TPF and was further stratified to concurrent chemoradiation based on tumor response. Similar to the DeCIDE trial, the study was halted midcourse secondary to poor accrual with only 145 of the 300 planned patients accrued. Patients with previously untreated, stage III or IV SCCHN were eligible. The majority (55%) had oropharyngeal primaries and 86% had stage IV disease. The primary end point was OS. After a median follow-up of 49 months, 3-year survival was better than expected in the chemoradiation arm (78%). Neither PFS nor OS favored the use of induction ($P$ = .82 and .77, respectively). Furthermore, there was no improvement in the rate of distant recurrence with induction. In terms of toxicity, patient deaths were again higher in the induction arm (4 patients died during the first year of treatment [2 during induction]) compared to those in the chemoradiation arm (1 death).

Based on these negative trials, concurrent chemoradiation remains the standard of care for locally advanced SCCHN, and the role of induction within the treatment paradigm remains investigational. Furthermore, TPF sequential regimens have primarily been studied in patients with SCC of the oropharynx, hypopharynx, or larynx. Additional studies are needed to determine if induction chemotherapy could benefit other head and neck tumor types.

## Adjuvant Chemotherapy

Adjuvant chemotherapy is not typically given in HNC, except for nasopharyngeal carcinoma because this tumor type is exquisitely sensitive to the effects of chemotherapy as well as radiation. The evidence for this is largely represented by several studies conducted in late 1990 to early 2000s. In the Intergroup Trial 0099, Al-Sarraf et al. compared radiation alone versus chemoradiation (including adjuvant chemotherapy) in 193 patients with advanced nasopharyngeal cancer (15). This study showed both a PFS and an OS advantage for patients in the chemoradiation arm, which included 3 cycles of adjuvant cisplatin–FU. The 3-year PFS was 69% versus 24% in the chemoradiation versus radiation-alone groups, respectively ($P < .001$). The 3-year OS was 78% versus 47% ($P = .005$). A conceptually similar trial was reported by Wee et al. in 221 patients with stage III–IV nasopharyngeal carcinoma (16). Disease-free survival (DFS) was better in chemotherapy-treated patients versus radiation-alone (HR for DFS was 0.57, $P = .0093$). The OS was also better in this group: HR for OS was 0.51 ($P = .0061$). The question that remains unanswered is the timing of chemotherapy in this setting: whether concurrent chemoradiation confers the observed benefit or the adjuvant chemotherapy explains the difference in outcomes, or a combination of both. Indeed, Chan et al. reported a trial of 350 patients with various stages of nasopharyngeal carcinoma and showed a similar benefit of concurrent-only chemoradiation versus radiation therapy alone in patients with stage III–IV disease (17). Similarly, OS was improved to a comparable extent by concurrent chemoradiation as compared to radiation alone in another trial reported by Lin et al. (18).

## Recurrent/Metastatic SCCHN

D.C. is a 63-year-old male who was diagnosed with a T2N2bM0 (stage IVA) SCC of the floor of the mouth 1 year prior to presentation. At that time, he underwent surgical extirpation including a unilateral neck dissection. Surgical margins were negative, but extracapsular extension and perineural invasion were noted. He then received adjuvant chemoradiation. Seven months following definitive therapy, he developed a cough. A CT scan of the chest revealed multiple, new pulmonary nodules. A biopsy was performed and confirmed SCC, consistent with metastatic disease.

D.C.'s medical history was otherwise positive for hypertension well controlled with lisinopril. He had developed mild neuropathy after treatment with cisplatin, manifesting as numbness in bilateral fingertips and toes. He had an 80-pack-year history of smoking and a remote history of excessive drinking (he quit both 2 years prior to his initial diagnosis). His family history was noncontributory. His physical examination was unremarkable with the exception of the stigmata related to his previous surgery and radiation therapy.

## Evidence-Based Case Discussion

### Single-Agent Chemotherapy

The aforementioned patient has metastatic cancer of the oral cavity. The extracapsular extension in his neck nodes attests to the aggressive nature of his cancer, portending a poor prognosis, despite aggressive surgery and chemoradiation. Survival in patients with recurrent or metastatic (R/M) SCCHN is approximately 6 months. Median survival rates, however, can be extended to 9–11 months with systemic chemotherapy.

Single-agent chemotherapy has been studied in metastatic HNC, but response rates are low, generally on the order of 10–30%. Traditional cytotoxic agents, including cisplatin, carboplatin, 5-FU, low-dose methotrexate, paclitaxel, docetaxel, ifosfamide, and bleomycin, have been tested as single agents in this setting. Given the improved tolerability of single-agent chemotherapy, such regimens are best suited for patients with a marginal performance status (i.e., ECOG PS 2). Combination regimens, on the other hand, improve response rates and are usually reserved for patients with an ECOG PS of 0–1.

### Targeted Therapies

Newer targeted therapies have also been tested as single-agent regimens for R/M SCCHN. Inhibition of the epidermal growth factor receptor (EGFR) pathway has been extensively studied due to the virtual overexpression of EGFR in >90% of SCCHN, as well as its strong correlation with poor prognostic outcomes (19,20). Cetuximab, a chimeric mouse–human monoclonal antibody against EGFR, is the only Food and Drug Administration (FDA)-approved molecularly targeted agent for HNC. In the R/M setting, it is approved as second-line therapy for patients with platinum-refractory disease, with a toxicity profile that is more tolerable compared to conventional, cytotoxic chemotherapy drugs. Vermorken et al. noted a response rate of 13%, and a disease stabilization rate of 46% (21).

Oral small tyrosine kinase inhibitors such as erlotinib and gefitinib have also been tested, with phase II trials in heavily pretreated patients with R/M demonstrating good tolerability and disease stabilization (22,23). A phase III study comparing the efficacy of gefitinib versus weekly methotrexate, however, showed no difference in survival outcome, although quality of life was better in the gefinitib arm (24).

Despite cetuximab's approval, its modest success underscores the need to better elucidate resistance mechanisms of EGFR inhibition, and to develop other targeted therapies. One strategy aimed at overcoming EGFR resistance includes the use of irreversible, pan-erythroblastic leukemia viral oncogene homolog (ErbB) receptor tyrosine kinase inhibitors (TKIs) such as afatinib. Phase II results of afatinib demonstrated at least comparable antitumor activity to cetuximab in platinum-refractory metastatic disease, with sequential EGFR/ErbB treatment providing sustained clinical benefit in a subset of patients, suggesting lack of cross-resistance (25).

## Combination Chemotherapy

Combination chemotherapy for R/M SCCHN with a platinum-based regimen remains standard of care and provides higher response rates compared to single-agent chemotherapy. A Southwest Oncology Group (SWOG) trial compared outcomes with combinations of cisplatin or carboplatin with 5-FU versus single-agent methotrexate (26). The response rates were higher for the combination regimens (32% for cisplatin plus 5-FU, 21% for carboplatin plus 5-FU, and 10% for methotrexate). There was, however, no significant difference in survival among the 3 treatment arms. Jacobs et al. reported similar results when cisplatin and 5-FU were administered either together or as single agents (27). Again, the response rate was higher in the combination arm, but no OS benefit was noted. Cisplatin in combination with a taxane has been evaluated and does not appear superior to other combination regimens. A phase III trial evaluating cisplatin with 5-FU versus cisplatin and paclitaxel demonstrated no difference in OS, although the quality-of-life scores were higher in the paclitaxel arm (28). Three-drug combinations of conventional cytotoxic agents have also been tested. However, these are more toxic and offer no survival advantage over doublet combinations.

Recently, the introduction of targeted agents with combination chemotherapy regimens has proven to be advantageous in the treatment of R/M SCCHN. Cetuximab was combined with either carboplatin plus 5-FU or cisplatin plus 5-FU in a large phase III trial (EXTREME trial) (29). The control group received a combination of either cisplatin or carboplatin with 5-FU. The patients in the cetuximab arm who attained stable disease continued to receive maintenance weekly cetuximab until disease progression or development of intolerable side effects. This study enrolled 442 previously untreated patients with R/M HNC. The addition of cetuximab increased the response rate from 20% to 36% ($P < .001$) and prolonged the median PFS from 3.3 to 5.6 months ($P < .001$) as well as OS (10.1 vs. 7.4 months, HR of death = 0.8, 0.64–0.99, $P = .04$). Quality of life was not adversely affected by the addition of cetuximab. The combination of platinum, 5-FU, and cetuximab is now considered an accepted, first-line, standard regimen for patients with R/M HNC. One remaining question, however, relates to the benefit of maintenance cetuximab therapy. Given its expense and potential for excessive toxicity, further evaluation of cetuximab in this setting is needed before such treatment is considered standard of care.

Cetuximab has also been combined with docetaxel in a regimen that may be promising for patients with platinum refractory R/M SCCHN. Knoedler et al. reported the results of a multicenter, phase II study of this combination in 84 patients (30). They noted a 12% partial response rate with a disease control rate (partial response plus stable disease) of 39%. The median OS was 7 months, with a satisfactory toxicity profile.

Erlotinib has also shown promising results when combined with cisplatin and docetaxel in a phase II trial in patients with untreated R/M HNC (31). The overall response rate for this study was 67% with a disease control rate of 95%. The median OS was 11 months and median PFS was 6 months.

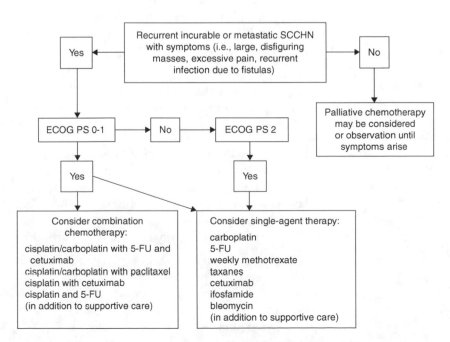

**Figure 1.1**

Palliative chemotherapy for recurrent/metastatic SCCHN. ECOG PS, Eastern Cooperative Oncology Group performance status; FU, fluorouracil; SCCHN, squamous cell carcinoma of the head and neck.

## SUMMARY

As shown in Figure 1.1, combination chemotherapy consisting of platinum plus 5-FU with or without cetuximab, or platinum combined with a taxane, are considered standard of care for patients with R/M HNC. Combination regimens are best suited for patients with ECOG PS 0–1 who have large bulky, disfiguring tumors or who have distant metastatic disease. Disease that is asymptomatic can be treated with best supportive care until symptoms arise. Patients with a marginal or limited performance status (PS = 2–3) are more likely to tolerate single-agent therapy.

## REVIEW QUESTIONS

1.  A 69-year-old otherwise healthy male presents with a 4.5-cm lateral tongue mass and multiple bilateral palpable neck nodes, with the largest node measuring 2 cm. Fine needle aspiration confirms squamous cell carcinoma. Imaging reveals no evidence of distant metastases. What would be the optimal treatment approach?

    (A) Primary surgical approach with adjuvant radiation with/without chemotherapy
    (B) Surgery alone
    (C) Radiation alone
    (D) Definitive chemoradiation

2.  The patient in Question 1 agrees to proceed with surgery. He undergoes surgical resection of the lateral tongue mass in addition to bilateral neck dissections. Final pathology reveals 5 of 44 lymph nodes positive with the presence of extracapsular extension. What would you recommend now?

    (A) Adjuvant chemotherapy
    (B) Adjuvant radiation
    (C) Adjuvant chemoradiation
    (D) No additional treatment recommended

3.  A 67-year-old female presents with a 6-month history of progressive odynophagia and dysphagia, and a 1-month history of a right neck lump. Clinical examination reveals a stage IVB oropharynx cancer. Fine needle aspiration confirms squamous cell carcinoma. Her medical history includes hypertension, diabetes mellitus, stage III chronic kidney disease, and severe painful neuropathy involving both hands and feet. Her status is Eastern Cooperative Oncology Group performance status 1. In addition to definitive radiation, which chemotherapy agent might you consider?

    (A) High-dose cisplatin
    (B) High-dose carboplatin
    (C) Carboplatin and paclitaxel
    (D) Cetuximab

4.  A 53-year-old male presents with a several month history of progressive hoarseness. He is diagnosed with a resectable, locally advanced laryngeal cancer. He works full time as a salesman, wishes to preserve his voice, and is not interested in surgery. He has a 60-pack-year smoking history (quit at time of diagnosis). He has no medical comorbidities and an excellent performance status. What would be the optimal treatment approach?

    (A) Induction with cisplatin, 5-fluorouracil (5-FU) (PF) followed by radiation
    (B) Induction with docetaxel, cisplatin, and 5-FU (TPF) followed by radiation
    (C) Induction with TPF followed by chemoradiation
    (D) Concurrent chemoradiation

5.  A 42-year-old female is diagnosed with a stage III squamous cell carcinoma of the left tonsil. She is a married homemaker with 2 children. She is a never smoker, only drinks alcohol on special occasions, and has no history of illicit drug use. She is concerned about what may have caused her cancer and asks you about potential etiologies. Which risk factor is most highly associated with cancer of the oropharynx?

    (A) Epstein-Barr virus
    (B) Human papillomavirus (HPV)
    (C) Human immunodeficiency virus
    (D) Tobacco and alcohol consumption

6.  A 59-year-old male with a history of squamous cell carcinoma of the floor of mouth status postsurgery and adjuvant radiation completed 9 months ago, now presents with a massive local recurrence that is unresectable and not amenable to further radiation therapy. He has received no prior chemotherapy. His performance status is excellent and he is otherwise healthy. He is interested in pursuing treatment, which may provide him the best chance at prolonged survival. What would be the optimal treatment approach?

    (A) Single-agent cetuximab
    (B) Single-agent methotrexate
    (C) Carboplatin/5-fluorouracil (5-FU) plus cetuximab
    (D) Carboplatin/5-FU

7.  A 41-year-old male presents with a 6-month history of nasal congestion, right ear fullness, and bilateral palpable neck masses. Clinicoradiologic assessment and biopsies confirm a stage IVB nasopharynx cancer. He is otherwise healthy with excellent performance status. What would be the optimal treatment approach?

    (A) Chemoradiation with/without adjuvant chemotherapy
    (B) Surgery with adjuvant radiation
    (C) Surgery alone
    (D) Radiation alone

# REFERENCES

1. National Comprehensive Cancer Network. Head and Neck Cancer (Version 2.2014). http://www.nccn.org/professionals/physician_gls/pdf/head-and-neck.pdf. Accessed May, 2014.

2. Veterans Affairs Laryngeal Cancer Study Group. Induction chemotherapy plus radiation compared with surgery plus radiation in patients with advanced laryngeal cancer. The Department of Veterans Affairs Laryngeal Cancer Study Group. N Engl J Med. 1991;324:1685–1690.

3. Pignon JP, Bourhis J, Domenge C, Designé L. Chemotherapy added to locoregional treatment for head and neck squamous-cell carcinoma: three meta-analyses of updated individual data. MACH-NC Collaborative Group. Meta-Analysis of Chemotherapy on Head and Neck Cancer. Lancet. 2000;355(9208):949–955.

4. Pignon JP, le Maître A, Maillard E, Bourhis J; MACH-NC Collaborative Group. Meta-analysis of chemotherapy in head and neck cancer (MACH-NC): an update on 93 randomised trials and 17,346 patients. Radiother Oncol. 2009;92(1):4–14.

5. Pointreau Y, Garaud P, Chapet S, et al. Randomized trial of induction chemotherapy with cisplatin and 5-fluorouracil with or without docetaxel for larynx preservation. J Natl Cancer Inst. 2009;101(7):498–506.

6. Posner MR, Hershock DM, Blajman CR, et al.; TAX 324 Study Group. Cisplatin and fluorouracil alone or with docetaxel in head and neck cancer. N Engl J Med. 2007;357(17):1705–1715.

7. Paccagnella A, Ghi MG, Loreggian L, et al.; Gruppo di Studio Tumori della Testa e del Collo XRP 6976 F/2501 Study. Concomitant chemoradiotherapy versus induction docetaxel, cisplatin and 5 fluorouracil (TPF) followed by concomitant chemoradiotherapy in locally advanced head and neck cancer: a phase II randomized study. Ann Oncol. 2010;21(7):1515–1522.

8. Paccagnella A, Orlando A, Marchiori C, et al. Phase III trial of initial chemotherapy in stage III or IV head and neck cancers: a study by the Gruppo di Studio sui Tumori della Testa e del Collo. J Natl Cancer Inst. 1994;86(4):265–272.

9. Zorat PL, Paccagnella A, Cavaniglia G, et al. Randomized phase III trial of neoadjuvant chemotherapy in head and neck cancer: 10-year follow-up. J Natl Cancer Inst. 2004;96(22):1714–1717.

10. Domenge C, Hill C, Lefebvre JL, et al.; French Groupe d'Etude des Tumeurs de la Tête et du Cou (GETTEC). Randomized trial of neoadjuvant chemotherapy in oropharyngeal carcinoma. French Groupe d'Etude des Tumeurs de la Tête et du Cou (GETTEC). Br J Cancer. 2000;83(12):1594–1598.

11. Vermorken JB, Remenar E, van Herpen C, et al.; EORTC 24971/TAX 323 Study Group. Cisplatin, fluorouracil, and docetaxel in unresectable head and neck cancer. N Engl J Med. 2007;357(17):1695–1704.

12. Hitt R, Grau JJ, López-Pousa A, et al.; Spanish Head and Neck Cancer Cooperative Group (TTCC). A randomized phase III trial comparing induction chemotherapy followed by chemoradiotherapy versus chemoradiotherapy alone as treatment of unresectable head and neck cancer. Ann Oncol. 2014;25(1):216–225.

13. Cohen EEW, Karrison T, Kocherginsky M, et al. DeCIDE: a phase III randomized trial of docetaxel (D), cisplatin (P), 5-fluorouracil (F) (TPF) induction chemotherapy (IC) in patients with N2/N3 locally advanced squamous cell carcinoma of the head and neck (SCCHN). J Clin Oncol. 2012;30(Suppl., Abstract.5500).

14. Haddad R, O'Neill A, Rabinowits G, et al. Induction chemotherapy followed by concurrent chemoradiotherapy (sequential chemoradiotherapy) versus concurrent chemoradiotherapy alone in locally advanced head and neck cancer (PARADIGM): a randomised phase 3 trial. Lancet Oncol. 2013;14:257–264.

15. Al-Sarraf M, LeBlanc M, Giri PG, et al. Chemoradiotherapy versus radiotherapy in patients with advanced nasopharyngeal cancer: phase III randomized Intergroup study 0099. J Clin Oncol. 1998;16(4):1310–1317.

16. Wee J, Tan EH, Tai BC, et al. Randomized trial of radiotherapy versus concurrent chemoradiotherapy followed by adjuvant chemotherapy in patients with American Joint Committee on Cancer/International Union against cancer stage III and IV nasopharyngeal cancer of the endemic variety. J Clin Oncol. 2005;23(27):6730–6738.

17. Chan AT, Leung SF, Ngan RK, et al. Overall survival after concurrent cisplatin-radiotherapy compared with radiotherapy alone in locoregionally advanced nasopharyngeal carcinoma. J Natl Cancer Inst. 2005;97(7):536–539.

18. Lin JC, Jan JS, Hsu CY, et al. Phase III study of concurrent chemoradiotherapy versus radiotherapy alone for advanced nasopharyngeal carcinoma: positive effect on overall and progression-free survival. J Clin Oncol. 2003;21(4):631–637.

19. Rubin Grandis J, Melhem MF, Gooding WE, et al. Levels of TGF-alpha and EGFR protein in head and neck squamous cell carcinoma and patient survival. J Natl Cancer Inst. 1998;90(11):824–832.

20. Ang KK, Berkey BA, Tu X, et al. Impact of epidermal growth factor receptor expression on survival and pattern of relapse in patients with advanced head and neck carcinoma. Cancer Res. 2002;62(24):7350–7356.

21. Vermorken JB, Trigo J, Hitt R, et al. Open-label, uncontrolled, multicenter phase II study to evaluate the efficacy and toxicity of cetuximab as a single agent in patients with recurrent and/or metastatic squamous cell carcinoma of the head and neck who failed to respond to platinum-based therapy. J Clin Oncol. 2007;25(16):2171–2177.

22. Soulieres D, Senzer NN, Vokes EE, et al. Multicenter phase II study of erlotinib, an oral epidermal growth factor receptor tyrosine kinase inhibitor, in patients with recurrent or metastatic squamous cell cancer of the head and neck. J Clin Oncol. 2004;22(1):77–85.

23. Cohen EE, Rosen F, Stadler WM, et al. Phase II trial of ZD1839 in recurrent or metastatic squamous cell carcinoma of the head and neck. J Clin Oncol. 2003;21(10):1980–1987.

24. Stewart JS, Cohen EE, Licitra L, et al. Phase III study of gefitinib compared with intravenous methotrexate for recurrent squamous cell carcinoma of the head and neck [corrected]. J Clin Oncol. 2009;27(11):1864–1871.

25. Seiwert TY, Fayette J, Cupissol D, et al. A randomized, phase II study of afatinib versus cetuximab in metastatic or recurrent squamous cell carcinoma of the head and neck†. Ann Oncol. 2014;25(9):1813–1820.

26. Forastiere AA, Metch B, Schuller DE, et al. Randomized comparison of cisplatin plus fluorouracil and carboplatin plus fluorouracil versus methotrexate in advanced squamous-cell carcinoma of the head and neck: a Southwest Oncology Group study. J Clin Oncol. 1992;10(8):1245–1251.

27. Jacobs C, Lyman G, Velez-García E, et al. A phase III randomized study comparing cisplatin and fluorouracil as single agents and in combination for advanced squamous cell carcinoma of the head and neck. J Clin Oncol. 1992;10(2):257–263.

28. Gibson MK, Li Y, Murphy B, et al.; Eastern Cooperative Oncology Group. Randomized phase III evaluation of cisplatin plus fluorouracil versus cisplatin plus paclitaxel in advanced head and neck cancer (E1395): an intergroup trial of the Eastern Cooperative Oncology Group. J Clin Oncol. 2005;23(15):3562–3567.

29. Vermorken JB, Mesia R, Rivera F, et al. Platinum-based chemotherapy plus cetuximab in head and neck cancer. N Engl J Med. 2008;359(11):1116–1127.

30. Knoedler M, Gauler TC, Matzdorff A, et al. Phase II trial to evaluate efficacy and toxicity of cetuximab plus docetaxel in platinum pretreated patients with recurrent and/or metastatic head and neck cancer. J Clin Oncol. 2008;26: Abstract 6066).

31. Kim ES, Kies MS, Glisson BS, et al. Final results of a phase II study of erlotinib, docetaxel and cisplatin in patients with recurrent/metastatic head and neck cancer. J Clin Oncol. 2007:6013.

# 2

# *Thyroid Cancer*

ALEXANDER T. PEARSON, KEVIN McDONNELL, AND MEGAN RIST HAYMART

## EPIDEMIOLOGY, RISK FACTORS, NATURAL HISTORY, AND PATHOLOGY

The incidence of thyroid cancer has tripled in the past 30 years (1–3). During the year 2014, it was estimated that 62,989 new cases of thyroid cancers would be diagnosed, with a female:male ratio of 3:1 (4). The median age at diagnosis for all thyroid cancers is 49 years. The majority (68%) of thyroid cancers present as localized disease at the time of diagnosis; regional lymph node disease and disseminated metastatic disease account for 24% and 5% of cases, respectively (5). The 5-year survival rates overall are 99.8%, 97.1%, and 58.1%, respectively, for localized, regional, and distant thyroid cancer (5). There are 3 primary histological subcategories of thyroid carcinoma: differentiated (comprising papillary, follicular, and Hürthle cells); medullary; and anaplastic.

Among the primary risk factors associated with the development of thyroid carcinoma is a family history of thyroid carcinoma and a history of exposure to ionizing radiation, particularly during childhood. An additional risk factor is iodine deficiency, especially relating to the development of follicular thyroid carcinomas.

## Differentiated Thyroid Carcinoma

### Papillary Thyroid Cancer

Papillary thyroid cancer accounts for over 80% of all thyroid cancers. Papillary carcinomas may present clinically as enlarged, palpable thyroid nodules; however, they are frequently incidentally discovered on imaging studies performed for other reasons (6). The incidence of papillary thyroid cancers peaks in the fourth or fifth decade of life, with a characteristic female predominance. The diagnosis of papillary thyroid cancer is typically made with an ultrasound-guided fine needle aspiration (FNA).

The growth and proliferation of papillary thyroid carcinomas are driven by mutations in a variety of molecular pathways, including the mitogen-activated protein kinase, RAS, BRAF, RET/PTC, and neurotrophic tyrosine kinase receptor type 1 molecular pathways (5,7). A cohort of patients with BRAF mutations had a somewhat worse clinical course than a comparable wild-type cohort (8). Characteristically, papillary thyroid carcinomas respond to therapeutic intervention, with only a small percentage of patients dying secondary to the cancer.

### Follicular Thyroid Carcinoma

Follicular thyroid carcinoma is estimated to account for 5–8% of thyroid cancers, but may be lower (9). Follicular thyroid cancer most often presents as a palpable nodule with peak incidence occurring in the fifth or sixth decade, later than papillary thyroid cancer. As with papillary cancer, there is a female predominance. Unlike papillary thyroid cancer, the diagnosis of follicular thyroid cancer cannot be achieved with a FNA. The FNA typically reveals a follicular neoplasm, but growth beyond the tumor capsule and vascular penetration cannot be assessed. An excisional biopsy or lobectomy is required to identify these features. Eighty percent of follicular neoplasms are benign and 20% are malignant follicular cancer or follicular variants of papillary thyroid cancer. On the molecular level, follicular thyroid carcinomas may express a PAX8 peroxisome proliferator-activated receptor gamma 1 (PPAR-γ1) fusion protein, which promotes cellular growth and prevents cellular differentiation. RAS mutations are also found not only in papillary thyroid carcinoma but also in the follicular cell carcinomas. More than three fourths of follicular thyroid carcinomas have either a PAX8 or RAS mutation. Epigenetic alterations, for example, hypermethylation of tumor suppressor genes such as RASSF1A, are thought to play a role in the tumor progression of follicular thyroid carcinoma (10). Overall, follicular thyroid carcinomas have a slightly worse prognosis relative to papillary thyroid carcinoma.

## Hürthle Cell Carcinoma

Hürthle cell carcinoma constitutes nearly 3% of thyroid cancers. The Hürthle cell carcinoma often manifests as a palpable nodule. As with follicular carcinoma, an FNA specimen of a suspected Hürthle cell carcinoma is insufficient to establish a diagnosis; thus, as with follicular cell carcinoma, the definitive diagnosis of Hürthle cell carcinoma is made following pathological assessment of a surgical specimen. Histologically, Hürthle cell carcinoma is variously classified as a variant of follicular thyroid carcinoma or as a separate independent subtype of differentiated thyroid carcinoma. Microanatomically, the Hürthle cell carcinoma is a tumor comprising at least 75% Hürthle cells, which are large, eosinophilic, oxyphilic, thyroglobulin-producing cells designated "oncocytes." The Hürthle cell carcinoma may present with either a papillary or follicular growth pattern. Genetic mutations harbored by these mitochondria underlie their increased proliferation and malignancy-promoting physiological dysfunction. A significant percentage of Hürthle cell carcinomas demonstrate the RET/PTC gene rearrangement, which may also be found in papillary thyroid carcinomas. Hürthle cell carcinoma demonstrates an increased incidence of metastatic disease as compared to either papillary or follicular thyroid carcinoma, and accordingly, it is considered to be a more aggressive disease with a higher mortality.

## Medullary Thyroid Carcinoma

Medullary thyroid carcinoma constitutes approximately 4% of the cases of thyroid cancer and is typically detected as a solitary nodule (11). There is a great propensity for medullary thyroid carcinoma to metastasize, so that at the time of diagnosis, the tumor has often spread to distant sites. Medullary thyroid carcinoma occurs with near equal frequency among men and women, and most often patients are in their 40s or 50s at the time of their presentation. FNA of the solitary nodule provides sufficient pathological information to establish the diagnosis of medullary thyroid carcinoma.

Medullary thyroid carcinoma, a type of neuroendocrine tumor, arises from the parafollicular C cell of the thyroid gland and characteristically produces calcitonin. Thus, at the time of diagnosis, the calcitonin levels are typically elevated molecularly, and mutations occur frequently in the RET proto-oncogene. Sporadic mutations in the RET proto-oncogene in medullary thyroid carcinoma represent the majority (>75%) of cases. Although most sporadic mutations are restricted to the tumor itself, the remainder of medullary thyroid cancer develops in the setting of an inherited germ-line mutation as part of

a hereditary cancer syndrome: either multiple endocrine neoplasia (MEN), 2A or 2B, or familial medullary thyroid cancer (FMTC). MEN2A, MEN2B, and FMTC are inherited in an autosomal dominant fashion. MEN2A is associated with medullary thyroid carcinoma, pheochromocytoma, and parathyroid hyperplasia. MEN2B tends to manifest clinically as medullary thyroid carcinoma and pheochromocytoma. Frequently, in MEN2B, there are additional clinical manifestations, including Marfanoid features and the development of neuroganglioneuromas. With FMTC, hereditary medullary thyroid cancer occurs in the absence of other endocrine manifestations observed in the MEN syndromes. Because of the propensity of the medullary thyroid carcinoma to derive from a germ-line genetic mutation, patients who are diagnosed with medullary thyroid carcinoma should be routinely tested for RET proto-oncogene mutation. Medullary thyroid cancer has a worse prognosis than either papillary or follicular thyroid cancers (12). Greater patient age, large tumors, presence of distant metastases, and number of positive regional lymph nodes were independently associated with decreased survival (13).

## Anaplastic Thyroid Carcinoma

Anaplastic thyroid carcinoma, which constitutes around 2% of thyroid cancers, is an extremely aggressive, undifferentiated carcinoma arising from the thyroid follicular epithelium. It typically presents as an enlarging neck mass or lymphadenopathy and tends to occur in older age, in the seventh or greater decades of life. FNA of the cervical mass or lymph node allows diagnosis of the anaplastic thyroid cancer. It is estimated that half of anaplastic thyroid carcinomas transform from an antecedent or synchronous differentiated thyroid carcinoma. Genetic alterations associated with anaplastic thyroid carcinoma include BRAF and RAS mutations. These same mutations can also be found in differentiated thyroid carcinomas and so are believed to represent foundational mutational events in the development of anaplastic thyroid carcinoma. Subsequent secondary mutations include alterations in p53, β-catenin, and PIK3CA, which confer upon anaplastic carcinoma its highly aggressive and deadly phenotype. Anaplastic thyroid carcinoma has expected median survival of <12 months (14).

## STAGING

Uniquely, the staging of differentiated thyroid carcinomas includes age as part of the staging schema, with age >45 years representing an independent risk factor associated with worse survival outcomes relative to younger patients (15). A summary of the American Joint Committee of Cancer (AJCC) cancer staging (12) for thyroid carcinoma is mentioned subsequently.

## Staging Thyroid Carcinomas

| Stage | Description |
|---|---|

**Staging Papillary and Follicular Thyroid Carcinomas**

**Under 45 Years of Age**

I — Primary tumor of any size with or without regional lymphatic spread (N0 or N1), but without distant metastases (M0)

II — Primary tumor of any size with or without regional lymphatic spread (N0 or N1), with distant metastases (M1)

**Over 45 Years of Age**

I — Primary tumor ≤2 cm in greatest dimension limited to the thyroid (T1), without regional lymphatic (N0) or distant metastatic spread (M0)

II — Primary tumor >2 cm but not >4 cm in greatest dimension limited to the thyroid (T2), without regional lymphatic (N0) or distant metastatic spread (M0)

III — Primary tumor ≤4 cm in greatest dimension limited to the thyroid (T1, T2), with regional lymph node metastases to level VI (pretracheal, paratracheal, and prelaryngeal/Delphian lymph nodes) (N1a) and without distant metastases (M0)

*or*

Primary tumor >4 cm in greatest dimension limited to the thyroid or any tumor with minimal extrathyroid extension (T3), with or without regional lymph node metastasis to level VI (pretracheal, paratracheal, and prelaryngeal/Delphian lymph nodes) (N0 or N1a) and without distant metastases (M0)

IVA — Primary tumor of any size limited to the thyroid or with minimal extrathyroid extension (T1, T2, or T3) with regional lymph node metastases to the unilateral, bilateral, or contralateral cervical or superior mediastinal lymph nodes (N1b) and without distant metastases (M0)

*or*

Primary tumor of any size extending beyond the thyroid capsule to invade subcutaneous soft tissues, larynx, trachea, esophagus, or recurrent laryngeal nerve, with any regional lymph node metastasis (N0, N1a, or N1b) and without distant metastases

IVB — Primary tumor of any size invading the prevertebral fascia or encasing the carotid artery or mediastinal vessels (T4b), with or without regional lymphatic spread (N0 or N1), and without distant metastases (M0)

IVC — Primary tumor of any size with or without regional lymphatic spread (N0 or N1), and with distant metastases (M1)

**Staging Medullary Thyroid Carcinoma**

I — Primary tumor ≤2 cm in greatest dimension limited to the thyroid (T1), without regional lymphatic (N0) or distant metastatic spread (M0)

II — Primary tumor >2 cm, but not >4 cm in greatest dimension limited to the thyroid (T2), without regional lymphatic (N0) or distant metastatic spread (M0)

III — Primary tumor ≤4 cm in greatest dimension limited to the thyroid (T1, T2), with regional lymph metastases to level VI (pretracheal, paratracheal, and prelaryngeal/Delphian lymph nodes) (N1a) and without distant metastases (M0)

*or*

Primary tumor >4 cm in greatest dimension limited to the thyroid or any tumor with minimal extrathyroid extension (T3), with or without regional lymph node metastasis to level VI (pretracheal, paratracheal, and prelaryngeal/Delphian lymph nodes) (N0 or N1a) and without distant metastases (M0)

IVA — Primary tumor of any size limited to the thyroid or with minimal extrathyroid extension (T1, T2, or T3) with regional lymph node metastases to the unilateral, bilateral, or contralateral cervical or superior mediastinal lymph nodes (N1b) and without distant metastases (M0)

*or*

Primary tumor of any size extending beyond the thyroid capsule to invade subcutaneous soft tissues, larynx, trachea, esophagus, or recurrent laryngeal nerve, with any regional lymph node metastases (N0, N1a, or N1b) and without distant metastases

IVB — Primary tumor of any size invading the prevertebral fascia or encasing the carotid artery or mediastinal vessels (T4b), with or without regional lymphatic spread (N0 or N1), and without distant metastases (M0)

IVC — Primary tumor of any size with or without regional lymphatic spread (N0 or N1), and with distant metastases (M1)

**Staging Anaplastic Thyroid Carcinoma (All Anaplastic Thyroid Carcinomas Are Stage IV)**

IVA — Primary tumor is intrathyroidal (T4a), with or without regional lymphatic spread (N0 or N1), and without distant metastases (M0)

IVB — Primary tumor is extrathyroidal (T4b), with or without regional lymphatic spread (N0 or N1), and without distant metastases (M0)

IVC — Primary tumor of any size with or without regional lymphatic spread (N0 or N1), and with distant metastases (M1)

## CASE SUMMARIES

### Early-Stage Papillary Thyroid Cancer: Stage I

A.M. is a 24-year-old woman who was involved in a low-speed motor vehicle accident. She developed neck pain for which she underwent a CT scan of the head and neck in the emergency department. These imaging studies did not demonstrate any acute pathology but did reveal, incidentally, a 2.5-cm solid mass in the right lobe of the thyroid. The emergency department physicians recommended that she have further evaluation as an outpatient, and the patient followed up with her primary care physician. She had no overt symptoms of a dysfunctional thyroid state and no compressive symptoms secondary to the nodule. There was no history of previous malignancy, prior irradiation, or family history of thyroid cancer. A thyroid-stimulating hormone (TSH) was obtained and was normal. The patient was directed to obtain a diagnostic ultrasound of the neck. The ultrasound confirmed the presence of a 2.3 × 1.7 cm² solid mass in the right lobe of the thyroid. There were no other nodules and no suspicious cervical lymph nodes were detected. Subsequently, a FNA of the nodule was performed, which revealed a well-differentiated papillary thyroid carcinoma.

## Evidence-Based Case Discussion

This case illustrates the evaluation of an incidentally discovered thyroid nodule with the establishment of early-stage papillary thyroid carcinoma.

The clinical approach to this patient begins with evaluation of the thyroid nodule. Frequently, as with this case, the thyroid nodule is discovered incidentally. Unless there exists a heightened suspicion for the occurrence of malignancy, such as the presence of a concomitant lymphadenopathy, a family history of thyroid cancer, a personal history of radiation exposure, high-risk features on a thyroid ultrasound, or the patient possesses a number of additional risk factors, only thyroid nodules >1 cm merit further evaluation. The history and physical examination initiate the evaluation of the thyroid nodule (see Figure 2.1) to assess for signs and symptoms consistent with the development of a thyroid cancer, including dysphonia secondary to impairment of the vocal cords or enlarged lymph nodes. A cervical ultrasound examination is recommended to further assess the thyroid nodule and assess for any additional neck pathology associated with the thyroid gland (16). Measurement of thyroid stimulating hormone (TSH) directs the further workup. With a high or normal TSH value, an FNA is indicated. With a low TSH value, thyroid scintigraphy

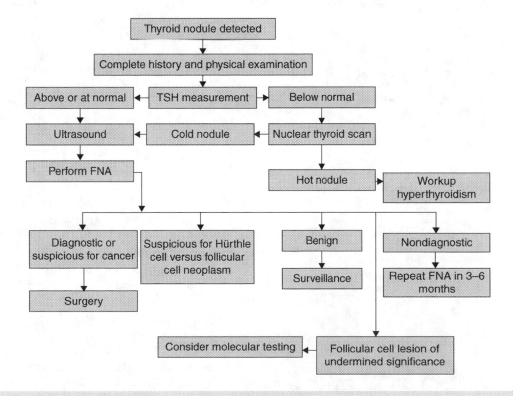

**Figure 2.1**

Algorithm: evaluation of the thyroid nodule. FNA, fine needle aspiration; TSH, thyroid-stimulating hormone. *Source:* Adapted from the American Thyroid Association Guidelines (16). Cooper DS, Doherty GM, Haugen BR, et al. Revised American Thyroid Association management guidelines for patients with thyroid nodules and differentiated thyroid cancer. *Thyroid.* 2009;19(11):1167–1214.

is recommended to determine whether the nodule shows avidity for radioactive iodine (RAI) and is therefore considered functioning, or does not incorporate the radiotracer and is nonfunctioning. The functioning thyroid nodule is rarely malignant, and in this case, no further evaluation for malignancy is required, though further clinical assessment for a hyperthyroid state would be indicated. With a nonfunctioning thyroid nodule, the suspicion for malignancy is increased and a tissue diagnosis by an FNA is indicated.

Even with pathological review of FNA samples, between 15% and 30% of aspirates yield an indeterminate histological result (16). Recent molecular diagnostic tests have leveraged the fact that 60–70% of thyroid cancers have at least 1 known genetic mutation (17) to develop a commercially available diagnostic test. A molecular testing based classifier has 92% sensitivity and 52% specificity at detecting malignant thyroid nodules from indeterminate histology specimens (18), and is now an option for evaluating indeterminate histology nodules following FNA.

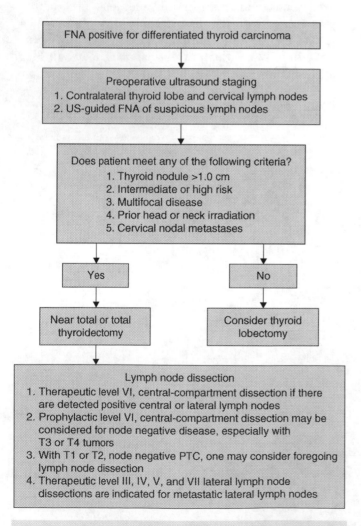

**Figure 2.2**

Algorithm: surgical management of the thyroid nodule in differentiated thyroid carcinoma. FNA, fine needle aspiration; PTC, papillary thyroid cancer.

In the case of an FNA diagnosis of papillary thyroid carcinoma, management entails surgical resection of the nodule either as a total or hemithyroidectomy (Figure 2.2). Prior to surgical intervention, a neck ultrasound is recommended to assess more carefully for thyroid pathology and involvement of lateral neck lymph nodes. If the patient demonstrates a thyroid nodule >1.0 cm, has intermediate- or high-risk features, multifocal disease, a history of prior head or neck irradiation, or cervical lymph node metastases are observed on the presurgical evaluation, then a near total or total thyroidectomy is recommended. In the case of A.M., because her nodule was 2.3 cm and her FNA was diagnostic for papillary thyroid carcinoma, she underwent a total thyroidectomy.

The question whether a lymph node dissection is required depends on the presence of detectable lymph node disease as well as the size of the thyroid nodule. Where lymph node metastases are found, a therapeutic lymph node dissection is indicated. Prophylactic lymph node dissection is controversial, but can be considered for T3 or T4 tumors. In the case of smaller T1 or T2 primaries without evidence of lymph node metastases, it is acceptable to forego the prophylactic lymph node dissection. Accordingly, A.M. did not undergo lymph node dissection.

The present case highlights the impact that the patient's age has on clinical staging. Because A.M. is younger than 45 years, she is considered having stage I disease. If she were older than 45 years, she would have had stage II disease.

Postoperatively, the clinician must decide whether to utilize RAI ablation and to what extent the TSH should be suppressed. While some studies provide conflicting evidence on the use of RAI, it is clinically beneficial in iodine-avid advanced disease. In view of this conflicting information, the American Thyroid Association (ATA) has generated consensus guidelines for the postoperative use of RAI in differentiated thyroid cancer (16). The ATA recommends the use of RAI if there is distant metastatic disease, extrathyroidal tumor extension, or the tumor exceeds 4 cm in size. The ATA does not recommend RAI ablation for patients with a single lesion <1 cm in size, unless there are also high-risk features present. However, there remains a large category of patients for whom the ATA leaves the use of RAI up to the provider's discretion because the available data are unclear. For thyroid nodules 1–4 cm in size, the ATA advocates the selective use of RAI ablation if there are lymph node metastases or other higher-risk features for recurrence such as microscopic invasion into the perithyroidal soft tissues. In the case of A.M., although the patient did not meet the criteria for high-risk disease, she was treated with RAI because of both the patient's and provider's preferences.

With well-differentiated thyroid cancers, the TSH receptor molecular signaling cascade remains intact and responsive to TSH. Reduction of TSH levels inhibits the proliferation of well-differentiated thyroid cancer. Postoperatively, administration of suppressive doses of levothyroxine acts in a negative feedback fashion to reduce TSH levels and can be used to decrease the growth and spread of remnant thyroid cancer. Clinical studies have demonstrated that in the postoperative setting, an association exists between levels of TSH and the risk of thyroid cancer recurrence and mortality (46). The clinical benefit of levothyroxine use to prevent thyroid cancer growth must, however, be balanced against the risks associated with the induction of subclinical hyperthyroidism, which may lead to the development of osteoporosis and exacerbation of cardiovascular disease (19). One clinical study (20) has demonstrated that for patients with advanced stage III or IV differentiated thyroid cancer, postoperative suppression of TSH to undetectable levels, or for patients with stage II disease, suppression below normal levels results in increased overall survival. In this same study, patients with early stage I disease did not benefit from TSH suppression. Reflecting these clinical observations, the ATA recommends that for high-risk postoperative patients (who are defined as having macroscopic tumor extension, metastatic disease to distant sites, or incomplete primary tumor resection) or for intermediate-risk patients (which includes patients with microscopic extension of their tumor into neighboring tissue, cervical lymph node involvement, or tumors with vascular invasion or aggressive histology), the TSH should be suppressed to below 0.1 mU/L. In low-risk patients (identified as those patients with complete macroscopic resection of their tumor and without metastatic disease, locoregional tumor invasion, aggressive histology, or vascular invasion), the TSH should be suppressed in the range 0.1–0.5 mU/L, which is below the lower normal limit. In the long term, patients are later risk stratified based on the presence or absence of residual disease and the TSH goal is adjusted appropriately. Other postoperative therapeutic modalities such as radiotherapy or chemotherapy are rarely, if ever, utilized in the postoperative setting to treat differentiated thyroid cancer. One exception involves the employment of palliative external beam radiation for inoperable localized disease.

In summary, in the present case, A.M. presented with an early-stage, differentiated papillary thyroid cancer. She was treated with total thyroidectomy followed by RAI and TSH suppression.

## Differentiated Follicular Thyroid Cancer: Late-Stage Follicular Thyroid Cancer

A.C. is a 78-year-old man with a history of chronic, progressive back pain who underwent an MRI of his lower spine, which revealed a 5-cm expansile mass at the L1 vertebral body. Additional CT imaging was performed, demonstrating an 8-cm mass at the T7 vertebral body invading through the posterior wall with extension to the adjacent rib, with possible left neuroforaminal involvement. In addition, hypodense nodular lesions were seen in both lobes of the thyroid. The patient underwent a biopsy of the rib lesion, the pathology of which documented metastatic follicular thyroid cancer. A total thyroidectomy with a central compartment (level VI) neck dissection was subsequently performed with pathological analysis identifying a 2.1 × 1.4 cm² follicular thyroid cancer.

### Evidence-Based Case Discussion

This is a 78-year-old man discovered to have metastatic follicular thyroid cancer in bone. Given the metastatic spread of the cancer and the patient's age, this thyroid cancer is pathologically classified as stage IVC disease. As with the previous case of papillary thyroid cancer, the age of the patient is a significant variable in the pathological classification of this differentiated thyroid cancer. The current patient has stage IV disease, but if he had been younger than 45 years, he would have been classified as having stage II disease.

Approximately 20% of patients with a diagnosis of follicular thyroid carcinoma develop distant metastatic disease. The initial therapeutic intervention for metastatic follicular thyroid cancer is RAI; however, this metastatic disease does not uniformly respond to this therapy. Important variables associated with response include whether the metastatic tumor takes up iodine (iodine avid) and the anatomic locus and size of the tumor. Patients with noniodine-avid metastatic tumors fare worse than patients with iodine-avid metastatic tumors, with cancer-specific 10-year survival of 67.9% versus 33.2%, respectively (13). In addition, among patients with iodine-avid disease, micrometastatic pulmonary follicular thyroid cancer demonstrates an excellent response to RAI with >90% 10-year survival (21). For larger (>1 cm), iodine-avid pulmonary metastatic tumors, patients often demonstrate a response to RAI, although survival is inferior to that of patients with micrometastatic disease. Similarly, patients with iodine-avid bone metastatic follicular thyroid cancer may respond to RAI but not as robustly as patients with pulmonary micrometastatic lesions (21).

A significant percentage of patients with metastatic follicular cancers are not iodine avid, thus presenting the clinician with the task of how best to treat these patients. Standard chemotherapy, which includes doxorubicin-based modalities, has proven to be suboptimal (22). Laboratory investigation has revealed, however, that RAI-resistant differentiated thyroid cancers constitute a unique genetic subgroup comprising tumors with frequent mutations of the BRAF (in the case of papillary thyroid cancer), RAS, and AKT molecular pathways (23). This observation raised the possibility that RAI-resistant tumors may be susceptible to biologic agents targeting these molecular pathways, specifically the tyrosine kinase inhibitors (TKIs).

Sorafenib, a TKI that acts on a variety of molecular targets, including BRAF, KIT, and RET, was approved in 2013 to treat RAI-resistant, metastatic, or locally recurrent well-differentiated thyroid cancer. Results of a randomized phase III, placebo-controlled, double-blinded, multisite clinical trial revealed a 12% overall response rate for the sorafenib arm compared to 1% in the control arm (24). The trial showed a 5-month increase in progression-free survival, but no significant difference in overall survival.

Additional clinical reports have documented benefit in upward of 80% of patients with RAI-resistant metastatic follicular or papillary thyroid cancer treated with sorafenib (25). As with RAI therapy, treatment response with sorafenib is variable. Pulmonary metastases demonstrate increased responsiveness to sorafenib relative to other sites of disease, including bone and lymph nodes (25). In addition to sorafenib, a number of other TKIs have demonstrated clinical promise for the treatment of RAI-resistant metastatic follicular thyroid cancers (26,27).

New options for well-differentiated thyroid cancer are being actively researched. Selumetinib is a MAPK kinase (MEK) 1 and MEK 2 inhibitor under active investigation. Selumetinib-induced MAPK inhibition reverses the constitutive activation of MAPK, caused by mutations in a group of genes including RET, NTRK1, RAS, and BRAF, which are present in approximately 70% of papillary thyroid cancers (28–31). MAPK activation inhibits thyroid hormone biosynthesis genes, and therefore MAPK inhibition may reverse RAI resistance (32). A small trial showed that selumetinib increased the uptake of iodine-124 in the majority of patients who received the drug, allowing treatment with RAI for patients who would not otherwise be candidates (33). Lenvantinib is an oral, small molecule inhibitor of tyrosine kinase receptors including vascular endothelial growth factor receptor (VEGFR) 1–3, F endothelial growth receptor (FEGR) 1–4, platelet-derived growth factor receptor (PDGFR)-β, CD 117 (KIT), and RET (34). The Study of E7080E lenvatinib in differentiated cancer of the thyroid (SELECT) trial, a randomized, placebo-controlled phase III study, showed improvement in progression-free survival of RAI-resistant, differentiated thyroid cancer patients over those treated with placebo.

In the present case, A.C. underwent a total thyroidectomy with a central lymph node dissection to assess for and surgically eliminate any regional metastatic lymph node disease. Given his metastatic disease and the high-risk categorization of his thyroid cancer, the patient thereafter underwent postoperative RAI with administration of suppressive levothyroxine therapy; the patient's TSH levels were maintained below 0.1 mU/L. In addition, because of the symptoms resulting from his metastases, he underwent palliative radiation therapy to the thoracic and vertebral lesions and received monthly zoledronic acid infusions. Should his disease progress, the patient is aware that TKI therapy remains an option.

## Medullary Thyroid Cancer

W.E. is a 50-year-old woman who detected a slight discomfort on the right side of her throat. She underwent a physical examination, which revealed a discrete nodule in the right lobe of the thyroid. A TSH level was determined to be normal. An ultrasound was performed revealing a 2.7-cm nodule in the right lobe of the thyroid gland. The patient then underwent an FNA and the cytopathology was consistent with medullary thyroid carcinoma. There was no history of thyroid cancer in her family or any history of other malignancies. The calcium level was normal, but the calcitonin and CEA levels were elevated. A RET mutational analysis from peripheral blood leukocytes was done, which identified an exon8 G533C activating RET germ-line mutation. A CT scan was performed of the neck, chest, and abdomen, which confirmed the mass in the right lobe of the thyroid, but otherwise revealed no pathology. Specifically, there were no adrenal masses to suggest the presence of a pheochromocytoma. The patient underwent a total thyroidectomy as well as a level VI compartment lymph node dissection. Pathological analysis documented a 2.7 × 2.1 cm$^2$ medullary thyroid carcinoma; the final pathological assessment was stage II disease.

## Evidence-Based Case Discussion

This is a case of a patient with a thyroid nodule diagnosed as an early-stage II medullary thyroid cancer. Imaging studies showed no evidence of metastatic spread or additional malignancies.

Because medullary thyroid cancer typically originates from an underlying RET mutation, genetic testing was performed. In this case, an exon8 G533C germ-line mutation was observed. A number of RET mutations have been identified and each of these is associated with a different mortality risk. The ATA has compiled a listing of the various RET mutations and their associated risk (35). In the present case, W.E.'s exon8 G533C mutation confers a relatively low risk.

Two new treatment options for medullary thyroid cancer have been approved by the Food and Drug Administration (FDA) in recent years. In 2011, the FDA approved vandetinib for locally advanced, unresectable, or metastatic medullary thyroid cancer. Vandetinib is an oral inhibitor of RET, EGFR, and VEGFR (36,37). A randomized, double-blind, phase III trial showed that vandetinib improved progression-free survival compared to placebo (38). Studies of vandetinib have revealed a significant potential cardiotoxicity of vandetinib, and prescribing information includes a boxed warning. In 2012, the FDA approved cabozantinib for medullary thyroid cancer. Cabozantinib was shown to increase progression free survivial (PFS) to 11.4 months compared to 4.0 months for placebo (39). Side effects of cabozantinib can include gastrointestinal (GI) bleeding, and severe hemorrhage is a contraindication to use.

Because medullary thyroid cancers are often associated with the MEN2 syndromes, patients diagnosed with medullary thyroid cancer with a RET mutation are screened for the presence of other neoplastic disease, most notably pheochromocytoma. In the current case, screening did not reveal evidence of an additional malignancy.

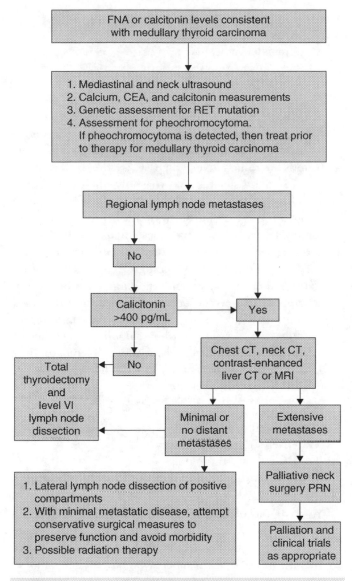

**Figure 2.3**

Diagnosis and management algorithm for medullary thyroid carcinoma. FNA, fine needle aspiration; PRN, if indicated. *Source:* Adapted from the American Thyroid Association Guidelines (16). Cooper DS, Doherty GM, Haugen BR, et al. Revised American Thyroid Association management guidelines for patients with thyroid nodules and differentiated thyroid cancer. *Thyroid.* 2009;19(11):1167–1214.

To assess for locoregional spread, the ATA also recommends neck ultrasound (see Figure 2.3) (35).

Laboratory testing should include calcitonin, CEA, and calcium measurements. Calcitonin doubling time is among the most prognostic studies for predicting survival in medullary thyroid cancer (40). If lymph node involvement is detected by ultrasound, further assessment for distant metastatic disease could be considered. In patients with lymph node involvement >2 cm and no distant metastatic disease, surgery results in a significant improvement in survival (41). A lateral compartment lymph node dissection is recommended if there is evidence of lateral neck disease or

extensive central neck disease. In some instances, radiation therapy is considered. With extensive distant metastatic disease, palliative measures and possible enrollment in a clinical trial can be implemented.

In the case of W.E., because of the early stage with no evidence of regional or distant metastatic spread, she underwent a total thyroidectomy with central (level VI) lymph node dissection.

## Anaplastic Thyroid Cancer

T.M. is a 78-year-old woman who noted the rapid development of a mass on the right side of her throat. She also reported some recent dyspnea, fatigue, and hoarseness. A physical examination performed by her primary care physician demonstrated a firm nodule in the right lobe of the thyroid gland. Laboratory testing was performed. An ultrasound of the thyroid was performed, which demonstrated 4 solid nodules in the right lobe of the thyroid, the largest measuring $3.5 \times 2.0$ cm$^2$. The remainder of the ultrasound examination did not demonstrate any abnormal findings on the left side; central and lateral compartment lymph nodes were assessed and were normal. An FNA biopsy was performed and demonstrated an undifferentiated malignancy consistent with anaplastic thyroid cancer. The patient proceeded to undergo a core biopsy of the mass, which confirmed the presence of the anaplastic thyroid cancer. Additional laboratory testing was accomplished including CBC and serum calcium, both of which were normal. CT scans of the head, neck, chest, abdomen, and pelvis revealed multiple pulmonary metastatic lesions in the middle lobe of the right lung. The CT scan of the neck confirmed the presence of the 4 nodules in the right lobe of the thyroid; one of the nodules, it was noted, was impinging on the right recurrent laryngeal nerve. A bone scan was also performed, which did not demonstrate any evidence of bony metastases.

### Evidence-Based Case Discussion

This patient is an older woman diagnosed with anaplastic thyroid carcinoma. All cases of anaplastic thyroid carcinoma are stage IV but in this case, because T.M. had distant pulmonary metastases, the anaplastic thyroid carcinoma is stage IVC.

Suspicion for anaplastic thyroid cancer on an FNA requires that a core or excisional biopsy be performed to confirm the diagnosis. Laboratory testing, including a CBC, TSH, and calcium levels, is recommended. Anaplastic thyroid cancer is a particularly aggressive neoplasm thought to arise from dedifferentiation of an antecedent differentiated thyroid carcinoma as a result of an accumulation of additional genetic mutations. Metastatic disease is common, with the vast majority of metastatic disease targeting the lungs. To assess for the extent of disease and to identify potential sites of metastatic disease, CT studies of the head, neck, chest, abdomen, and pelvis; PET imaging; and a bone scan are performed.

Anaplastic thyroid carcinoma commonly extends beyond local control at the time of diagnosis. Surgical resection is typically performed only when indicated for palliative relief of symptoms. In those infrequent clinical cases where the primary anaplastic thyroid carcinoma is amenable to local resection (stage IVA disease), thyroidectomy and resection of local and regional metastatic lymph node disease are indicated. Most typically, anaplastic thyroid cancer is stage IVB or IVC. At these late stages, radiation may be employed with the aim of achieving local control (42). Radiation therapy may also be combined with doxorubicin employed as a sensitizing agent (43). There is some evidence that doxorubicin combined with cisplatin may be more effective than doxorubicin alone (22). The use of $I^{131}$ as a therapeutic modality is not effective because the anaplastic carcinoma is dedifferentiated and remains incapable of iodine uptake or processing. Novel agents, including antiangiogenic agents, RET inhibitors, and PPAR agonists, are currently being evaluated as therapeutic agents for anaplastic thyroid cancer (44). All patients should be encouraged to consider participation in a clinical trial. Optimization of current therapeutic modalities and investigational efforts notwithstanding anaplastic thyroid cancer has a dismal prognosis with the vast majority of patients succumbing to the disease in <12 months' time (45). Multimodality therapy involving chemotherapy, radiation, and surgery results in only a marginal improvement in survival time of months (14).

## REVIEW QUESTIONS

1.  Your patient is a 45-year-old woman who presents with a palpable thyroid nodule. She reports that she feels well and has no specific complaints. Physical examination reveals no other abnormalities. She sees her primary physician regularly and has no previous medical history. Laboratory examination reveals a white blood cell count of $3.5 \times 10^9$/L with normal distribution. Hemoglobin is 14 g/dL and platelets are $210 \times 10^9$/L. Thyroid-stimulating hormone level is 0.1 U/mL. Which one of the following is the best next step?

    (A) Nuclear thyroid scan
    (B) Evaluation for causes of hyperthyroidism
    (C) Ultrasound-guided fine needle aspiration
    (D) Surveillance
    (E) Surgery

2.  Your patient is a 49-year-old woman who had a fine needle aspiration (FNA) performed on a thyroid nodule. The biopsy pathology returned as follicular cell lesion of undetermined significance. Laboratory examination revealed a thyroid-stimulating hormone level of 3.1 U/mL. Which one of the following is the best next step?

    (A) Thyroidectomy
    (B) Reassurance
    (C) Consider molecular testing
    (D) Repeat FNA in 3–6 months
    (E) C and D

3.  Your patient is a 72-year-old man with biopsy-confirmed metastatic follicular thyroid cancer. He has bone and lymph node involvement. He has received multiple rounds of radioactive iodine (RAI) therapy over the last 18 months. He failed to show clinical response with his last round of RAI therapy and has had disease progression by response evaluation criteria in solid tumors (RECIST) criteria. The patient is otherwise in good health with no other medical comorbidities. He is Eastern Cooperative Oncology Group performance status 1 due to occasional bone pain, controlled with acetaminophen as needed. He has been prescribed zolendronic acid for his bony metastases. Laboratory examination reveals a white blood cell count of $5.5 \times 10^9$/L with normal distribution. Hemoglobin is 13.5 g/dL and platelets are $260 \times 10^9$/L. Which one of the following is the best next step?

    (A) Referral to surgery
    (B) Referral to hospice
    (C) Offer sorafanib
    (D) Offer cabozantanib
    (E) Offer carboplatin-based couplet chemotherapy

4.  Your patient is a 35-year-old man with recently diagnosed medullary thyroid carcinoma. During his initial history and physical examination, the patient reports that there are numerous family members who have been diagnosed with thyroid cancer and pheochromocytoma. Mutations of which of the following genes are most likely to be identified in this patient with genetic testing?

    (A) *RAS*
    (B) *RET*
    (C) *PPAR-γ1*
    (D) *BRAF*

5.  Your patient is a 38-year-old woman with recently diagnosed papillary thyroid carcinoma with nodal involvement, but no evidence of metastatic disease. Which of the following factors is the most important prognostic factor for overall survival in a patient with differentiated thyroid cancer?

    (A) Nodal involvement
    (B) Distant metastases
    (C) Sex
    (D) Age

6.  Your patient is a 55-year-old man with medullary thyroid cancer. Serial imaging examinations reveal

progression by RECIST criteria of metastases to regional lymph nodes and 4 lung nodules between 1 cm and 2 cm. The patient is otherwise in good health with no other medical comorbidities. He is Eastern Cooperative Oncology Group performance status 0. Laboratory examination reveals a white blood cell count of $5.5 \times 10^9$/L with normal distribution. Hemoglobin is 15.5 g/dL and platelets are $300 \times 10^9$/L. Which one of the following is the most appropriate next treatment option?

(A) Offer hospice
(B) Offer sorafanib
(C) Offer carboplatin/paclitaxel
(D) Offer cabozantinib

7. Your patient is a 65-year-old man with anaplastic thyroid cancer. Imaging examination reveals distant metastases to lung and liver. He was treated with combination therapy including surgery, chemotherapy, and radiation. His most recent CT scans show progression of disease in liver and lung. The patient reports no other medical comorbidities. He is Eastern Cooperative Oncology Group performance status 2 due to fatigue. Laboratory examination reveals a white blood cell count of $5.0 \times 10^9$/L with normal distribution. Hemoglobin is 14.0 g/dL and platelets are $300 \times 10^9$/L. Which one of the following is the best next treatment option?

(A) Offer hospice
(B) Offer sorafanib
(C) Offer gemcitabine-based chemotherapy
(D) Offer cabozantinib

## REFERENCES

1. Davies MA, Stemke-Hale K, Lin E, et al. Integrated molecular and clinical analysis of AKT activation in metastatic melanoma. *Clin Cancer Res.* 2009;15(24):7538–7546.
2. Altekruse SF, Krapcho M, Neyman N, et al. *SEER Cancer Statistics Review, 1975–2007.* Bethesda, MD: National Cancer Institute; 2010.
3. American Cancer Society. *Cancer Facts and Figures 2010.* Atlanta, GA: American Cancer Society; 2010.
4. Siegel R, Ma J, Zou Z, et al. Cancer statistics, 2014. *CA Cancer J Clin.* 2014;64(1):9–29.
5. Xing M. BRAF mutation in papillary thyroid microcarcinoma: the promise of better risk management. *Ann Surg Oncol.* 2009;16(4):801–803.
6. Davies L, Welch HG. Increasing incidence of thyroid cancer in the United States, 1973–2002. *JAMA.* 2006;295(18):2164–2167.
7. Fagin JA, Mitsiades N. Molecular pathology of thyroid cancer: diagnostic and clinical implications. *Best Pract Res Clin Endocrinol Metab.* 2008;22(6):955–969.
8. Xing M, Alzahrani AS, Carson KA, et al. Association between BRAF V600E mutation and mortality in patients with papillary thyroid cancer. *JAMA.* 2013;309(14):1493–1501.
9. Otto KJ, Lam JS, MacMillan C, et al. Diminishing diagnosis of follicular thyroid carcinoma. *Head Neck.* 2010;32(12):1629–1634.
10. Kondo T, Ezzat S, Asa SL. Pathogenetic mechanisms in thyroid follicular-cell neoplasia. *Nat Rev Cancer.* 2006;6(4):292–306.
11. *American Cancer Society: Thyroid cancer detailed guide.* www.cancer.org. Accessed May 1, 2014.
12. Edge S, Byrd DR, Compton CC, eds., et al. *AJCC Cancer Staging Manual.* 7th ed. New York, NY: Springer Science + Business Media; 2010.
13. Lang BH, Wong KP, Cheung CY, et al. Evaluating the prognostic factors associated with cancer-specific survival of differentiated thyroid carcinoma presenting with distant metastasis. *Ann Surg Oncol.* 2013;20(4):1329–1335.
14. Haymart MR, Banerjee M, Yin H, et al. Marginal treatment benefit in anaplastic thyroid cancer. *Cancer.* 2013;119(17):3133–3139.
15. Haymart MR. Understanding the relationship between age and thyroid cancer. *Oncologist.* 2009;14(3):216–221.
16. Cooper DS, Doherty GM, Haugen BR, et al. Revised American Thyroid Association management guidelines for patients with thyroid nodules and differentiated thyroid cancer. *Thyroid.* 2009;19(11):1167–1214.
17. Moses W, Weng J, Sansano I, et al. Molecular testing for somatic mutations improves the accuracy of thyroid fine-needle aspiration biopsy. *World J Surg.* 2010;34(11):2589–2594.
18. Alexander EK, Kennedy GC, Baloch ZW, et al. Preoperative diagnosis of benign thyroid nodules with indeterminate cytology. *N Engl J Med.* 2012;367(8):705–715.
19. Toft AD. Clinical practice. Subclinical hyperthyroidism. *N Engl J Med.* 2001;345(7):512–516.
20. Jonklaas J, Sarlis NJ, Litofsky D, et al. Outcomes of patients with differentiated thyroid carcinoma following initial therapy. *Thyroid.* 2006;16(12):1229–1242.
21. Durante C, Haddy N, Baudin E, et al. Long-term outcome of 444 patients with distant metastases from papillary and follicular thyroid carcinoma: benefits and limits of radioiodine therapy. *J Clin Endocrinol Metab.* 2006;91(8):2892–2899.
22. Shimaoka K, Schoenfeld DA, DeWys WD, et al. A randomized trial of doxorubicin versus doxorubicin plus cisplatin in patients with advanced thyroid carcinoma. *Cancer.* 1985;56(9):2155–2160.
23. Ricarte-Filho JC, Ryder M, Chitale DA, et al. Mutational profile of advanced primary and metastatic radioactive iodine-refractory thyroid cancers reveals distinct pathogenetic roles for BRAF, PIK3CA, and AKT1. *Cancer Res.* 2009;69(11):4885–4893.
24. Brose MS, Nutting C, Jarzab B, et al. Sorafenib in locally advanced or metastatic patients with radioactive iodine-refractory differentiated thyroid cancer: the phase III DECISION trial. *J Clin Oncol.* 2013;31(suppl; abstr 4).
25. Cabanillas ME, Waguespack SG, Bronstein Y, et al. Treatment with tyrosine kinase inhibitors for patients with differentiated thyroid cancer: the M.D. Anderson experience. *J Clin Endocrinol Metab.* 2010;95(6):2588–2595.
26. Sherman SI, Wirth LJ, Droz JP, et al.; Motesanib Thyroid Cancer Study Group. Motesanib diphosphate in progressive differentiated thyroid cancer. *N Engl J Med.* 2008;359(1):31–42.
27. Cohen EE, Rosen LS, Vokes EE, et al. Axitinib is an active treatment for all histologic subtypes of advanced thyroid cancer: results from a phase II study. *J Clin Oncol.* 2008;26(29):4708–4713.
28. Kimura ET, Nikiforova MN, Zhu Z, et al. High prevalence of BRAF mutations in thyroid cancer: genetic evidence for constitutive activation of the RET/PTC-RAS-BRAF signaling pathway in papillary thyroid carcinoma. *Cancer Res.* 2003;63(7):1454–1457.
29. Cohen Y, Xing M, Mambo E, et al. BRAF mutation in papillary thyroid carcinoma. *J Natl Cancer Inst.* 2003;95(8):625–627.
30. Knauf JA, Fagin JA. Role of MAPK pathway oncoproteins in thyroid cancer pathogenesis and as drug targets. *Curr Opin Cell Biol.* 2009;21(2):296–303.
31. Soares P, Trovisco V, Rocha AS, et al. BRAF mutations and RET/PTC rearrangements are alternative events in the etiopathogenesis of PTC. *Oncogene.* 2003;22(29):4578–4580.
32. Liu D, Hu S, Hou P, et al. Suppression of BRAF/MEK/MAP kinase pathway restores expression of iodide-metabolizing genes in thyroid cells expressing the V600E BRAF mutant. *Clin Cancer Res.* 2007;13(4):1341–1349.

33. Ho AL, Grewal RK, Leboeuf R, et al. Selumetinib-enhanced radioiodine uptake in advanced thyroid cancer. *N Engl J Med.* 2013;368(7):623–632.

34. Matsui J, Yamamoto Y, Funahashi Y, et al. E7080, a novel inhibitor that targets multiple kinases, has potent antitumor activities against stem cell factor producing human small cell lung cancer H146, based on angiogenesis inhibition. *Int J Cancer.* 2008;122(3):664–671.

35. Kloos RT, Eng C, Evans DB, et al. Medullary thyroid cancer: management guidelines of the American Thyroid Association. *Thyroid.* 2009;19(6):565–612.

36. Carlomagno F, Vitagliano D, Guida T, et al. ZD6474, an orally available inhibitor of KDR tyrosine kinase activity, efficiently blocks oncogenic RET kinases. *Cancer Res.* 2002;62(24): 7284–7290.

37. Wedge SR, Ogilvie DJ, Dukes M, et al. ZD6474 inhibits vascular endothelial growth factor signaling, angiogenesis, and tumor growth following oral administration. *Cancer Res.* 2002;62(16):4645–4655.

38. Wells SA Jr, Robinson BG, Gagel RF, et al. Vandetanib in patients with locally advanced or metastatic medullary thyroid cancer: a randomized, double-blind phase III trial. *J Clin Oncol.* 2012;30(2):134–141.

39. Elisei R, Schlumberger MJ, Müller SP, et al. Cabozantinib in progressive medullary thyroid cancer. *J Clin Oncol.* 2013;31(29): 3639–3646.

40. Barbet J, Campion L, Kraeber-Bodéré F, et al.; GTE Study Group. Prognostic impact of serum calcitonin and carcinoembryonic antigen doubling-times in patients with medullary thyroid carcinoma. *J Clin Endocrinol Metab.* 2005;90(11):6077–6084.

41. Esfandiari NH, Hughes DT, Yin H, et al. The effect of extent of surgery and number of lymph node metastases on overall survival in patients with medullary thyroid cancer. *J Clin Endocrinol Metab.* 2014;99(2):448–454.

42. Wang Y, Tsang R, Asa S, et al. Clinical outcome of anaplastic thyroid carcinoma treated with radiotherapy of once- and twice-daily fractionation regimens. *Cancer.* 2006;107(8): 1786–1792.

43. Kim JH, Leeper RD. Treatment of locally advanced thyroid carcinoma with combination doxorubicin and radiation therapy. *Cancer.* 1987;60(10):2372–2375.

44. Tuttle RM, Leboeuf R. Investigational therapies for metastatic thyroid carcinoma. *J Natl Compr Canc Netw.* 2007;5(6): 641–646.

45. Neff RL, Farrar WB, Kloos RT, et al. Anaplastic thyroid cancer. *Endocrinol Metab Clin North Am.* 2008;37(2):525–38, xi.

46. Hovens GC, Stokkel MP, Kievit J, et al. Associations of serum thyrotropin concentrations with recurrence and death in differentiated thyroid cancer. *J Clin Endocrinol Metab.* 2007;92(7):2610–2615.

# 3

# Non-Small-Cell Lung Cancer

KUNAL C. KADAKIA AND NITHYA RAMNATH

## EPIDEMIOLOGY, RISK FACTORS, NATURAL HISTORY, AND PATHOLOGY

Lung cancer, including non-small-cell lung cancer (NSCLC) and small cell lung cancer (SCLC), is the leading cause of cancer death among men and women in the United States. In 2014, there were an estimated 224,210 new cases of lung cancer (116,000 men and 108,210 women) with an estimated 159,260 attributable deaths (1). The 5-year survival rate for all lung cancers combined is 15%, with disease stage at diagnosis the most important prognostic indicator. Other poor prognostic factors include poor performance status (PS), male gender, older age, and African American heritage (2). In the United States, as many men die from lung cancer as from prostate and colon cancers combined. Also, as many women die from lung cancer as from breast, ovarian, and uterine cancers combined (1). The incidence has plateaued since 2003, but the lung cancer death rate in women is still slowly increasing (2). In men, both the incidence and the death rates are slowly decreasing. The trends in incidence and mortality tend to parallel smoking rates, with a 20-year latency. The diverse smoking prevalence from state to state results in large variations in lung cancer incidence, with the lowest rate (per 100,000) in Utah (34.1 male and 23.3 female) and the highest rate in Kentucky (125.9 male and 80.3 female) (1).

Most lung cancers are attributable to cigarette smoking (90%) (3). Other risk factors include exposure to radon, radiation, asbestos, arsenic, chromium, nickel, chloromethyl ethers, and cadmium (3–5). Cigarette smoke contains >300 chemicals, 40 of which are known carcinogens.

Two of the major carcinogens, $N$-nitrosamine ketones (NNKs) and polycyclic aromatic hydrocarbons, cause DNA adduct formation, resulting in mutations. Nicotine and NNK also activate Akt signal transduction, causing apoptotic inhibition and increased cellular proliferation. Lung cancer risk increases with smoking duration and daily number of cigarettes smoked. The risk in smokers is about 20-fold more than that in nonsmokers. Changing to cigarettes marked as "light," menthol, or improved filtering, does not decrease risk. Risk decreases with smoking cessation and approaches that of a nonsmoker after 15–20 years of abstinence. About 30% of lung cancers in nonsmokers may be related to passive smoke exposure (3). The risk from electronic cigarettes is not established yet, but preliminary studies demonstrated detectable levels of known carcinogens and toxins (6,7).

Radon is a radioactive gas produced by uranium and radium decay, emitting alpha particles, which can damage cells. Uranium miners have the greatest occupational exposure, but residential exposure may cause up to 10% of NSCLC (4). There is a dose–response effect, and the risk is synergistic with smoking. Asbestos exposure is also synergistic with smoking due to impaired bronchial clearance of asbestos. For example, if the relative risk is 2–4 in a nonsmoker exposed to asbestos, it would be 40–100 in a smoker. After asbestos exposure, lung cancer incidence peaks 25–35 years later and is much higher than the mesothelioma incidence. Prior radiation treatments for breast cancer and lymphoma also increase lung cancer risk, especially in smokers. The latency is typically 5–10 years, and the tumors are often more aggressive.

Given the large high-risk population, there were several randomized, double-blinded, placebo-controlled lung cancer chemoprevention trials. However, supplementation with vitamin A, beta-carotene, their derivatives, or selenium provided no benefit (8–10). Lung cancer risk was increased in smokers who were given extra beta-carotene (8,9). Smoking's confounding effect has made it difficult to elucidate any genetic hereditary factors.

Genome-wide association studies have identified lung cancer susceptibility loci at chromosome 6q, 15q25 5p15, 13q31, and 6p21 (11–16). The single nucleotide polymorphisms involved in the 5p15.33 region map to TERT, a telomerase extension reverse transcriptase. TERT is activated in many cancers and increases cellular proliferation through abnormal telomere maintenance. The 5p15 locus has an association with adenocarcinoma (AC), regardless of smoking status. However, the 15q25 locus, which maps to the nicotinic acetylcholine receptor, appears to be only associated with smokers.

Most patients present with signs and symptoms related to the primary mass, locoregional spread, metastasis, or paraneoplastic syndromes (Table 3.1). About 10% of patients are asymptomatic, often diagnosed after a chest x-ray or CT scan obtained for other reasons. Lung AC has surpassed squamous cell carcinoma (SCC) as the most common histologic subtype in the United States. These tumors tend to be peripherally located, and may not cause significant early symptoms. They also tend toward early lymph node metastasis, hematogenous spread, and appearance near old scars. Histologically, ACs exhibit glandular differentiation and evidence of mucin production, often with cytoplasmic vacuoles. There are 4 major types: acinar, papillary, solid with mucin formation, and bronchioalveolar (BAC).

SCC currently accounts for about 25% of NSCLC in the United States and is exclusively related to tobacco smoke exposure. Typically, SCCs are larger and centrally located, forming in the segmental bronchi and extending to involve the lobar and main-stem bronchi. Central necrosis and cavitation are common. Histologically, SCCs are characterized by intercellular bridging, squamous pearl formation, and individual cell keratinization.

Large cell carcinomas account for about 10% of NSCLC and are clinically similar to ACs. Histologically, the cells are larger, with abundant, minimally differentiated cytoplasm. Some large cell carcinomas can have a partial neuroendocrine phenotype, staining positive for chromogranin A and/or synaptophysin. A poor prognosis is associated with a subtype showing increased mitotic figures and necrosis with neuroendocrine features. Large cell neuroendocrine carcinoma is a rarer subtype that also includes evidence of palisading or rosette-like morphology.

Lung cancer develops over time, through a series of genetic and epigenetic changes in bronchial epithelial cells. Three known premalignant morphologies, namely, squamous dysplasia, atypical adenomatous hyperplasia, and diffuse idiopathic pulmonary neuroendocrine hyperplasia, can develop into SCC, AC, and carcinoid tumors, respectively. Multiple chromosomal alterations occur during tumor pathogenesis, including loss of 3p, 4q, 9p, and 17p. Loss of 1 copy of 3p is an early event, found in 96% of lung tumors. Multiple tumor suppressor genes, including fragile histidine triad (FHIT), have been

**Table 3.1**  Clinical Signs and Symptoms of Lung Cancer

| Primary Central/Endobronchial Tumor | Primary Peripheral Tumor |
| --- | --- |
| Cough (+/– sputum production) | Cough |
| Hemoptysis | Pain—pleural or chest wall involvement |
| Dyspnea (related to obstruction) | Dyspnea (more restrictive basis) |
| Wheezing (often unilateral) or stridor | Pleural effusion |
| Postobstructive pneumonia | Pneumonitis |

**Locally Advanced Disease (direct or metastatic spread)**
Hoarseness (recurrent laryngeal nerve paralysis)
Phrenic nerve paralysis (elevated hemidiaphragm and dyspnea)
Dysphagia (esophageal compression)
Stridor (tracheal obstruction)
Superior vena cava (SVC) syndrome
Pancost/Horner's syndromes (apical tumor)
Dyspnea (pleural effusions, trachea/bronchial obstruction, pericardial effusion, phrenic nerve palsey, SVC obstruction, lymphangitic spread

**Metastatic Disease**
Brain (altered mental status, seizures, headache, nausea/emesis, motor or sensory deficits)
Bone (pain, exacerbated by movement or weight bearing)
Spine (extremity weakness, pain)
Liver (right upper quadrant and/or epigastric pain, nausea/emesis, icterus)

**Paraneoplastic Syndromes** *(more common in small cell lung cancer)*
Hypercalcemia (most common in squamous cell)
Pulmonary hypertrophic osteoarthropathy (clubbing, painful arthralgias)
Trousseau's syndrome/hypercoagulability
*Syndrome of inappropriate secretion of antidiuretic hormone (SIADH)*
*Cushing's syndrome—ectopic adrenocortiotropic hormone production*
*Eaton-Lambert syndrome*
*Dermatomyositis*

*Note:* Text in italics indicates findings more common in small-cell lung cancer.

mapped to 3p. Other alterations have been noted in oncogenes and tumor suppressor genes including mutations, amplification, loss of protein expression or overexpression, gene hypermethylation, and increased telomerase activity (Table 3.2).

Epidermal growth factor receptor (EGFR) is an epithelial cell surface transmembrane receptor of the ErbB family of tyrosine kinase receptors. When activated, the resulting signal transduction cascade leads to decreased apoptosis along with increased cellular proliferation, angiogenesis, and invasiveness. The EGFR gene mutational status is most predictive of response to small molecule inhibitors. EGFR mutations are most common (approximately 40%) in never

**Table 3.2** Selected Molecular Alterations in NSCLC

| Description | All NSCLC (%) | Adenocarcinoma (%) | Squamous Cell Carcinoma (%) |
|---|---|---|---|
| **Tumor Suppressor Genes** | | | |
| Rb mutations (13q14) | 20–40 | | |
| Rb loss of protein expression | 15–60 | 23–57 | 6–14 |
| p16/CDKN2A mutations (9p21) | 10–40 | | |
| p16/CDKN2A hypermethylation | 15–41 | 21–36 | 24–33 |
| p53 mutations (17p13) | 50–60 | 50–70 | 60–70 |
| **Oncogenes** | | | |
| EFGR mutations | 20 | <10 (West) ~40 (Asia) | Rare |
| EFGR protein overexpression | 50–90 | 40–65 | 60–85 |
| Her-2 protein overexpression | 20–35 | 16–38 | 6–16 |
| K-ras mutation | 10–30 | 15–35 | <5 |
| B-raf mutation | 1–3 | | |
| Myc family gene amplication | 8–22 | | |
| EML4-ALK fusion oncogene | 1–4 | 1–4 | Rare |
| Bcl-2 protein overexpression | 10–35 | | |

NSCLC, non-small-cell lung cancer.
*Source*: Adapted from Ref. (17). Larsen JE, Spinola M, Gazdar AF, et al. *An Overview of the Molecular Biology of Lung Cancer*. Philadelphia, PA: Lippincott Williams & Wilkins; 2010.

or light-smoking Asian women with AC. These mutations are seen in 10% or less of non-Asian populations and almost never in SCC. Located in the tyrosine kinase domain, the mutations cause constitutive receptor activation. The small molecule inhibitors (erlotinib, gefitinib, and afatinib) bind to the tyrosine kinase domain, turning off the downstream signaling cascade. Although the inhibitors were designed against wild-type EGFR receptors, they more potently inhibit mutated receptors. About 45% of EGFR mutations are small in-frame deletions in exon 19 and another 40–45% are an exon 21 point mutation, L858R. A rare intrinsic or frequently acquired point mutation in exon 20, T790M confers resistance to erlotinib or gefitinib.

Ras family gene members encode cell membrane-associated GTPases involved in cellular signal transduction. The most common K-ras mutation (90%) in NSCLC is a G → T transversion in codon 12 causing constitutive activation, but mutations can also occur in codons 13 and 61. When K-ras is mutated in nonsmokers, a G → A transition is more common. K-ras mutations are typically seen in AC and are associated with tobacco smoke exposure. They are mutually exclusive from EGFR mutations and the echinoderm microtubule-associated protein like 4 (EML4)–anaplastic lymphoma kinase (ALK) fusion. There is no clear evidence of a difference in survival between patients with K-ras mutated versus K-ras wild-type tumors, particularly if the tumors also have wild-type EGFR. Tumors with K-ras mutations are less likely than those with wild-type K-ras to respond to treatment with the small molecule inhibitors erlotinib or gefitinib, but this was not noted with the EGFR monoclonal antibody, cetuximab.

p53 is the most frequently mutated gene in human cancer. In NSCLC, these mutations are smoking related. Again, G → T transversions are most common. Without functional p53, there is no G1 arrest in the cell cycle to allow for DNA repair. Instead, the cells continue to divide and propagate damaged DNA. Retrospectively, p53 overexpression in NSCLC has been related to poor prognosis and decreased overall survival (OS). However, prospectively, p53 mutations only predicted decreased survival in surgically resected stage I tumors.

Some ACs contain a chromosome 2p inversion, Inv(2) (p21p32), forming the EML4–ALK fusion oncogene. The resulting protein has an N-terminus derived from EML4 and a C-terminus with the tyrosine kinase domain of ALK. This fusion tends to be mutually exclusive from EGFR and K-ras mutations, occurs in about 4% of NSCLC, and is associated with AC in younger patients with little or no smoking history. Tumors with this alteration have a significant response to crizotinib (a small molecule inhibitor of c-MET and the ALK fusion protein).

Additional molecular markers examined as potential prognostic and/or predictive markers include ERCC1 (excision repair cross-complementing rodent repair deficiency group 1) and RRM1 (ribonucleotide reductase M1). ERCC1 contributes to a rate-limiting step in the nucleotide excision repair pathway used to overcome the DNA crosslinks formed by platinum agents. RRM1 is the regulatory unit of ribonucleotide reductase needed for DNA synthesis and repair. Gemcitabine is a cytidine analog that inhibits RRM1 and thereby DNA production. Retrospective data suggested that in advanced NSCLC, a high ERCC1 level

| Non-Small-Cell Lung Cancer Staging | | | | | |
| --- | --- | --- | --- | --- | --- |
| Sixth Edition T/M Descriptor | Seventh Edition T/M | N0 | N1 | N2 | N3 |
| T1 (≤2 cm) | T1a | IA | IIA | IIIA | IIIB |
| T1 (>2–3 cm) | T1b | IA | IIA | IIIA | IIIB |
| T2 (≤5 cm) | T2a | IB | **IIA** | IIIA | IIIB |
| T2 (>5–7 cm) | T2b | **IIA** | IIB | IIIA | IIIB |
| T2 (>7 cm) | T3 | **IIB** | **IIIA** | IIIA | IIIB |
| T3 invasion | | IIB | IIIA | IIIA | IIIB |
| T4 (same lobe nodules) | | **IIB** | **IIIA** | **IIIA** | IIIB |
| T4 (extension) | T4 | **IIIA** | **IIIA** | IIIB | IIIB |
| M1 (ipsilateral lung) | | **IIIA** | **IIIA** | **IIIB** | **IIIB** |
| T4 (pleural effusion) | M1a | IV | IV | IV | IV |
| M1 (contralateral lung) | | IV | IV | IV | IV |
| M1 (distant) | M1b | IV | IV | IV | IV |

N1 is consistent with metastasis in ipsilateral peribronchial and/or ipsilateral hilar lymph nodes and intrapulmonary nodes, including involvement by direct extension. N2 is consistent with metastasis in ipsilateral mediastinal and/or subcarinal lymph node/nodes. N3 is consistent with metastasis in contralateral mediastinal, contralateral hilar, ipsilateral or contralateral scalene, or supraclavicular lymph node/nodes; items in boldface indicate a change from the sixth edition for a particular TNM category.
*Source*: Adapted from Ref. (18). Goldstraw P, Crowley J, Chansky K, et al. The IASLC Lung Cancer Staging Project: proposals for the revision of the TNM stage groupings in the forthcoming (seventh) edition of the TNM Classification of malignant tumours. *J Thorac Oncol.* 2007;2(8):706–714.

was associated with decreased survival and decreased tumor response to platinum-based therapies. Similarly, a high RRM1 level was associated with decreased tumor response to gemcitabine. However, in stage I disease treated with surgical resection alone, high levels of RRM1 and ERCC1 correlated with improved survival. There is no clear consensus on the quantification method of these markers, for example, mRNA expression or immunohistochemistry (IHC), and these markers can change in metastatic or previously treated disease. Thus, large-scale prospective studies are still needed to validate RRM1, ERCC1, K-ras, p53, and EGFR, or others as predictive or prognostic markers.

## STAGING

The International Association for the Study of Lung Cancer (IASCLC) staging for NSCLC is shown previously.

## CASE SUMMARIES

### Early-Stage NSCLC

M.E. is a 68-year-old man with a 60-pack-year smoking history and a persistent cough, recently treated for community-acquired pneumonia, who was found to have a 3.2 × 2.4 cm left lower lobe mass on CT scan. A CT-guided biopsy revealed SCC. He had a history of well-controlled hypertension and hyperlipidemia and is a retired construction worker. He is active and likes to go mountain climbing. A PET-CT scan was negative for involvement of

lymph nodes or distant metastases. He is enquiring about his treatment options.

## Evidence-Based Case Discussion

### Surgery Alone in Early-Stage NSCLC

In this otherwise healthy patient with a good PS, surgical resection of a clinical stage I or II NSCLC provides the greatest chance of cure. The type of procedure depends on the extent of disease and the patient's cardiopulmonary reserve. On the basis of pulmonary function testing, a patient with a pre-resection forced expiratory volume in 1 second (FEV1) ≥2 L or 80% of predicted is able to tolerate pneumonectomy, and generally, an FEV1 of 1.5 L is required for lobectomy. If either the FEV1 or the diffusion lung capacity for carbon monoxide (DLCO) is <60% of that predicted, then quantitative ventilation–perfusion scans can be used to predict the postoperative lung function. If the FEV1 and/or DLCO is <40% of the predicted value, then exercise testing is needed. Patients with a maximal oxygen consumption ($Vo_{2max}$) of 15 mL/kg/min or greater can still be considered for resection.

Mediastinal lymph node evaluation is important in staging, as the treatments for stage IIIA disease and stage I disease differ. Traditionally, mediastinoscopy is the gold standard and is recommended for any enlarged (>1 cm) mediastinal lymph nodes on CT scan, regardless of the PET scan. In prospective studies, PET detected mediastinal lymph node metastases more accurately than CT alone, and PET or PET-CT is now frequently used to evaluate new lung nodules. However, PET is more costly, has limited availability, and cannot detect lesions <8 mm. Inflammatory processes can cause false-positive results, and some low metabolic tumors, such as BAC or carcinoid, can have false-negative results. Therefore, PET positive lymph nodes still require tissue confirmation. Mediastinal lymph node sampling can be performed by mediastinoscopy, endobronchial ultrasound (EBUS), transesophageal endoscopic ultrasound (EUS), or CT-guided or blind transbronchial needle aspiration or biopsy. A randomized controlled study showed that there is no difference in sensitivity between mediastinoscopy and EBUS plus EUS approach (79% vs. 85%, respectively). Blind transbronchial needle aspiration has much lower sensitivity. Choice of diagnostic modality also depends on nodal location, locally available resources, and practitioner experience. The American College of Chest Physician (ACCP) guideline recommends a nonsurgical approach as a first choice. If nodal involvement is highly suspected after negative result with a nonsurgical method, mediastinoscopy or video-assisted thoracic surgery (VATS) can be used (19). Also, the test result is influenced by thoroughness of the procedure rather than which modality is used. On the basis of the guideline, further preoperative mediastinal lymph node evaluation would not be necessary in our patient M.E., as he has nonenlarged, PET-negative mediastinal lymph nodes.

The extent of intraoperative lymph node sampling has been widely studied, but the results are unclear. A Cochrane meta-analysis concluded that systematic mediastinal nodal dissection in patients resected for stage I–IIIA NSCLC improved overall survival (OS), compared to using only lymph node sampling (hazard ratio [HR] = 0.63, 95% CI [0.51–0.58], $P \leq .0001$). However, a trial conducted by the American College of Surgeons Oncology Group, randomizing patients to mediastinal lymph node dissection, or to sampling only, showed no difference in OS or time to recurrence. Adequate mediastinal lymphadenectomy should include stations 2R, 4R, 7, 8, and 9 for right-sided cancers and stations 4L, 5, 6, 7, 8, and 9 for left-sided cancers.

Lobectomy, a single-lobe surgical resection, became the standard treatment for early-stage NSCLC, on the basis of a Lung Cancer Study Group trial that randomized 276 stage T1N0 NSCLC patients to either lobectomy or to limited resection. In the limited resection arm, the overall recurrence rate increased by 75% ($P = .04$), and the local recurrence rate tripled ($P = .008$), with a trend toward increased overall and cancer-specific death rates. Because the study's tumor size limit was ≤3 cm, trials are now examining the same question with tumors ≤2 cm. In patients with decreased cardiopulmonary reserve and single tumors ≤2–3 cm, retrospective data suggest that surgical morbidity and mortality are similar or improved when receiving a sublobar resection versus a lobectomy, partly due to the smaller postoperative drop in pulmonary function.

VATS is an option in early-stage lung cancer, but there is not yet any definitive data to prove that VATS delivers an equivalent oncologic resection to open lobectomy. Patients undergoing VATS have a similar operative mortality, but with a shorter hospital stay, fewer postoperative complications, and less pain-related issues than with open lobectomy. In more proximally located tumors, where lobectomy may not be an option, a lung-sparing sleeve resection is preferred over pneumonectomy, when possible. Although OS is fairly similar, sleeve lobectomy in stage-appropriate patients can better preserve pulmonary function and avoid pneumonectomy-related complications. Meanwhile, T3 tumors invading the chest wall or mediastinum often require an en bloc resection for clear margins.

It is of note that given the size of M.E.'s tumor (>3 cm) and his smoking history, the suspicion of cancer is high enough that he could have proceeded directly to resection without a tissue diagnosis. The evidence is less clear for tumors <3 cm. On the basis of the tumor size, pretest probability of malignancy, potential for surgical resection, available resources, and patient preferences, a useful algorithm has been suggested by the ACCP (see Figure 3.1). When patients are not good surgical candidates, a tissue diagnosis prior to treatment is preferred.

Options for patients with limited cardiopulmonary reserve include definitive thoracic radiation therapy (60 Gy in 30 daily fractions), continuous hyperfractionated accelerated radiotherapy (CHART, 1.5 Gy, 3 times a day for 12 days, total dose of 54 Gy), stereotactic body radiation therapy (SBRT), radiofrequency ablation (RFA), and cryoablation. Radiation therapy alone for stages I–II NSCLC has a 10–25% survival rate at 5 years. The randomized phase III trial comparing CHART to conventional therapy had 169 (of 563 total) patients with stage I–IIA NSCLC. In this subset, the 2-year OS rate was 24% in the traditional arm versus 37% in the CHART arm, with 4-year OS rates of 12% and 18%, respectively. The data on SBRT, RFA, and cryoablation are currently limited to phase I or II studies, and no comparisons have been made between modalities or to surgical resection. Any option could be considered for a nonsurgical candidate with a peripheral tumor ≤3 cm. SBRT can be used for tumors up to 5 cm. A recent meta-analysis showed better 2-year and 5-year OS with SBRT than with conventional radiation therapy (CRT), but the CRT studies were older, and the SBRT studies had shorter follow-up.

## Surgery and Adjuvant Chemotherapy in Early-Stage NSCLC

Despite adequate surgery, cancer often recurs in patients with stage II disease, with a 5-year OS of about 30–40%. Thus, adjuvant treatment has been evaluated in stage I–III disease. The meta-analyses by the LACE (lung adjuvant

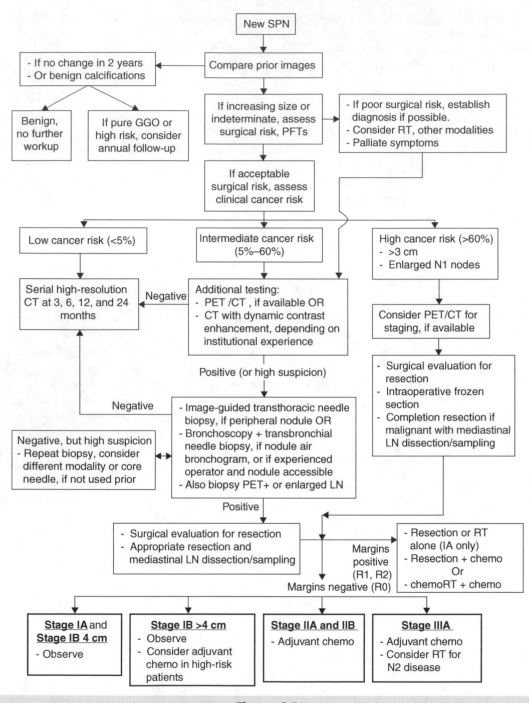

**Figure 3.1**

Pathway for diagnosis and clinical decision making in early-stage non-small-cell lung cancer. Chemo, chemotherapy; chemoRT, chemoradiotherapy; GGO, ground glass opacity; LN, lymph node; PFTs, pulmonary function tests; pts, patients; R0, no residual tumor; R1, microscopic residual tumor; R2, macroscopic residual tumor; RT, radiotherapy; SPN, solitary pulmonary nodule. *Source*: Adapted from Ref. (20). Gould MK, Fletcher J, Iannettoni MD, et al. Evaluation of patients with pulmonary nodules: when is it lung cancer? ACCP evidence-based clinical practice guidelines (2nd ed.). *Chest*. 2007;132(suppl 3):108S–130S.

cisplatin evaluation) and NSCLC collaborative groups indicate that adjuvant chemotherapy provides a 5-year OS benefit of about 4–5% in stage II–III disease. In the LACE study, the HR was 0.89 (95% CI [0.82–0.96], $P = .005$), corresponding to a 5-year survival benefit of 5.4% (21). In the NSCLC collaborative group meta-analysis, the HR was 0.86 (95% CI [0.81–0.92], $P < .0001$), corresponding to a 5-year survival benefit of 4%, an increase from 60% to 64% overall (22). In a separate analysis of trials using adjuvant chemotherapy with/and without radiation, the overall HR was 0.88 (95% CI [0.81–0.97], $P = .009$), corresponding to a 5-year survival benefit of 4%, increase from 29%

to 33% overall. The patients in this second group were mostly men with a median age of 59 years, good PS, and stage III disease. An exploratory analysis showed no difference between combination chemoradiotherapy and chemotherapy followed by radiation. Cisplatin plus vinorelbine showed slightly more benefit than other combinations, but the cisplatin doses were also higher. Although never compared head-to-head in the adjuvant setting, cisplatin plus either etoposide, gemcitabine, docetaxel, or pemetrexed are all acceptable adjuvant regimens, based on their relative equivalence in the advanced setting. If cisplatin cannot be used, carboplatin and paclitaxel are recommended.

Although adjuvant chemotherapy for stage IA patients is not helpful, and may actually decrease OS, the data for stage IB patients are less clear. Nodal metastases and increased size are the biggest risk factors for relapse in early-stage disease. Visceral pleural invasion and vascular invasion are also independent prognostic factors. Until recently, the stage IB patient population was more heterogeneous, including primary N0 tumors >5 cm, without direct invasion beyond the visceral pleura, and those ≤5 cm with N1 disease. The Cancer and Leukemia Group B (CALGB) 9663 trial, which specifically examined adjuvant chemotherapy in stage IB (old classification), only showed a survival benefit for patients with tumors ≥4 cm

(HR = 0.69, 95% CI [0.48–0.99], $P$ = .043). However, this study was criticized for its use of carboplatin/paclitaxel instead of a cisplatin doublet, early stopping due to initial positive results, and being underpowered to detect a small difference. The updated survival analysis of the JBR-10 adjuvant trial provides additional evidence, showing a trend toward benefit for tumors >4 cm (HR = 0.66, 95% CI [0.39–1.14], $P$ = .13) and lack of benefit for tumors <4 cm (HR = 1.73, 95% CI [0.98–0.34], $P$ = .06). As previously discussed, various molecular markers and gene expression profiles are being evaluated to determine which specific subgroups would benefit most from adjuvant chemotherapy, but this is not a routine clinical practice. Given M.E.'s tumor location, he may have evidence of visceral pleural invasion at surgery, and thus may want to consider adjuvant chemotherapy, after an informed discussion about risks and benefits.

Adjuvant radiation has also been examined in early-stage lung cancer, but several meta-analyses indicate that postoperative radiation has an adverse effect on OS for N0 and N1 disease. The best evidence is for N2 disease (HR = 0.855, 95% CI [0.762–0.959]; $P$ = .0077) (23). Therefore, unless this patient has pathological N2 nodal involvement or positive margins, adjuvant radiation therapy would not be recommended (see Figure 3.2).

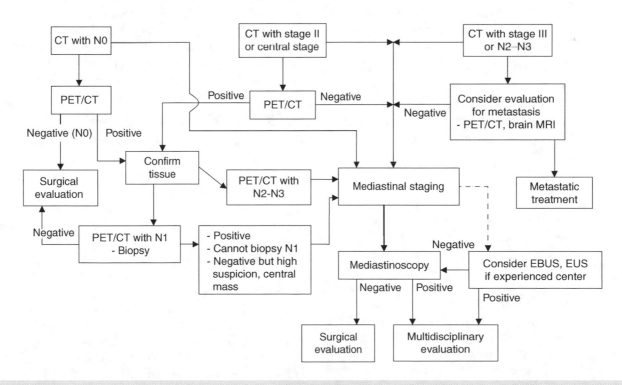

## Figure 3.2

Guidelines for locoregional lymph node staging in non-small-cell lung cancer. PET/CT positive nodes must have tissue confirmation. Mediastinal staging with mediastinoscopy is still the gold standard for all but peripheral PET/CT node negative tumors. EBUS, endobronchial ultrasound guided biopsy; EUS, esophageal ultrasound guided biopsy; Neg, negative; Pos, positive. *Source:* Adapted from Ref. (24). Vansteenkiste J, Dooms C, De Leyn P. Early stage non-small-cell lung cancer: challenges in staging and adjuvant treatment: evidence-based staging. *Ann Oncol* 2010;21(suppl 7):vii189–195.

## Neoadjuvant Chemotherapy in Early-Stage NSCLC

Multiple smaller studies have suggested that chemotherapy can also be given neoadjuvantly. However, many studies were stopped early as the adjuvant data became available or because of slow accrual. A Cochrane meta-analysis revealed a benefit of platinum-based neoadjuvant chemotherapy over surgery alone with an HR of 0.82 (95% CI [0.69–0.97], $P = .022$), corresponding to an absolute benefit of 6–7% in stages IB–IIIA, and 3–5% in IIIB. When the data from the European intergroup trial were added to this meta-analysis, the statistical significance was no longer present (HR = 0.88, 95% CI [0.76–1.01], $P = .07$). However, this trial had 61% stage I patients and allowed any 1 of the 6 adjuvant chemotherapy regimens. The only trial to compare neoadjuvant and adjuvant chemotherapy to date is the NATCH trial. This trial also had mostly stage I patients (75%) and used 3 cycles of carboplatin/aclitaxel. Patients with T1N0 to T3N1 disease were randomized to surgery alone, neoadjuvant, or adjuvant chemotherapy. Notably, 97% of the patients in the neoadjuvant arm received the planned chemotherapy versus 66.2% in the adjuvant arm, but there was no statistical difference in progression-free survival or OS. Although the strong adjuvant data may limit further studies, neoadjuvant chemotherapy with 3 cycles of a cisplatin-based doublet seems reasonable in stages IB–IIIA (N0–1), especially if there is a concern about ability to tolerate postoperative chemotherapy.

## Treatment of Superior Sulcus Tumors

The approach to superior sulcus tumors, even in the earlier stages, has been slightly different, given the tumor type and the risk to, or involvement of, adjacent structures. The classic presentation includes shoulder/arm pain or paresthesias, Horner's syndrome, and intrinsic arm muscle atrophy, caused by extrinsic tumor compression or direct brachial plexus involvement. Brachial plexus MRI imaging helps to determine resectability and extent of disease, as an MRI provides better resolution than a CT scan of the vascular and neurologic structures in this region. As these are relatively rare tumors (about 5% of all NSCLC), there is limited evidence-based data to guide treatment. The largest multi-institutional study, the Southwest Oncology Group (SWOG) Trial 9416, was a phase II trial to evaluate induction cisplatin/etoposide combined with radiation to 45 Gy, followed by surgery and 2 cycles of consolidation chemotherapy. With an 82-month median follow-up, the 5-year OS was 54% after an R0 resection, versus 44% for all patients. The median OS was not reached for those with a complete pathological response at surgery (R0), but the median OS was 30 months for patients with minimal microscopic disease (R1) and 29 months for those with gross residual disease (R2). Institutional protocols differ, but cisplatin-based induction chemoradiation followed by surgery is the standard of care in the United States for resectable superior sulcus tumors. Microscopic residual

disease clearly has a worse prognosis, but the protocols of additional chemotherapy and/or radiation also vary.

## Treatment of Positive Margins

There are no data on the most effective treatment for positive surgical margins. In stage I and II disease, re-resection (with adjuvant chemotherapy in stage II) is preferred, because surgery is still the most definitive modality in early-stage disease. When re-resection is not possible, combination chemoradiation followed by chemotherapy is recommended, depending on patient PS and ability to tolerate treatment postoperatively.

## Regional (Stage III) NSCLC

S.S. is a 55-year-old woman with a history of mitral valve prolapse and anxiety, who presents with a persistent cough. A chest x-ray revealed a 3.5-cm right upper lobe mass. A subsequent chest CT showed a spiculated $3.5 \times 3.3$ cm$^2$ right upper lobe mass with right hilar lymphadenopathy and an enlarged 1.9-cm right paratracheal lymph node. A subsequent PET/CT demonstrated $^{18}$F-fludeoxyglucose (FDG) uptake in the lung mass and the paratracheal lymph node. A transbronchial core needle aspiration of both the mass and the 4R lymph node were both positive for poorly differentiated carcinoma, consistent with a lung primary. She has never smoked, but did have exposure working as a bartender for many years. She cares for her 2 young sons and teaches Pilates at the local gym. Her sister was diagnosed with breast cancer at the age of 33 years. Her brain MRI was negative and she had normal pulmonary function testing.

### Evidence-Based Case Discussion

Stage III disease is heterogeneous, ranging from nonbulky, incidental N2 disease at resection to bulky, unresectable T4N3 disease. Definitive evidence regarding treatment, if available, does not necessarily apply to all patient populations. Varied imaging and diagnostic techniques, changes in staging, improvements in chemotherapy and radiation delivery, and small or underpowered studies further complicate the interpretation of available data. In general, primary tumor location, mediastinal lymph node involvement, patient PS, and lung function are all considered in treatment planning. For most patients, the treatment goal is cure, but about 80% of patients recur, frequently locally or in the brain. Although there are limited retrospective data regarding routine screening for asymptomatic brain metastases, it is a general practice that patients with stage III disease have either a head CT with IV contrast or an MRI.

### Microscopic N2 Disease or Pathological N2 Disease After Resection

Although not the case in S.S., if M.E. had incidental N2 disease at surgical resection, radiation after completion of adjuvant chemotherapy is recommended, based on the previously mentioned Surveillance, Epidemiology and End Results (SEER) Medicare study, suggesting a benefit of postoperative radiotherapy (PORT) in patients with pN2 disease (23). There are also data from an unplanned subgroup analysis of patients on the Adjuvant Navelbine International Trialist Association (ANITA) trial. The data are only descriptive, as the allocation was not randomized. Patients with pN2 disease who received PORT after adjuvant chemotherapy had a median OS of 47 versus 24 months for patients receiving only adjuvant chemotherapy. Corresponding 5-year OS values were 47.4% and 34%, respectively. Adjuvant radiation typically follows chemotherapy, but the outcome is not clearly different if this sequencing is reversed (22).

## Definitive Chemoradiotherapy

The standard of care in stage III disease is cisplatin-based chemotherapy with etoposide or vinblastine and concurrent radiation. This is the primary treatment for patients who are not operative candidates due to tumor size, location, or PS. Multiple studies have indicated the benefit of concomitant chemoradiation over sequential chemotherapy and radiation or over radiation alone. A Cochrane meta-analysis of concurrent versus sequential chemotherapy and radiation had an HR of 0.74 (95% CI [0.62–0.89]) and a 10% absolute survival benefit at 2 years (25). An NSCLC Collaborative Group meta-analysis found a significant but smaller absolute survival benefit of 5.7% at 3 years and 4.5% at 5 years (HR = 0.84, 95% CI [0.74–0.95], $P = .004$) (26). Some of the difference in the latter analysis may be explained by the longer median follow-up (6 years) and the inclusion of 3 trials with single-agent cisplatin or carboplatin and 2 trials with split course radiation. All of the Cochrane analysis trials used cisplatin-based doublets and continuous radiation. Concomitant chemoradiation improved locoregional control, but distant progression was similar to sequential therapy. Chemoradiation also increased acute esophageal toxicity (grades 3–4) from 4% to 18% ($P < .001$), but acute pulmonary toxicity was similar. In poor PS patients, weekly low-dose carboplatin/paclitaxel with concurrent thoracic radiation to 63 Gy, followed by 2 cycles of standard carboplatin/paclitaxel have been used, but not compared with full-dose chemoradiotherapy in a randomized trial.

The optimal chemotherapy combination for chemoradiation is not clear and other agents, including pemetrexed, taxanes, and EGFR inhibitors, are also being examined. The radiation dose is typically 60–70 Gy. Newer 3-D and 4-D conformal techniques and respiratory gating have decreased the off-target delivery to the lungs, spinal cord, and esophagus. Various protocols have also used hyperfractionated radiation or intensity-modulated radiotherapy (IMRT) to optimize radiation dosing. In IMRT, the radiation beam is modulated to increase the primary tumor radiation dose and decrease the normal tissue dose.

Early results are promising. However, neither IMRT nor hyperfractionation should be used outside of a clinical protocol. For patients with very large radiation ports or significantly decreased PS, sequential chemotherapy followed by radiation or radiation alone can still be used.

Both induction and consolidation chemotherapy have been used with chemoradiation in phase II studies, but have not been of proven benefit in randomized phase III studies. The CALGB 39801 study randomized patients to receive 2 induction cycles of carboplatin and paclitaxel followed by chemoradiation or to chemoradiation alone, but there was no survival benefit to induction. Initial SWOG phase II data were promising for docetaxel consolidation. However, a randomized phase III study showed increased toxicity in the consolidation docetaxel arm, without a difference in median OS. Therefore, neither induction nor consolidation chemotherapy is recommended with definitive chemoradiation outside of a clinical trial.

## Multimodality Treatment

Because of the high incidence of locoregional failure (up to 83%) with chemoradiation, many have questioned if including surgery would provide any additional benefit. There has also been interest in trying to control micrometastatic disease and therefore distant recurrence with neoadjuvant chemotherapy. Most of the initial data for neoadjuvant chemotherapy relates to smaller trials, frequently with surgery alone as the comparison arm, which is inferior in stage III disease. Again, the analysis of these trials is complicated by mixed tumor burden, varied mediastinal disease assessment, and varied protocols. This topic was recently reviewed in depth (27), and several trials are still accruing data. The reader is encouraged to keep in mind that some patients designated as stage IIIB in these trials may now be classified as stage IIB (T4 same lobe nodule N0) or stage IIIA (T4 same lobe nodule N1-2, T4 ipsilateral lobe nodule N0-1).

Limited data suggest the emergence of 2 important classes of current stage IIIA patients that are often considered for multimodality therapy, T4N0-1 disease, and potentially resectable T3N2 disease. The interest in limited T4 disease began with SWOG 8805, a phase II study of 2 cycles of cisplatin/etoposide with 45 Gy of concurrent radiation, followed by surgery. Remarkably, 19 patients achieved complete pathological response with a 50% 6-year survival. An exploratory multivariate analysis indicated that T4 non-N2 disease was the only independent predictor of long-term survival. SWOG 9019 was a phase II study evaluating only T4N0-3 patients, with the same induction regimen as 8805, but with completion to definitive radiation without interruption if there was no progressive disease. The median OS in this poor prognostic group was 15 months, but the prior improved response in the T4 N0-1 group was not seen (5-year OS = 15%). Combined, these trials suggest that surgery after neoadjuvant chemoradiation may be beneficial in the T4 N0-1 group. Using neoadjuvant chemotherapy alone, the Spanish Lung Cancer Group Trial 9901 was a phase II study of 3 cycles of induction cisplatin, gemcitabine, and docetaxel, followed by surgery in 67 patients with T4N0-1 disease and 69 with T1-3N2 disease. The median OS was 15.9 months and not significantly different between T4 and N2 disease. The median OS was 48.5 months for all with a complete (R0) resection (33 stage IIIA and 29 stage IIIB), but was 60.6 months for the 29 T4N0-1 patients (53.2% 5-year survival rate). Interestingly, of the 9 patients with complete pathological response at surgery, 8 had T4N0-1 disease, and the median OS was not reached after a median follow-up of 53.5 months (5-year OS = 57%). Given these small numbers, it remains in question whether induction chemotherapy truly provides benefit for T4N0-1 disease, or if these tumors are less invasive by nature.

A recent summary of 15 cohort studies of patients who underwent primary surgery for T4 disease suggests that the 5-year OS in T4N0-N1 disease may be as high as 43–74% versus a 15–18% 5-year OS in T4N2 disease (28). Complete resection (5-year OS = 38–46%) and T4 stage due to satellite nodules (5-year OS = 48–57%) were also significant predictors of improved outcome. The improved prognosis of those with T4N0 ipsilateral tumor nodules who had an R0 resection (5-year OS = 48%) was also seen in the data for the seventh edition of the American Joint Committee on Cancer (AJCC) staging criteria for NSCLC. However, the low prevalence makes a randomized trial determining the benefit of neoadjuvant or adjuvant chemotherapy in resectable T4N0-1 disease rather unlikely. Thus, complete surgical resection with or without additional chemotherapy and radiation could be considered in T4N0-1 disease (see Figure 3.3).

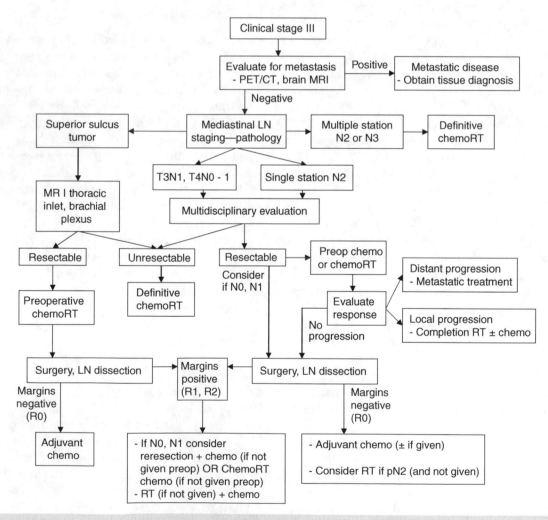

**Figure 3.3**

Pathway for diagnosis and clinical decision making in clinical stage III non-small-cell lung cancer. Head CT with contrast is an acceptable alternative to brain MRI. ChemoRT, chemoradiotherapy; LN, lymph node; pN2, pathological N2; Preop, preoperative; R0, no residual tumor; R1, microscopic residual tumor; R2, macroscopic residual tumor; RT, radiotherapy. *Source:* Adapted from National Comprehensive Cancer Network (29). Network. National Comprehensive Cancer. Practice guidelines in oncology— v. 3.2014. Non-small cell lung cancer, 2014.

In patients, such as S.S., with potentially resectable T3N2 disease, multiple phase II and retrospective cohort studies suggest that nodal downstaging with neoadjuvant treatment is both predictive and prognostic. The European Organization for Research and Treatment of Cancer (EORTC) 08941 trial comparing sequential chemotherapy followed by radiation versus the same chemotherapy followed by surgery in surgically unresectable, stage IIIA N2 patients had 41.4% nodal downstaging to N0/1. This nodal downstaging group had a median OS of 22.7 months, compared to the OS of the radiation and surgery arms (17.5 and 16.4 months, respectively). Also, nodal downstaging, complete pathological clearance, and no pneumonectomy were significant predictors of OS in the surgical arm. The phase III intergroup 0139 trial hoped for more definitive data. Patients with biopsy-proven T1–3N2 disease received chemoradiation to 45 Gy with 2 cycles of cisplatin/etoposide. If there was no progression on CT scan, patients then proceeded to either completion radiation up to 61 Gy or surgical resection, followed by 2 additional cycles of cisplatin and etoposide in both arms. The surgical group had a statistically improved progression-free survival (PFS) (12.8 vs. 10.5 months; HR = 0.77, 95% CI [0.62–0.96], P = .017), but the OS was similar (23.6 vs. 22.2 months; HR = 0.87, 95% CI [0.70–1.10], P = .24). The surgical group also had fewer local-only relapses, with similar rates of distant metastases. Survival was complicated by a 26% perioperative mortality in pneumonectomy patients. Notably, the T0N0 and TanyN0 groups had a higher median and 5-year OS (39.8 months and 42%, and 34.4 months and 41%, respectively). However, the recurrence pattern of these groups is not described, and these groups might have responded well to any treatment. No comparison could be made to the nonsurgical arm, as it has been documented that in NSCLC, CT scans do not accurately evaluate nodal response to chemotherapy and/or radiation. Surgical mediastinal staging has not been done in any nonsurgical arm to date, and it is unknown if PET/CT or staging by EUS could be an accurate alternative. Data from the seventh edition of AJCC NSCLC staging had a similar OS in patients who had primary surgical resection in multistation N1 disease and in single-station N2 disease.

In comparison to the trial's mortality, retrospective reports of pneumonectomies after neoadjuvant treatment have shown a 90-day postoperative mortality rate as low as 3% at major tertiary care centers. Although a right-sided pneumonectomy can have increased early perioperative mortality related to bronchial stump covering, the long-term survival of right and left pneumonectomy patients is similar in experienced centers. Thus, induction chemotherapy or chemoradiation followed by surgery could be considered for selected patients with excellent PS and nonbulky, stage IIIA N2 disease, especially those with single-station N2 disease and not requiring a right pneumonectomy. In summary, S.S. should have multidisciplinary evaluation to determine resectability and the type of surgery, followed by a risks-and-benefits discussion of standard definitive chemoradiation versus a trimodality treatment.

## Prophylactic Cranial Irradiation

Although commonly used in SCLC, there is no indication for prophylactic cranial irradiation (PCI) in locally advanced NSCLC, as a survival benefit has not been shown. The Radiation Therapy Oncology Group (RTOG) 0214 trial randomizing 340 stage IIIA and IIIB patients to PCI or observation closed early due to slow accrual. There were no differences in OS or PFS, but the observation arm patients were 2.52 times more likely to develop central nervous system (CNS) metastases than those in the PCI arm. Final recommendations regarding PCI may depend on whether significant differences in quality of life (QOL) measures are observed.

## Metastatic NSCLC, Case 1

L.A. is a 55-year-old nonsmoking Asian woman from Hong Kong who was visiting her daughter in the United States. She reported an unrelenting cough productive of clear sputum associated with shortness of breath. A chest x-ray revealed a large right upper lobe lung mass and an elevated right hemidiaphragm. A subsequent chest CT revealed a $4.5 \times 5$ cm$^2$ right upper lobe mass, diffuse mediastinal lymphadenopathy, multiple subcentimeter lung nodules, and a 3.5-cm mass in the right anterior lobe of the liver. A bronchoscopy with biopsy and a liver mass biopsy both demonstrated AC. She never smoked, but frequently inhaled cooking oil fumes in China. She is small, frail, and has dropped from 100 to 95 pounds in the past month.

## Evidence-Based Case Discussion

### EGFR Inhibitor

L.A.'s clinical characteristics, being female, Asian, a nonsmoker, and having AC, increases the likelihood that her tumor has an EGFR mutation. However, clinical characteristics should not replace formal mutational testing. The most common sensitizing EGFR mutations include exon 19 deletion and exon 21 L858R mutation (30). As previously mentioned, the incidence of this mutation in NSCLC is 30–50% in those of Asian descent and 10–15% in non-Asian populations. The Iressa Pan-Asia Study (IPASS) trial was a phase III study of 1217 treatment-naive Asian, nonsmokers (80% women) with advanced NSCLC that were randomized to either first-line gefitinib or to carboplatin/paclitaxel (31). The study met its primary objective, illustrating noninferior PFS (HR = 0.74, 95% CI [0.65–0.85], P < .001). An exploratory subgroup analysis revealed that gefitinib-treated patients with EGFR-mutated tumors had a significantly higher PFS (HR = 0.48, 95% CI [0.36–0.64], $P < .001$), whereas gefitinib-treated patients with EGFR wild-type tumors had a significant decrease in PFS (HR = 2.85, 95% CI [0.36–0.64], $P < .001$). Two subsequent randomized phase III trials included only patients with EGFR-mutated tumors. The North-East Japan (NEJ) 002 trial randomized patients to gefitinib or to carboplatin/paclitaxel. The gefitinib arm had a significantly better PFS, 10.8 versus 5.4 months (HR = 0.30, 95% CI [0.22–0.41], $P < .001$) and objective response rate (ORR) (73.7% vs. 30.7%, $P < .001$). Ninety-five percent of the chemotherapy arm patients received second-line gefitinib, but only 58.5% had an objective response. The West Japan Trial Oncology Group (WJTOG) 3405 trial included a higher number of patients with postoperative relapses than in the NEJ002 trial (41% vs. 9%). Patients were randomized to gefitinib or to cisplatin/docetaxel. The gefitinib arm had significantly better PFS, 9.2 versus 6.3 months (HR = 0.49, 95% CI [0.34–0.71], $P < .001$) and ORR (62.1% vs. 32.2%, $P < .0001$). Although not a part of the preplanned analysis, a difference in PFS was not statistically significant between the 2 arms in the postoperative subgroup (13.7 vs. 8.1 months, $P = .069$). No OS benefit was observed in any of the aforementioned trials; however, this lack of benefit is most certainly related to the high degree of crossover (i.e., subsequent EGFR tyrosine kinase inhibitor [TKI] therapy) in the cohorts that were randomized to chemotherapy (32,33). Erlotinib has also shown superior PFS compared with chemotherapy in 2 separate phase III trials in the first-line setting. The larger of these studies, the EURTAC trial, assigned 174 patients to erlotinib or a platinum doublet with PFS that nearly doubled in the erlotinib arm, median PFS of 9.7 versus 5.2 months (HR = 0.37, 95% CI [0.25–0.54], $P < .0001$) (34). Afatinib, a second-generation irreversible EGFR TKI, has also shown similar improved PFS compared to chemotherapy in 2 randomized phase III trials. The most recent of these, the Lux-Lung 6 trial, included 364 Asian patients and showed an increased PFS with afatinib compared to gemcitabine–cisplatin combination, median PFS of 11.0 versus 5.6 months (HR = 0.28, $P < .0001$) (35).

Nearly all patients with activating EGFR mutations responding to EGFR TKI therapy will eventually progress. The etiology of acquired resistance remains to be fully elucidated; however, secondary mutations in EGFR (most commonly the T790M mutation) and amplification of the MET oncogene have been established. The management of patients who develop resistance on EGFR TKI is dependent on the underlying molecular phenotype. Patients with T790M mutations or those with a MET amplification may be considered for ongoing clinical trials with therapies directed against these specific targets. In the absence of such actionable targets, it is reasonable to consider chemotherapy, as would be done in EGFR wild-type patients.

Previous studies did not support combined EGFR TKIs along with chemotherapy (36); however, this question has been revisited with the publication of results from the FASTACT-2 study. In this phase III study, patients with advanced NSCLC were given a platinum and gemcitabine with or without erlotinib in an intercalated fashion (the TKI was only given on days 15–28 of each cycle). There was an improved PFS with combination therapy (median PFS of 7.6 vs. 6.0 months, HR = 0.57, 95% CI [0.47–0.69]; $P < .0001$) (37). The reason for the positive findings in the study compared to previous combination studies remains unknown but one hypothesis is that using concurrent daily dosing of EGFR TKI might have an antagonistic rather than a synergistic effect as EGFR TKIs causes G1 cell-cycle arrest, thereby inhibiting cell cycle-dependent cytotoxic effects of chemotherapy, which can be abrogated by using therapy in an intercalated fashion as done in FASTACT-2 (38). Moreover, the most pronounced benefit with combination therapy was observed in patients with an EGFR mutation (median PFS = 16.8 vs. 6.9 months, HR = 0.25, 95% CI [0.16–0.39]), suggesting that patients with known EGFR-activating mutations could be considered for chemotherapy with EFGR TKI given in an intercalated fashion.

The most common toxicities associated with EGFR TKI can vary in severity and include rash (dry skin to acneiform rash) and diarrhea. Rare but serious toxicities include lung toxicity (interstitial lung disease) and hepatic toxicity.

Based on the preceding data, the National Comprehensive Cancer Network (NCCN) recommends (Category 1) testing for driver mutations including EFGR, ALK, and ROS1 (see later) in patients with non-squamous NSCLC. L.A. should be tested for EGFR, ALK, and ROS1 mutational status and if EGFR mutation is found, she should be treated with single-agent EGFR TKI (see Figure 3.4). In the United States, only erlotinib and afatinib are available.

## ALK Inhibitors

If L.A. were observed to harbor an ALK fusion gene, the ALK-inhibitor crizotinib would be indicated. The ALK gene encodes for a transmembrane receptor tyrosine kinase. The normal physiological role of ALK is poorly understood but is proposed to be involved in nervous system development; however, ALK-knockout mice are viable and exhibit no apparent developmental or tissue abnormalities. In a seminal study published in 2007, researchers in Japan first observed the novel ALK fusion of EML4 and ALK as a somatic gene rearrangement resulting from a small inversion within chromosome 2p in NSCLC (39). With this inversion, constitutive activation of the ALK tyrosine kinase occurs and leads to downstream effects on cellular proliferation and cell survival pathways. Since the discovery of the EML4–ALK fusion oncogene in NSCLC, it has been found that a number of less-common inversions and translocations also lead to ALK-mediated constitutive activation in

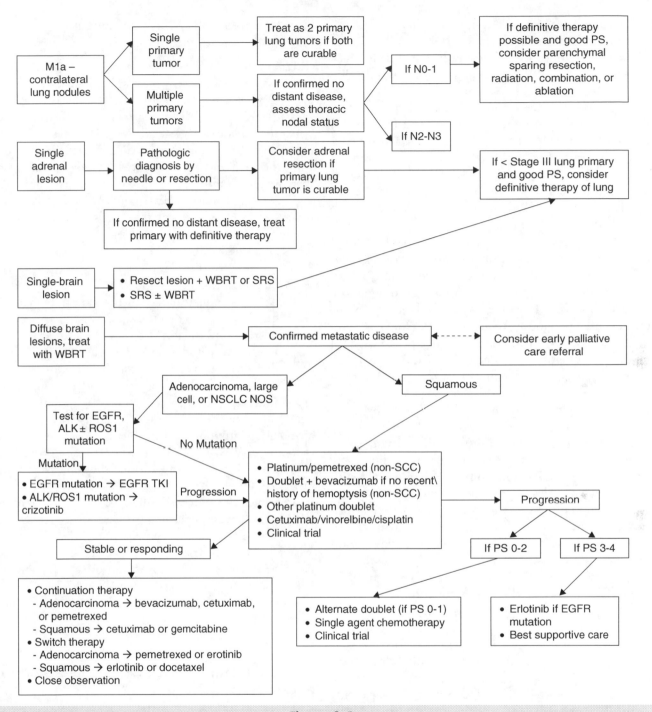

**Figure 3.4**

Pathway for clinical decision making in metastatic NSCLC. Obtain brain MRI or head CT with contrast, if not already done. Consider PET/CT and/or CT of the abdomen/pelvis if not already done. If bone pain, and no clear findings on CT or PET are available, consider a bone scan. If treating with surgery, recommend mediastinal staging evaluation. ALK, anaplastic lymphoma kinase; EGFR, epidermal growth factor receptor; N, node; Non-SCC, non-squamous cell carcinoma; NSCLC, non-small-cell lung cancer; PS, performance status; SRS, stereotactic radiosurgery; TKI, tyrosine kinase inhibitor; WBRT, whole-brain radiotherapy.
*Source*: Adapted from National Comprehensive Cancer Network (29). Network. National Comprehensive Cancer. Practice guidelines in oncology—v. 3.2014. Non-small cell lung cancer, 2014.

NSCLC. ALK gene rearrangements are identified by a Food and Drug Administration (FDA)-approved fluorescence in situ hybridization (FISH) assay and observed in approximately 3–5% of NSCLC. These rearrangements occur primarily in ACs and are more common in nonsmokers.

Crizotinib is an oral selective inhibitor of the ALK and MET tyrosine kinases and underwent accelerated FDA approval in 2011 based on the findings from the phase I Study 1001 and the phase II PROFILE 1005 trial. The updated analysis of the phase I Study 1001 showed an overall response rate of 60% with a median PFS of 9.7 months in 149 patients with stage III or IV ALK-positive NSCLC with crizotinib 250 mg orally twice daily given on a 28-day cycle (40). In the phase II PROFILE 1005 trial, 255 heavily pretreated ALK-positive NSCLC patients (85% with ≥2 previous chemotherapies) were noted to have an overall response rate of 50% with a median PFS of 8.5 months (41). Most recently, a phase III study confirmed the superiority of crizotinib over chemotherapy in 347 patients with ALK-positive NSCLC who had received at least 1 prior platinum-based regimen. In this study, the median PFS was 7.7 months in the crizotinib group compared to 3 months in the chemotherapy group (HR for progression or death with ctizotinib = 0.49, 95% CI [0.37–0.64]; P < .001) (42). Importantly, statistically significant improvements in symptom burden and overall QOL were observed in the crizotinib arm. No difference in OS was observed; however, as observed in the EGFR TKI trials noted previously, the majority of patients (64%) in this trial crossed over to crizotinib after progression on chemotherapy. Ongoing trials, such as PROFILE 1014, in the first-line setting have completed accrual and results are pending.

Treatment with crizotinib is generally well tolerated. The most common toxicity observed in 60–65% of patients is visual disturbances that manifests as difficulty adjusting from light to dark. These symptoms occur within a few weeks and improve over time and are not associated with objective abnormalities on ophthalmological assessment. Another common clinical adverse effect is gastrointestinal toxicity and occurs in around 25% of patients and manifests as nausea, vomiting, diarrhea, and constipation and is only rarely dose limiting. Elevated transaminases can be observed in up to 70% of patients with rare fatal hepatotoxicity reported; thus, liver function tests should be monitored during therapy. Rare pneumonitis could herald life-threatening respiratory failure and should prompt discontinuation of the medication. Other reported toxicities include sinus bradycardia, QTc interval prolongation, and reduction in serum testosterone in men.

As observed with EGFR TKIs, nearly all patients on crizotinib will eventually have progressive disease. Overcoming mechanisms of resistance are being elucidated and phase I data have shown promise with ceritinib (LDK378), a more potent inhibitor of ALK, in patients who have progressed on crizotinib and phase III trials are being planned (43). Another recently defined molecular subgroup of NSCLC that is responsive to ALK inhibition includes those patients with chromosomal rearrangements in the ROS1 gene (44). These data support the use of crizotinib 250 mg twice daily in patients with advanced or metastatic NSCLC whose tumors harbor an ALK fusion oncogene or ROS1 gene rearrangement. At the time of progression for these patients, participation in a clinical trial or standard chemotherapy is recommended.

## Standard Treatment, Platinum Versus Non-Platinum Chemotherapy

Alternatively, if L.A. tests negative for the EGFR mutation as well as ALK and ROS1 gene rearrangements, a platinum-based chemotherapy doublet would be indicated, provided her PS is 0–2. Some debate the benefits of cisplatin over carboplatin in metastatic NSCLC. A meta-analysis of individual patient data from 9 trials (2968 patients) showed that while the ORR was higher in patients treated with cisplatin, there was no significant OS difference between carboplatin and cisplatin regimens (HR = 1.07, 95% CI [0.99–1.15], P = .10) (45). However, when the analysis was restricted to third-generation platinum-based regimens, the survival difference became significant (HR = 1.11, 95% CI [1.01–1.21]). Patients treated with cisplatin were more likely to have nausea, vomiting, and renal dysfunction. Patients treated with carboplatin were more likely to have thrombocytopenia. Given the importance of QOL in metastatic disease, the potential risks of cisplatin use should be taken into consideration, along with the small benefit. There is currently no evidence that 1 particular third-generation platinum-based doublet is better than another, and a 3-drug regimen (excluding targeted therapies) provides no additional benefit. If a patient cannot tolerate platinum-based chemotherapy, a non-platinum-based doublet is recommended, but it is controversial whether this treatment is inferior. A meta-analysis of 37 phase I and II trials showed a significantly increased ORR with platinum-based treatment, with an improvement in 1-year survival by 5% (P = .0003). However, when only third-generation agents were used, the survival difference was no longer apparent. In a separate meta-analysis of 11 phase III trials, all with newer agents, platinum-based treatment provided a 2.9% absolute reduction in the risk of death at 1 year (HR = 0.88, 95% CI [0.78–0.99], P = .044), but with a higher risk of toxicity (46). Thus, a nonplatinum combination could be considered first line, if platinum agents are contraindicated.

## Standard Treatment With/Without Bevacizumab or Cetuximab

Two targeted agents combined with standard chemotherapy doublets have shown improved response in metastatic disease. Bevacizumab and cetuximab are monoclonal antibodies targeted against the vascular endothelial growth factor and EGFR, respectively. In a randomized phase III trial, Eastern Cooperative Oncology Group (ECOG) 4599 compared carboplatin/paclitaxel with or without bevacizumab dosed at 15 mg/kg every 3 weeks in patients with newly diagnosed metastatic or recurrent NSCLC. Patients randomized to the bevacizumab arm continued bevacizumab alone after the initial 6 cycles, until disease progression or toxicity (47). The bevacizumab arm had significantly improved OS (12.3 vs. 10.3 months, HR = 0.79, 95% CI [0.67–0.92], P = .003), PFS, and ORR, but higher toxicity rates, including clinically significant bleeding (4.4% vs. 0.7%) and arterial thrombosis. AVAiL was a 3-arm phase III trial comparing cisplatin/gemcitabine with or without bevacizumab at 7.5 mg/kg or 15 mg/kg every 3 weeks (48). In the updated analysis, PFS and ORR were improved in the bevacizumab-containing arms compared to chemotherapy alone, but no survival benefit was observed. There were no major differences in outcomes between the low versus high-dose bevacizumab arms. The reason why no survival advantage was observed remains unknown but it has been suggested that, in part, it was due to the relatively high proportion (65%) of patients who were able to proceed to second-line therapy as well as the better outcomes observed in the chemotherapy alone arm of 13.1 months compared to historical controls, which has been attributed to the high rate of nonsmokers (24%) in this trial. Most recently, a meta-analysis including 2194 patients from 4 trials suggested that the addition of bevacizumab significantly increased OS and PFS compared to chemotherapy alone (for OS, HR = 0.90, 95% CI [0.81–0.99]) (49).

Absolute contraindications to bevacizumab include squamous histology, major vessel involvement, untreated brain metastases, and active hemoptysis or other bleeding. Based on the phase II PASSPORT trial, patients who have had a treated and stable prior brain metastasis appear to tolerate bevacizumab without an increased risk of intracranial hemorrhage (50). Those on stable long-term anticoagulation could also be considered for treatment with bevacizumab after an informed discussion of the risks and benefits.

The First-Line ErbituX (FLEX) trial was an open-label phase III trial of cisplatin/vinorelbine with or without cetuximab in advanced lung cancer patients who had at least 1 tumor cell with EGFR expression by IHC. The patients in this arm had a significantly improved OS (11.3 vs. 10.1 months; HR = 0.87, 95% CI [0.762–0.996], $P = .044$). The BMS099 trial used carboplatin/paclitaxel or docetaxel, with or without cetuximab, but did not require EGFR status for enrollment, and saw no difference in DFS or OS. A meta-analysis combining the data from these 2 phase III trials and 2 phase II trials suggested an improvement in OS with a pooled HR of 0.87 (95% CI [0.79–0.96], $P = .004$) (20), but showed no benefit in PFS or 1-year survival. In the most recent trial of 939 patients assigned to single-agent chemotherapy (pemetrexed or docetaxel) either alone or in combination with cetuximab as second-line therapy after progression on a platinum-based regimen, no difference in PFS was observed (51). Given these data, cetuximab is not FDA approved for use in advanced NSCLC.

## Length of Treatment and Maintenance

To date, guidelines recommend that first-line chemotherapy be stopped after 4 cycles in patients who are not responding to treatment, or after a maximum of 6 cycles (29). A meta-analysis of 13 trials comparing a shorter versus a longer duration of chemotherapy found that longer chemotherapy durations improved both PFS (HR = 0.75, 95% CI [0.69–0.81], $P < .001$) and OS (HR = 0.92, 95% CI [0.86–0.99], $P = .03$) but also increased toxicity (52). In a meta-analysis of a more uniform set of 7 trials with third-generation platinum doublets, only PFS was improved in patients who received >4 cycles of therapy (53). These data support limiting combination platinum-based chemotherapy in the metastatic setting to a maximum of 4–6 cycles.

For patients who have a responding or stable disease following 4–6 cycles of combination chemotherapy, continuing therapy with either a cytotoxic agent or a targeted therapy can be considered. Two such maintenance approaches have been studied and include continuation maintenance and switch maintenance. Continuation maintenance refers to using a part of the initial regimen, whereas switch maintenance refers to the initiation of a different agent that was not utilized in the first-line regimen.

Three cytotoxic therapies (pemetrexed, docetaxel, and gemcitabine) have shown improved PFS when used as single-agent maintenance therapies. In the JMEN trial (switch maintenance), patients who had responding or stable disease after 4 cycles of a non-pemetrexed containing platinum doublet were randomized 2:1 to pemetrexed or placebo (54). Both PFS (HR = 0.5, 95% CI [0.42–0.61], $P < .0001$) and OS (HR = 0.79, 95% CI [0.65–0.95], $P = .12$) were significantly improved in the pemetrexed arm; this benefit was limited to patients with non-squamous histology. The PARAMOUNT trial included 939 patients with non-squamous histology who were treated with cisplatin/pemetrexed and randomized to pemetrexed or placebo (continuation maintenance). Similar to the JMEN trial, both PFS and OS were improved in the maintenance pemetrexed arm. Pemetrexed in combination with bevacizumab has also shown to improve PFS as maintenance and will be described subsequently. Docetaxel was observed to improve PFS and OS in a randomized phase III trial of 566 patients who received 4 cycles of gemcitabine/carboplatin followed by maintenance docetaxel for 6 cycles (switch maintenance) or docetaxel at the time of progression. Although a PFS and OS benefit was observed, it was noted that the patients who did receive docetaxel at the time of progression had comparable outcomes to the immediate treatment group (55). Gemcitabine used as continuation maintenance therapy was compared to erlotinib in a French phase III trial in 464 patients after 4 cycles of cisplatin/gemcitabine and a PFS benefit was observed (3.8 vs. 1.9 months, HF = 0.56) and a trend toward OS benefit (median survival = 12.1 vs. 10.6 months, HF = 0.89, 95% CI [0.69–1.15] (56).

Studies of EGFR TKIs and bevacizumab as maintenance therapy have also been extensively tested. In the SATURN trial, 889 patients who had not progressed after

4 cycles of a platinum doublet were randomized 1:1 to erlotinib or placebo (57). Patients were stratified for EGFR IHC and not for EGFR mutations, but EGFR mutations were similar between the groups. Both PFS (HR = 0.71, 95% CI [0.62–0.82], $P < .0001$) and OS (HR = 0.81, 95% CI [0.70–0.95], $P = .0088$) were significantly improved in the erlotinib arm. Notably, an OS benefit was observed in the erlotinib arm patients with wild-type EGFR tumors (HR = 0.77, 95% CI [0.61–0.97], $P = .0243$). The ATLAS trial randomized 768 patients (who had stable or responding disease to platinum doublets combined with bevacizumab) to erlotinib or placebo. Although PFS was improved in the erlotinib/bevacizumab arm, no statistically significant difference was observed in OS (median = 14.4 vs. 13.3 months, HR = 0.92, 95% CI [0.70–1.21]) (58).

Bevacizumab is commonly used in combination with platinum doublet in patients with advanced non-squamous NSCLC based on the aforementioned data (see the Standard Treatment With/Without Bevacizumab or Cetuximab section). Based on 2 large trials, bevacizumab utilized as continuation maintenance therapy remains a standard of care in select patients. In the PointBreak trial, 939 patients with advanced non-squamous NSCLC were randomized to first-line therapy with pemetrexed/carboplatin/bevacizumab or paclitaxel/carboplatin/bevacizumab and if stable or responding disease after 4 cycles, continuation therapy with either pemetrexed/bevacizumab or bevacizumab alone. Five hundred ninety patients received continuation therapy and there was no difference in OS (13 months in each arm) although PFS was slightly improved in the combination arm (median = 6.0 vs. 5.6 months, HR = 0.83, 95% CI [0.71–0.96]) (59). Similarly, in the AVAPERL trial, 253 patients with stable or responding disease treated with cisplatin/pemetrexed/bevacizumab were randomized to continuation therapy with either pemetrexed/bevacizumab or bevacizumab alone and a PFS was observed in the combination arm (median = 7.4 vs. 3.7 months following randomization, HR = 0.48, 95% CI [0.35–0.66]) but no OS benefit was noted (60).

Based on the previously mentioned data, for patients with an objective response (stable or responding disease) following a maximum of 4–6 cycles of initial therapy with a platinum doublet, it is reasonable to consider maintenance therapy. For those patients treated with bevacizumab as part of their initial therapy, continuing bevacizumab until progression or toxicity is reasonable. For patients with non-squamous NSCLC, switch or continuation maintenance with pemetrexed can be considered.

## Metastatic NSCLC, Case 2

H.P. is a 60-year-old man with a smoking history of 2 packs a day, who presented to his physician with a month-long history of persistent headaches, blurry vision, and cough after having been treated for community-acquired pneumonia. A head CT revealed a 2.5-cm right occipital lobe mass. Subsequent PET-CT showed a 4-cm left hilar lung mass with 2 FDG positive hilar lymph nodes and uptake in the occipital mass. A bronchoscopy and hilar lymph node biopsy were positive for SCC. Both EUS-guided sampling of mediastinal lymph nodes and mediastinoscopy were negative for evidence of N2 involvement. He had since quit smoking and has had improvement of his headaches and vision with steroids. He is the primary caretaker of his 85-year-old mother with dementia and has a good PS.

## Evidence-Based Case Discussion

### SCC Versus AC

The standard first-line treatment for metastatic SCC is a platinum-based doublet. The small molecule EGFR inhibitors (erlotinib and gefitinib) are not used because SCCs rarely carry EGFR mutations, and do not respond to these drugs. Bevacizumab is not used due to the increased bleeding risk seen with this tumor type. Pemetrexed is also not indicated for use in SCC, based on data from 2 phase III trials (61). One was a front-line non-inferiority trial in patients with stage IIIB or IV NSCLC, randomized to either cisplatin/gemcitabine or cisplatin/pemetrexed. The other trial compared pemetrexed to docetaxel in the second-line setting. Nonsquamous patients in both trials had a longer survival when treated with pemetrexed (HR = 0.84, 95% CI [0.74–0.96], $P = .011$; HR = 0.78, 95% CI [0.61–1.00], $P = .47$, respectively). It is hypothesized that this histological difference in efficacy may be related to higher expression of thymidylate synthase (the primary target of pemetrexed) in SCC.

### Treatment of Isolated Metastasis

In a patient with good PS and favorable prognostic factors (age <65 years, controlled primary tumor in the prior 3 months, and absence of extracranial metastases), treatment of a solitary brain metastasis with either surgical resection followed by whole-brain radiotherapy (WBRT) or with WBRT and stereotactic radiosurgery (SRS) can improve OS and PFS (62), with a 5-year survival rate of 11–30%. SRS has been shown to be equivalent to surgery for single lesions <3 cm and without extensive edema or mass effect (63). Surgery should be considered with posterior fossa lesions, due to the risk of fourth ventricle compression and subsequent increased intracranial pressure. Limited data, largely based on cases series, suggest that SRS for up to 3 small brain lesions might still have a survival benefit over WBRT alone. Standard WBRT is given as 30 Gy in 10 fractions and can be used alone in cases where surgery or SRS are not indicated. However, there are limited data if WBRT provides any significant benefit to patients with poor PS or advanced systemic disease with possible adverse effects on PS, QOL, and neurologic function. On completion of cranial treatment, systemic palliative chemotherapy or local radiation can be considered for the remaining extracranial disease, as tolerated.

However, in the case of H.P., a relatively young patient with good PS, aggressive treatment of both the lung primary and the solitary brain metastasis could be considered, based on retrospective analyses showing improved outcome in such patients (64). There are insufficient data to recommend concurrent chemotherapy and radiation with brain metastases. Therefore, the most aggressive treatment that could be offered would be surgical resection followed by WBRT or SRS, and definitive treatment of his lung lesion with surgery and adjuvant chemotherapy. Less aggressive options should also be discussed, given the higher risks of side effects (see Figure 3.4).

## Elderly or Poor PS

If instead of being a healthy 60-year-old, the patient described is a 76-year-old gentleman who is wheelchair bound from a recent stroke, the treatment options become much different. The median age of patients with newly diagnosed NSCLC is about 68 years; up to 40% of patients are older than 70 years. However, the vast majority of trials are conducted in nonelderly patients with a good PS. The American Society of Clinical Oncology consensus statement from 2011 recommends single agent rather than combination chemotherapy in patients with a PS of 2 (65). Three of the largest trials in the elderly suggest possible benefit with combination chemotherapy; however, patients with a PS of 2 made up a small subset in these trials and showed minimal to no benefit. In the French IFCT-0501 trial, 451 patients aged 70–89 years (30% with PS of 2) were treated with carboplatin/paclitaxel for 4 cycles versus single-agent therapy with either gemcitabine or vinorelbine followed by erlotinib in all patients after progression (66). At 30 months of follow-up, OS was prolonged in the combination chemotherapy arm (median OS = 10.3 vs. 6.2 months, HR = 0.64, 95% CI [0.52–0.78]); however, there was a greater risk of treatment-related death in the combination arm (4.4% vs. 1.3%). In a German phase III trial of 251 patients aged ≥65 years, there was only a nonsignificant trend toward improved PFS with pemetrexed/carboplatin/bevacizumab compared to pemetrexed/carboplatin (67). Importantly, the 13 patients with a PS of 2 did not demonstrate any benefit. Finally, the MILES trial randomized 698 patients to a non-platinum combination with gemcitabineor vinorelbine versus either drug as a single agent in patients aged ≥70 years (20% with PS of 2) with no significant difference in ORR or median survival in the combination arms (68). Given these data, age alone should not be used to guide treatment decisions in patients with NSCLC without a driver mutation, as older patients with good PS and minimal comorbidities can derive similar benefit from treatment as younger patients. However, patients with PS of 2 are exceedingly underrepresented in clinical

trials and caution should be exercised before pursuing palliative intent chemotherapy.

If a driver mutation (i.e., EGFR mutation) is found in an elderly patient with a PS of ≥2, single-agent EGFR TKI can be considered based on a small Japanese study in which 15 of 22 patients (68%) with a PS of 3 and an EGFR mutation improved to a PS ≤ 1, with a median OS of 18 months for the entire 29-patient group (69). However, other patients with a PS of 3–4 should be offered best supportive care, including palliative radiation for symptom control.

## Recurrent NSCLC

Our first patient, M.E., had an uneventful left lower lobectomy and lymph node dissection. After an informed discussion, he opted not to have adjuvant chemotherapy. Two years later, he presented with chest pain and dyspnea. A chest CT showed multiple bilateral lung nodules, concerning for metastatic disease. A bronchoscopy and a fine-needle aspirate revealed AC, consistent with a lung primary. He had a good partial response to carboplatin and pemetrexed, but 6 months later had progression.

### Evidence-Based Case Discussion

#### Isolated Recurrence

If he presented with a single isolated recurrence, he could be considered for additional local therapy, including resection. Alternatively, if he presented with an isolated distant metastasis, such as an adrenal or brain metastasis, consideration for definitive treatment of the lesion with surgery or SRS ± WBRT could be entertained. However, there is no evidence for additional adjuvant chemotherapy for a treated isolated metastasis with no other evidence of disease. Though recurrences of the primary cancer make up the vast majority of recurrences and most often occur in the first 2 years, patients with previously treated NSCLC have a 3–4% risk of developing a new primary lung cancer each year. As such, if the presentation, such as a late recurrence, suggests a new primary lung cancer, stage-appropriate treatment with histologic confirmation and molecular testing (EGFR, ALK, ROS1) would be indicated as the new primary may be molecularly distinct and offer novel therapeutic targets.

#### Multiple Areas of Recurrence

Utilizing non-cross-resistant chemotherapy or an EGFR, TKI in patients who have progressed after first-line platinum-based treatment has shown to improve outcomes in patients with recurrent NSCLC (65). Docetaxel initially demonstrated benefit in a randomized trial versus placebo and showed OS benefit (median = 7.5 vs. 4.6 months) when given at 75 m/m$^2$ every 3 weeks (70). Docetaxel can be given weekly at 33.3 mg/m$^2$ and appears to be better tolerated than the 3-week schedule with similar survival rates. Pemetrexed was established as an alternative following a phase III trial of 571 patients randomized to docetaxel or pemetrexed every 3 weeks in the second-line setting (71). Although the ORR was similar in both arms (≈10%), pemetrexed was associated with less neutropenia, need for granulocyte colony-stimulating factor support, and alopecia. As in other trials with pemetrexed, patients with non-squamous histology achieved the most benefit from pemetrexed. These data suggest that docetaxel or pemetrexed (in non-SCC NSCLC) can be used as second-line therapy.

EGFR TKI therapy in both wild-type and EGFR-mutated NSCLC has been shown to improve outcomes in recurrent NSCLC. The initial phase III trial that compared erlotinib to placebo provided evidence that erlotinib as second-line treatment can improve OS (median = 6.7 vs. 4.7 months, HR = 0.70, 95% CI [0.58–0.85]) (72). Multiple trials have compared EGFR TKIs to single-agent chemotherapy in patients with wild-type EGFR NSCLC. Overall, these trials support that cytotoxic chemotherapy has improved ORR and PFS compared to EGFR TKIs. In patients who progress on second-line chemotherapy, it is reasonable to consider EGFR TKI though there is no definitive evidence of benefit with third-line treatment.

If EGFR TKI was given first line, a platinum doublet could be considered in the second-line setting. However, there is no evidence to suggest benefit in switching from a cisplatin-based doublet to a carboplatin-based doublet, switching from erlotinib to gefitinib, or vice versa. Survival and response rates tend to decrease with each subsequent regimen, with increasing risk of toxicities. Best supportive care, including palliative care or hospice, is always reasonable to discuss in the metastatic setting. Alternatively, additional clinical trials could be considered for patients who maintain a good PS (see Figure 3.5).

## Emerging Therapy for NSCLC

Beyond newer combinations of cytotoxic chemotherapy regimens and the more recently defined actionable driver mutations (EGFR, ALK, ROS1 as described previously), immunotherapies along with novel combinations of targeted agents with cytotoxics are being developed for NSCLC. Improved understanding of the immune system's role in tumorogenesis, as observed and targeted in melanoma and renal cell carcinoma, continues to evolve in

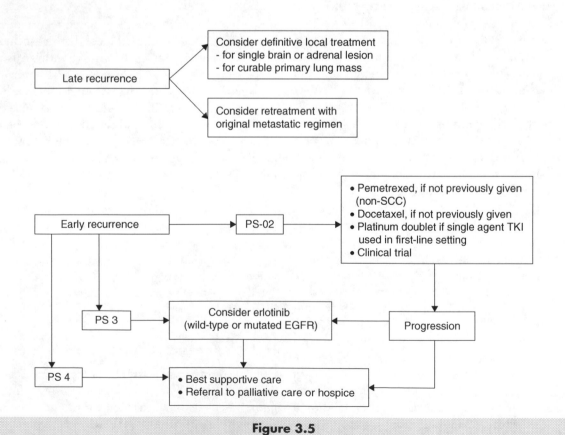

**Figure 3.5**

Pathway for clinical decision making in recurrent non-small-cell lung cancer. EGFR, epidermal growth factor receptor; non-SCC, non-squamous cell carcinoma; PS, performance status; TKI, tyrosine kinase inhibitor. *Source*: Adapted from National Comprehensive Cancer Network (29). National Comprehensive Cancer. Practice guidelines in oncology—v. 3.2014. Non-small cell lung cancer, 2014.

NSCLC. Programmed death receptor (PD1) has emerged as an innovative immunotherapy. Nivolumab, an IgG4 monoclonal antibody to PD1, has shown efficacy in early phase trials and many other immunotherapies are currently being evaluated (73).

The improved understanding of the genomic landscape involved in NSCLC has increased the awareness of potential actionable mutations. Multiple early phase trials have attempted to target some of these oncogenic pathways such as PIK3CA, AKT1, HER2, RET, PDGFRA, BRAF among others (74). Although a detailed discussion of these emerging therapies is beyond the scope of this chapter, multiple studies are currently in preclinical development or clinical trial stage. Patients should be informed of and offered clinical trial participation throughout their cancer trajectory.

## REVIEW QUESTIONS

1. A 48-year-old man with no medical history presents to your clinic to discuss decreasing his lung cancer risk and the role of chemoprevention. He does not smoke tobacco. His family history is significant for non-small-cell lung cancer diagnosed at age 61 years in his father, who had a tobacco-use history (25 pack-years). Which one of the below agents has shown benefit as a chemoprevention agent in lung cancer?

   (A) Vitamin A
   (B) Beta-carotene
   (C) Selenium
   (D) None of the above

2. A 61-year-old nonsmoking man is found to have a 4-cm right upper-lobe lesion that is biopsied and found to be adenocarcinoma (AC). A CT of the chest showed enlarged ipsilateral mediastinal and subcarinal lymphadenopathy with subsequent biopsy confirming AC. CT of the head and abdomen showed no evidence of distant metastases. You stage his cancer as stage IIIA (T2N2). He has no other comorbidities and his Eastern Cooperative Oncology Group performance status is 0. Which is the most appropriate recommendation?

   (A) Concurrent chemoradiotherapy followed by consolidation erlotinib
   (B) Induction therapy with platinum doublet followed by surgery and then radiation
   (C) Carboplatin with paclitaxel and bevacizumab for 4–6 cycles and then observation
   (D) Concurrent chemotherapy plus radiation therapy

3. A 52-year-old Asian nonsmoking woman presents with persistent cough and is found to have bilateral pulmonary nodules. Biopsy confirms adenocarcinoma of the lung with mutational analysis confirming epidermal growth factor receptor exon 19 deletions. She has no other comorbidities and her Eastern Cooperative Oncology Group performance status is 1. Which is the most appropriate first-line anticancer agent?

   (A) Carboplatin with paclitaxel
   (B) Erlotinib
   (C) Erlotinib with carboplatin and paclitaxel
   (D) Carboplatin with paclitaxel and bevacizumab

4. A 67-year-old man with known epidermal growth factor receptor (EGFR) exon 19 mutated non-small-cell lung cancer (NSCLC) was placed on afatinib as first-line therapy for metastatic disease at presentation. After 1.2 years of treatment, serial imaging shows disease progression in the lung and new lesions in the liver. Liver biopsy confirms the presence of NSCLC. Which is the most common mechanism of resistance in patients who progress after first-line EGFR tyrosine kinase inhibitor therapy?

   (A) Secondary T790M mutations in EGFR
   (B) Bypass signaling via c-MET amplification
   (C) Histologic transformation, NSCLC to small-cell lung cancer
   (D) Secondary L747S mutation in EGFR

5. The patient described in Question 2 returns for follow-up after biopsy confirmed metastatic non-small-cell lung cancer. He has pain in his right upper quadrant abdomen from tumor burden, but otherwise has no significant comorbidities and his Eastern Cooperative Oncology Group performance status is 1. Among the available choices, which is the most appropriate second-line therapy?

   (A) Increase the dose of afatinib
   (B) Continue afatinib and add erlotinib
   (C) Stop afatinib and start carboplatin/paclitaxel/docetaxel
   (D) Stop afatinib and start carboplatin/paclitaxel

6. A 71-year-old woman with a past medical history of insulin-dependent diabetes presents with dyspnea on exertion. CT of the chest shows bilateral nodules with mediastinal lymphadenopathy. A bronchoscopy with biopsy of the mediastinal lymph nodes and of a pulmonary nodule returns positive for adenocarcinoma. Molecular testing is completed and EML4-ALK translocations are found. The patient is initiated on crizotinib 250 mg twice daily and has a near complete response after 3 months of therapy. Nine months into therapy, she begins complaining of increasing exertional dyspnea. Repeated CT of chest shows patchy bilateral interstitial opacities with no increase in lymphadenopathy and no distant metastases. Her Eastern Cooperative

Oncology Group performance status is 1. Which is the next best step in management?

(A) Hold crizotinib and restart in 2 weeks
(B) Increase dose of crizotinib
(C) Stop crizotinib indefinitely
(D) Continue crizotinib and add carboplatin/pemetrexed

7. A 58-year-old man with a past medical history of hypertension and tobacco abuse (30 pack-years) presents with persistent cough and intermittent hemoptysis of 2 months' duration. CT of the chest shows a large 7-cm central mass partially obstructing the right pulmonary bronchus with bilateral pleural effusions and bilateral supraclavicular lymphadenopathy. A biopsy of the right supraclavicular lymph node along with bronchoscopy of the primary central mass returns positive for squamous cell carcinoma (SCC). During the bronchoscopy, a stent is placed in the right pulmonary bronchus. Diagnostic thoracentesis is completed and cytology returns positive for SCC. Patient has improvement in his cough following stent placement though intermittent hemoptysis persists. CT of the brain and abdomen reveals no other evidence of metastases. His Eastern Cooperative Oncology Group performance status is 1. Which is the next best step in management?

(A) Refer to hospice
(B) Start carboplatin/pemetrexed
(C) Start cisplatin/gemcitabine/bevacizumab
(D) Start cisplatin/paclitaxel

8. A 48-year-old female with a medical history significant for tobacco abuse (25 pack-years) but no other comorbidities presents with mild dyspnea on exertion and intermittent headaches. CT of the chest, abdomen, and pelvis reveals multiple pulmonary nodules along with 3 liver lesions. MRI of the brain confirms an isolated temporal lesion consistent with metastases with minimal peritumoral edema. Liver biopsy confirms poorly differentiated adenocarcinoma with immunohistochemistry consistent with a lung primary. Molecular studies including mutations of epidermal growth factor receptor and anaplastic lymphoma kinase return negative. She undergoes surgical resection of the brain metastasis without complications and declines whole-brain radiotherapy. Four weeks after surgery, a repeat MRI of the brain shows expected postsurgical changes without evidence of disease progression. Patient continues to have mild dyspnea on exertion but otherwise feels well. Her Eastern Cooperative Oncology Group performance status is 0. Which is the next best step in management?

(A) Start carboplatin/pemetrexed/bevacizumab for 4–6 cycles and if stable or responding disease, switch to maintenance pemetrexed
(B) Start carboplatin/pemetrexed for 2 cycles and if stable or responding disease, switch to maintenance pemetrexed
(C) Start carboplatin/pemetrexed/bevacizumab for 8 cycles followed by observation
(D) Start carboplatin/docetaxel/pemetrexed for 4–6 cycles and if stable or responding disease, switch to maintenance docetaxel

9. A 79-year-old man with a past medical history of tobacco abuse (40 pack-years) and well-controlled hypertension and mild chronic obstructive pulmonary disease presents with a 2-month history of fatigue and a 35-lb weight loss. Prior to the onset of these symptoms, the patient was able to golf 18 holes with a pull-cart and independently manage all of his activities of daily living and instrumental activities of daily living. CT of the chest and abdomen reveals right central pulmonary mass with multiple liver lesions. Biopsy of the liver confirms poorly differentiated squamous cell carcinoma with immunohistochemistry consistent with a lung primary. On physical examination, the patient is a frail-appearing man who can slowly get to the examining table without assistance along with scattered expiratory wheezes but is otherwise unremarkable. His Eastern Cooperative Oncology Group performance status is 3. What is the next best step in management?

(A) Start carboplatin/pemetrexed
(B) Start erlotinib and refer to palliative care
(C) Start pemetrexed alone
(D) Start carboplatin/bevacizumab

## REFERENCES

1. Society AC. *Cancer Facts & Figures*; 2014.
2. Prevention CfDCa. National Vital Statistics Reports. 2013;61(4).
3. Alberg AJ, Samet JM. Epidemiology of lung cancer. *Chest.* 2003;123(suppl 1):21S–49S.
4. Leuraud K, Schnelzer M, Tomasek L, et al. Radon, smoking and lung cancer risk: results of a joint analysis of three European case-control studies among uranium miners. *Radiat Res.* 2011;176(3):375–387.
5. Gottschall EB. Occupational and environmental thoracic malignancies. *J Thorac Imag.* 2002;17(3):189–197.
6. Release FN. FDA and public health experts warn about electronic cigarettes. http://www.fda.gov/newsevents/newsroom/pressannouncements/ucm173222.htm.
7. News F. Summary of results: laboratory analysis of electronic cigarettes conducted by FDA. http://www.fda.gov/newsevents/publichealthfocus/ucm173146.htm. Accessed April 22, 2014.
8. The Alpha-Tocopherol, Beta Carotene Cancer Prevention Study Group. The effect of vitamin E and beta carotene on the incidence of lung cancer and other cancers in male smokers. *N Engl J Med.* 1994;330(15):1029–1035.
9. Omenn GS, Goodman GE, Thornquist MD, et al. Effects of a combination of beta carotene and vitamin A on lung cancer and cardiovascular disease. *N Engl J Med.* 1996;334(18):1150–1155.
10. Hennekens CH, Buring JE, Manson JE, et al. Lack of effect of long-term supplementation with beta carotene on the incidence of

malignant neoplasms and cardiovascular disease. *N Engl J Med.* 1996;334(18):1145–1149.

11. Amos CI, Pinney SM, Li Y, et al. A susceptibility locus on chromosome 6q greatly increases lung cancer risk among light and never smokers. *Cancer Res* 2010;70(6):2359–2367.

12. Wang Y, Broderick P, Webb E, et al. Common 5p15.33 and 6p21.33 variants influence lung cancer risk. *Nat Genet* 2008;40(12):1407–1409.

13. Wang Y, Broderick P, Matakidou A, et al. Role of 5p15.33 (TERT-CLPTM1L), 6p21.33 and 15q25.1 (CHRNA5-CHRNA3) variation and lung cancer risk in never-smokers. *Carcinogenesis.* 2010;31(2):234–238.

14. Hsiung CA, Lan Q, Hong YC, et al. The 5p15.33 locus is associated with risk of lung adenocarcinoma in never-smoking females in Asia. *PLoS Genet.* 2010;6(8).

15. Li Y, Sheu CC, Ye Y, et al. Genetic variants and risk of lung cancer in never smokers: a genome-wide association study. *Lancet Oncol.* 2010;11(4):321–330.

16. Truong T, Hung RJ, Amos CI, et al. Replication of lung cancer susceptibility loci at chromosomes 15q25, 5p15, and 6p21: a pooled analysis from the International Lung Cancer Consortium. *J Natl Cancer Inst.* 2010;102(13):959–971.

17. Larsen JE, Spinola M, Gazdar AF, et al. *An Overview of the Molecular Biology of Lung Cancer.* Philadelphia, PA: Lippincott Williams & Wilkins; 2010.

18. Goldstraw P, Crowley J, Chansky K, et al. The IASLC Lung Cancer Staging Project: proposals for the revision of the TNM stage groupings in the forthcoming (seventh) edition of the TNM Classification of malignant tumours. *J Thorac Oncol.* 2007;2(8):706–714.

19. National Guideline C. *Methods for Staging Non-small Cell Lung Cancer: Diagnosis and Management of Lung Cancer.* 3rd ed. American College of Chest Physicians evidence-based clinical practice guidelines. http://www.guideline.gov/content.aspx?id=4 6169&search=mediastinal. Accessed May 18, 2014.

20. Gould MK, Fletcher J, Iannettoni MD, et al. Evaluation of patients with pulmonary nodules: when is it lung cancer? ACCP evidence-based clinical practice guidelines (2nd ed.). *Chest.* 2007;132(suppl 3):108S–130S.

21. Pignon JP, Tribodet H, Scagliotti GV, et al. Lung adjuvant cisplatin evaluation: a pooled analysis by the LACE Collaborative Group. *J Clin Oncol.* 2008;26(21):3552–3559.

22. Arriagada R, Auperin A, Burdett S, et al. Adjuvant chemotherapy, with or without postoperative radiotherapy, in operable non-small-cell lung cancer: two meta-analyses of individual patient data. *Lancet.* 2010;375(9722):1267–1277.

23. Lally BE, Zelterman D, Colasanto JM, et al. Postoperative radiotherapy for stage II or III non-small-cell lung cancer using the surveillance, epidemiology, and end results database. *J Clin Oncol.* 2006;24(19):2998–3006.

24. Vansteenkiste J, Dooms C, De Leyn P. Early stage non-small-cell lung cancer: challenges in staging and adjuvant treatment: evidence-based staging. *Ann Oncol* 2010;21(suppl 7):vii189–195.

25. O'Rourke N, Roque IFM, Farre Bernado N, et al. Concurrent chemoradiotherapy in non-small cell lung cancer. *The Cochrane Database of Systematic Reviews* 2010(6):CD002140.

26. Auperin A, Le Pechoux C, Rolland E, et al. Meta-analysis of concomitant versus sequential radiochemotherapy in locally advanced non-small-cell lung cancer. *J Clin Oncol.* 2010;28(13):2181–2190.

27. Ramnath N, Dilling TJ, Harris LJ, et al. Treatment of stage III non-small cell lung cancer: diagnosis and management of lung cancer (3rd ed.). American College of Chest Physicians evidence-based clinical practice guidelines. *Chest.* 2013;143(suppl 5):e314S–e340S.

28. Chambers A, Routledge T, Bille A, et al. Does surgery have a role in T4N0 and T4N1 lung cancer? *Interact Cardiovasc Thorac Surg.* 2010;11(4):473–479.

29. Network. National Comprehensive Cancer. Practice guidelines in oncology—v. 3.2014. Non-small cell lung cancer, 2014.

30. Riely GJ, Politi KA, Miller VA, et al. Update on epidermal growth factor receptor mutations in non-small cell lung cancer. *Clin Cancer Res.* 2006;12(24):7232–7241.

31. Mok TS, Wu YL, Thongprasert S, et al. Gefitinib or carboplatin-paclitaxel in pulmonary adenocarcinoma. *New Engl J Med.* 2009;361(10):947–957.

32. Fukuoka M, Wu YL, Thongprasert S, et al. Biomarker analyses and final overall survival results from a phase III, randomized, open-label, first-line study of gefitinib versus carboplatin/paclitaxel in clinically selected patients with advanced non-small-cell lung cancer in Asia (IPASS). *J Clin Oncol.* 2011;29(21):2866–2874.

33. Inoue A, Kobayashi K, Maemondo M, et al. Updated overall survival results from a randomized phase III trial comparing gefitinib with carboplatin-paclitaxel for chemo-naive non-small cell lung cancer with sensitive EGFR gene mutations (NEJ002). *Ann Oncol.* 2013;24(1):54–59.

34. Rosell R, Carcereny E, Gervais R, et al. Erlotinib versus standard chemotherapy as first-line treatment for European patients with advanced EGFR mutation-positive non-small-cell lung cancer (EURTAC): a multicentre, open-label, randomised phase 3 trial. *Lancet Oncol.* 2012;13(3):239–246.

35. Wu YL, Zhou C, Hu CP, et al. Afatinib versus cisplatin plus gemcitabine for first-line treatment of Asian patients with advanced non-small-cell lung cancer harbouring EGFR mutations (LUX-Lung 6): an open-label, randomised phase 3 trial. *Lancet Oncol.* 2014;15(2):213–222.

36. OuYang PY, Su Z, Mao YP, et al. Combination of EGFR-TKIs and chemotherapy as first-line therapy for advanced NSCLC: a meta-analysis. *PloS ONE.* 2013;8(11):e79000.

37. Wu YL, Lee JS, Thongprasert S, et al. Intercalated combination of chemotherapy and erlotinib for patients with advanced stage non-small-cell lung cancer (FASTACT-2): a randomised, double-blind trial. *Lancet Oncol.* 2013;14(8):777–786.

38. Gandara DR, Gumerlock PH. Epidermal growth factor receptor tyrosine kinase inhibitors plus chemotherapy: case closed or is the jury still out? *J Clin Oncol.* 2005;23(25):5856–5858.

39. Soda M, Choi YL, Enomoto M, et al. Identification of the transforming EML4-ALK fusion gene in non-small-cell lung cancer. *Nature.* 2007;448(7153):561–566.

40. Camidge DR, Bang YJ, Kwak EL, et al. Activity and safety of crizotinib in patients with ALK-positive non-small-cell lung cancer: updated results from a phase 1 study. *Lancet Oncol.* 2012;13(10):1011–1019.

41. Kim Dea. Results of a global phase II study with crizotinib in advanced ALK-positive non-small cell lung cancer (NSCLC). *J Clin Oncol.* 2012 (suppl; abstr 7533).

42. Shaw AT, Kim DW, Nakagawa K, et al. Crizotinib versus chemotherapy in advanced ALK-positive lung cancer. *New Engl J Med.* 2013;368(25):2385–2394.

43. Shaw AT, Kim DW, Mehra R, et al. Ceritinib in ALK-rearranged non-small-cell lung cancer. *New Engl J Med.* 2014;370(13):1189–1197.

44. Bergethon K, Shaw AT, Ou SH, et al. ROS1 rearrangements define a unique molecular class of lung cancers. *J Clin Oncol.* 2012;30(8):863–870.

45. Ardizzoni A, Boni L, Tiseo M, et al. Cisplatin- versus carboplatin-based chemotherapy in first-line treatment of advanced non-small-cell lung cancer: an individual patient data meta-analysis. *J Natl Cancer Inst.* 2007;99(11):847–857.

46. Pujol JL, Barlesi F, Daures JP. Should chemotherapy combinations for advanced non-small cell lung cancer be platinum-based? A meta-analysis of phase III randomized trials. *Lung Cancer* 2006;51(3):335–345.

47. Sandler A, Gray R, Perry MC, et al. Paclitaxel-carboplatin alone or with bevacizumab for non-small-cell lung cancer. *New Engl J Med.* 2006;355(24):2542–2550.

48. Reck M, von Pawel J, Zatloukal P, et al. Overall survival with cisplatin-gemcitabine and bevacizumab or placebo as first-line therapy for nonsquamous non-small-cell lung cancer: results from a randomised phase III trial (AVAiL). *Ann Oncol.* 2010;21(9):1804–1809.

49. Soria JC, Mauguen A, Reck M, et al. Systematic review and meta-analysis of randomised, phase II/III trials adding bevacizumab to platinum-based chemotherapy as first-line treatment in patients with advanced non-small-cell lung cancer. *Ann Oncol.* 2013;24(1):20–30.

50. Socinski MA, Langer CJ, Huang JE, et al. Safety of bevacizumab in patients with non-small-cell lung cancer and brain metastases. *J Clin Oncol.* 2009;27(31):5255–5261.

51. Kim ES, Neubauer M, Cohn A, et al. Docetaxel or pemetrexed with or without cetuximab in recurrent or progressive non-small-cell lung cancer after platinum-based therapy: a phase 3, open-label, randomised trial. *Lancet Oncol.* 2013;14(13):1326–1336.

52. Soon YY, Stockler MR, Askie LM, et al. Duration of chemotherapy for advanced non-small-cell lung cancer: a systematic review and meta-analysis of randomized trials. *J Clin Oncol.* 2009;27(20):3277–3283.

53. Lima JP, dos Santos LV, Sasse EC, et al. Optimal duration of first-line chemotherapy for advanced non-small cell lung cancer: a systematic review with meta-analysis. *Eur J Cancer.* 2009;45(4):601–607.

54. Ciuleanu T, Brodowicz T, Zielinski C, et al. Maintenance pemetrexed plus best supportive care versus placebo plus best supportive care for non-small-cell lung cancer: a randomised, double-blind, phase 3 study. *Lancet* 2009;374(9699):1432–1440.

55. Fidias PM, Dakhil SR, Lyss AP, et al. Phase III study of immediate compared with delayed docetaxel after front-line therapy with gemcitabine plus carboplatin in advanced non-small-cell lung cancer. *J Clin Oncol.* 2009;27(4):591–598.

56. Perol M, Chouaid C, Perol D, et al. Randomized, phase III study of gemcitabine or erlotinib maintenance therapy versus observation, with predefined second-line treatment, after cisplatin-gemcitabine induction chemotherapy in advanced non-small-cell lung cancer. *J Clin Oncol.* 2012;30(28):3516–3524.

57. Cappuzzo F, Ciuleanu T, Stelmakh L, et al. Erlotinib as maintenance treatment in advanced non-small-cell lung cancer: a multicentre, randomised, placebo-controlled phase 3 study. *Lancet Oncol.* 2010;11(6):521–529.

58. Johnson BE, Kabbinavar F, Fehrenbacher L, et al. ATLAS: randomized, double-blind, placebo-controlled, phase IIIB trial comparing bevacizumab therapy with or without erlotinib, after completion of chemotherapy, with bevacizumab for first-line treatment of advanced non-small-cell lung cancer. *J Clin Oncol.* 2013;31(31):3926–3934.

59. Patel JD, Socinski MA, Garon EB, et al. PointBreak: a randomized phase III study of pemetrexed plus carboplatin and bevacizumab followed by maintenance pemetrexed and bevacizumab versus paclitaxel plus carboplatin and bevacizumab followed by maintenance bevacizumab in patients with stage IIIB or IV nonsquamous non-small-cell lung cancer. *J Clin Oncol.* 2013;31(34):4349–4357.

60. Barlesi F, Scherpereel A, Rittmeyer A, et al. Randomized phase III trial of maintenance bevacizumab with or without pemetrexed after first-line induction with bevacizumab, cisplatin, and pemetrexed in advanced nonsquamous non-small-cell lung cancer: AVAPERL (MO22089). *J Clin Oncol.* 2013;31(24):3004–3011.

61. Scagliotti G, Hanna N, Fossella F, et al. The differential efficacy of pemetrexed according to NSCLC histology: a review of two Phase III studies. *The Oncologist.* 2009;14(3):253–263.

62. Kalkanis SN, Kondziolka D, Gaspar LE, et al. The role of surgical resection in the management of newly diagnosed brain metastases: a systematic review and evidence-based clinical practice guideline. *J Neuro-oncol* 2010;96(1):33–43.

63. Linskey ME, Andrews DW, Asher AL, et al. The role of stereotactic radiosurgery in the management of patients with newly diagnosed brain metastases: a systematic review and evidence-based clinical practice guideline. *J Neuro-oncol.* 2010;96(1):45–68.

64. Pfannschmidt J, Dienemann H. Surgical treatment of oligometastatic non-small cell lung cancer. *Lung Cancer.* 2010;69(3):251–258.

65. Azzoli CG, Temin S, Aliff T, et al. Focused update of 2009 American Society of Clinical Oncology Clinical Practice Guideline update on chemotherapy for stage IV non-small-cell lung cancer. *J Clin Oncol.* 2011;29(28):3825–3831.

66. Quoix E, Zalcman G, Oster JP, et al. Carboplatin and weekly paclitaxel doublet chemotherapy compared with monotherapy in elderly patients with advanced non-small-cell lung cancer: IFCT-0501 randomised, phase 3 trial. *Lancet.* 2011;378(9796):1079–1088.

67. Schuette Wea. 65 plus: a randomized phase III trial of pemetrexed and bevacizumab versus pemetrexed, bevacizumab, and carboplatin as first-line treatment for elderly patients with advanced nonsquamous, non-small cell lung cancer (NSCLC). *J Clin Oncol.* 2013;31(suppl; abstr 8013).

68. Gridelli C, Perrone F, Gallo C, et al. Chemotherapy for elderly patients with advanced non-small-cell lung cancer: the Multicenter Italian Lung Cancer in the Elderly Study (MILES) phase III randomized trial. *J Natl Cancer Inst.* 2003;95(5):362–372.

69. Inoue A, Kobayashi K, Usui K, et al. First-line gefitinib for patients with advanced non-small-cell lung cancer harboring epidermal growth factor receptor mutations without indication for chemotherapy. *J Clin Oncol.* 2009;27(9):1394–1400.

70. Shepherd FA, Dancey J, Ramlau R, et al. Prospective randomized trial of docetaxel versus best supportive care in patients with non-small-cell lung cancer previously treated with platinum-based chemotherapy. *J Clin Oncol.* 2000;18(10):2095–2103.

71. Hanna N, Shepherd FA, Fossella FV, et al. Randomized phase III trial of pemetrexed versus docetaxel in patients with non-small-cell lung cancer previously treated with chemotherapy. *J Clin Oncol.* 2004;22(9):1589–1597.

72. Shepherd FA, Rodrigues Pereira J, Ciuleanu T, et al. Erlotinib in previously treated non-small-cell lung cancer. *New Engl J Med.* 2005;353(2):123–132.

73. Topalian SL, Hodi FS, Brahmer JR, et al. Safety, activity, and immune correlates of anti-PD-1 antibody in cancer. *New Engl J Med.* 2012;366(26):2443–2454.

74. Pikor LA, Ramnarine VR, Lam S, et al. Genetic alterations defining NSCLC subtypes and their therapeutic implications. *Lung Cancer.* 2013;82(2):179–189.

# 4

# Small Cell Lung Cancer

IGOR I. RYBKIN, BINU MALHOTRA, AND GREGORY P. KALEMKERIAN

## EPIDEMIOLOGY, RISK FACTORS, NATURAL HISTORY, AND PATHOLOGY

Small cell lung cancer (SCLC) is a distinct subtype of lung cancer that is characterized by neuroendocrine differentiation, early metastatic spread, and initial responsiveness to therapy. The incidence rate of SCLC peaked in the 1980s and has since been declining. The proportional incidence of SCLC as a fraction of all lung cancer cases has also decreased from 17–20% in the 1980s to 13–15% in 2002. Among patients with SCLC, the percentage of women has steadily increased from 28% in 1973 to 50% in 2002. These temporal trends in SCLC incidence directly reflect the prevalence of tobacco use among men and women over the past few decades.

The major risk factor for SCLC is a history of tobacco smoking, with >95% of patients being current or former smokers. The degree of risk is proportional to the overall exposure to tobacco smoke and to the tar and nicotine content of the tobacco smoked. Other less common risk factors include exposure to secondhand smoke, radon, ionizing radiation, and bis(chloromethyl)ether (an industrial solvent). Although screening with annual CT scans has been shown to decrease the mortality from non-small-cell lung cancer (NSCLC) in high-risk people, this screening strategy does not seem to impact on the early detection or outcome of SCLC (1,2).

SCLC typically presents as a large mass arising from a central airway with bulky hilar and mediastinal lymph node involvement. Most patients present with shortness of breath, cough, fatigue, and a variety of symptoms related to metastatic disease, such as weight loss, bone pain, and neurological dysfunction. Bronchoscopic biopsy and brushings are usually diagnostic, though the bulk of the tumor is often submucosal, requiring a deeper biopsy or aspiration of the central mass or lymph nodes to obtain adequate diagnostic tissue.

SCLC is an aggressive disease with a high growth fraction and early metastatic spread, with more than two-thirds of patients presenting with hematogenous metastases. Historically, patients with SCLC who did not receive therapy had a very poor prognosis, with a median survival of 7 weeks for those in the extensive stage (ES) and 14 weeks for those in the limited stage (LS). The use of combination chemotherapy and radiation therapy has dramatically altered the course of SCLC due to the remarkable initial responsiveness of the disease. However, despite initial responses, most patients relapse and die with treatment-resistant disease. For patients with LS-SCLC, median survival is 18–24 months with a 5-year survival rate of 20–25%, and for those with ES-SCLC, median survival is 9–10 months with a 2-year survival rate of <10%.

SCLC is a highly proliferative and invasive malignancy made up of small cells with a high nuclear-to-cytoplasmic ratio, frequent mitoses, nuclear molding, finely granular chromatin, and inconspicuous nucleoli. Usually, SCLC can be diagnosed by histology alone. However, in some cases, immunohistochemical studies can provide important supporting data. As with NSCLC, SCLC usually expresses thyroid transcription factor-1 (TTF-1) and cytokeratin, but can be differentially characterized by the expression of neuroendocrine markers, such as synaptophysin, neural cell adhesion molecule (NCAM, CD56), chromogranin A, neuron-specific enolase (NSE), and Leu-7 (CD57). SCLC exhibits extensive cytogenetic abnormalities, including defects that cluster on chromosomes 1, 3 (particularly 3p), 5, and 17. In addition, many specific genetic abnormalities have been implicated in the pathogenesis of SCLC, including mutations of *p53*, *p16*, and *RB1*, and overexpression of *bcl-2*, *c-kit*, and *myc* family genes. Microarray expression analysis of lung cancers has revealed substantial differences in the expression profiles of SCLC and NSCLC. However, thus far, none of these cytogenetic or molecular markers has proven to be of additional diagnostic, prognostic, or therapeutic use in the clinical setting.

## STAGING

| Veterans' Administration Lung Study Group Staging for Small Cell Lung Cancer | |
|---|---|
| **Stage** | **Description** |
| Limited | Tumor confined to 1 hemithorax, with or without regional lymph node involvement (including contralateral hilar and medi-astinal and ipsilateral supraclavicular lymph nodes), and all disease can be safely contained within a tolerable radiation field |
| Extensive | Disease that has spread beyond limited stage, including contralateral supraclavicular lymph nodes, malignant pleural or pericardial effusion, and distant metastases |

| TNM Staging for Small Cell Lung Cancer | |
|---|---|
| **Stage** | **Description** |
| IA | Primary tumor ≤3 cm (T1a, T1b) surrounded by lung or visceral pleura, without bronchoscopic invasion to the main bronchus, and no nodal or distant metastases (N0 M0) |
| IB | Primary tumor >3 cm, but ≤5 cm (T2a) and no nodal or distant metastases (N0 M0) |
| | Primary tumor ≤5 cm (T1a, T1b, T2a) that invades visceral pleura, involves the main bronchus (≥2 cm distal to the carina), or is associated with atelectasis or obstructive pneumonitis extending to the hilar region, but not involving the entire lung, and no nodal or distant metastases (N0 M0) |
| IIA | Primary tumor ≤5 cm (T1a, T1b, T2a) and metastasis in ipsilateral peribronchial, hilar, and/or intrapulmonary lymph node(s) (N1), and no distant metastasis (M0) |
| | Primary tumor >5 cm, but ≤7 cm (T2b) and no nodal or distant metastases (N0 M0) |
| IIB | Primary tumor >5 cm, but ≤7 cm (T2b), and metastasis in ipsilateral peribronchial, hilar, and/or intrapulmonary lymph node(s) (N1), and no distant metastasis (M0) |
| | Primary tumor >7 cm (T3) *or* one directly invading the chest wall, diaphragm, phrenic nerve, mediastinal pleura, or parietal pericardium, or in the main bronchus <2 cm distal to the carina without involving the carina, or associated with atelectasis or obstructive pneumonitis of the entire lung (T3), *or* separate tumor nodule(s) in the same lobe as the primary tumor (T3), and no nodal or distant metastases (N0 M0) |
| IIIA | Primary tumor of any size that invades the mediastinum, heart, great vessels, trachea, recurrent laryngeal nerve, esophagus, vertebral body, or carina (T4), *or* separate tumor nodule(s) in a different lobe ipsilateral to that of the primary (T4), and no nodal or distant metastases (N0 M0) |
| | Primary tumor (T3, T4), and metastasis in ipsilateral peribronchial, hilar, and/or intrapulmonary lymph node(s) (N1), and no distant metastasis (M0) |
| | Primary tumor (T1–T3), and metastasis in the ipsilateral mediastinal and/or subcarinal lymph nodes(s) (N2), and no distant metastasis (M0) |
| IIIB | Primary tumor (T4), and metastasis in the ipsilateral mediastinal and/or subcarinal lymph nodes(s) (N2), and no distant metastasis (M0) |
| | Primary tumor of any size or invasion (T1–T4), and metastasis in the contralateral mediastinal, contralateral hilar, or ipsilateral or contralateral scalene or supraclavicular lymph node(s) (N3), and no distant metastasis (M0) |
| IV | Primary tumor of any size or invasion (T1–T4), with or without any lymph node metastasis (N0–N3) and separate tumor nodule(s) in a contralateral lobe *or* pleural nodules, *or* malignant pleural or pericardial effusion (M1a) or distant metastasis (M1b) |

TNM, tumor, node, and metastasis.
*Source*: Edge SB, Byrd DR, Compton CC, et al. (eds). *AJCC Cancer Staging Handbook. 7th ed.* New York: Springer Science + Business Media, 2010, pp 299–323.

## CASE SUMMARIES

### LS-SCLC: Combined Modality Therapy

M.R. is a 52-year-old woman who presents with progressive dyspnea on exertion over the past 4 weeks. She has also noted weight loss, fatigue, anterior chest pain, fever, and a nonproductive cough, although she continues to work full time. She is a current smoker with a 30-pack-year history. Her past medical history is otherwise unremarkable. Her physical examination reveals mild tachycardia and low-grade fever with decreased breath sounds over the right lower lung field and no cervical or supraclavicular lymphadenopathy. Laboratory studies are remarkable for a slightly elevated WBC count, normal electrolytes, normal renal and hepatic function, and a serum lactate dehydrogenase (LDH) of 240 IU/L. Chest radiography shows right hilar fullness and a large right lower lobe density. A chest CT reveals a 4-cm right hilar mass with obstruction of the right lower lobe bronchus and partial atelectasis of the right lower lobe, as well as bulky lymphadenopathy in the right paratracheal, precarinal, and subcarinal regions. A PET-CT reveals intense [18]F-fludeoxyglucose (FDG) uptake in the right hilar mass and numerous mediastinal lymph nodes, but only mild uptake in the right lower lobe corresponding to the area of atelectasis and no abnormal FDG uptake elsewhere. An MRI of the brain reveals no suspicious lesions. Endobronchial biopsy of the right hilar mass and transbronchial aspiration of a subcarinal lymph node reveals SCLC.

## Evidence-Based Case Discussion

The patient presented here is a middle-aged woman with a good Eastern Cooperative Oncology Group performance status (ECOG PS 1) and no comorbid medical problems. Her staging workup appropriately included both an MRI of the brain, which can detect asymptomatic brain metastases in about 10% of patients, and a PET scan, which can upstage 17% of patients with apparent LS-SCLC per conventional imaging studies (3). After a complete staging evaluation, she is found to have LS-SCLC with a central primary tumor mass and mediastinal lymph node involvement that can all be safely treated with thoracic radiation. The right hilar mass is causing atelectasis and she has clinical evidence of mild postobstructive pneumonia for which initiation of oral, broad-spectrum antibiotics (e.g., amoxicillin-clavulanate) would be appropriate. Assistance with smoking cessation through aggressive counseling and pharmacological means is also indicated to improve lung function, decrease the risks of treatment-related complications, and reduce the risk of second primary malignancy. She requires immediate referral to medical and radiation oncology in order to initiate treatment with curative intent in a timely manner.

## Chemotherapy

The current standard-of-care for patients with LS-SCLC consists of 4–6 cycles of etoposide plus cisplatin (EP) along with early, concurrent thoracic radiotherapy. One randomized trial has suggested that carboplatin can be safely substituted for cisplatin in patients with LS-SCLC with statistically similar outcomes. However, due to the paucity of comparative data, cisplatin should be used unless it is contraindicated (e.g., neuropathy, hearing loss, renal insufficiency). There are no data in the literature to justify the use of combinations other than platinum plus etoposide in patients with LS-SCLC. After completion of chemoradiotherapy, prophylactic cranial irradiation (PCI) should be strongly considered for those achieving a good response. It is important to remember that LS-SCLC is a curable disease and, as such, all patients should be offered optimal treatment as established by years of clinical research.

## Thoracic Radiotherapy

Over the past 3 decades, most of the progress in the treatment of LS-SCLC has been due to advances in the use of radiotherapy. Two meta-analyses demonstrated that the addition of definitive thoracic radiation to chemotherapy significantly improved overall survival in patients with LS-SCLC by 5.4% at 2–3 years (P = .001), largely due to a decrease in the local recurrence rate (4,5). Subsequent studies demonstrated that early thoracic radiotherapy (initiated within 9 weeks of starting chemotherapy or during the first 2 cycles of chemotherapy) improved local control and afforded a 5% overall survival benefit at 2 years when compared to late radiotherapy (P = .03) (6).

Despite the fact that a large, randomized trial reported a significant survival benefit with the use of hyperfractionated thoracic radiotherapy, this strategy remains controversial. Turrisi et al. randomized 417 patients with LS-SCLC to receive standard EP along with 45 Gy of early, concurrent thoracic radiotherapy given either once daily over 5 weeks or twice daily over 3 weeks (7). Patients receiving the twice-daily regimen had a significant improvement in overall survival compared to those receiving once-daily therapy (median = 23 vs. 19 months; 5-year, 26% vs. 16%; P = .04). Not surprisingly, twice-daily radiation also increased the risk of developing severe esophagitis (7). This study has been criticized for the relatively low total dose of radiation given to patients receiving once-daily therapy, resulting in a lack of biological equivalence between the radiation doses administered on the 2 arms. Therefore, the potential benefit of hyperfractionated radiation in LS-SCLC remains open to debate pending the results of ongoing, well-designed, confirmatory trials. However, based on the available data, early, hyperfractionated, twice-daily radiation to 45 Gy should be strongly considered for patients in whom the potential toxicity of this approach is deemed acceptable by the treating physicians. Alternatively, in patients with poorer performance status or bulky disease that would require an excessively large treatment field, thoracic radiation may be administered once daily to a total dose of 60–70 Gy.

In patients with LS-SCLC, standard chemoradiotherapy yields an overall response rate of 80–95% and a complete response rate of 40% with median survival of 18–24 months and a 5-year survival rate of 20–25% (8). Owing to the high degree of responsiveness to therapy, even patients with impaired performance status should be considered for standard therapy with curative intent.

## Prophylactic Cranial Irradiation

More than 50% of patients with SCLC will develop brain metastases during the course of their illness. A meta-analysis of 7 randomized trials evaluating PCI versus no PCI reported a 25% absolute decrease in the incidence of brain metastases at 3 years (control = 58.6% vs. PCI = 33.3%; P < .001) and a 5.4% increase in 3-year overall survival (control = 15.3% vs. PCI = 20.7%; P = .01) (9). In this meta-analysis, 86% of patients had LS-SCLC and had achieved a complete or near-complete response to initial

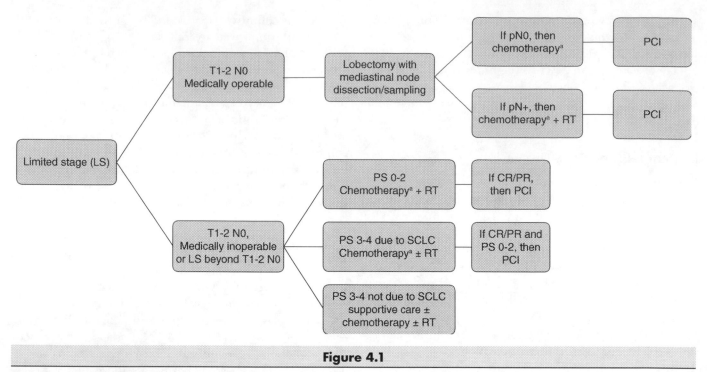

**Figure 4.1**

Treatment algorithm for LS-SCLC. CR, complete response; LS-SCLC, limited-stage-small cell lung cancer; PCI, prophylactic cranial irradiation; PR, partial response; PS, Zubrod performance status. ªChemotherapy = cisplatin plus etoposide (recommended) or carboplatin plus etoposide.

therapy. On the basis of these data, PCI at 25 Gy in 10 fractions is recommended for patients with LS-SCLC who have good performance status, intact neurological function, and complete or partial response to initial therapy.

## Surgery

Less than 5% of all patients with SCLC present with clinical stage I (T1–2 N0 M0) disease. However, these patients comprise a special case in which surgical resection followed by adjuvant chemotherapy is the preferred treatment option. Prior to resection, all such patients should undergo surgical or endoscopic mediastinal staging to rule out occult nodal disease. If mediastinal staging shows no lymph node involvement, then patients should undergo lobectomy with further mediastinal lymph node dissection followed by adjuvant chemotherapy with 4 cycles of cisplatin plus etoposide (10). Patients with pathologic stage I disease (T1–2 N0 M0) should receive adjuvant chemotherapy alone, while those with nodal metastases should undergo concurrent chemotherapy and postoperative hilar/mediastinal radiation. After complete resection and adjuvant therapy, PCI should also be considered.

Figure 4.1 shows the treatment algorithm for LS-SCLC.

## ES-SCLC: Systemic Palliative Therapy

D.F. is a 72-year-old man who presents with a 3-week history of worsening shortness of breath, abdominal fullness,

weight loss, fatigue, right anterior chest pain, and swelling of his face and neck. He has also noted recent onset of difficulty standing up from a chair and walking upstairs. He has smoked 1 pack a day for 50 years. His past medical history is remarkable for chronic obstructive pulmonary disease, hypertension, and coronary artery disease. His physical examination reveals an elderly man who appears fatigued, but has an ECOG performance status of 1. There is moderate swelling of his face and neck and a palpable, hard, 3-cm right supraclavicular lymph node. His breath sounds are diminished in all lung fields with coarse rhonchi in the right upper lung field. Abdominal examination reveals a firm, nodular, mildly tender liver edge 8 cm below the costal margin in the midline. Neurological examination reveals symmetrical proximal muscle weakness in upper and lower extremities. Laboratory studies are remarkable for normal electrolytes and blood counts: creatinine = 1.3 mg/dL; LDH = 450 IU/L; alkaline phosphatase = 270 IU/L; aspartate aminotransferase (AST) = 45 IU/L; alanine aminotransferase (ALT) = 56 IU/L; and total bilirubin = 1.2 mg/dL. The paraneoplastic antibody panel reveals the presence of antibodies against voltage-gated calcium channels. Chest radiography reveals a widened mediastinum, a large right suprahilar mass, and emphysema. A CT of the chest and upper abdomen shows a 3.5-cm right supraclavicular lymph node, bilateral bulky mediastinal lymph nodes, a 7 × 5 cm right suprahilar mass with marked narrowing of the superior vena cava and the right upper lobe bronchus, multiple bilateral lung nodules ranging in size from 0.4 to 2.5 cm, postobstructive atelectasis in the right upper lobe, a 4.2-cm left adrenal mass, multiple liver nodules ranging in size from 1.2 to 5.7 cm, and numerous lytic bone lesions involving the vertebral bodies and ribs. An MRI of the brain is negative for metastatic lesions. A biopsy of a liver lesion shows metastatic SCLC.

## Evidence-Based Case Discussion

The patient presented is an elderly man with widely metastatic ES-SCLC causing superior vena cava syndrome and paraneoplastic Lambert–Eaton myasthenic syndrome. His staging workup did not include a PET scan since his conventional imaging studies strongly suggested ES disease and a biopsy confirmed liver metastases. If left untreated, he would likely succumb to his disease in a few weeks. Although treatment with combination chemotherapy should afford him good palliation of symptoms, improved quality of life (QOL), and prolongation of survival, his prospects for long-term survival are limited. Owing to the high likelihood of achieving a brisk response and relief of symptoms with standard chemotherapy, palliative radiation is generally not indicated for the management of superior vena cava syndrome in patients with SCLC unless they have severe symptoms, such as confusion (due to cerebral edema) or stridor (due to laryngeal edema).

## Chemotherapy

Many classes of chemotherapy agents have demonstrated relatively high response rates in patients with ES-SCLC, including platinums (cisplatin, carboplatin); epipodophyllotoxins (etoposide, tenoposide); camptothecin analogs (irinotecan, topotecan); alkylating agents (isofosfamide, cyclophosphamide); anthracyclines (doxorubicin, epirubicin); taxanes (paclitaxel, docetaxel); antimetabolites (methotrexate, gemcitabine); and vinca alkaloids (vincristine, vinblastine, vinorelbine). Alkylator-based combination chemotherapy regimens, such as cyclophosphamide, doxorubicin, and vincristine (CAV), were developed in the 1970s and resulted in significant improvements in response rate (60–80%) and overall survival (median = 7–10 months) (11). During the 1980s, the combination of etoposide and cisplatin (EP) was found to yield response and survival rates similar to those of older alkylator-based regimens, with a relatively favorable toxicity profile (12). Randomized trials directly comparing CAV to EP failed to demonstrate the superiority of either regimen, and, recently, a phase III study comparing EP to cyclophosphamide, epirubicin, and vincristine (CEV) reported that overall survival was significantly better in patients assigned to the EP arm of the trial (10.2 vs. 7.8 months, $P = .0004$), with most of the difference noted in patients with LS-SCLC (13). Meta-analyses have also demonstrated a modest

survival advantage for cisplatin-based therapy (14), and an analysis of randomized clinical trials performed over 20 years in patients with ES-SCLC revealed a 2-month survival improvement during the latter time interval when cisplatin-based trials predominated (15). EP has become the standard of care for both ES- and LS-SCLC because it results in less myelotoxicity and is relatively well tolerated in combination with thoracic irradiation in patients with LS-SCLC.

Phase II trials of several newer regimens have reported reasonable efficacy in patients with ES-SCLC. The combination of irinotecan plus cisplatin (IP) is one of the few regimens that has undergone phase III evaluation. The Japanese Clinical Oncology Group (JCOG) randomized 154 patients with previously untreated ES-SCLC to either EP or IP and reported that IP resulted in a significantly better response rate, progression-free survival, and overall survival (16). IP also induced significantly more severe diarrhea, while EP caused greater hematologic toxicity. Two randomized trials in Western patients have failed to confirm the superiority of IP over EP. A North American/Australian trial that compared a modified IP regimen to EP in 331 patients with previously untreated ES-SCLC reported similar efficacy in both arms in terms of response rate, progression-free survival, and overall survival (17). As in the JCOG trial, there was more myelosuppression and febrile neutropenia associated with EP and more diarrhea with IP. A Southwest Oncology Group (SWOG) trial in the United States randomized 651 patients with previously untreated ES-SCLC to receive IP or EP using the same regimens and schedules as reported by JCOG, and again found no significant difference in efficacy between the 2 arms (18). The combination of cisplatin plus oral topotecan, a topoisomerase 1 inhibitor related to irinotecan, was also compared to EP in 784 patients with previously untreated ES-SCLC with the finding that efficacy was similar in both arms (19). Quality of life (QOL) analysis on this trial favored EP ($P = .049$).

Although most of the randomized studies in ES-SCLC have utilized cisplatin-based combinations, there is evidence that carboplatin-based regimens yield similar response rates and survival. A meta-analysis of studies comparing cisplatin- to carboplatin-based regimens has demonstrated equivalent efficacy in patients with ES-SCLC (20). Depending on the degree of response, a maximum of 4–6 cycles of initial chemotherapy should be administered. Elderly patients older than 70 years have similar survival rates when compared with younger patients if they have a good performance status. Therefore, performance status and comorbidities, rather than age, should guide therapy. Overall, the combination of a platinum plus etoposide results in an objective response rate of 60–70%, complete response rate of 10%, median survival of 8–10 months, and a 2-year survival rate of 5%. Despite these dismal long-term survival rates, platinum plus etoposide combinations remain the standard-of-care for patients with SCLC.

Encouraging data have been reported from phase II trials in patients with ES-SCLC with a variety of other doublet and triplet regimens incorporating newer chemotherapy agents, such as carboplatin plus paclitaxel and paclitaxel plus topotecan. However, it is highly unlikely that any of these empiric regimens will result in dramatic improvements in long-term survival. Numerous chemotherapy-based strategies, including dose-intensification, weekly administration, triplet therapy, high-dose consolidation, alternating or sequential non-cross-resistant regimens, and maintenance therapy, have failed to yield consistent or convincing improvements in survival, and several of these approaches have resulted in unacceptable toxicity.

## Prophylactic Cranial Irradiation

The role of PCI in patients with ES-SCLC was evaluated by the European Organisation for Research and Treatment of Cancer (EORTC) in a trial in which 286 patients with ES-SCLC who had responded to initial chemotherapy were randomized to receive PCI or no PCI (21). In this trial, PCI significantly decreased the incidence of symptomatic brain metastases (14.6% vs. 40.4%; $P < .001$) and increased the 1-year survival rate (27.1% vs. 13.3%; $P = .003$). Although PCI did have a negative effect on QOL within the first 3 months of treatment, by 6 months there was no significant difference in global QOL scores between patients who did or did not receive PCI (22). Importantly, this trial excluded patients older than 75 years due to an increased risk of neurocognitive toxicity; so the benefits of PCI in elderly patients remain unclear. PCI is now recommended for patients with ES-SCLC who have responded to initial therapy along the same guidelines as those noted for patients with LS-SCLC.

## Paraneoplastic Syndromes

The neuroendocrine nature of SCLC cells is responsible for the relatively common occurrence of neurological and endocrine paraneoplastic syndromes in this disease. Hyponatremia, due to ectopic secretion of antidiuretic hormone (ADH) or atrial natiuretic peptide (ANP), is observed in up to 15% of patients with SCLC. Cushing syndrome, due to ectopic ACTH secretion, occurs in 2–5% of patients (23). Both of these syndromes are reversible with successful treatment of the disease, although the metabolic derangements should be medically managed and controlled before initiating anticancer therapy. Neurological paraneoplastic syndromes typically caused by antibodies that cross-react between antigens on SCLC cells and neurons, occur less frequently, but are generally more debilitating. Most of these neurological syndromes, such as subacute cerebellar degeneration and limbic encephalopathy, are irreversible because they are caused by antibodies that are cytotoxic to specific types of neurons. One notable exception is Lambert–Eaton myasthenic syndrome in which the proximal myopathy may improve as the disease is treated and the causative antibodies that interfere with presynaptic voltage-gated calcium channels are suppressed. Clinical recognition of paraneoplastic syndromes is important as it may allow for detection of SCLC at an earlier stage of disease.

## Recurrent Disease

The majority of patients with SCLC will develop recurrent disease, which has been divided into 2 categories: refractory/resistant (primary progression or recurrence <3 months after initial therapy) and relapsed/sensitive (recurrence ≥3 months after initial therapy), with much lower responses to second-line therapy in patients with refractory/resistant disease. Trials have suggested that reinitiation of the initial chemotherapy regimen results in response rates of 50–60% in patients whose initial response duration was greater than 6–8 months (24). Therefore, reinduction with the initial chemotherapy regimen is recommended for patients relapsing ≥6 months after the initial therapy, while single-agent second-line therapy, such as topotecan or paclitaxel, is more appropriate for those relapsing within 6 months.

The survival benefit of second-line chemotherapy was demonstrated in a randomized trial comparing oral topotecan to best supportive care in 141 patients with recurrent SCLC. Although the response rate to oral topotecan was only 7%, overall survival was significantly better in patients receiving chemotherapy (median = 26 vs. 14 weeks; 6 months, 49% vs. 26%; $P = .01$) (25). In phase II trials, combination chemotherapy regimens generally demonstrate higher response rates than single agents, but overall survival does not appear to be improved and the toxicity of combination regimens can be challenging. One randomized phase III trial directly compared single-agent topotecan to the combination of CAV in 211 patients with SCLC who had relapsed >60 days after initial therapy (26). This trial reported no significant difference in response rate (24% vs. 18%; $P = .29$), time to progression (13 vs. 12 weeks; $P = .55$), or overall survival (median = 25 vs. 25 weeks; $P = .79$) between patients treated with topotecan versus CAV, although toxicity was significantly greater with CAV (26). On the basis of these results, single-agent chemotherapy is considered the standard approach for patients with relapsed SCLC. Figure 4.2 is an algorithm for the treatment of patients with ES-SCLS.

## Investigational Agents

Amrubicin is an investigational anthracycline with promising activity in early phase studies in patients with SCLC; however, results from 2 phase III trials have recently tempered enthusiasm. In the first phase III trial, 637 patients with recurrent SCLC were randomized to receive either amrubicin or topotecan (27). Although there was a significant improvement in response rate with amrubicin (31% vs. 17%, $P = .0002$), there was no difference in median progression-free survival (4.1 vs. 4.0 months, $P = .98$) or overall survival (7.5 vs. 7.8 months, $P = .17$). Interestingly,

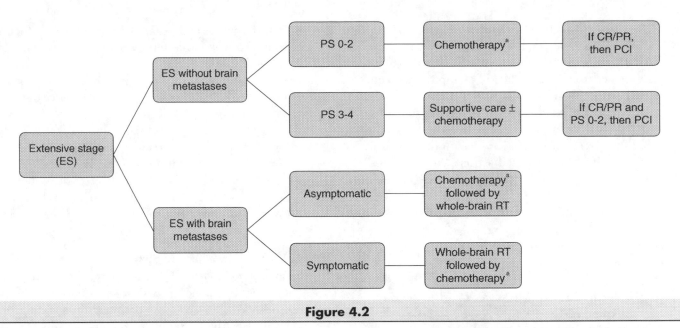

**Figure 4.2**

Treatment algorithm for ES-SCLC. CR, complete response; ES-SCLC, extensive-stage small cell lung cancer; PCI, prophylactic cranial irradiation; PR, partial response; PS, Zubrod performance status. ᵃChemotherapy = platinum-based 2-drug regimen (carboplatin plus etoposide preferred).

in the subgroup of patients with refractory/resistant disease, the 1-year overall survival rate was significantly better with amrubicin (17% vs. 8%, *P* = .019). In the second phase III trial, 248 patients with ES-SCLC were randomized to receive amrubicin plus cisplatin or IP (28). The study was stopped early due to futility with significantly worse overall survival for amrubicin plus cisplatin (median = 15 vs. 17.7 months, hazard ratio [HR] = 1.43, 95% confidence interval [CI] [1.10–1.85]).

Over the past 30 years, we have gained extensive knowledge of the biology of SCLC, and preclinical studies have identified a plethora of molecular therapeutic targets. Many therapeutic agents aimed at these targets have been evaluated in phase II and III clinical trials in patients with SCLC, but thus far, none has demonstrated promising clinical activity. Among these failed approaches are anti-angiogenic agents (e.g., vandetinib, cediranib); metalloproteinase inhibitors (e.g., marimastat); growth factor inhibitors (e.g., dasatinib, imatinib); signal transduction pathway inhibitors (e.g., everolimus); retinoids (e.g., fenretinide); and pro-apoptotic agents (e.g., oblimersen). Despite these setbacks, an unprecedented number of novel, rational, molecular strategies are now being evaluated in preclinical and clinical trials in SCLC, including those targeting angiogenesis (e.g., bevacizumab); apoptotic pathways (e.g., small molecule Bcl-2 inhibitors); immune surveillance (e.g., PD1 and PDL1 antagonists); and cancer stem cells (e.g., Notch and hedgehog signaling). It is unlikely that empiric chemotherapy will lead to further significant improvements in patients with SCLC. Future advances will rely on ongoing efforts to identify molecular targets that drive the survival, proliferation, and metastatic potential of cancer cells.

## REVIEW QUESTIONS

1. A 53-year-old male smoker presents with a cough, fatigue, and progressive dyspnea on exertion of 3 weeks' duration. Physical examination shows a thin man in no distress with tachycardia, normal respiratory rate at rest, and wheezing throughout the left lung field. Blood counts and serum electrolytes are normal. Chest radiography reveals a left hilar mass. CT scan shows a 4-cm left hilar mass that is narrowing the left main stem bronchus and enlarged left hilar, left paratracheal, aortopulmonary window, and subcarinal lymph nodes. Bronchoscopy with transbronchial biopsy of the subcarinal lymph node reveals sheets of poorly differentiated cells with a high nuclear-to-cytoplasmic ratio, nuclear molding, and absent nucleoli. Immunohistochemistry reveals that the malignant cells are positive for pancytokeratin, chromogranin A, and CD56, and negative for CD20 and common leukocyte antigen. Which of the following is the most appropriate statement regarding this man's disease?

   (A) Two-thirds of patients have hematogenous metastases at time of diagnosis
   (B) One-third of patients have myasthenia gravis
   (C) Half of patients have the syndrome of inappropriate antidiuretic hormone secretion
   (D) One-third of patients have a neurological paraneoplastic syndrome
   (E) Half of patients can be cured with surgical resection

2. A 58-year-old woman is found to have a 1.5-cm left lower lobe nodule on chest radiography obtained as part of an executive physical. Chest radiography 1 year earlier was normal. She is asymptomatic and has no other significant medical problems. She smoked 1 pack of cigarettes a day for 30 years, but quit 10 years ago. Physical examination is unremarkable. CT scan shows a 1.3-cm peripheral left lower lobe mass with no enlargement of hilar or mediastinal lymph nodes. PET scan shows abnormal $^{18}$F-fludeoxyglucose-avidity only in the left lower lobe nodule without any evidence of metastases. Pulmonary function testing shows a mild obstructive deficit. She undergoes video-assisted thoracoscopic left lower lobectomy with mediastinal lymph node sampling without complications. Pathology reveals a 1.8-cm small cell carcinoma with negative surgical margins and no metastases in 15 hilar and mediastinal lymph nodes. Postoperative MRI of the brain is normal. Which of the following is the most appropriate next step in the management of this patient?

(A) Surveillance with annual CT scan of the chest
(B) Cisplatin plus etoposide for 4 cycles
(C) Oral topotecan for 4 cycles
(D) Thoracic radiotherapy
(E) Cisplatin plus etoposide with concurrent thoracic radiotherapy

*Questions 3 and 4 are coupled*

3. A 64-year-old man presents with fatigue and shortness of breath, which has progressed over the past 4 weeks. He has a 90-pack-year smoking history. Physical examination reveals a thin, tired man who is oriented × 3 but slow in responding to questions. Sensation and motor strength are normal. Lung examination reveals decreased breath sounds with rhonchi in the left lower lung field. Laboratory evaluation reveals a serum sodium of 116 mg/L with normal renal and hepatic function. Chest radiography reveals a left infrahilar mass. CT scan shows a 4-cm central left lower lobe mass narrowing the left lower lobe airway with early atelectatic changes and enlarged left hilar, paratracheal, and subcarinal lymph nodes. PET scan shows intense $^{18}$F-fludeoxyglucose (FDG)-avidity in the left lower lobe mass and the enlarged left hilar and mediastinal lymph nodes, but there are no other FDG-avid foci. Endobronchial ultrasound-guided biopsy of a left paratracheal lymph node reveals small cell carcinoma. MRI scan of the head is normal. His sodium increases to 131 mg/L with normal saline, free-water restriction, and demeclocycline, and his mental status improves. His Zubrod performance status is 1. Which of the following is the most appropriate next step in the management of this patient?

(A) Cisplatin plus etoposide for 4 cycles followed by thoracic radiotherapy delivered once daily to a total dose of 66 Gy

(B) Cisplatin plus irinotecan for 4 cycles with concurrent thoracic radiotherapy delivered once daily to a total dose of 45 Gy
(C) Cisplatin plus etoposide for 4 cycles with concurrent thoracic radiotherapy delivered twice daily to a total dose of 45 Gy
(D) Carboplatin plus paclitaxel administered weekly with concurrent thoracic radiotherapy delivered once daily to a total dose of 66 Gy
(E) Carboplatin plus paclitaxel for 2 cycles followed by carboplatin plus paclitaxed administered weekly with thoracic radiotherapy delivered twice daily to a total dose of 45 Gy

4. On completion of chemotherapy and thoracic radiotherapy, the patient in Question 3 recovers with mild residual peripheral neuropathy. He continues to have a Zubrod performance status of 1. Serum sodium normalized after the initiation of therapy and he is now off demeclocycline and fluid restriction with a serum sodium of 135 mg/L. Repeat CT scans of the chest and abdomen 4 weeks after completion of therapy reveal mild left infrahilar soft-tissue thickening with no residual mass, no enlarged lymph nodes, and no evidence of systemic metastases. Repeat MRI scan of the brain is normal. Which of the following is the most appropriate next step in the management of this patient?

(A) Clinical and radiographic surveillance
(B) Topotecan 1.5 mg/m$^2$/d IV × 5 days every 3 weeks for 4 cycles
(C) Bevacizumab 15 mg/kg IV every 3 weeks until progression of disease
(D) Prophylactic cranial irradiation
(E) Left lower lobectomy with mediastinal lymph node dissection

5. A 56-year-old man presents with cough, dyspnea, abdominal discomfort, and weight loss. Over the past 3 weeks, he has been spending over half of his day sitting in a chair or lying in bed due to dyspnea and pain. He has been taking ibuprofen with mild, transient relief of abdominal pain. He has a 60-pack-year smoking history and drinks a 6-pack of beer per day, but has no chronic medical problems. Physical examination reveals a man in moderate painful distress who is short of breath on minimal exertion. Lung examination shows decreased breath sounds and rhonchi throughout the left lung. Palpation of the right upper quadrant reveals firm, nodular hepatomegaly with moderate tenderness. He is neurologically intact. CT scans of the chest and abdomen show a 5-cm left hilar mass with critical narrowing of the left main-stem bronchus, bulky bilateral mediastinal and hilar lymphadenopathy, and numerous enhancing lesions in the liver measuring up to 4.6 cm in diameter. Core biopsy of a liver lesion reveals small cell carcinoma. Laboratory studies

reveal hemoglobin of 11.5 g/dL, white blood cell count of 8.4 K/mm³, platelet count of 100,000/mm³, peripheral reticulocytes and teardrop erythrocytes, normal renal function, alkaline phosphatase of 481 IU/L, alanine aminotransferase of 54 IU/L, aspartate aminotransferase of 76 IU/L, and total bilirubin of 1.4 mg/dL. CT scan of the head shows no brain metastases. Which of the following is the most appropriate next step in the management of this patient?

(A) Cisplatin plus etoposide with concurrent thoracic radiotherapy
(B) Topotecan
(C) Carboplatin plus etoposide
(D) Oral etoposide
(E) Palliative care with hospice support

6. A 59-year-old man presents with shortness of breath, cough, and fatigue. He has an 80-pack-year smoking history, but no significant past medical history. A chest x-ray reveals a large right hilar mass and several lung nodules. CT scans of the chest and abdomen show a 5-cm right hilar mass, bulky bilateral hilar and mediastinal lymph nodes, bilateral lung nodules, multiple ring-enhancing liver lesions, and a 3-cm left adrenal nodule. Core biopsy of one of the liver lesions reveals small cell carcinoma. MRI scan of the brain is normal as are renal and liver function tests. He receives 4 cycles of chemotherapy with carboplatin plus etoposide, which he tolerates well with relief of his presenting symptoms. Repeat CT scans show a resolution of hilar and mediastinal lymph nodes and adrenal mass, and near complete response of the right hilar mass and liver metastases. Repeat MRI of the brain remains normal. Which of the following is the most appropriate next step in the management of this patient?

(A) Resection of residual right hilar mass
(B) Stereotactic body radiotherapy to residual right hilar mass and liver metastases
(C) Four cycles of topotecan
(D) Two additional cycles of carboplatin and etoposide
(E) Prophylactic cranial irradiation

7. A 68-year-old woman returns for a follow-up examination 4 months after completing 4 cycles of cisplatin and etoposide for extensive-stage small cell lung cancer. CT scan performed after completion of therapy showed a near-complete response. She then underwent prophylactic cranial irradiation. She has persistent grade 2 peripheral sensory neuropathy that developed after her fourth cycle of cisplatin-based chemotherapy. She otherwise feels well with a Zubrod performance status of 1. On neurological examination, deep tendon reflexes are absent in the upper and lower extremities and sensation to light touch is diminished in her hands and below the knees bilaterally. Results of laboratory

studies are within normal limits. CT scan of the chest and abdomen shows progression of bilateral lung nodules, mediastinal lymph nodes, and liver and adrenal metastases. Which of the following is the most appropriate next step in the management of this patient?

(A) Palliative care with hospice support
(B) Topotecan
(C) Vinorelbine
(D) Cyclophosphamide, doxorubicin, and vincristine
(E) Carboplatin plus paclitaxel

## REFERENCES

1. Aberle DR, Adams AM, Berg CD, et al. Reduced lung-cancer mortality with low-dose computed tomographic screening. *N Engl J Med.* 2011;365:395–409.
2. Cuffe S, Moua T, Summerfield R, Roberts H, Jett J, Shepherd FA. Characteristics and outcomes of small cell lung cancer patients diagnosed during two lung cancer computed tomographic screening programs in heavy smokers. *J Thorac Oncol.* 2011;6(4):818–822.
3. Jett JR, Schild SE, Kesler KA, Kalemkerian GP. Treatment of small cell lung cancer: diagnosis and management of lung cancer, 3rd ed: American College of Chest Physicians evidence-based clinical practice guidelines. *Chest* 2013;143(5 Suppl):e400S–e419S.
4. Pignon JP, Arriagada R, Ihde DC, et al. A meta-analysis of thoracic radiotherapy for small-cell lung cancer. *N Engl J Med.* 1992;327(23):1618–1624.
5. Warde P, Payne D. Does thoracic irradiation improve survival and local control in limited-stage small-cell carcinoma of the lung? A meta-analysis. *J Clin Oncol.* 1992;10(6):890–895.
6. Fried DB, Morris DE, Poole C, et al. Systematic review evaluating the timing of thoracic radiation therapy in combined modality therapy for limited-stage small-cell lung cancer. *J Clin Oncol.* 2004;22(23):4837–4845.
7. Turrisi AT 3rd, Kim K, Blum R, et al. Twice-daily compared with once-daily thoracic radiotherapy in limited small-cell lung cancer treated concurrently with cisplatin and etoposide. *N Engl J Med.* 1999;340(4):265–271.
8. Hann CL, Rudin CM. Management of small-cell lung cancer: incremental changes but hope for the future. *Oncology.* 2008;22(13):1486–1492.
9. Aupérin A, Arriagada R, Pignon JP, et al. Prophylactic cranial irradiation for patients with small-cell lung cancer in complete remission. Prophylactic Cranial Irradiation Overview Collaborative Group. *N Engl J Med.* 1999;341(7):476–484.
10. Tsuchiya R, Suzuki K, Ichinose Y, et al. Phase II trial of postoperative adjuvant cisplatin and etoposide in patients with completely resected stage I-IIIa small cell lung cancer: the Japan Clinical Oncology Lung Cancer Study Group Trial (JCOG9101). *J Thorac Cardiovasc Surg.* 2005;129(5):977–983.
11. Lowenbraun S, Bartolucci A, Smalley RV, et al. The superiority of combination chemotherapy over single agent chemotherapy in small cell lung carcinoma. *Cancer.* 1979;44(2):406–413.
12. Evans WK, Shepherd FA, Feld R, et al. VP-16 and cisplatin as first-line therapy for small-cell lung cancer. *J Clin Oncol.* 1985;3(11):1471–1477.
13. Sundstrøm S, Bremnes RM, Kaasa S, et al.; Norwegian Lung Cancer Study Group. Cisplatin and etoposide regimen is superior to cyclophosphamide, epirubicin, and vincristine regimen in small-cell lung cancer: results from a randomized phase III trial with 5 years' follow-up. *J Clin Oncol.* 2002;20(24):4665–4672.
14. Pujol JL, Carestia L, Daurès JP. Is there a case for cisplatin in the treatment of small-cell lung cancer? A meta-analysis of randomized trials of a cisplatin-containing regimen versus a regimen without this alkylating agent. *Br J Cancer.* 2000;83(1):8–15.

15. Chute JP, Chen T, Feigal E, et al. Twenty years of phase III trials for patients with extensive-stage small-cell lung cancer: perceptible progress. *J Clin Oncol.* 1999;17(6):1794–1801.

16. Noda K, Nishiwaki Y, Kawahara M, et al.; Japan Clinical Oncology Group. Irinotecan plus cisplatin compared with etoposide plus cisplatin for extensive small-cell lung cancer. *N Engl J Med.* 2002;346(2):85–91.

17. Hanna N, Bunn PA Jr, Langer C, et al. Randomized phase III trial comparing irinotecan/cisplatin with etoposide/cisplatin in patients with previously untreated extensive-stage disease small-cell lung cancer. *J Clin Oncol.* 2006;24(13):2038–2043.

18. Lara PN Jr, Natale R, Crowley J, et al. Phase III trial of irinotecan/cisplatin compared with etoposide/cisplatin in extensive-stage small-cell lung cancer: clinical and pharmacogenomic results from SWOG S0124. *J Clin Oncol.* 2009;27(15):2530–2535.

19. Eckardt JR, von Pawel J, Papai Z, et al. Open-label, multicenter, randomized, phase III study comparing oral topotecan/cisplatin versus etoposide/cisplatin as treatment for chemotherapy-naive patients with extensive-disease small-cell lung cancer. *J Clin Oncol.* 2006;24(13):2044–2051.

20. Rossi A, Di Maio M, Chiodini P, et al. Carboplatin- or cisplatin-based chemotherapy in first-line treatment of small-cell lung cancer: the COCIS meta-analysis of individual patient data. *J Clin Oncol.* 2012;30(14):1692–1698.

21. Slotman B, Faivre-Finn C, Kramer G, et al.; EORTC Radiation Oncology Group and Lung Cancer Group. Prophylactic cranial irradiation in extensive small-cell lung cancer. *N Engl J Med.* 2007;357(7):664–672.

22. Slotman BJ, Mauer ME, Bottomley A, et al. Prophylactic cranial irradiation in extensive disease small-cell lung cancer: short-term health-related quality of life and patient reported symptoms: results of an international Phase III randomized controlled trial by the EORTC Radiation Oncology and Lung Cancer Groups. *J Clin Oncol.* 2009;27(1):78–84.

23. Marchioli CC, Graziano SL. Paraneoplastic syndromes associated with small cell lung cancer. *Chest Surg Clin N Am.* 1997;7(1):65–80.

24. Postmus PE, Berendsen HH, van Zandwijk N, et al. Retreatment with the induction regimen in small cell lung cancer relapsing after an initial response to short term chemotherapy. *Eur J Cancer Clin Oncol.* 1987;23(9):1409–1411.

25. O'Brien ME, Ciuleanu TE, Tsekov H, et al. Phase III trial comparing supportive care alone with supportive care with oral topotecan in patients with relapsed small-cell lung cancer. *J Clin Oncol.* 2006;24(34):5441–5447.

26. von Pawel J, Schiller JH, Shepherd FA, et al. Topotecan versus cyclophosphamide, doxorubicin, and vincristine for the treatment of recurrent small-cell lung cancer. *J Clin Oncol.* 1999;17(2):658–667.

27. Jotte R, Von Pawel J, Spigel DR, et al. Randomized phase III trial of amrubicin versus topotecan as second-line treatment for small cell lung cancer. *J Clin Oncol.* 2011;29(15S):453s.

28. Satouchi M, Kotani Y, Shibata T, et al. Phase III study comparing amrubicin plus cisplatin with irinotecan plus cisplatin in the treatment of extensive-disease small-cell lung cancer: JCOG 0509. *J Clin Oncol.* 2014;32(12):1262–1268.

# 5

## Breast Cancer

PRIYA GOMATHI KUMARAVELU, AIHUA EDWARD YEN, MICHELINA M. CAIRO,
MOTHAFFAR F. RIMAWI, AND POLLY A. NIRAVATH

## EPIDEMIOLOGY, RISK FACTORS, NATURAL HISTORY, AND PATHOLOGY

Breast cancer is the leading cause of cancer in women in the United States, with 232,340 new cases diagnosed each year, representing 29% of all new cancer cases. It comprises 15% of all cancer deaths in women in the United States, second only to lung cancer. The lifetime risk of developing breast cancer for an American woman is 12.3%, or 1 in 8.

There are several known risk factors for breast cancer. Some of these factors are not modifiable such as age, family history of breast cancer, age at first full-term pregnancy, early menarche, late menopause, breast density, and personal history of atypical breast biopsies. However, postmenopausal obesity, use of menopausal hormones, alcohol consumption, and physical inactivity are also associated with significantly increased breast cancer risk, and lifestyle modifications can potentially reduce these risks. Breast cancer survivors with a body mass index (BMI) of 30 and above have upto a 1.4-fold increased risk of contralateral breast cancer, as compared to patients with BMI <25. Likewise, patients consuming 7 alcoholic beverages per week have a 1.9-fold increased risk of contralateral breast cancer, compared to patients consuming <7 alcoholic beverages per week; this risk escalated to 7.2-fold if they were smokers as well. This increased risk is commonly attributed to endogenous estrogens produced by adipose tissue in obese and alcoholic patients. In a prospective study of breast cancer survivors, physical activity, equivalent to 3 hours of walking each week, and healthy consumption of vegetables and fruits reduced the risk of death by 50% in both obese and nonobese patients, more so in hormone receptor–positive breast cancer patients (1).

Women with a family history of breast cancer are at an increased risk of developing breast cancer. Having >1 first-degree relatives with breast cancer confers higher risk, and the risk increases further if the relatives are premenopausal at the time of diagnosis. A history of ovarian cancer in first-degree relatives may be associated with certain breast cancer syndromes and increased breast cancer risk. Approximately 5–10% of breast cancer cases result from inherited mutations in the breast cancer susceptibility genes *BRCA1* or *BRCA2*. In a combined analysis of 22 studies, women with *BRCA1* mutations are estimated to have a cumulative breast cancer risk of 65% by age 70 years. Those with *BRCA2* mutations have a 45% breast cancer risk (2). Breast cancer may also result from other less common syndromes such as Li-Fraumeni or Cowden syndrome (see Table 5.1). Identified mutations only account for about 50% of heritable breast cancer.

Long-term exposure to hormones may contribute to the increased risk of developing breast cancer with increased age. Early menarche (<12 years) and older age at menopause (>55 years) increase the risk of breast cancer, most likely due to longer exposure of breast tissue to reproductive hormones. For example, younger age at first full-term pregnancy (<30 years), greater number of pregnancies, and longer duration of breastfeeding decrease the risk of breast cancer over the long term. Recent use of hormones also appears to be a risk factor. Oral contraceptive (OC) use may slightly increase breast cancer risk, but it falls to normal risk after 10 years of stopping use. Hormone replacement therapy (HRT) in postmenopausal women, on the other hand, likely carries a greater risk of breast cancer.

Although the incidence of breast cancer is highest in white women, black women are more likely to die of the disease. The 5-year survival for white women is 90%, compared to only 79% for black women. Younger age at diagnosis, more advanced stage at diagnosis, higher probability of triple-negative cancer, and less access to quality health care for black women may, in part, explain this discrepancy.

**Table 5.1** Hereditary Breast Cancer Syndromes

| Gene | Mutation | Inheritance | Other Cancers |
|---|---|---|---|
| BRCA 1 | 17q21 | AD | Ovarian cancer |
| BRCA 2 | Chr 13 | AD | Male breast, prostate, and pancreatic cancer |
| Li-Fraumeni syndrome | P53 | AD | Soft-tissue sarcomas, osteosarcomas, brain, leukemia, lung, and adrenocortical cancer |
| Cowden syndrome | PTEN | AD | Multiple hamartomas, benign skin tumors, thyroid, and endometrium carcinoma and macrocephaly |
| Ataxia-telangiectasia | ATM | AR | Cerebellar ataxia, telangiectasia, growth retardation, and leukemia |
| Hereditary diffuse gastric cancer | CDH1 | AD | Diffuse gastric and invasive lobular breast carcinoma |
| CHEK2 | Chr 22q | | Low-penetrance breast cancer |

AD, autosomal dominant; AR, autosomal recessive.

Increased breast density also increases the risk of breast cancer. Women with dense breasts by breast imaging-reporting and data system (BIRADS) criteria have a 4- to 6-fold increase in breast cancer risk. Increased bone mineral density in postmenopausal women is also associated with increased risk of breast cancer, which may be mediated by hormonal effects.

Atypical proliferative lesions including atypical ductal hyperplasia (ADH) and atypical lobular hyperplasia (ALH) are associated with 4–5 times increased risk of breast cancer. Radiation exposure is also a breast cancer risk factor. In a study conducted at 15 institutions in female children <16 years old treated for Hodgkin lymphoma, up to 35% of these survivors developed breast cancer by age 40 years. Breast cancer risk was higher among those aged 10–16 years, as opposed to <10 years old (RR = 1.9). Similarly, higher radiation dose is associated with increased breast cancer risk (3).

Early-stage breast cancer has a high probability of cure. Women with localized breast cancer that has not spread to locoregional lymph nodes have a 98% 5-year relative overall survival (OS), compared with women who do not have cancer. Once the tumor spreads to regional lymph nodes, survival falls to 83%. The number of positive axillary lymph nodes is the most powerful poor prognostic indicator, and risk increases with the number of lymph nodes involved. Metastatic breast cancer (MBC), on the other hand, is not curable, but it may be very treatable, with a 5-year average survival of 23.4%.

Although rare pathological subtypes can be seen, most breast cancers are adenocarcinomas that are subdivided into noninvasive (carcinoma in situ) and invasive. Among invasive adenocarcinomas, there are 2 dominant subtypes, invasive ductal carcinoma (IDC) and invasive lobular carcinoma (ILC), which carry a similar prognosis, stage for stage. Ductal carcinomas account for about 90% of all breast cancers. Tubular and mucinous carcinomas are special subtypes of ductal carcinomas and account for 5–8%. They are almost universally estrogen receptor (ER) positive, and they have an excellent prognosis. Medullary carcinomas represent another special type of breast cancer and include 3–5% of ductal carcinomas. They tend to be negative for ER, progesterone receptor (PR), and human epidermal growth factor-2 (HER2; triple negative). Medullary carcinoma is found more commonly in patients with *BRCA1* gene mutations. Any breast cancer with poorly differentiated histology and higher nuclear grade has a worse prognosis than a well-differentiated, low-grade tumor.

Certain biomarkers have emerged as important factors affecting the natural history and treatment of breast cancer. The 3 most validated biomarkers in breast cancer are ER, PR, and HER2. They are valuable prognostic markers and also predict response to therapy. The majority of breast cancers (70% or more) is positive for the hormone receptors (ER and/or PR), and 20–25% are HER2-amplified or overexpressing (HER2+). ER-positive and/or PR-positive breast cancer has a better prognosis, and is also responsive to hormonal therapy. HER2 overexpressing breast cancer correlates to a more aggressive tumor subtype, but it also presents a valuable target for HER2-directed therapy.

In the last decade, molecular expression profiling has led to the identification of molecular subtypes of breast cancer, namely, luminal A and B, basal type, and HER2+. Luminal epithelial cells play a role in milk production in response to hormones. Basal myoepithelial cells are involved in milk ejection and are, hence, hormone receptor negative. Phenotypically, luminal A and B are usually lower grade and ER+. Luminal B can be higher grade and either HER2+ or HER2–. Basal type is usually high-grade triple-negative breast cancer (TNBC). These molecular subtypes shed light on the heterogeneity of breast cancer and are the subjects of ongoing research to characterize clinical and biological behavior and develop new therapeutics.

## STAGING

The American Joint Committee on Cancer (AJCC) staging system for breast cancer is shown as follows:

### Breast Cancer Clinical Staging

| Stage | Definition |
|---|---|
| 0 | Ductal carcinoma in situ |
| IA | Tumor <2 cm in greatest dimension (T1); no regional lymph node metastases |
| IB | No evidence of primary tumor (T0) *or* a T1 tumor with microscopic invasion of 1–3 ipsilateral axillary lymph nodes (N1 mic) |
| IIA | No evidence of primary tumor (T0) *or* a T1 tumor with metastases in 1–3 ipsilateral, mobile axillary lymph nodes (N1); *or* a tumor of >2 cm but <5 cm (T2) with no axillary lymph nodes (N0) |
| IIB | Tumor 2–5 cm (T2) with invasion in 1–3 ipsilateral, mobile axillary lymph nodes (N1) *or* a tumor >5 cm (T3) with no axillary lymph node metastases (N0) |
| IIIA | Tumor of any size (T0, T1, T2, or T3) with invasion into ipsilateral fixed or matted axillary lymph nodes, clinically apparent internal mammary lymph nodes, *or* Pathological involvement of 4–9 axillary lymph nodes (N2) *or* Tumor >5 cm (T3) with metastases in 1–9 ipsilateral, mobile, or fixed axillary lymph nodes (N1, N2) |
| IIIB | Tumor of any size with direct extension to the chest wall or the skin (T4) with *or* without metastases to ipsilateral, axillary lymph nodes (N0 to N2) |
| IIIC | Tumor of any size with metastases to ipsilateral infraclavicular and axillary, ipsilateral internal mammary and axillary, or ipsilateral supraclavicular lymph nodes *or* Pathological involvement of >10 axillary lymph nodes (N3) |
| IV | Tumor of any size, with distant metastatic disease (M1) |

## CASE SUMMARIES

### Ductal Carcinoma In Situ

L.P. is a healthy 48-year-old woman who was found to have an abnormal screening mammogram, with a cluster of pleomorphic calcifications in the left breast. Her physical examination showed no palpable masses, dimpling, nipple discharge, or lymphadenopathy. A stereotactic core biopsy showed ductal carcinoma in situ (DCIS), ER+ and PR+. She was referred to a multidisciplinary breast care clinic seeking treatment recommendations.

### Evidence-Based Case Discussion

L.P. has DCIS, or stage 0 breast cancer. Annually in the United States, >50,000 patients are diagnosed with DCIS. By definition, it is noninvasive, meaning that the basement membrane of the ductal unit is preserved. However, recurrences may rarely present even after 15 years, and half of those recurrences become invasive cancer. DCIS represents a heterogeneous group, and various treatment options exist. Surgery is the primary treatment modality for this localized breast cancer and may be offered as mastectomy or breast conservation surgery.

Regarding the choice of surgery, lumpectomy followed by radiation therapy is equivalent to mastectomy, as shown by the National Surgical Adjuvant Breast and Bowel Project (NSABP) B-06 trial. For patients who had breast-conserving surgery, the omission of post-lumpectomy radiation increased the risk of local recurrence (39% chance of ipsilateral breast tumor vs. 14.3%; $P < .001$). After 20 years of follow-up, there continues to be no significant difference in OS or disease-free survival (DFS) between the group of patients who underwent total mastectomy and the group treated with lumpectomy and breast radiation (4). In the landmark Milan trial, patients with tumors <2 cm and no palpable axillary lymph nodes were randomized to mastectomy versus breast conservation surgery followed by radiation. At 8 years, OS (83.7% vs. 85%) and DFS (77% vs. 80%) were not statistically different between the 2 groups (5).

Adjuvant radiotherapy is beneficial for DCIS, but experts do not agree on its use across all cases. Large prospective trials such as NSABP B-17 and European Organisation for Research and Treatment of Cancer (EORTC) 10853 showed that radiation following breast conservation therapy significantly reduced local recurrences, but did not translate to an OS benefit (6, 7). These findings are limited by the trial design. In NSABP B-17, 80% of the patients had DCIS measuring <1.0 cm, and margin widths were not quantified in either study. In addition, successful surgical resection was not confirmed with a post-lumpectomy mammogram.

Increased tumor size, higher pathological grade, presence of necrosis, younger patient age, and smaller margin width are each associated with higher risk of recurrence. Four risk factors, including pathological classification, margin size, tumor size, and age, were incorporated into the Van Nuys Prospective Index (VNPI) for use as a risk-adapted clinical tool for adjuvant management (7). A scoring number is assigned to each risk factor, and the resulting sum is then classified as low, intermediate, or high risk for local recurrence. Risk-dependent management decisions may include breast conservation therapy and observation

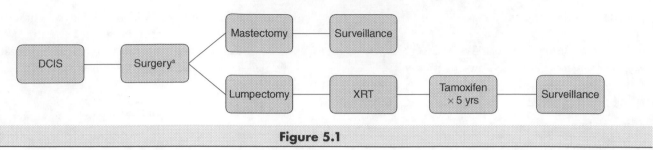

**Figure 5.1**

Treatment algorithm for DCIS. [a]Patients with any evidence of invasive breast cancer on surgical specimen should undergo complete staging with sentinel lymph node biopsy, and treatment should proceed according to the appropriate breast cancer treatment algorithm. DCIS, ductal carcinoma in situ; XRT, radiation therapy.

alone, breast conservation therapy and radiotherapy, or mastectomy. Unfortunately, subsequent prospective trials using the VNPI have produced conflicting results, and there has not yet been a large prospective, randomized trial validating the VNPI. It should thus be used only with caution and in selected patients. The 12-gene *Oncotype* DX DCIS score identifies a subset of DCIS patients with lower risk of local recurrence and invasive local recurrence. Lower score may indicate a patient who could avoid adjuvant radiation after surgical excision, although this test also needs further validation before it can be recommended for routine use.

Adjuvant hormonal therapy is another important aspect of adjuvant treatment. The NSABP B-24 trial, a prospective, randomized study, evaluated adjuvant tamoxifen after lumpectomy and radiation in women with extensive DCIS, or those with close margins. At 7 years, the tamoxifen-treated group had a 10.3% recurrence rate in breast cancer events compared with 16.9% in the placebo arm. Furthermore, in the tamoxifen arm, invasive breast cancer events were reduced by 48% and contralateral breast cancer events were reduced from 3.2% to 1.8% (9). The investigators did not initially evaluate ER status, but a post hoc analysis did report that in those women with ER+ DCIS, tamoxifen significantly reduced incidence of breast cancer by 59% versus 20% in those who were ER–.

ADH, ALH, lobular carcinoma in situ (LCIS), and flat epithelial atypia (FEA) are considered as non-premalignant high-risk breast lesions, because they increase future risk of breast cancer. ADH and ALH increased the relative risk (RR) by 4-fold, and LCIS by 10-fold. These lesions should be treated with surgical excision followed by surveillance. Five years of tamoxifen chemoprevention is also indicated for these women. In the future, aromatase inhibitors (AIs) may also be a standard option for chemoprevention. MAP.3 and IBIS-II were large trials in which high-risk, postmenopausal women were randomized to receive either placebo or AI for breast cancer prevention. In both trials, the AI more than halved the incidence of breast cancer compared to placebo (10,11). AIs are not currently Food and Drug Administration (FDA) approved for prevention of breast cancer.

For L.P., the recommendations should include breast conservation surgery and adjuvant radiation. Tamoxifen should be offered to further decrease the chance of contralateral breast cancer or ipsilateral recurrence. Figure 5.1 provides a treatment algorithm for patients with DCIS.

## Early-Stage ER+ Breast Cancer

J.S. is a 51-year-old perimenopausal woman, for whom routine screening mammogram detected a 1.3 × 1.4 cm spiculated mass in the left breast. On physical and ultrasound examination, her axillary lymph nodes were not found enlarged. An ultrasound-guided core needle biopsy revealed grade 2 IDC, ER+, PR+, and HER2– by immunohistochemistry (IHC).

After multidisciplinary clinical evaluation, J.S. opted for breast conservation. She underwent left breast lumpectomy with sentinel lymph node biopsy. The surgical pathology revealed IDC, 1.9 cm in greatest diameter, histological grade 2, Ki67 31%, ER+ (90% staining, 3+ intensity), PR+ (50% staining, 2+ intensity), and HER2– (2+ IHC, fluorescence in situ hybridization [FISH] ratio = 1.3). Surgical margins were free of tumor. None of the 3 sentinel lymph nodes was involved with cancer.

### Evidence-Based Case Discussion

J.S. has a T1 N0 (stage IA) left breast IDC. Regarding the choice of surgery, lumpectomy followed by radiation therapy is equivalent to mastectomy as shown by the NSABP B-06 and Milan trials discussed earlier (4,5). However, it should be noted that if J.S. were older, she could reasonably choose lumpectomy alone, without radiation. In the Cancer and Leukemia Group B (CALGB) 9343 trial, women 70 years or older with stage I (T1N0M0) ER+ breast cancer after lumpectomy were randomized to receive tamoxifen plus radiation or tamoxifen alone. Although the local recurrence was significantly higher without radiation (4% vs. 1%), OS was not significantly different (87% vs. 86%) (12).

Sentinel lymph node biopsy provides adequate axillary lymph node staging when negative. In fact, even when 1–2 sentinel nodes are positive, the results of the American College of Surgeons Oncology Group (ACOSOG) Z0011 suggested that there is no survival advantage to completing an axillary lymph node dissection (ALND) (13). It is noteworthy that this study was done in patients with clinically negative axillary nodes and tumors <5 cm. No study patients received neoadjuvant therapy, and they all underwent lumpectomy and postoperative radiation. In this select group of patients, it is possible to rely on sentinel lymph node biopsy only, and spare patients the potential morbidity of ALND. This conclusion is supported by the results of the phase III IBCSG 23–0 trial involving patients with ≤5-cm breast cancers and clinically non-palpable axillary lymph nodes, with 1 or more micro metastatic (≤2 mm) sentinel nodes. Patients were randomized to have ALND or no further surgery. At 5 years, DFS and OS for those without ALND were noninferior to ALND, 84.4% versus 87.8% and 97.5% versus 97.6%, respectively (14). Nearly identical results were reported in the phase III After Mapping of the Axilla: Radiotherapy or Surgery (AMAROS) trial of similar design with the risk of short- and long-term lymphedema significantly decreased in the non-ALND radiotherapy arm (15).

After completion of her lumpectomy and sentinel lymph node biopsy, the question then arises as to whether or not J.S. would benefit from systemic adjuvant therapy. Adjuvant systemic therapy for hormone receptor positive, HER2– breast tumors can include endocrine therapy alone or chemotherapy followed by endocrine therapy. When considering chemotherapy, one must take into account the factors relating to the patient's general health and factors relating to the disease. Competing comorbidities need to be weighed against the potential benefits of therapy. First, we consider the patient factors. J.S. is an otherwise healthy woman who has no contraindications to adjuvant therapy.

When we consider factors related to her tumor, J.S. has multiple favorable features, including a small tumor that is node negative. Her tumor is ER+ and PR+, which predicts better outcome and response to hormone therapy. ER content is reported as positive or negative based on the Allred score (see Table 5.2). The tumor cells are stained with the hormone receptor antibody; both the percentage of positively staining tumor cells and the average intensity of the staining are independently graded. The resulting ER proportion score and intensity score are added together, resulting in the Allred score. The Allred score has been prospectively validated to correlate with endocrine therapy responsiveness. In prospectively validated clinical trials, patients with Allred scores of 3–8 derive additional benefit from endocrine therapy. Allred scores of 0–2 are reported as negative because patients with these scores did not derive additional benefit from adjuvant endocrine therapy. J.S. has an Allred score of 8 given the 90% ER staining and strong intensity; so she would be expected to have a favorable response to endocrine therapy. In some patients, the progesterone content may not correlate to the estrogen content. Retrospective analysis of endocrine therapy treatment for ER+ and PR– tumors revealed that these patients had worse outcomes than those who had ER+ and PR+ tumors. The Adjuvant! Online (AOL) tool uses age, menopausal status, comorbidity, tumor size, number of

**Table 5.2** Allred Score

| Proportion | Percentage of Positive Staining Cells | Intensity | Average Intensity of Stained Cells |
|---|---|---|---|
| 0 | None | 0 | None |
| 1 | <1 | 1 | Weak |
| 2 | 1–10 | 2 | Intermediate |
| 3 | 10–33 | 3 | Strong |
| 4 | 33–66 | | |
| 5 | 66–100 | | |

| Sum of Proportion and Intensity Score | Interpretation |
|---|---|
| 0–2 | Negative |
| 3–8 | Positive |

*Source*: Derived from Ref. (16). Harvey JM, Clark GM, Osborne CK, Allred DC. Estrogen receptor status by immunohistochemistry is superior to the ligand-binding assay for predicting response to adjuvant endocrine therapy in breast cancer. *J Clin Oncol*. 1999;17(5):1474–1481.

positive axillary nodes, and ER status to estimate the risk of breast cancer recurrence and related death at 10 years. All of these factors should be considered in combination to determine the best adjuvant therapy for any individual patient.

J.S.'s tumor also has 2 less favorable pathological features. The tumor grade, a measure of aggressiveness derived from the degree of cellular atypia, is intermediate. In addition, the proliferation index, Ki67, is high, suggesting rapid growth. Considering J.S.'s tumor being ER+ and HER2–, which portends a good prognosis, but intermediate grade with a high Ki67, which suggests poor prognosis, we conclude that this is an intermediate-risk case based on the clinical and pathological features.

As illustrated by this case, it can be difficult to determine recurrence risk and chemotherapy benefit from clinical and pathological features alone. Therefore, molecular tests have been developed to provide additional information about the risk of recurrence. These include the MammaPrint and Oncotype DX assays. MammaPrint (FDA approved as the Symphony assay) is a 70-gene signature DNA microarray assay, which stratifies women with node-negative breast cancer into 2 groups: those who are at low risk and high risk of distant recurrence. MammaPrint low-risk patients, 85% of whom chose not to have adjuvant chemotherapy, had a 97% distant recurrence–free interval (DRFI) of 5 years; conversely, high-risk patients (among whom 81% chose not to have chemotherapy) had a 92% DRFI at 5 years (17). The MammaPrint assay does not predict chemosensitivity for high-risk patients (18). Oncotype DX is a 21-gene assay, which is performed on stored tumor tissue blocks and which provides a "recurrence score" (10–100) with scores <18 being low risk (with benefits of chemotherapy being low), 18–31 being intermediate risk (with unclear benefit of adjuvant therapy), and >31 being high risk (with the benefit of adjuvant therapy likely being greater than the risk of side effects (8). The current TAILORx trial is designed to determine the potential benefit of adjuvant endocrine or chemotherapy for ER+, node-negative patients in the Oncotype DX intermediate-risk group.

Large randomized studies have shown that the adjuvant use of tamoxifen for 5 years decreases the risk of recurrence of breast cancer by 45–50% and the risk of death by 31%, and the benefit persists for years after therapy is discontinued (17). Tamoxifen is effective in both premenopausal and postmenopausal women, although a greater benefit was seen in postmenopausal patients. Does adjuvant tamoxifen treatment offer more? (aTTom) trial in ER+ early breast cancer patients who had completed 4+ years of adjuvant tamoxifen, randomized patients to either continue tamoxifen for another 5 years or to stop. Compared to the patients who took tamoxifen for only 5 years, those who continued for 10 years had 15% reduction in the risk of recurrence ($P = .003$), and 23% reduction in the risk of breast cancer death ($P = .007$). There was an absolute increase in endometrial cancer of 0.5% ($P = .02$), without increase in mortality from endometrial cancer (19). Nearly identical results favoring longer-term tamoxifen adjuvant therapy were reported in the Adjuvant Tamoxifen: Longer Against Shorter (ATLAS) trial involving 12,894 women and showed that 10 years of tamoxifen therapy reduced both breast cancer recurrence ($P = .002$) and breast cancer mortality ($P = .01$) as compared to 5 years (20). The RR of having a pulmonary embolus, stroke, and endometrial cancer was higher while ischemic heart disease was lower, with the absolute mortality from endometrial cancer increased only by 0.2%.

Several trials have assessed the utility of AIs in postmenopausal women with ER+ or PR+ breast cancer (Table 5.3). These agents have a different mechanism of action and a distinct side-effect profile compared to the selective ER modulators (SERM). AIs are less likely than tamoxifen to increase the risk for thrombotic events or endometrial cancer; however, they are more likely to be associated with arthralgia and osteoporosis. In the largest clinical trials, joint pains were reported in 5–36% of patients taking AIs compared with 4–29% of patients on tamoxifen. Bone mineral density is also more likely to be affected by AIs with a 2- to 3-fold decrease in bone mineral density, a 1.5-fold increased risk of osteoporosis, and a 1.5-fold increased risk of fracture when compared with tamoxifen. Tamoxifen use was associated with an increased risk of venous thrombotic events (3.9% vs. 1.7% in BIG 1–98) compared to AIs, but no increased incidence of cerebrovascular events. In addition, the risk of endometrial cancer was increased in patients taking tamoxifen compared to AIs (0.8% vs. 0.2% in the Arimidex, Tamoxifen, alone

**Table 5.3** Adjuvant Endocrine Therapy in Postmenopausal Women With ER+ Tumors

| Trial Design | Median Follow-Up (Months) | Aromatase Inhibitor | Disease-Free Survival | | Overall Survival | |
|---|---|---|---|---|---|---|
| | | | Hazard Ratio | P Value | Hazard Ratio | P Value |
| *Sequential* | | | | | | |
| ABCSG 8 | 72 | Anastrozole | 0.85 | .067 | 0.78 | .032 |
| ARNO 95 | 30 | Anastrozole | 0.66 | .049 | 0.53 | .045 |
| IES | 55.7 | Exemestane | 0.76 | <.001 | 0.85 | .08 |
| ITA | 64 | Anastrozole | 0.57 | .005 | 0.56 | .1 |
| TEAM[a] | 61 | Exemestane | 0.97 | .604 | 1 | .999 |
| BIG 1–98[a] | 71 | Letrozole | 0.96 | NR | 0.9 | NR |
| *Upfront* | | | | | | |
| ATAC | 100 | Anastrozole | 0.9 | .025 | 1 | .99 |
| BIG 1–98 | 76 | Letrozole | 0.88 | .030 | 0.81 | .08 |
| ABCSG 12 | 47.8 | Anastrozole | 1.1 | .590 | 1.8 | .7 |
| *Extended* | | | | | | |
| ABCSG 6a | 62 | Anastrozole | 0.62 | .031 | 0.89 | .57 |
| MA-17 | 30 | Letrozole | 0.68 | <.001 | 0.98 | .853 |
| NSABP B-33 | 30 | Exemestane | 0.68 | .070 | NR | NR |

[a]In TEAM and BIG 1–98, hazard ratio is reported for sequential therapy compared to AI alone, rather than to tamoxifen alone.
*Extended* refers to treatment with an aromatase inhibitor after 5 years of tamoxifen therapy; *sequential* refers to treatment with an aromatase inhibitor before or after 2–3 years of tamoxifen therapy; *upfront* refers to initial treatment with an aromatase inhibitor. NR is not reported.
*Source*: Adapted from ASCO Clinical Practice Guidelines (21). ASCO Clinical Practice Guidelines: updates on adjuvant endocrine therapy for women with hormone receptor positive breast cancer. July 12, 2010.

or in combination [ATAC] trial). There were no reported deaths from endometrial cancer in either group.

In several clinical studies, including the ATAC, BIG 1–98, and Intergroup Exemestane Study (IES) trials, there was a small but significant (2–5%) absolute DFS advantage associated with the use of AIs as compared to tamoxifen alone when the former were used in postmenopausal patients either upfront for 5 years or after 2 to 3 years of initial tamoxifen, but improvement in OS has not been demonstrated. Many studies have sought to determine the optimal sequence of adjuvant endocrine therapy (see Table 5.3).

On the basis of these data, the choice of hormone therapy in a postmenopausal woman should include at least 2 years of an AI, either upfront or after initial therapy with tamoxifen. Studies are underway comparing ovarian suppression therapy plus AIs versus tamoxifen in premenopausal women. At this time, this strategy is reserved for patients with relative contraindications to tamoxifen therapy such as previous venous thromboembolic events.

In summary, in the case of J.S., a perimenopausal woman with a 1.9-cm, node-negative, ER+, PR+, HER2– IDC, who underwent breast conservation therapy, the decision to administer systemic chemotherapy can be made based on clinical and pathologic features alone. Alternatively, additional testing with a gene signature may be pursued. Should the result show high-risk disease, the patient may benefit from adjuvant systemic chemotherapy. If it shows low-risk disease, chemotherapy can be forgone as it offers little or no benefit to the patient. Evidence of benefit in patients with an intermediate risk is inconclusive, and participation on a clinical trial may be appropriate where available. Otherwise, the decision needs to be based on the available clinicopathological features, while incorporating the patient's preferences.

If the patient has had spontaneous amenorrhea for 12 months (24 months for chemotherapy-induced amenorrhea, preferably with a hormone profile consistent with postmenopausal status in either case), her therapy can be switched to

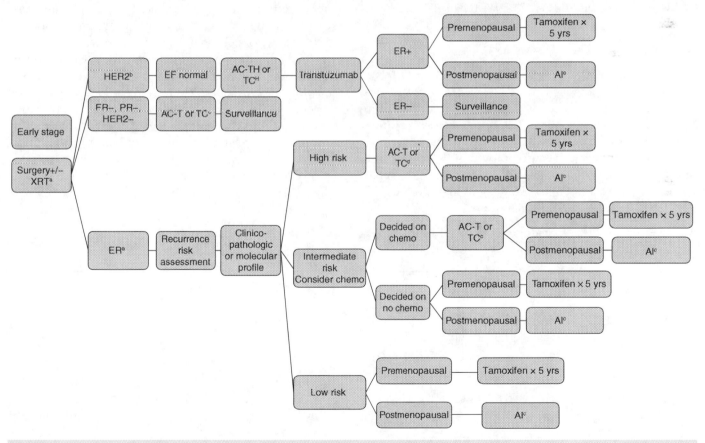

**Figure 5.2**

Treatment algorithm for early-stage breast cancer. [a]Radiotherapy (XRT) is given to appropriately selected patients after the completion of adjuvant chemotherapy. It may be given concurrently with adjuvant HER2 targeted therapy or endocrine therapy. [b]In the case of HER2+ tumors, trastuzumab (H) is added in combination with a taxane most commonly after AC. [c]AI, aromatase inhibitor, may be given for 5 years or for 2–3 years followed by tamoxifen to complete 5 years of adjuvant endocrine therapy. If tamoxifen was started when a patient was premenopausal it may be switched to AI when she is verifiably postmenopausal. [d]Adjuvant chemotherapy for breast cancer involves a combination of A (doxorubicin), C (cyclophosphamide), and T (taxane, either docetaxel or paclitaxel). In clinical trials, they have been administered: sequentially AC-T, or concurrently TAC, or without anthracyclines (TC). TCH refers to docetaxel, carboplatin, and trastuzumab. AC, adenocarcinoma; AI, aromatase inhibitors; ER, estrogen receptor; HER2, human epidermal growth factor-2; PR, progesterone receptor; XRT, radiation therapy.

an AI after 2 to 3 years of tamoxifen for a total treatment time of 5 years. Figure 5.2 includes a suggested treatment algorithm for ER+, early-stage breast cancer. Alternatively, she could take either take tamoxifen for 10 years, or take tamoxifen for 5 years and then an AI for an additional 5 years, for a total of 10 years of anti-estrogen therapy.

## Early-Stage ER+ Breast Cancer, Stage I or II

T.J. is a 48-year-old woman who underwent a yearly screening mammogram and was found to have an abnormal 1.3 × 1.0 cm mass in the right breast. No palpable axillary masses were found on examination, and ultrasound-guided core needle biopsy showed IDC, ER weakly positive, PR–, and HER2– (1+ by IHC). She had lumpectomy and sentinel lymph node biopsy, and the pathological review of the surgical specimen showed IDC, 1.1 cm in greatest diameter, intermediate ER staining in 10% of the specimen, PR–, HER2–, grade 3, Ki-67 of 46%, with 2 sentinel lymph nodes negative for malignancy. All margins were free of cancer.

### Evidence-Based Case Discussion

T.J. has right breast IDC, pathological stage I (T1 N0). Although the staging is identical to the previous case, it is important to note that T.J. is younger and that the pathological characteristics suggest a more aggressive tumor biology. Several features in this case speak toward a greater benefit from adjuvant chemotherapy than hormonal therapy: the patient's young age, the weak hormone receptor status, the high pathological grade, and high proliferation

rate. Oncotype DX testing may be performed to confirm her high risk, but it is reasonable to recommend adjuvant chemotherapy solely based on the characteristics described earlier. Because patients with high-risk disease generally benefit from adjuvant chemotherapy regardless of their lymph node status, the following discussion will apply to both lymph node-negative and -positive patients.

Adjuvant chemotherapy may prolong survival and decrease the risk of relapse in early breast cancer. A large meta-analysis by the Early Breast Cancer Trialists' Collaborative Group (EBCTCG) pooled the results of 194 randomized trials for adjuvant chemotherapy and hormonal therapy initiated before or in 1995 (18). Overall, adjuvant chemotherapy reduced recurrences and improved mortality after 15 years of follow-up, particularly in patients younger than 50 years compared with those 50–69 years old (12.3% vs. 4.5% recurrence rate, and 10% vs. 3% death rate, respectively). The use of an anthracycline-containing, polychemotherapy regimen showed significantly superior efficacy (0.89 recurrence rate ratio and 0.84 breast cancer death rate ratio) over non-anthracycline regimens (e.g., cyclophosphamide, methotrexate, and fluorouracil [CMF]). The benefit of chemotherapy was greater in ER– disease compared with that in ER+ disease, with RR reductions in those 50–69 years old of 33% versus 14%, respectively. These cumulative results provided the rationale for anthracycline-containing regimens to be a standard of care for adjuvant treatment of breast cancer.

The use of taxanes in adjuvant chemotherapy has been explored in many trials (Table 5.4). Adding paclitaxel sequentially after an anthracycline-containing chemotherapy

**Table 5.4** Prospective Randomized Controlled Trials for Adjuvant Chemotherapy for HER2– Breast Cancer

| Reference | Trial Name | N | Comparative Arms | DFS (%)[a] | OS (%)[a] |
|---|---|---|---|---|---|
| Mamounas et al., *JCO* 2005 | NSABP B-28 | 3060 | AC vs. AC—paclitaxel | 72 | NS |
| | | | | 76 | |
| Henderson et al., *JCO* 2003 | CALGB 9344 (Intergroup 148) | 3121 | AC vs. AC—paclitaxel | 65 | 77 |
| | | | | 70 | 80 |
| Sparano et al., *NEJM* 2008 | ECOG 1199 | 4950 | AC—paclitaxel every wk vs. docetaxel every 3 wk vs. paclitaxel every 3 wk | 81.5 | 89.7 |
| | | | | 81.2 | 86.2 |
| | | | | 76.9 | 86.5 |
| Citron et al., *JCO* 2003 (24) | CALGB 9741 | 2005 | Dose-dense schedule vs. conventional schedule | 82 | 92 |
| | | | | 75 | 90 |
| Martin et al., *NEJM* 2005 | BCIRG 001 | 1491 | TAC vs. FAC | 62 | 76 |
| | | | | 55 | 69 |
| Martin et al., *NEJM* 2010 | GEICAM 9805 | 1060 | TAC vs. FAC | 87.8 | NS |
| | | | | 81.8 | |
| Jones et al., *JCO* 2009 (42) | US oncology 9735 | 1016 | TC vs. AC | 81 | 87 |
| | | | | 75 | 82 |
| Joensuu et al., *Lancet* 2009 | FinXX | 1500 | DX-CEX vs. D-FEC | NS | NS |

AC, adriamycin and cyclophosphamide; BCIRG, Breast Cancer Research International Group; CALGB, Cancer and Leukemia Group B; DFS, disease-free survival; DX-CEX, docetaxel and capecitabine, followed by cyclophosphamide, epirubicin, and capecitabine; FAC, fluorouracil, adriamycin, cyclophosphamide; D-FEC, docetaxel followed by fluorouracil, epirubicin, and cyclophosphamide; GEICAM, Grupo Espanol de Investigacion en Cancer de mama; HER2, human epidermal growth factor-2; OS, overall survival; NS, not significant; TAC, docetaxel, doxorubicin, cyclophosphamide.
[a]Unless indicated by NS, the DFS and OS differences in the comparison groups were statistically significant.

combination was shown to improve DFS (NSABP B-28 and CALGB 9344), with 1 trial (CALGB 9344) demonstrating improved OS as well. The E1199 trial evaluated two different taxanes, paclitaxel and docetaxel, each in two different schedules. After treatment with 4 cycles of standard doxorubicin (adriamycin) and cyclophosphamide (AC) chemotherapy, patients were randomized in a 2-by-2 factorial design to receive either paclitaxel or docetaxel administered on either a weekly or every 3-week regimen for 3 months. Approximately 10% of the study group had no nodes involved, and two-thirds had <4 lymph nodes involved. A small but significant benefit in 5-year OS was shown when paclitaxel was administered weekly as compared to every 3 weeks (89.7% vs. 86.5%; $P = .01$). Five-year DFS was also greatest in the same arm (81.5% vs. 76.9%; $P = .006$). Docetaxel given every 3 weeks was equivalent to weekly paclitaxel. Peripheral neuropathy was more frequently associated with weekly paclitaxel, although myelosuppression was more severe in the every-3-week-docetaxel arm.

The BCIRG 001 and the GEICAM 9805 trials demonstrated the feasibility and efficacy of combining a taxane with an anthracycline in the adjuvant therapy of node-positive and node-negative breast cancers, respectively (Table 5.4). In BCIRG 001, 6 cycles of TAC (docetaxel, doxorubicin, and cyclophosphamide) showed superior efficacy over fluorouracil, adriamycin, cyclophosphamide (FAC) in node-positive patients at 10 years, with an improved DFS (62% vs. 55%; $P = .004$). TAC was associated with a significantly higher incidence of grade 3 and 4 neutropenia as compared to FAC, because primary prophylaxis with granulocyte colony–stimulating factor (G-CSF) was not allowed. Patients in the TAC arm also demonstrated an improved OS at 10 years (76% vs. 69%; $P = .002$). Similar findings were observed in the GEICAM 9805 trial at first interim analysis, which randomized node-negative patients to TAC versus FAC (87.8% vs. 81.8%; hazard ratio [HR] = 0.68, 95% confidence interval [CI] [0.49–0.93], $P = .01$) but this did not translate into a benefit in OS (HR = 0.76, 95% CI [0.45–1.26]).

The role of anthracycline-based chemotherapy as a stand-alone regimen was challenged in the U.S. Oncology Research Trial 9735 (Table 5.4). After 7 years' follow-up, this study, which included node-positive and node-negative patients, confirmed that 4 cycles of docetaxel and cyclophosphamide (TC) were superior to 4 cycles of doxorubicin (adriamycin) and cyclophosphamide (AC) not only in DFS (81% vs. 75%; $P = .033$) but also in OS (87% vs. 82%; $P = .032$). Approximately half of the cases were node negative, and most cases had <4 nodes involved. Superior DFS and OS were seen in both older and younger patients. Although febrile neutropenia occurred twice as frequently in the TC group, 3 deaths in the AC group were attributed to cardiomyopathy, congestive heart failure, myelodysplasia, and myelofibrosis. This trial provided a rationale for

TC as an attractive non-anthracycline-containing alternative regimen as a standard of care.

However, the TC regimen has not yet been compared to sequential AC followed by taxane. NSABP B-49, a randomized phase III trial in HER2−, locally advanced breast cancer (LABC), will compare docetaxel and cyclophosphamide (TC) to doxorubicin, cyclophosphamide, and taxane (TAC or AC followed by T) in terms of invasive DFS. The study recently completed accrual, and results are awaited.

Agents other than taxanes and anthracyclines have been tested in the adjuvant setting. Recently, capecitabine in combination with docetaxel, epirubicin, and cyclophosphamide was evaluated in the FinXX trial, which demonstrated no benefit to the addition of capecitabine. In NSABP B-38, the following adjuvant regimens were compared: (a) concurrent docetaxel, doxorubicin, and cyclophosphamide for 6 cycles; (b) dose-dense doxorubicin and cyclophosphamide (AC) followed by dose-dense paclitaxel; and (c) dose-dense AC followed by dose-dense paclitaxel and gemcitabine. There was no significant difference in 5-year DFS and OS among the 3 groups, leading the investigators to conclude that there is no role for adding gemcitabine to adjuvant chemotherapy.

For T.J., with her higher-risk, node-negative, stage I IDC, the rationale of adjuvant therapy should be explained, and treatment recommendations should begin with adjuvant combination chemotherapy, with a regimen containing taxane and anthracycline. After completing subsequent radiotherapy, further treatment with hormonal therapy should be recommended. Figure 5.2 features a treatment algorithm for patients with high-risk node-negative cancer (which is also applicable to patients with node-positive disease).

## Early-Stage TNBC

P.L. is a 39-year-old African American woman who presented to her physician with a 4-cm left breast mass. Her mother and older sister had premenopausal breast cancer, and she is worried about having it as well. Mammogram and ultrasound showed a 3.8 × 2.6 × 3.6 cm left breast mass, and core biopsy revealed an ER−, PR−, and HER2− IDC. A diagnostic MRI showed the mass to be 3.5 × 3.2 × 3.0 cm with no other lesions in either breast.

### Evidence-Based Case Discussion

P.L. has clinically stage IIA (cT2 N0 M0) TNBC. TNBC is a molecularly heterogeneous category of aggressive breast cancer, comprising approximately 10–15% of breast cancers. Unlike other types of breast cancer, it lacks the advantage of having hormone receptor targets for treatment, and the backbone of medical treatment for this group is cytotoxic chemotherapy.

The clinicopathological features and behavior of TNBC are distinct from other breast cancers. Epidemiological associations include younger age, Hispanic or African American background, obesity, and lower socioeconomic level. Tumors tend to be larger at presentation and are known to sometimes arise in between yearly screening mammograms (interim cancers). Unlike other breast cancer types, tumor size and node status do not always reliably predict the prognosis of TNBC. Histopathological characteristics and receptor status dominate the prognostic picture.

Trials with neoadjuvant single-agent and combination chemotherapy regimens for TNBC have shown pathological complete response (pCR) rates ranging from 20 to 66%. However, despite the responsiveness of TNBC to initial chemotherapy, recurrence and survival rates are worse— an observation coined the "triple-negative paradox." This was best demonstrated in a study by Liedtke et al. that examined 1118 patients, including 255 who had TNBC. The TNBC group demonstrated a trend toward a higher incidence of pCR after neoadjuvant chemotherapy (22% vs. 11%; $P = .34$) compared to the non-TNBC group, but the 3-year DFS (63% vs. 76%) and OS (74% vs. 89%, HR = 2.53, 95% CI [1.77–3.57]; $P < .0001$) were significantly worse (22). However, patients with TNBC who achieved pCR with neoadjuvant chemotherapy had similar OS as non-TNBC cohorts (94% vs. 95%; $P = .24$). Research is ongoing toward finding more efficient treatment for chemotherapy-resistant TNBC.

Although poly ADP ribose polymerase (PARP) inhibitors initially showed promise in TNBC, further studies have since cast doubt on their effectiveness. In contrast to the results of an earlier phase II study, a randomized phase III trial in which patients were randomized to receive chemotherapy (carboplatin plus gemcitabine) with or without the addition of the PARP inhibitor, BSI-201 (Iniparib) failed to demonstrate an improvement in DFS and OS (23). However, a planned subgroup analysis showed that there was a significant benefit in patients receiving the PARP inhibitor regimen as second- or third-line therapy. These disappointing results could be due to initial misclassification of Iniparib as a PARP inhibitor; additional research is ongoing with more effective PARP inhibition agents.

P.L. would likely benefit from neoadjuvant therapy followed by surgery. In patients with palpable masses, neoadjuvant therapy may provide good locoregional response, and thus improve surgical outcomes. Dose-dense chemotherapy may be considered for this young, healthy patient with TNBC. CALGB 9471, a randomized trial conducted in node-positive breast cancer, compared to (a) sequential adjuvant doxorubicin, paclitaxel, and cyclophosphamide; (b) sequential dose-dense doxorubicin, paclitaxel, and cyclophosphamide; (c) concurrent doxorubicin and cyclophosphamide (AC) followed by paclitaxel (T); and (d) dose-dense AC followed by paclitaxel. Filgrastim was used in the dose-dense regimens, which led to decreased neutropenic complications. Dose-dense treatment improved DFS (RR = 0.74; $P = .010$), and

OS (RR = 0.69; $P = .013$) (24). The benefit of dose-dense therapy was most marked in ER$^-$ patients. The addition of carboplatin, but not bevacizumab, to neoadjuvant regimens for TNBC is gaining popularity based on recent phase II trials, which have demonstrated improvements in the rate of pCR.

Figure 5.2 includes a treatment algorithm for patients like P.L. who have triple negative, early-stage breast cancer.

Given her strong family history of breast cancer and her diagnosis at a young age, genetic evaluation of *BRCA1* and *BRCA2* mutations is warranted. If P.L. is found to be a carrier of a mutation, genetic testing should be offered to her first-degree relatives. Several risk reduction strategies exist, but the most effective is prophylactic surgery with bilateral mastectomy and bilateral oophorectomy. Mutation carriers (affected and unaffected) should be counseled extensively on these surgeries and their timing by a multidisciplinary team, and issues such as fertility, reconstructive surgeries, and psychological impact need to be taken into consideration as well.

## Locally Advanced HER2+ Breast Cancer

S.R. is a 58-year-old postmenopausal woman who presents with a 5 × 7 cm right breast mass along with matted right axillary lymphadenopathy (3.5 × 4 cm), both of which have been increasing in size since the patient first noticed these 9 months ago. She has no palpable cervical, supraclavicular, or contralateral axillary lymph nodes. One-third of the breast is erythematous, and the surrounding tissue is indurated. A mammogram showed a 5.1 × 4.3 cm right breast mass without other suspicious lesions in either breast, and ultrasound revealed right axillary lymphadenopathy. A core needle biopsy of the breast mass and the lymph node revealed grade 3 IDC, with Ki-67 of 74%. Tumor markers were ER+, PR+, and HER2+. The patient was concerned that the tumor was going to extrude through the skin in the near future and was anxious about starting therapy as soon as possible to remove the tumor.

### Evidence-Based Case Discussion

S.R. has presented with stage III, ER+, PR+, and HER2+ LABC. Regarding the interpretation of her pathology results, it is important to be familiar with the recently updated 2013 ASCO-CAP recommendations for HER2 measurement. Immunohistochemical HER2 staining of 3+ (circumferential membrane staining that is complete, intense, and within >10% of tumor cells) is considered positive. IHC 2+ staining is equivocal and requires retesting the same specimen using in-situ hybridization (ISH), or testing a new specimen using IHC or ISH. HER2 gene amplification test using dual-probe ISH, HER2/CEP17 ratio of ≥2.0 is considered positive, and single-probe ISH with an average HER2 copy number of ≥6.0 signals/cell is also considered positive. When average HER2 copy number is ≥4.0 and <6.0 signals/cell, it is considered equivocal, and the test should be repeated with the same specimen using dual-probe ISH or IHC.

In terms of her clinical evaluation, further basic staging studies are indicated to rule out metastatic disease at presentation. A complete physical examination looking for signs of metastatic disease is always indicated but particularly important in this case, given her clinical stage III disease. Laboratory studies including blood counts and chemistries should be ordered. A bone scan and CT of the chest and abdomen to assess for systemic metastases in the lungs and liver should be performed as well.

In the case of S.R., these studies showed no evidence of metastatic disease. Although HER2+ disease has a tendency to metastasize to the brain, routine imaging with MRI or CT scan is not indicated unless the patient presents with symptoms of central nervous system (CNS) metastases.

Certain features of S.R.'s physical examination could raise concern for inflammatory breast cancer (IBC). IBC is a clinically aggressive subtype of breast cancer found in 2% of breast cancer patients marked by rapid onset, diffuse erythema and edema over one-third of the breast, peau d'orange, tenderness, warmth, enlargement of the breast, and diffuseness or even absence of identifiable tumor on palpation. On microscopic examination of a skin biopsy, tumor infiltration of the dermal lymphatics may also be observed, but IBC is ultimately a clinical diagnosis. The aggressive clinical features of IBC correlate to a poor prognosis with a 5-year survival of only 20–50%. In the case of S.R., she does not meet criteria for diagnosis of IBC because her symptoms have developed over 9 months, and IBC must have a history of <6 months at the time of diagnosis.

Although the patient's first inclination may be to proceed directly to surgery, she may be better served by starting with neoadjuvant therapy. Several neoadjuvant combination regimens have been shown to produce significant tumor shrinkage (>50% by World Health Organization [WHO] criteria) in >70% of patients; however, complete clinical response and pCR are less frequent. Tumor progression is very uncommon (1–2%) so that operable patients rarely become inoperable. In up to 63% of patients who have undergone neoadjuvant chemotherapy, it may be possible to consider breast conservation therapy, depending on the tumor-to-breast ratio. In an EORTC 10902 study, neoadjuvant therapy with a combination of 5-FU, epirubicin, and cyclophosphamide (FEC) reduced the size of locally advanced breast tumors such that 23% of patients were downstaged at surgery and 16% of previously unresectable tumors became resectable (25). Similar results were observed in the NSABP B-18 trial in which neoadjuvant chemotherapy with anthracyclines increased the possibility of breast-conserving therapy, although there was no significant increase in OS. Patients who achieved a pCR had significantly better DFS and OS than those who did not.

The results of NSABP B-27 showed that adding docetaxel to neoadjuvant doxorubicin and cyclophosphamide (AC) in women with surgically resectable tumors doubled the pCR rate from 13 to 26% (P > .00001) (26). In both NSABP trials, patients who achieved a pCR had significantly better DFS and OS than those who did not.

In HER2+ tumors, the results may be even more dramatic with pCR rates up to 40% as observed in the GeparQuattro trial. When the pCR rates of IBCs and LABCs treated with neoadjuvant chemotherapy were compared with that of (smaller) operable breast cancers, there was no difference between the groups, suggesting that tumor size does not predict the probability of pCR. Very large tumors should not be excluded from neoadjuvant therapy because it is the chemosensitivity of the tumor rather than the size that determines the response to therapy.

Neoadjuvant treatment can include cytotoxic chemotherapy, hormonal therapy, and targeted biological agents. Although potentially as effective, hormonal therapy is not as commonly used as neoadjuvant chemotherapy. Hormonally sensitive tumors are usually lower grade and slower growing; therefore, their rate of shrinkage in response to treatment is usually slower. Carefully selected patients may receive neoadjuvant hormonal therapy if their tumor type is likely to respond (high ER content, low-grade, postmenopausal age) or if their comorbidities prohibit the use of more toxic chemotherapy.

The rationale for administering HER2 targeted therapy is based on its dramatic survival benefit over that of chemotherapy alone. The NSABP B-31 trial compared adjuvant doxorubicin and cyclophosphamide followed by paclitaxel with the same regimen plus 52 weeks of trastuzumab. At 3 years, the trastuzumab group had an absolute difference in DFS of 12% over the control group, and trastuzumab therapy was associated with a 33% reduction in the risk of death (P = .015) (27). Another trial, the BCIRG 006, used a non-anthracyline-containing regimen (docetaxel, carboplatin, and trastuzumab) and compared it to AC followed by docetaxel with or without trastuzumab. This trial also showed that the trastuzumab-containing arms had a superior outcome (28). These findings changed the standard of care to include 12 months of treatment with trastuzumab as part of the adjuvant therapy of patients with HER2+ breast cancer.

One concern with this strategy was a 3% increase in heart failure symptoms in patients on anthracycline-containing regimens who then received trastuzumab. However, subsequent safety analysis both on and off trial have found no significant increase in clinically significant heart failure. Cardiac monitoring at baseline and periodically during therapy is advised as a means of identifying early cardiac toxicity prior to clinical manifestations.

Mounting clinical and preclinical evidence suggests that combination targeted anti-HER2 therapy may be a superior therapeutic strategy to single-agent targeted therapy. Several neoadjuvant clinical trials were designed to assess the relative efficacy of anti-HER2 agents (including trastuzumab, pertuzumab, and lapatinib) used singly or in combination with each other. In the GeparQuinto study, patients received neoadjuvant chemotherapy with epirubucin and cyclophosphamide followed by docetaxel combined with trastuzumab or lapatinib. The primary end point, pCR, was significantly higher in the trastuzumab arm as compared to the lapatinib arm (31.3% vs. 21.7 %; $P < .05$) (29). Similarly, the neoadjuvant lapatinib and/or trastuzumab treatment optimisation trial was a phase III neoadjuvant study of lapatinib, trastuzumab, or their combination along with paclitaxel. The pCR rate in the combination lapatinib, trastuzumab, and paclitaxel arm was significantly higher than that in the trastuzumab and paclitaxel arm (51.3% vs. 29.5%; $P = .001$) (30). However, lapatinib is currently only approved in the metastatic setting.

In the Neosphere trial, patients were treated with neoadjuvant pertuzumab, trastuzumab, or their combination, with or without docetaxel. The combination targeted therapy arm of trastuzumab, pertuzumab, and docetaxel had a 45% pCR rate, which was significantly higher than that seen in the docetaxel and trastuzumab arm (29%; $P = .014$), which was in turn significantly higher than that observed in the trastuzumab and pertuzumab arm (16.8%; $P = .019$) (31). The combination of trastuzumab and pertuzumab did not cause an increased risk of serious adverse events. Based on the results of this trial, pertuzumab, in combination with docetaxel and trastuzumab, is now FDA approved for neoadjuvant HER2+ breast cancer treatment. However, we still lack long-term overall and DFS data from Neosphere. In contrast to the efficacy of combined anti-HER2 therapy in the neoadjuvant setting, the recently reported results of the ALLTO trial failed to show a benefit for combined targeted therapy when combined with chemotherapy in the adjuvant treatment of HER2+ breast cancer (32).

S.R. underwent neoadjuvant therapy with docetaxel, trastuzumab, and pertuzumab for 4 cycles followed by 4 cycles of doxorubicin and cyclophosphamide, with a complete clinical response. She elected to have a modified radical mastectomy, and the pathology assessment revealed a pCR with no residual carcinoma in the breast or lymph nodes.

S.R. was advised to undergo adjuvant radiation to the breast and axilla, which could be administered concurrently with trastuzumab. Post-mastectomy radiation therapy is indicated in women with tumors >5 cm (T3), involvement of skin or chest wall (T4), and involvement of >4 lymph nodes (N2–N3). She will continue trastuzumab beyond radiation, for a total treatment duration of 12 months. Because her tumor was ER+ and PR+, subsequent hormonal therapy with upfront AIs or sequential therapy with tamoxifen followed by an AI are appropriate strategies for this postmenopausal woman.

Surveillance during the 5 years of hormonal therapy includes yearly mammography. There is no evidence supporting surveillance with whole-body imaging at this time. Figure 5.3 represents a treatment algorithm for LABC.

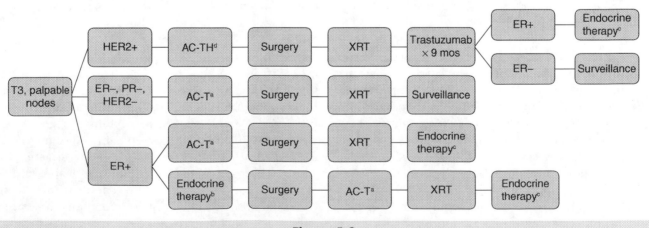

## Figure 5.3

Treatment algorithm for locally advanced breast cancer. [a]Neoadjuvant chemotherapy for breast cancer involves a combination of A (doxorubicin), C (cyclophosphamide), and T (taxane, either docetaxel or paclitaxel). The optimal sequence has not yet been determined. In clinical trials, they have been administered: sequentially AC-T, concurrently TAC, or before and after surgery AC-surgery-T, or T-surgery-AC. [b]The optimal neoadjuvant endocrine therapy regimen has not yet been defined. With low pathological complete response rates, neoadjuvant endocrine therapy is uncommon and reserved for a specific subset of patients. [c]For details of adjuvant endocrine therapy treatment by menopausal status, please see the endocrine therapy section of the early-stage breast cancer treatment algorithm. [d]In the case of HER2+ tumors, trastuzumab (H) is added in combination with a taxane most commonly after AC. ER, estrogen receptor; HER2, human epidermal growth factor-2; PR, progesterone receptor; XRT, radiation therapy.

## Metastatic Breast Cancer

G.T. is a 62-year-old woman with a prior history of a T2 N0 M0 IDC of the left breast (ER+, PR+, and HER2–) that was diagnosed 7 years ago and treated with partial mastectomy and radiation followed by adjuvant hormonal therapy with a nonsteroidal AI for 5 years. She came to her oncologist complaining of shortness of breath for 3 months. She had previously been physically active until she experienced left leg pain for 3 weeks, and a swollen painful right underarm, both interfering with her ability to work. Physical examination revealed no breast masses bilaterally. However, right axillary lymphadenopathy and point tenderness at the lumbar spine (L5) were detected.

CT scans confirmed the axillary mass and also demonstrated the presence of 3 subcentimeter nodules in the upper lobe of the right lung, but showed no evidence of metastasis in the liver. A bone scan revealed technetium uptake in the lumbar vertebrae, ribs, and pelvis. An MRI showed a compression fracture of the involved vertebrae, with >50% loss of height, and also T2 flair signal along the spinal cord.

## Evidence-Based Case Discussion

G.T. has now developed a metastatic (Stage IV) recurrence of her breast cancer to bone, lymph nodes, and possibly lungs. MBC is an incurable group of cancers, with widely ranging survival times. With the advent of effective screening for early-stage breast cancer, most cases of MBC are recurrences of earlier breast cancers treated with curative intent. Of the women with invasive breast cancer, 20–30% will develop metastases, most frequently in the first 5–10 years after diagnosis. Once metastases arise, the median OS is approximately 2 years but this varies by tumor subtype.

The goals of treatment are to prolong life, optimize quality of life, control symptoms, and control the disease burden. Treatment modalities include chemotherapy, hormonal therapy, radiation, and palliative surgery. Breast cancer recurrence may occur locally or distantly. Involvement of almost every known organ by metastatic lesions has been described in the literature. Disease progression represents a growing population of resistant cells from the original tumor, and the pattern of progression is influenced by the histology of the cancer. For example, IDC recurs more commonly in lungs ($P < .05$), pleura ($P < .05$), and brain ($P < .05$), when compared with ILC, which more commonly spreads to the bone marrow ($P < .01$) and peritoneum ($P < .01$). Bone involvement as the initial presentation of distant metastases occurred in significantly more women with ILC than with IDC (50% vs. 34%, $P < .01$) (33,34).

Histology also influences prognosis. In a 2009 study, patients with IDC had poorer 5-year (80%) and 10-year (61%) survival compared with patients with ILC (87% and 68%) and mixed (84% and 69%) cancers ($P = .029$) (35).

### Hormonal Therapy for MBC

Hormonal therapy is the preferred initial treatment for metastatic, hormone-responsive breast cancer without visceral metastases and associated organ dysfunction. Advantages of hormonal therapy include a milder side-effect profile, ease of administration, and a proven survival benefit. Ovarian suppression or ablation, antiestrogens, ER modulators, and AIs are among the hormonal treatment strategies used.

Twenty to thirty-five percent of patients may have a clinical response to initial hormonal therapy, with an additional 30–35% experiencing stable disease. Clinical response may take 2–3 months to achieve maximum benefit, and the mean response duration may extend to 2 years or longer. If there is a response to first-line treatment, the likelihood of response to second-line treatment is 50%. If both ER and PR are positive, the response rate may be up to 70–80%, but may be slightly less if only 1 receptor is positive. Other positive predictive factors include postmenopausal status, longer DFS, no liver involvement, slower tumor growth, and older age. The menopausal status influences the initial choice of hormonal treatment. Tamoxifen, a SERM, has been the standard endocrine therapy for premenopausal women since it was approved by the FDA in 1977. It offers approximately 50% clinical benefit (combined objective response and stable disease) for an average duration of 12 months. A tumor flare is possible with initiation of tamoxifen and predicts an excellent response. The flare symptoms, if they occur, generally resolve spontaneously after a few weeks but may be attenuated by steroids.

When compared to oophorectomy in a phase III trial, there was an insignificant trend favoring tamoxifen. However, tamoxifen failure does not preclude response to oophorectomy. Chemical ablation with GnRH analogs has also been compared to oophorectomy in premenopausal women. Compared to oophorectomy, monthly, low-dose goserelin showed similar failure-free survival and OS in patients with hormone receptor–positive, metastatic disease. Tamoxifen added to hormonal ablation demonstrated superiority over ablation alone. In a meta-analysis of 4 trials, this combination suggested better response rates, median response duration, progression-free survival (PFS), and OS. After progression, AIs (with ovarian ablation), progestins, and high-dose estrogen can still be utilized.

Unlike premenopausal women, the principal source of estrogen in postmenopausal women is from peripheral tissue conversion of adrenal hormones by the aromatase enzyme, rather than from ovarian production. Third- and fourth-generation AIs are commonly used in the adjuvant and metastatic settings for postmenopausal women. AI has proven superior to tamoxifen in a multicenter, phase III study of 900 metastatic postmenopausal women, in which letrozole demonstrated superior median time to progression (9.4 vs. 6 months; $P < .0001$) and overall objective response (32% vs. 21%; $P = .0002$) as compared to tamoxifen (35). Headaches, arthralgia, bone loss, vaginal dryness, fatigue, and hot flashes are common side effects of AIs. After progression with AI, fulvestrant and exemestane have shown clinical benefit. AIs should not be used as single-agent therapy in premenopausal women.

The mTOR inhibitor, everolimus, was recently approved by the FDA for use in metastatic ER$^+$ breast cancer. The phase II trial, Tamrad, randomized postmenopausal ER+ breast cancer patients to receive everolimus and tamoxifen, or tamoxifen alone. At 6 months, clinical benefit rate (complete response (CR) + partial response (PR) + stable disease (SD)) and time to progression were superior with tamoxifen plus everolimus (61%, 8.6 months), compared to tamoxifen alone (42%, 4.5 months) (36). Similarly, BOLERO-2 was a large trial studying ER$^+$ MBC patients who had recurrence or progression after nonsteroidal AIs. Patients were randomized to everolimus and exemestane or exemestane and placebo. The median PFS was significantly higher for those on the everolimus arm, at 10.6 versus 4.1 months, HR = 0.36 ($P < .001$) (37). Everolimus is now approved for metastatic ER+ breast cancer, in combination with AI therapy.

Preclinical studies have shown that resistant ER$^+$ breast cancer exhibits increased expression of CDK-4/6 and cyclin-D1, which regulate the cell cycle. Palbociclib (PD 0332991) is a selective CDK-4/6 inhibitor. A randomized phase II study conducted in ER+/HER2– MBC compared palbociclib plus letrozole with letrozole alone. It showed improved PFS of 20.2 months in the combination arm, and only 10.2 months in the letrozole-only arm (HR = 0.488, $P = .0004$) (38). Palbociclib is not yet approved by the FDA, and further trials are ongoing.

### Non-Hormonal Therapy for MBC

Data analyzed from 12 randomized controlled trials in women with MBC compared combination chemotherapy to the same drugs used sequentially, and showed no difference in OS ($P = .45$), despite higher risk of febrile neutropenia in the combination arm (RR = 1.32; $P = .01$) (39). Thus, sequential single-agent chemotherapy is generally preferred for metastatic patients, because disease stabilization, symptom palliation, and maintenance of quality of life are the main goals.

The choice of agents in the treatment of MBC is based on extensive clinical trial experience. Anthracyclines, such as doxorubicin and epirubicin, are among the most active agents. When used in first-line combination regimens, response rates range from 50 to 80% with associated response duration of 8–15 months. Myelosuppression can be a dose-limiting factor, though dose reductions can improve tolerability. Dose-related cardiotoxicity is well described and can result in permanent cardiac dysfunction, which has been associated with poor prognosis. The incidence of clinically apparent congestive heart failure with cumulative doses of 400 mg/m$^2$ is 3%, and it increases to 7% at 550 mg/m$^2$. For metastatic patients who respond well to anthracyclines, pegylated liposomal doxorubicin is also a viable option, and it may be less cardiotoxic over a long period of time, although it has increased hematological toxicities.

Taxanes are also active in MBC, initially finding their role in anthracycline-resistant cancers, with response rates of 20–30%. As first-line treatment, paclitaxel response rates are 32–62% with response durations of approximately 6 months in phase III trials. In patients with MBC, a randomized study compared paclitaxel alone with CMF plus Prednisone as first-line therapy. Median survival was significantly improved with paclitaxel (17.3 vs. 13.9 months; $P = .025$) without compromising quality of life (40). Docetaxel is another active taxane. When compared to doxorubicin salvage therapy in a phase III randomized multicenter trial of women whose MBC progressed after previous alkylating therapy, docetaxel demonstrated a significantly higher overall response rate (47.8% vs. 33.3%; $P = .008$) and median time to treatment failure (22 vs. 18 weeks; $P = .01$) (41). Early data from the TAX 311 trial also showed a significantly improved median OS of 15.4 versus 12.7 months ($P = .03$) favoring docetaxel over paclitaxel (42). Important toxicities to consider when using taxanes include edema, hypersensitivity, and neuropathy. Early success with nab-paclitaxel, a second-generation taxane that eliminates cremaphor from its preparation, led to its FDA approval in 2005 for use in relapsed MBC.

After disease progression on anthracyclines and taxanes, several other options for palliative chemotherapy exist including capecitabine, gemcitabine, vinorelbine, or eribulin. Capecitabine is an oral prodrug of 5-FU that has activity and utility as a salvage treatment after anthracycline and taxane therapy. In a phase III trial, the addition of capecitabine to docetaxel extended survival from 11.5 to 14.5 months ($P < .01$) with improvements in both response and time to disease progression as well (43). A phase III open-label randomized study conducted in locally recurrent or MBC compared eribulin mesilate, a microtubule inhibitor, with treatment of physician's choice (TPC). In this group of heavily pretreated metastatic patients, eribulin significantly increased OS (13.1 vs. 10.6 months, HR = 0.81, $P$ = .041) (44).

For patients with HER2+ MBC, HER2-directed therapy has proven effective in either second- or first-line settings. EGF104900, a phase III study conducted in patients with in heavily pretreated HER2+ MBC, compared the efficacy of lapatinib plus trastuzumab versus lapatinib alone. The lapatinib and trastuzumab combination significantly increased absolute OS by 10% at 6 months and 15% at 12 months as compared to lapatinib alone (45). Thus, lapatinib and trastuzumab are approved for use in MBC.

In previously untreated patients with HER2+ MBC, the phase III clinical evaluation of pertuzumab and trastuzumab (CLEOPATRA) trial randomized patients to pertuzumab, trastuzumab, and docetaxel versus placebo, trastuzumab, and docetaxel. At a median follow-up of 30 months, the number of deaths in the placebo group (38%) was higher than that in the pertuzumab group (28%), and median OS was 37.6 months for the placebo group, which was not reached by the pertuzumab group (46). Based on these results, pertuzumab, trastuzumab, and docetaxel are FDA approved for first-line treatment of metastatic HER2+ breast cancer.

The efficacy of a novel HER2-directed agent trastuzumab emtasine (TDM-1, consisting of trastuzumab as a targeting agent linked to the cytotoxic agent emtasine) was tested in the trastuzumab emtansine (T-DM1) vs. capecitabine + lapatinib in patients with HER2+ locally advanced or metastatic breast cancer (EMILIA) study, which compared TDM-1 versus the combination of lapatinib and capecitabine in women with HER2+ MBC who progressed after treatment with trastuzumab and a taxane. Patients receiving TDM-1 showed an improved PFS of 9.6 months and an improved median OS of 30.9 versus 25.1 months as compared to those who received the capecitabine and lapatinib combination (47). Thus, TDM-1 is a reasonable option for the second-line (or later) treatment of patients with HER2+ MBC.

In addition to trastuzumab, which targets the HER2 pathway, anti-angiogenesis agents such as bevacizumab have also been tested in combination with conventional chemotherapy. However, results have been conflicting, resulting in retraction of prior FDA approval.

For patients with bone metastases, intravenous bisphosphonates can improve quality of life and pain control, reduce incidence of fractures, and treat hypercalcemia of malignancy. Accordingly, the ASCO consensus statement supports the administration of pamidronate, zoledronate, or denosumab every 4 weeks for metastatic bone lesions. When compared with pamidronate, zoledronate significantly improved skeletal-related events (SRE, including incidence of pathological fracture, cord compression, or need for radiation or surgical treatment) by an additional 20% ($P$ = .025) and by an additional 30% in patients receiving hormonal therapy ($P$ = .009) (48). Side effects include osteonecrosis of the jaw, renal insufficiency, and ocular inflammation. A randomized study showed denosumab (human monoclonal RANKL antibody) was superior to zoledronic acid in delaying or preventing SRE in MBC patients ($P$ = .01) and time to first and subsequent SRE ($P$ = .001) but with increased incidence of hypocalcemia (49).

The CNS is a known site of metastasis for breast cancer. The management of CNS metastases in breast cancer is similar to that in other tumors. Selected solitary metastases may be removed surgically followed by whole-brain or stereotactic radiotherapy. Alternatively, stereotactic radiotherapy alone may be an option for select patients with 3 or less brain lesions with minimal edema. Treatment of multiple metastases and leptomeningeal disease is outlined in Figure 5.4. Participation in a clinical trial should be considered because the optimal management of brain metastases is still being defined.

In summary, G.T. has hormone receptor-positive, MBC to the lymph nodes, bone, and lung, with a long disease-free interval. Surgical stabilization of her spine should be considered. Once addressed and treated, her breast cancer can be treated with a palliative intent. The burden of disease in the lungs is small and not eliciting symptoms; therefore, a reasonable initial approach may be to administer hormonal therapy with close monitoring. Exemestane, a steroidal AI, is a reasonable option given evidence of its efficacy after progression on a nonsteroidal AI.

Once refractory to hormone therapy (she may benefit from the use of sequential hormonal agents), G.T.'s chemotherapy management may include use of anthracycline, taxane, and perhaps capecitabine, as determined by her performance status, cardiac function, and comorbidities. Bisphosphonates should be included in her plan of care.

## A Special Note on Breast Cancer in Pregnancy

Patients are sometimes diagnosed with breast cancer during pregnancy. Termination of pregnancy does not improve the outcome of breast cancer. Chest x-ray, liver ultrasound, and routine lab work should be used for staging, but CT and bone scans should be avoided. Anthracyclines, 5-FU, and cyclophosphamide can be used in the second and third trimesters. However, taxanes, trastuzumab, hormonal treatment, and radiation are all highly teratogenic and should be avoided during pregnancy. Women diagnosed with breast cancer in the postpartum period have a poorer prognosis. Breast cancer survivors may have decreased fertility after chemotherapy, but future pregnancy does not impact negatively on recurrence risk and OS.

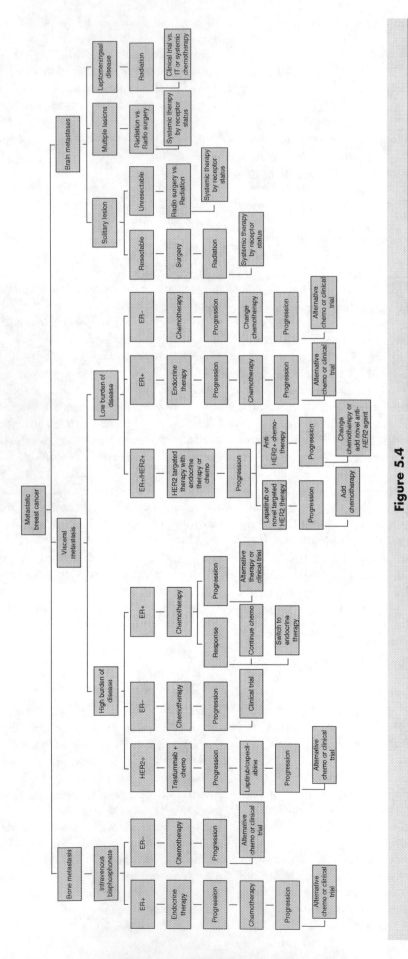

**Figure 5.4**

Treatment algorithm for metastatic breast cancer. ER, estrogen receptor; HER2, human epidermal growth factor-2; PR, progesterone receptor.

# REVIEW QUESTIONS

1. A 52-year-old woman underwent her routine yearly screening mammogram and was found to have a cluster of abnormal calcifications in her right breast. Her physical examination was unremarkable without a palpable breast mass or any enlarged lymph nodes in the right axillary or supraclavicular regions. A stereotactic breast biopsy demonstrated ductal carcinoma in situ (DCIS), which was ER+ and PR+. She undergoes a lumpectomy, which confirmed extensive DCIS with a narrow but negative margin of resection. Which of the following would you recommend to her as appropriate next step(s) in her breast cancer management?

   (A) Reexcision to gain a wider margin
   (B) Breast radiotherapy
   (C) Tamoxifen adjuvant therapy for 5 years
   (D) Chemotherapy with doxorubicin and taxol
   (E) B plus C
   (F) A plus D

2. A 75-year-old, otherwise healthy, woman is found to have a 1.9 × 1.8 cm invasive ductal carcinoma in her right breast for which she has a lumpectomy (with clear margins) and a sentinel lymph node biopsy, which is negative. On pathology, her tumor is found to be grade 2, Ki-67 20%, ER+ (80% staining; 3+ intensity); PR+ (60% staining, 2+ intensity); and HER2–. Her tumor is subjected to Oncotype Dx analysis with a score of 12. She asks your opinion about the next course of action to prevent a recurrence of her breast cancer. Which of the following would you recommend?

   (A) Completion mastectomy
   (B) Adjuvant aromatase inhibitor therapy, with or without radiotherapy
   (C) Adjuvant chemotherapy with doxorubicin and cyclophosphamide
   (D) Surveillance
   (E) Axillary lymph node dissection to confirm N0 status

3. A 45-year-old premenopausal woman discovers a small lump in her left breast and a diagnostic mammogram shows a 3-cm spiculated mass. A core biopsy demonstrates a grade 3, Ki-67 59%, ER-weakly positive, PR–, and HER2– invasive ductal carcinoma (IDC). She subsequently has a lumpectomy, which confirms a 2.9-cm IDC with the same histological and immunohistochemistry staining features. A sentinel lymph node biopsy is negative. You would recommend all of the following in the subsequent management of her breast cancer, *except*:

   (A) Breast radiotherapy
   (B) Adjuvant chemotherapy to include a taxane and an anthracycline

   (C) Adjuvant aromatase inhibitor hormonal therapy
   (D) Adjuvant tamoxifen hormonal therapy

4. A 41-year-old premenopausal woman reports to her physician a 5.0-cm right breast mass, which on core biopsy is an ER–, PR–, and HER2– invasive ductal carcinoma. She wishes to preserve her breast and seeks your recommendations on next steps. Which of the following would you advise as a first step?

   (A) Immediate lumpectomy and sentinel lymph node biopsy
   (B) Initial breast radiotherapy to reduce the size of the tumor prior to surgery
   (C) Neoadjuvant "dose dense" chemotherapy consisting of doxorubicin, cyclophosphamide, and paclitaxel
   (D) A trial of neoadjuvant tamoxifen

5. A 64-year-old, otherwise healthy, woman presents with a 5.5-cm right breast mass and right axillary lymphadenopathy. A biopsy of the mass and axillary lymph node shows grade 1 invasive ductal carcinoma, which is strongly ER+, PR+, and HER2– with a Ki-67 of 4%. Staging scans show no evidence of metastatic disease elsewhere. She hopes to avoid mastectomy. Which initial therapy would you recommend?

   (A) Neoadjuvant anastrozole for 4–6 months
   (B) Neoadjuvant capecitabine for 4 cycles
   (C) Neoadjuvant doxorubicin and cyclophosphamide, followed by bilateral mastectomies with sentinel lymph node biopsy on the left
   (D) Radiation to the breast and axilla

6. The patient in Question 5 undergoes initial neoadjuvant therapy and the breast mass shrinks to 1 cm and the axillary lymph nodes are no longer palpable. She subsequently has a right lumpectomy and an axillary lymph node dissection demonstrating a 1.2-cm invasive ductal carcinoma (with a Ki-67 of 18%) and 4 of 12 axillary lymph nodes positive for tumor. Which of the following would be an appropriate course of therapy at this point?

   (A) Send an Oncotype Dx on the surgical specimen, and give chemotherapy if this indicates a high risk, or give hormonal therapy if low risk
   (B) Administer doxorubicin and cyclophosphamide for 4 cycles, followed by weekly paclitaxel for 12 weeks, followed by breast radiotherapy, followed by 5 years of anastrozole
   (C) Start the same adjuvant chemotherapy as in (B) followed by anastrozole hormonal therapy
   (D) Administer adjuvant anastozole for 5 years

7. A 69-year-old woman has prior history of a T2N0M0 invasive ductal carcinoma, which was ER+, PR+, and HER2–. She had been treated with a lumpectomy,

breast radiotherapy, and 5 years of adjuvant aromatase inhibitor therapy. Now, 7 years from the time of her initial cancer diagnosis, she presents with new and gradually worsening back pain of 6 weeks' duration. A restaging CT scan of the chest, abdomen, and pelvis shows no evidence of visceral metastatic disease, but a bone scan is positive in multiple vertebrae, ribs, and pelvis. A follow-up MRI scan of these affected areas is consistent with metastatic disease. Low-dose narcotic pain medications achieve good pain control. With the goal of prolonging survival and achieving the highest quality of life, which of the following would you recommend as initial therapy for her stage IV disease?

(A) Systemic hormonal therapy with letrozole
(B) Systemic chemotherapy with an anthracycline and a taxane combination
(C) Systemic chemotherapy with a single agent capecitabine
(D) Radiotherapy to the dominant sites of boney metastases

8. A 40-year-old woman presents with a 4-cm right breast mass, right axillary lymphadenopathy, a persistent cough with left chest wall pain along with mild dyspnea on exertion, and right upper quadrant pain. A core needle biopsy of the breast mass demonstrates invasive ductal carcinoma, which is ER– and PR–, but HER2+; Ki-67 70%. A CT scan of the chest, abdomen, and pelvis demonstrates several bilateral lung nodules (the largest being 2.3 cm), a moderate-sized right pleural effusion, and multiple enhancing liver lesions consistent with metastases. Cytology of the pleural fluid demonstrates malignant cells with the same immunohistochemistry staining pattern as the breast mass. Her performance status is 0–1. Which of the following would you *not* consider in her initial disease management?

(A) Capecitabine plus trastuzumab
(B) Docetaxel, trastuzumab, and pertuzumab
(C) Cycles of cyclophosphamide, doxorubicin, and 5-fluorouracil; alternating with cycles of docetaxel
(D) Docetaxel plus trastuzumab

9. The patient in Question 8 demonstrates a durable response for 8 months to the initial therapy recommended, but then develops progressive disease in both liver and lung. What options would you advise in the setting of relapsed disease?

(A) Lapatinib plus trastuzumab
(B) Trastuzumab emtasine
(C) Capecitabine plus bevacizumab
(D) Tamoxifen
(E) A or B
(F) C or D

10. A 47-year-old premenopausal woman with a history of stage II, ER+, PR+, and HER2+ breast cancer 2 years ago is treated with neoadjuvant chemotherapy followed by mastectomy and subsequent adjuvant chemotherapy plus HER2-directed therapy. While on adjuvant tamoxifen (which she has been taking for the past year), she develops persistent headache and blurry vision. An MRI of the brain reveals a 2-cm lesion in the right frontal lobe associated with vasogenic edema. A restaging CT and bone scan show no evidence of metastatic disease elsewhere. What would you recommend now?

(A) Whole-brain radiotherapy
(B) Resection of the brain lesion followed by whole-brain radiotherapy
(C) Start capecitabine plus lapatinib chemotherapy
(D) Start an aromatase inhibitor

11. A pregnant 33-year-old African American woman at 11 weeks' gestation presents with a 6-cm fixed, left breast mass, associated with left axillary lymphadenopathy. Biopsy of the mass demonstrates a grade 3 IDC, which is ER+, PR+, and HER2+, with a Ki-67 of 75%. Which of the following is advisable regarding the subsequent staging of her disease?

(A) She should have a mammogram, breast ultrasound, CT scan, and bone scan
(B) She should have a mammogram, breast ultrasound, axillary lymph node fine needle aspiration, chest x-ray, labwork, and an abdominal ultrasound
(C) She should have a mammogram, breast ultrasound, and a PET-CT scan
(D) She should have a breast MRI with contrast, labwork, and an abdominal ultrasound

## REFERENCES

1. Pierce JP, Stefanick ML, Flatt SW, et al. Greater survival after breast cancer in physically active women with high vegetable-fruit intake regardless of obesity. *J Clin Oncol.* 2007;25(17):2345–2351.
2. Antoniou A, Pharoah PD, Narod S, et al. Average risks of breast and ovarian cancer associated with BRCA1 or BRCA2 mutations detected in case series unselected for family history: a combined analysis of 22 studies. *Am J Hum Genet.* 2003;72(5):1117–1130.
3. Hodgson DC, Gilbert ES, Dores GM, et al. Long-term solid cancer risk among 5-year survivors of Hodgkin's lymphoma. *J Clin Oncol.* 2007;25(12):1489–1497.
4. Fisher B, Anderson S, Bryant J, et al. Twenty-year follow-up of a randomized trial comparing total mastectomy, lumpectomy, and lumpectomy plus irradiation for the treatment of invasive breast cancer. *N Engl J Med.* 2002;347(16):1233–1241.
5. Veronesi U, Zucali R, Luini A. Local control and survival in early breast cancer: the Milan trial. *Int J Radiat Oncol Biol Phys.* 1986;12(5):717–720.
6. Bijker N, Meijnen P, Peterse JL, et al. Breast-conserving treatment with or without radiotherapy in ductal carcinoma-in-situ: ten-year results of European Organization for Research and Treatment of

Cancer randomized phase III trial 10853? Study by the EORTC Breast Cancer Cooperative group and EORTC Radiotherapy Group. *J Clin Oncol.* 2006;24:3381–3387.

7. Silverstein MJ. The University of Southern California/Van Nuys prognostic index for ductal carcinoma in situ of the breast. *Am J Surg.* 2003;186(4):337–343.

8. Solin LJ, Gray R, Baehner FL, et al. A multigene expression assay to predict local recurrence risk for ductal carcinoma in situ of the breast. *J Natl Cancer Inst.* 2013;105(10):701–710.

9. Fisher B, Dignam J, Wolmark N, et al. Tamoxifen in treatment of intraductal breast cancer: National Surgical Adjuvant Breast and Bowel Project B-24 randomised controlled trial. *Lancet.* 1999;353(9169):1993–2000.

10. Cuzick J, Sestak I, Forbes JF, et al.; IBIS-II investigators. Anastrozole for prevention of breast cancer in high-risk postmenopausal women (IBIS-II): an international, double-blind, randomised placebo-controlled trial. *Lancet.* 2014;383(9922):1041–1048.

11. Goss PE, Ingle JN, Alés-Martínez JE, et al.; NCIC CTG MAP.3 Study Investigators. Exemestane for breast-cancer prevention in postmenopausal women. *N Engl J Med.* 2011;364(25):2381–2391.

12. Hughes KS, Schnaper LA, Berry D, et al.; Cancer and Leukemia Group B; Radiation Therapy Oncology Group; Eastern Cooperative Oncology Group. Lumpectomy plus tamoxifen with or without irradiation in women 70 years of age or older with early breast cancer. *N Engl J Med.* 2004;351(10):971–977.

13. Giuliano AE, Hunt KK, Ballman KV, et al. Axillary dissection vs no axillary dissection in women with invasive breast cancer and sentinel node metastasis: a randomized clinical trial. *JAMA.* 2011;305(6):569–575.

14. Galimberti V, Cole BF, Zurrida S, et al.; International Breast Cancer Study Group Trial 23–01 investigators. Axillary dissection versus no axillary dissection in patients with sentinel-node micrometastases (IBCSG 23–01): a phase 3 randomised controlled trial. *Lancet Oncol.* 2013;14(4):297–305.

15. Rutgers EJ, Donker M, Straver ME, et al. Radiotherapy or surgery of the axilla after a positive sentinel node in breast cancer patients: final analysis of the EORTC AMAROS trial (10981/22023). *J Clin Oncol.* 2013;31s:abstr LBA1001.

16. Harvey JM, Clark GM, Osborne CK, Allred DC. Estrogen receptor status by immunohistochemistry is superior to the ligand-binding assay for predicting response to adjuvant endocrine therapy in breast cancer. *J Clin Oncol.* 1999;17(5):1474–1481.

17. Early Breast Cancer Trialists Collaborative Group (EBCTCG). Effects of chemotherapy and hormonal therapy for early breast cancer on recurrence and 15-year survival: an overview of the randomized trials. *Lancet.* 2005;365(9472):1687–1717.

18. Drukker CA, Bueno-de-Mesquita JM, Retèl VP, et al. A prospective evaluation of a breast cancer prognosis signature in the observational RASTER study. *Int J Cancer.* 2013;133(4):929–936.

19. Gray RG, Rea DW, Handley K, et al. aTTom: long-term effects of continuing adjuvant tamoxifen to 10 years versus stopping at 5 years in 6,953 women with early breast cancer. *J Clin Oncol.* 2013;31(suppl;abstr 5).

20. Davies C, Pan H, Godwin J, et al.; Adjuvant Tamoxifen: Longer Against Shorter (ATLAS) Collaborative Group. Long-term effects of continuing adjuvant tamoxifen to 10 years versus stopping at 5 years after diagnosis of oestrogen receptor-positive breast cancer: ATLAS, a randomised trial. *Lancet.* 2013;381(9869):805–816.

21. Burstein HJ, Prestrud AA, Seidenfeld J, et al. ASCO Clinical Practice Guidelines: updates on adjuvant endocrine therapy for women with hormone receptor positive breast cancer. *J Clin Oncol.* 2010; 28(23):3784–3796.

22. Liedtke C, Mazouni C, Hess KR, et al. Response to neoadjuvant therapy and long-term survival in patients with triple-negative breast cancer. *J Clin Oncol.* 2008;26(8):1275–1281.

23. O'Shaughnessy J, Schwartzberg LS, Danso MA, et al. A randomized phase III study of iniparib (BSI-201) in combination with

gemcitabine/carboplatin (G/C) in metastatic triple-negative breast cancer (TNBC). *J Clin Oncol.* 2011;29(suppl;abstr 1007).

24. Citron ML, Berry DA, Cirrincione C, et al. Randomized trial of dose-dense versus conventionally scheduled and sequential versus concurrent combination chemotherapy as postoperative adjuvant treatment of node-positive primary breast cancer: first report of Intergroup Trial C9741/Cancer and Leukemia Group B Trial 9741. *J Clin Oncol.* 2003;21(8):1431–1439.

25. van der Hage JA, van de Velde CJ, Julien JP, et al. Preoperative chemotherapy in primary operable breast cancer: results from the European Organization for Research and Treatment of Cancer trial 10902. *J Clin Oncol.* 2001;19(22):4224–4237.

26. Bear HD, Anderson S, Smith RE, et al. Sequential preoperative or postoperative docetaxel added to preoperative doxorubicin plus cyclophosphamide for operable breast cancer: National Surgical Adjuvant Breast and Bowel Project Protocol B-27. *J Clin Oncol.* 2006;24(13):2019–2027.

27. Romond EH, Perez EA, Bryant J, et al. Trastuzumab plus adjuvant chemotherapy for operable HER2-positive breast cancer. *N Engl J Med.* 2005;353(16):1673–1684.

28. Slamon D, Eiermann W, Robert N, et al. Phase III randomized trial comparing doxorubicin and cyclophosphamide followed by docetaxel (ACT) with doxorubicin and cyclophosphamide followed by docetaxel and trastuzumab (ACTH) with docetaxel, carboplatin and trastuzumab (TCH) in Her2neu positive early breast cancer patients: BCIRG 006 study. *Cancer Res.* 2009;69(24 suppl.):62.

29. Untch M, Loibl S, Bischoff J, et al. Lapatinib vs trastuzumab in combination with neoadjuvant anthracycline-taxane-based chemotherapy: primary efficacy endpoint analysis of the GEPARQUINTO study (GBG 44). *SABCS.* 2010; abstract S3.

30. Baselga J, Bradbury I, Eidtmann H, et al.; NeoALTTO Study Team. Lapatinib with trastuzumab for HER2-positive early breast cancer (NeoALTTO): a randomised, open-label, multicentre, phase 3 trial. *Lancet.* 2012;379(9816):633–640.

31. Gianni L, Pienkowski T, Im YH, et al. Efficacy and safety of neoadjuvant pertuzumab and trastuzumab in women with locally advanced, inflammatory, or early HER2-positive breast cancer (NeoSphere): a randomised multicentre, open-label, phase 2 trial. *Lancet Oncol.* 2012;13(1):25–32.

32. Piccart-Gebhart MJ, Holmes, AP, Baselga J, et al. First results from the phase III ALTTO trial comparing one year of anti-HER2 therapy with lapatinib alone, trastuzumab alone, their sequence, or their combination in the adjuvant treatment of HER2-positive early breast cancer [abstract]. In: ASCO Annual Meeting, May 30 to June 3, 2014, Chicago, IL. Abstract LBA4.

33. Jain S, Fisher C, Smith P, et al. Patterns of metastatic breast cancer in relation to histological type. *Eur J Cancer.* 1993;29A(15):2155–2157.

34. Bharat A, Gao F, Margenthaler JA. Tumor characteristics and patient outcomes are similar between invasive lobular and mixed invasive ductal/lobular breast cancers but differ from pure invasive ductal breast cancers. *Am J Surg.* 2009;198(4):516–519.

35. Mouridsen H, Gershanovich M, Sun Y, et al. Phase III study of letrozole versus tamoxifen as first-line therapy of advanced breast cancer in postmenopausal women: analysis of survival and update of efficacy from the International Letrozole Breast Cancer Group. *J Clin Oncol.* 2003;21(11):2101–2109.

36. Bachelot T, Bourgier C, Cropet C, et al. Randomized phase II trial of everolimus in combination with tamoxifen in patients with hormone receptor-positive, human epidermal growth factor receptor 2-negative metastatic breast cancer with prior exposure to aromatase inhibitors: a GINECO study. *J Clin Oncol.* 2012;30(22):2718–2724.

37. Baselga J, Campone M, Piccart M, et al. Everolimus in postmenopausal hormone-receptor-positive advanced breast cancer. *N Engl J Med.* 2012;366(6):520–529.

38. Finn RS, Crown JP, Lang I, et al. Final results of a randomized phase II study of PD 0332991, a cyclin-dependent kinase

(CDK)-4/6 inhibitor, in combination with letrozole vs letrozole alone for first-line treatment of ER⁺/HER2⁻ advanced breast cancer (PALOMA-1; TRIO-18) *AACR*. 2014;(abstract CT101).

39. Dear RF, McGeechan K, Jenkins MC, et al. Combination versus sequential single agent chemotherapy for metastatic breast cancer. *Cochrane Database Syst Rev*. 2013;12:CD008792.

40. Bishop JF, Dewar J, Toner GC, et al. Initial paclitaxel improves outcome compared with CMFP combination chemotherapy as front-line therapy in untreated metastatic breast cancer. *J Clin Oncol*. 1999;17(8):2355–2364.

41. Chan S, Friedrichs K, Noel D, et al.; 303 Study Group. Prospective randomized trial of docetaxel versus doxorubicin in patients with metastatic breast cancer. *J Clin Oncol*. 1999;17(8): 2341–2354.

42. Jones SE, Erban J, Overmoyer B, et al. Randomized phase III study of docetaxel compared with paclitaxel in metastatic breast cancer. *J Clin Oncol*. 2005;23(24):5542–5551.

43. O'Shaughnessy J, Miles D, Vukelja S, et al. Superior survival with capecitabine plus docetaxel combination therapy in anthracycline-pretreated patients with advanced breast cancer: phase III trial results. *J Clin Oncol*. 2002;20(12):2812–2823.

44. Cortes J, O'Shaughnessy J, Loesch D, et al.; EMBRACE (Eisai Metastatic Breast Cancer Study Assessing Physician's Choice Versus E7389) investigators. Eribulin monotherapy versus treatment of physician's choice in patients with metastatic breast cancer (EMBRACE): a phase 3 open-label randomised study. *Lancet*. 2011;377(9769):914–923.

45. Blackwell KL, Burstein HJ, Storniolo AM, et al. Overall survival benefit with lapatinib in combination with trastuzumab for patients with human epidermal growth factor receptor 2-positive metastatic breast cancer: final results from the EGF104900 Study. *J Clin Oncol*. 2012;30(21):2585–2592.

46. Swain SM, Kim SB, Cortés J, et al. Pertuzumab, trastuzumab, and docetaxel for HER2-positive metastatic breast cancer (CLEOPATRA study): overall survival results from a randomised, double-blind, placebo-controlled, phase 3 study. *Lancet Oncol*. 2013;14(6):461–471.

47. Verma S, Miles D, Gianni L, et al.; EMILIA Study Group. Trastuzumab emtansine for HER2-positive advanced breast cancer. *N Engl J Med*. 2012;367(19):1783–1791.

48. Rosen LS, Gordon D, Kaminski M, et al. Long-term efficacy and safety of zoledronic acid compared with pamidronate disodium in the treatment of skeletal complications in patients with advanced multiple myeloma or breast carcinoma: a randomized, double-blind, multicenter, comparative trial. *Cancer*. 2003;98(8):1735–1744.

49. Stopeck AT, Lipton A, Body JJ, et al. Denosumab compared with zoledronic acid for the treatment of bone metastases in patients with advanced breast cancer: a randomized, double-blind study. *J Clin Oncol*. 2010;28(35):5132–5139.

# 6

# Esophageal Cancer

RAY ESPER AND SUSAN G. URBA

## EPIDEMIOLOGY, RISK FACTORS, NATURAL HISTORY, AND PATHOLOGY

Despite advances in staging and treatment, esophageal cancer continues to be associated with a high mortality rate. Among all forms of cancer, it ranks eighth in incidence throughout the world. Based on Surveillance, Epidemiology, and End Results (SEER) data, the National Cancer Institute estimates that in 2014 there will be 18,170 new diagnoses of esophageal cancer, comprising 1.1% of all cancers. At the same time, 15,450 deaths from esophagus cancer are expected in the United States, which is about 2.6% of all cancer-related deaths. In parallel with the increased prevalence of obesity and acid reflux disease, the incidence of esophageal cancer has been increasing in the United States. There has been a marked increase in diagnoses of esophageal adenocarcinoma in young white males, a population whose incidence rate rose 463% since the late 1970s (1). In contrast, the incidence of squamous cell carcinoma of the esophagus has declined slightly, possibly due to decreased smoking rates. It is unclear if the rise in human papillomavirus (HPV) infections in young people will lead to an increased incidence of esophageal squamous cell carcinoma.

Esophageal cancers are seen far more frequently in men than in women with a median age at diagnosis of 67 years. There are predominantly 2 types of esophageal cancer: adenocarcinoma and squamous cell carcinoma. Adenocarcinoma is now the most common histological subtype of esophageal cancer in the United States and the Western world, accounting for approximately 75–80% of patients. Conversely, squamous cell carcinoma of the esophagus has decreased in incidence, but still remains the most common histological subtype seen in African Americans.

Strong risk factors for squamous cell cancer are alcohol and tobacco. Other relatively rare predisposing conditions are long-standing achalasia, tylosis, esophageal webs, and HPV. For adenocarcinoma of the esophagus, gastroesophageal (GE) reflux and intestinal metaplasia of the lower esophagus (Barrett's esophagus) are well-recognized risk factors, with approximately 1% of patients with Barrett's esophagus progressing to adenocarcinoma annually. Obesity is clearly an independent risk factor for esophageal adenocarcinoma, with a relative risk of 2.0 associated with being overweight (body mass index [BMI] = 25–30), and increasing to 3.0 for obese persons (BMI > 30). *Helicobacter pylori* is a type of bacterium that is found in the stomach in about two-thirds of the world's population. Although it is a risk factor for gastric cancer and mucosa-associated lymphoid tissue (MALT) lymphoma, it has not been demonstrated to be a risk factor for esophageal cancer. Approximately 0.5% of men and women will be diagnosed with esophageal cancer at some point during their lifetime, based on 2008–2010 SEER data.

Dysphagia and weight loss are the most common presenting symptoms. Patients who are deconditioned at presentation with >10% of body weight loss have a worse overall prognosis. Swallowing difficulties are typically worst with meats and breads, and often a patient eats primarily soft foods and liquids when seeking medical attention. Pain may also occur with swallowing. Anemia secondary to gastrointestinal (GI) blood loss, or frank GI bleeding, may be the first sign of esophageal cancer. Patients who have cough associated with swallowing may have a tracheoesophageal fistula and should undergo bronchoscopy as part of the evaluation. Unfortunately, because the esophagus has a rich lymphatic network, the cancer has an early tendency to metastasize, and approximately two-thirds of patients have metastatic disease at the time of diagnosis. As of 2014, the expected 5-year overall survival (OS) rate for esophageal cancer is 17.5%, with 39.6% of those diagnosed with localized disease and only 3.8% of those with distant metastasis being alive at 5 years.

## STAGING

The American Joint Committee on Cancer (AJCC) staging of esophagus and esophagogastric junction cancer is shown as follows.

### Squamous Cell Carcinoma of the Esophagus

| Stage | Description |
| --- | --- |
| IA | Well-differentiated (G1) tumor invades the lamina propria, muscularis mucosa, or submucosa (T1), no lymph nodes (N0), no metastases (M0) |
| IB | Moderate to poorly differentiated (G2–G3) tumor invades the lamina propria, muscularis mucosa, or submucosa (T1), no lymph nodes (N0), no metastases (M0)<br>*or*<br>Well-differentiated (G1) tumor invades the muscularis propria or adventitia (T2–T3) of lower esophagus, no lymph nodes (N0), no metastases (M0) |
| IIA | Well-differentiated (G1) tumor invades the muscularis propria or adventitia (T2–T3) of upper or middle esophagus, no lymph nodes (N0), no metastases (M0)<br>*or*<br>Moderate to poorly differentiated (G2–G3) tumor invades muscularis propria or adventitia (T2–T3) of lower esophagus, no lymph nodes (N0), no metastases (M0) |
| IIB | Moderate to poorly differentiated (G2–G3) tumor invades muscularis propria or adventitia (T2–T3) of upper or middle esophagus, no lymph nodes (N0), no metastases (M0)<br>*or*<br>Any grade (G1–G4) tumor invades the lamina propria, muscularis mucosa, submucosa, or muscularis propria (T1–T2), 1–2 regional lymph nodes involved (N1), no metastases (M0) |
| IIIA | Any grade (G1–G4) tumor invades the lamina propria, muscularis mucosa, submucosa, or muscularis propria (T1–T2), 3–6 regional lymph nodes involved (N2), no metastases (M0)<br>*or*<br>Any grade (G1–G4) tumor invades adventitia (T3), 1–2 regional lymph nodes involved (N1), no metastases (M0)<br>*or*<br>Any grade (G1–G4) resectable tumor invades pleura, pericardium, or diaphragm (T4a), no lymph nodes (N0), no metastases (M0) |
| IIIB | Any grade (G1–G4) tumor invades adventitia (T3), 3–6 regional lymph nodes involved (N2), no metastases (M0) |
| IIIC | Any grade (G1–G4) resectable tumor involves pleura, pericardium, or diaphragm (T4a), 1–6 regional lymph nodes involved (N1–N2), no metastases (M0)<br>*or*<br>Any grade (G1–G4) unresectable tumor invades other adjacent structures, such as aorta, vertebral body, trachea (T4b), any lymph node involvement (N0–N3), no metastases (M0)<br>*or*<br>Any grade (G1–G4) tumor with invasion to any depth (T1–T4b), 7 or more regional lymph nodes involved (N3), no metastases (M0) |
| IV | Any grade (G1–G4) tumor with invasion to any depth (T1–T4b), any regional lymph node involvement (N0–N3), distant metastasis (M1) |

### Adenocarcinoma of the Distal Esophagus and Esophagogastric Junction

| Stage | Description |
| --- | --- |
| IA | Well to moderately differentiated (G1–G2) tumor invades the lamina propria, muscularis mucosa, or submucosa (T1), no lymph nodes (N0), no metastases (M0) |
| IB | Poorly differentiated (G3) tumor invades the lamina propria, muscularis mucosa, or submucosa (T1), no lymph nodes (N0), no metastases (M0)<br>*or*<br>Well to moderately differentiated (G1–G2) tumor invades the muscularis propria (T2), no lymph nodes (N0), no metastases (M0) |
| IIA | Poorly differentiated (G3) tumor invades the muscularis propria (T2), no lymph nodes (N0), no metastases (M0) |
| IIB | Any grade (G1–G4) tumor invades the adventitia (T3), no lymph nodes (N0), no metastases (M0)<br>*or*<br>Any grade (G1–G4) tumor invades the lamina propria, muscularis mucosa, submucosa, or muscularis propria (T1–T2), 1–2 regional lymph nodes involved (N1), no metastases (M0) |

| IIIA | Any grade (G1–G4) tumor invades the lamina propria, muscularis mucosa, submucosa, or muscularis propria (T1–T2), 3–6 regional lymph nodes involved (N2), no metastases (M0) |
| | *or* |
| | Any grade (G1–G4) tumor invades adventitia (T3), 1–2 regional lymph nodes involved (N1), no metastases (M0) |
| | *or* |
| | Any grade (G1–G4) resectable tumor invades pleura, pericardium, or diaphragm (T4a), no lymph nodes (N0), no metastases (M0) |

## CASE SUMMARIES

### Locally Advanced Resectable Esophageal Cancer

J.D. is a 53-year-old man with a past medical history significant for tobacco use, obesity, and GE reflux disease (GERD). His reflux had become progressively worse over the past 2 years, but for the most part he responded to an over-the-counter proton pump inhibitor. He began to have difficulty swallowing and presented to his primary care physician complaining of solid food getting stuck in his throat. He stated that his appetite had decreased and he believed that this was secondary to nervousness regarding pain with swallowing. He had not been to see a doctor recently but believed his weight was stable. He reported that he was very active, working as a carpenter without any limitations. His physical examination was negative with no palpable masses or adenopathy in the neck or abdomen. He was surprised that his weight had dropped approximately 5 pounds from his usual weight. Laboratory studies including a complete blood cell count and a comprehensive metabolic panel were within normal limits.

He was referred to a gastroenterologist for further evaluation and an upper endoscopy revealed a partially obstructing mass in the distal portion of the thoracic esophagus. The lesion was biopsied and the pathology review revealed a grade 2 adenocarcinoma. On receiving the diagnosis, his primary care physician ordered a CT of the chest, abdomen, and pelvis to rule out metastatic disease. The only abnormalities identified were the known esophageal mass that measured 2.8 cm and a suspiciously enlarged paraesophageal lymph node. A PET scan was performed that did not identify any other worrisome lesions. An endoscopic ultrasound (EUS) showed that the tumor invaded the muscularispropria and demonstrated an enlarged hypoechoic node measuring approximately 1.8 cm. On the basis of this staging evaluation, J.D. was judged to have T2 N1 M0, stage IIB disease. The gastroenterologist referred J.D. to an oncologist for treatment discussion.

### Evidence-Based Case Discussion

To assess the appropriate treatment options, a staging workup begins with a CT scan. If there is no obvious metastatic disease, the full workup includes a PET-CT to rule out distant metastasis and an EUS to determine tumor depth and node involvement. Biopsies of suspicious nodes can be obtained during the EUS. Once staging was completed for this patient, he needed to be seen by 3 major disciplines: thoracic surgery, radiation oncology, and medical oncology. This is done most expeditiously in a tumor board setting, if one exists. Ideally, the surgeon would see J.D. first to make sure that he is a surgical candidate, both from the standpoint of extent of disease and medical comorbidities. The surgeon met J.D. and determined that he had locally advanced esophageal cancer that appeared amenable to resection, and he had no medical conditions that would preclude him going through surgery. Therefore, the next step would be referral to the medical oncologist and radiation oncologist for evaluation.

J.D.'s risk factors include GERD and obesity. His tumor, having penetrated the submucosa into the muscularis, significantly increased the chance of spreading to the lymphatics as well as distant metastases. Survival with surgical treatment alone in this setting is poor, 20–30% at 2 years (2). Recent evidence supports the use of multimodality therapy. However, there are several possible standards of care for management of stage II and III disease. They include preoperative (neoadjuvant) chemoradiation, perioperative chemoradiation, and surgery followed by chemoradiation. The decision regarding which is the best treatment for this patient depends on his performance status, his personal wishes, and the level of expertise of participating specialists.

### Preoperative (Neoadjuvant) Chemoradiation

Preoperative chemoradiation followed by surgery is the most common treatment approach in the United States for patients with resectable locally advanced esophageal cancer. For the rare patients who present with very early disease, it is not necessary to give trimodality therapy. For instance, patients with T1a disease (tumor limited to the mucosa) may be treated with endoscopic mucosal resection or esophagectomy, and those with T1b (tumor invades the submucosa) may be treated with esophagectomy. However, most patients present with locally advanced disease, T2 or higher tumors, and often with lymph nodes that are involved with cancer. It is for this group that combination therapy is a major consideration. Several randomized trials have shown to benefit from this approach (Table 6.1).

**Table 6.1** Select Randomized Preoperative Chemoradiation Trials for Potentially Resectable Esophageal Cancer

| Author (Ref. No.) | No. of Patients | Histology | Regimen | Survival | P Values |
|---|---|---|---|---|---|
| Walsh et al. (3) | 113 | AC: 100% | Cisplatin/5-FU/40 Gy XRT + surgery | 3 yr: 32% | |
| | | | Surgery alone | 6% | (P = .01) |
| Urba et al. (4) | 100 | AC: 75% | Cisplatin/5-FU/vinblastine/45 Gy XRT +surgery | 3 yr: 30% | |
| | | SCC: 25% | Surgery alone | 16% | (P = .15) |
| Tepper et al. (5) | 56 | AC: 75% | Cisplatin/5-FU/50.4 Gy XRT + surgery | 5 yr: 39% | |
| | | SCC: 25% | Surgery alone | 16% | (P = .002) |
| Stahl et al. (6) | 172 | SCC: 100% | Induct: cisplatin/5-FU/Leucovorin/ Etoposide | 3 yr: 31% | |
| | | | Concurrent: Cisplatin/Etoposide/40 Gy XRT + surgery | 25% | (P = .02) |
| Gaast et al. (CROSS) (7) | 363 | AC: 74% | Carboplatin/paclitaxel/41.4 Gy XRT + surgery | 3 yr: 59% | |
| | | SCC: 23% | Surgery alone | 48% | (P = .011) |

AC, adenocarcinoma; 5-FU, 5-fluorouracil; SCC, squamous cell carcinoma; XRT, radiation therapy.

Historically, cisplatin plus 5-fluorouracil (5-FU) has been the chemotherapy regimen most frequently given in the neoadjuvant setting with concurrent radiation. More recently, other chemotherapy agents have been used, including carboplatin, paclitaxel, irinotecan, oxaliplatin, and capecitabine.

One of the first trials showing a survival benefit was an Irish trial reported in 1996 by Walsh et al., in which 113 patients with adenocarcinoma were randomized to either surgery alone or concurrent cisplatin, 5-FU, and radiation therapy (40 Gy) followed by surgery (3). A statistically significant survival benefit was shown favoring the combined modality arm: 32% versus 6% of patients alive at 3 years. While this survival benefit was promising, the data were interpreted with some caution because of the unexpectedly low survival rate for the patients treated with surgery alone on the standard arm.

At the University of Michigan, an aggressive neoadjuvant regimen was evaluated, in which 100 patients with esophageal cancer were randomized to either preoperative chemoradiation consisting of cisplatin, 5-FU, and vinblastine versus surgery alone (4). Median survival was similar between the 2 groups, and although the 3-year survival was 30% with multimodality therapy compared with 16% in the surgery-only arm, this did not meet statistical significance. Interestingly, the survival rate for patients treated with trimodality therapy was similar for this trial and the Irish trial described earlier—30% and 32%. However, the survival in the surgical arm was different in each of the studies—16% in the Michigan trial and 6% in the Irish trial.

More recently, the Cancer and Leukemia Group B (CALGB) designed a large randomized trial conducted by the Intergroup to compare surgery alone to preoperative cisplatin, 5-FU, and radiation (5). Unfortunately, the trial had to close early after only 56 of the projected 500 patients were enrolled, due to poor accrual. Surprisingly, even with such small numbers, the median survival was superior for the group treated with multimodality therapy, 4.5 versus 1.8 years (P = .02).

A pressing question is whether surgery really has to be added to a patient's regimen after chemoradiation. A group from Germany enrolled 172 patients with squamous cell carcinoma of the esophagus in a trial that directed them to receive induction chemotherapy followed by chemoradiation followed by surgery, or the same induction chemotherapy followed by chemoradiation without surgery (6). The induction chemotherapy was 3 cycles of cisplatin, 5-FU, leucovorin, and etoposide, and the chemotherapy given concurrently with radiation was cisplatin and etoposide. Three-year survival was similar between the 2 arms—31% with surgery versus 24% with chemoradiation only. Local progression-free survival (PFS) at 2 years was better in the surgery group—64.3% versus 40.7%, P = .003. However, this trial only included patients with squamous cell carcinoma, and it is not clear if these results can be extrapolated to patients with the more commonly seen adenocarcinoma of the distal esophagus or gastroesophageal junction (GEJ). Also, only 66% of the patients randomized to surgery actually underwent resection of their tumor. While surgery is still typically added to most patients' treatment plan if possible, there are circumstances where a surgeon skilled in performing an esophagectomy may not be available, and definitive chemoradiation is therefore administered to these patients.

The Chemoradiotherapy for Oesophageal Cancer Followed by Surgery (CROSS) study group from the Netherlands demonstrated the benefit of preoperative combined modality therapy (7). Three hundred

**Table 6.2** Select Randomized Preoperative Chemotherapy Trials for Resectable Esophageal Cancer

| Author (Ref. No.) | No. of Patients | Histology | Regimen | Survival | P Values |
|---|---|---|---|---|---|
| Medical Research Council Oesophageal Cancer Working Party (9) | 802 | AC: 66% | Cisplatin/5-FU + surgery | 2 yr: 43% | |
| | | SCC: 31% | Surgery alone | 34% | (P = .004) |
| Cunningham et al. (MAGIC) (10) | 503 (75% gastric, 25% esophageal) | AC: 100% | Epirubicin/cisplatin/ 5-FU + surgery | 5 yr: 36% | |
| | | | Surgery alone | 23% | (P = .008) |
| Kelsen et al. (11) | 440 | AC: 54% | Cisplatin/5-FU + surgery | 3 yr: 23% | |
| | | SCC: 46% | Surgery alone | 26% | (P = .74) |

AC, adenocarcinoma; 5-FU, 5-fluorouracil; MAGIC, Medical Research Council Adjuvant Gastric Infusional Chemotherapy trial; SCC, squamous cell carcinoma.

sixty-three patients with resectable T2–3 N0–1 M0 esophageal cancers were randomized to receive either surgical resection alone or preoperative paclitaxel and carboplatin given concurrently with 41.4 Gy of radiation over 23 fractions, followed by surgery 6 weeks later. The median age of the patients was 60 years, and the median World Health Organization (WHO) performance status was 0. Three-fourths of the patients had adenocarcinoma, reflecting the national average. Chemotherapy consisted of paclitaxel 50 mg/m$^2$ and carboplatin area under the curve (AUC) = 2 mg/mL·min, which was administered weekly on days 1, 8, 15, 22, and 29 of radiation. The treatment was extremely tolerable, and resection was performed in a high percentage of patients: 90% of patients in the combined modality arm, and 86% of patients in the surgery-alone arm. Complete (R0) resections were possible in 92.3% of patients in the trimodality arm compared to 67% of the patients in the surgery-alone arm (P < .002). This was an important factor in the results, because unless patients have an R0 resection (microscopic negative margins) the chance of disease recurrence is high. The 3-year OS favored the multimodality arm: 59% versus 48% alive at 3 years. The median survival was 49 versus 26 months (P = .011, hazard ratio [HR] = 0.67).

The Australasian Gastrointestinal Trials Group published a meta-analysis of 10 trials and 1209 patients that assessed preoperative chemoradiotherapy versus surgery alone (8). The results showed a 2-year absolute survival benefit of 13% for chemoradiation (HR = 0.81, P = .002). At present, preoperative chemoradiation followed by surgery is the most common approach used by physicians in the United States. Chemotherapy doublets that are used most commonly contain a platinum agent or a fluoropyrimidine, coupled with a taxane, irinotecan, or oxaliplatin.

The National Comprehensive Center Network Guidelines for Esophageal and Esophagogastric Junction Cancers affirm preoperative chemoradiation as a standard treatment approach to localized esophageal cancer. The guidelines list a sample of 18 possible chemotherapy combinations that have been utilized and reported in this setting. This underscores the fact that the final choice of the chemotherapy agents can be determined by the oncologist, taking into consideration factors related to the patient's medical condition and the physician's own interpretation of reported data.

## Preoperative or Perioperative Chemotherapy

Another possible approach to the treatment of esophageal cancer is preoperative chemotherapy. Because the most common site of disease recurrence after surgery is distant disease, theoretically it would be very important to deliver chemotherapy to a patient as soon as possible after diagnosis to minimize the chance of micrometastatic disease. Three large randomized trials tested this concept (Table 6.2). Two showed survival benefit for preoperative chemotherapy before esophagectomy, and 1 did not.

The Medical Research Council in the United Kingdom showed evidence for the superiority of giving 2 cycles of preoperative epirubicin, cisplatin, and fluorouracil versus surgery alone for 802 patients (9). Median survival was 16.8 months in the combined modality arm and 13.3 months in the surgery-alone arm. The results of this trial were updated in 2007, and the difference in OS at 5 years persisted—23% for the dual modality arm versus 17% for the surgery-alone arm.

In addition, the Medical Research Council Adjuvant Gastric Infusional Chemotherapy (MAGIC) trial provided more evidence for the benefit of 3 cycles of preoperative chemotherapy with a triplet regimen consisting of epirubicin, cisplatin, and infused fluorouracil, with an additional 3 cycles of the same triplet postoperation (10). The study randomized 503 patients with resectable adenocarcinoma of the lower esophagus, GEJ, or stomach to perioperative therapy and surgery versus surgery alone. All patients had an Eastern Cooperative Oncology Group (ECOG) performance status of 0 or 1. Although gastric cancers were the predominant tumor type (74%), the remaining 26% of patients in the trial had cancer of the esophagus or GEJ. Chemotherapy was well tolerated and rates of postoperative complications were similar between the 2 groups. With a median follow-up of 4 years, the perioperative chemotherapy group had a 5-year OS of 36% versus 23% for those treated with surgery ($P = .009$). This difference was observed despite the fact that only 42% of the patients in the perioperative treatment group completed all protocol treatment, and 34% of patients who completed the preoperative chemotherapy and surgery did not go on to receive any postoperative treatment.

In contrast, the results and conclusions were different in an American Intergroup trial in which Kelsen et al. randomized 440 patients with esophageal cancer to either surgery alone or 3 cycles of cisplatin and 5-FU given preoperatively, followed by 2 additional cycles in the postoperative setting (11). There was no significant survival difference between the 2 arms: 2-year survival was 35% for patients treated with preoperative chemotherapy and 37% for those treated with surgery alone. This trial also demonstrated that for patients with localized esophageal cancer, whether or not preoperative chemotherapy is given, an R0 resection plays a crucial role in long-term survival. Even a microscopically positive margin is a poor prognostic factor. This negative trial possibly contributed to the bias of American physicians against preoperative chemotherapy and in favor of preoperative chemoradiation.

In 2007, 2 meta-analyses reported some benefit for preoperative chemotherapy compared to surgery alone. The Australasian Gastrointestinal Trials Group, with a sample of 8 trials and 1724 patients reported a 2-year absolute survival benefit of 7% favoring preoperative systemic therapy (8). The Meta-Analysis of Chemotherapy in Esophagus Cancer Collaborative Group with a sample size of 9 trials containing 2012 patients reported a 5-year absolute survival increase of 4% in preoperative chemotherapy arms (12). Accordingly, the National Comprehensive Cancer Network (NCCN) guidelines currently include perioperative chemotherapy as an acceptable treatment option for adenocarcinoma of the distal esophagus and GEJ. The suggested chemotherapy regimen is epirubicin, cisplatin, and 5-FU, and possible modifications include substituting oxaliplatin for cisplatin, or substituting capecitabine for 5-FU.

## Postoperative Chemoradiation

Another approach to the treatment of locally advanced esophageal cancer is to perform surgery first, and then to follow up with chemoradiation in some patients. Reasons for starting with surgery may include patient preference, a borderline medical condition of the patient that causes concern about the ability to deliver trimodality therapy, a very elderly patient who may not tolerate long periods of aggressive treatment, or the occasional rare instance when an esophageal perforation occurs during a diagnostic endoscopy and necessitates immediate surgery.

Patients with stage II or III esophageal cancer should be considered for postoperative chemoradiation if no neoadjuvant therapy was administered. An Intergroup trial that included 556 patients with surgically resected adenocarcinoma of the stomach or GEJ demonstrated a 9-month median survival advantage favoring postoperative chemoradiation compared with surgery alone (13). Patients were randomized to either surgery alone or postoperative chemoradiation. The adjuvant therapy was 5-FU 425 mg/$m^2$ daily for 5 days, followed by 45 Gy of radiation over 5 weeks with 2 more cycles of chemotherapy delivered concurrently, and then 2 more 5-day cycles of 5-FU. T3 tumors predominated in both groups, with similar representation of patients having more than 4 positive lymph nodes. With a median follow-up of 5 years, the median duration of survival was 36 months in the chemoradiation group and 27 months in the control arm. At 3 years, 50% of patients in the chemoradiation arm were alive versus 41% in the surgery-alone arm ($P = .005$).

The NCCN guidelines recognize postoperative chemoradiation as a standard of care for patients with adenocarcinoma of the stomach or GEJ, particularly for those patients who either have T3 tumors, are node positive, or had an R1 (microscopic positive margins) or R2 (macroscopic positive margins) resection. Because the trial that generated this recommendation used 5-FU and leucovorin, those agents are the ones listed in the guidelines as the major recommendation. However, it is acceptable to substitute capecitabine for 5-FU, or to use the regimen of paclitaxel and 5-FU.

## Summary

With 3 reasonable therapeutic options (see Figure 6.1), how does a physician choose the appropriate treatment? The selection and dosing of anticancer treatment is complex, and must take into account patient variability, comorbidities, and nutritional status. If a patient has a very good performance status and wants aggressive treatment, then preoperative chemoradiation is a very reasonable choice. This practice is particularly common in the United States, and is supported by a substantial survival difference compared to surgery alone in meta-analyses. Occasionally, there might be some concern about a compromised patient being able to tolerate full-dose chemoradiation and its accompanying toxicities, or a patient may have had prior radiation for another cancer in the past, which would make current administration of radiation difficult or impossible. This type of patient could be treated with perioperative chemotherapy to give some additional benefit over surgery alone. This approach is supported by meta-analyses comparing perioperative chemotherapy to surgery, although the survival benefit noted was slightly lower than that observed in the meta-analyses done for preoperative chemoradiation. Lastly, some patients may get surgery first for a variety of

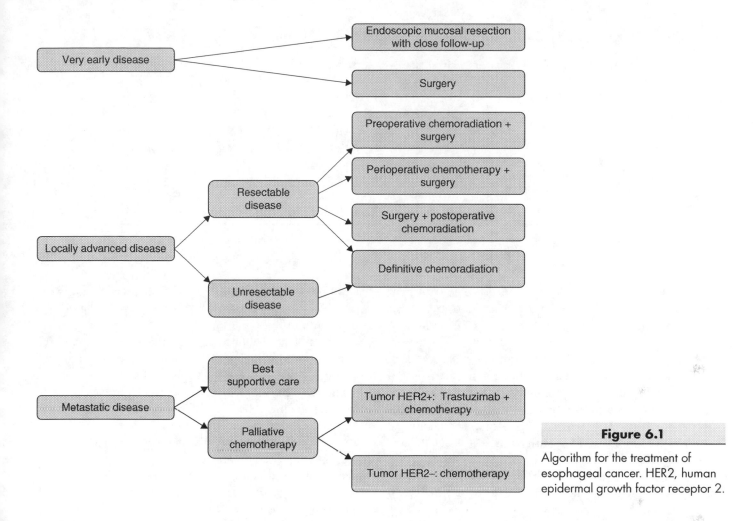

**Figure 6.1**

Algorithm for the treatment of esophageal cancer. HER2, human epidermal growth factor receptor 2.

reasons. In that case, if the surgery was well tolerated and the patient's disease was T3 tumor, lymph node positive, or had positive surgical margins, evaluation should be done to determine if postoperative chemoradiation would be appropriate for that patient to improve the his or her overall and disease-free survival (DFS). In the case of J.D., his relatively young age, good performance status, and desire for aggressive treatment would lead to treatment with preoperative chemoradiation. The chemotherapy agents would most likely include a doublet of platinum, or a fluoropyrimidine, or a taxane.

## Locally Advanced Unresectable Esophageal Cancer

M.W. is a 68-year-old man who has been a heavy smoker for most of his life. He was also an alcoholic who has been sober for the past 2 years. He developed throat and neck pain and was seen by an otolaryngologist who did not find any abnormality during an office examination. He was then referred on for an upper endoscopy, and a fungating tumor was noted <25 cm from the incisors. The biopsy was positive for squamous cell carcinoma. CT scan of the neck, chest, and abdomen showed no visceral metastases but did suggest that the tumor was growing posteriorly

to involve a cervical vertebral body. His tumor stage was therefore IIIC (T4b N0 M0). He was evaluated by a thoracic surgeon who deemed his tumor to be unresectable. He was referred to medical oncology and radiation oncology for possible concurrent chemoradiation.

### Evidence-Based Case Discussion

This patient's tumor is surgically unresectable for 2 reasons. First, the lesion appears to invade the vertebral body, making it technically difficult or impossible to achieve clear margins. Second, even if there was no bony involvement, the tumor is very high in the upper esophagus and would require a pharyngo-laryngo-esophagectomy, which would be too morbid with too little chance of cure. Therefore, definitive chemoradiation is the best choice for this patient. Evidence shows that patients who will not receive surgery should be treated with chemoradiation rather than radiation alone, if they can tolerate the side effects of combined modality treatment.

The Intergroup conducted a trial that was reported by Herskovic et al. (14). This was a phase III prospective, randomized trial that enrolled 121 patients and randomized them to either radiation alone or a combination of radiation with concurrent cisplatin and 5-FU. The dose of

**Table 6.3** Select Randomized Definitive Chemoradiation Trials for Unresectable Esophageal Cancer

| Author (Ref. No.) | No. of Patients | Histology | Regimen | Survival |
|---|---|---|---|---|
| Herskovic et al. (14) | 121 | AC: 13% | Cisplatin/5-FU + 50 Gy XRT | 2 yr: 38% |
| | | SCC: 87% | 64 Gy XRT | 10% ($P$ =.001) |
| Minsky et al. (15) | 218 | AC: 14% | Cisplatin/5-FU + 50.4 Gy XRT | 2 yr: 40% |
| | | SCC: 86% | Cisplatin/5-FU + 64.5 Gy XRT | 31% (NSD) |
| Crosby et al. (16) | 258 | AC: 26% | Cisplatin/capecitabine + 50 Gy XRT | Median: 22.1 mo |
| | | SCC: 74% | Cisplatin/capecitabine/cetuximab + 50 Gy XRT | 25.4 mo |

AC, adenocarcinoma; 5-FU, 5-fluorouracil; NSD, no significant difference; SCC, squamous cell carcinoma; XRT, radiation therapy.

radiation as a single modality was 64 Gy. The treatment in the combination therapy arm consisted of 50 Gy of radiation given concurrently with cisplatin 75 mg/m² and 5-FU 1000 mg/m²/d over 4 days for 4 cycles. The majority of patients in both arms had squamous cell cancers: 84% in the chemoradiation arm and 92% in the radiation alone/control arm. Most patients were between the ages of 60 and 69 years and the Karnofsky performance status (KPS) was >80 in 92–95% of all patients. The combined treatment was more toxic overall with severe side effects in 44% and life threatening in 20% of patients receiving chemoradiation compared with 25% and 3%, respectively, in the radiation alone arm. The median survival was 12.5 months for patients in the combined modality arm, compared with 8.9 months for patients treated with single-agent radiation. Five-year survival rates for chemoradiotherapy versus radiotherapy were 26% and 0%. The authors concluded that concurrent therapy with cisplatin, 5-FU, and radiation is superior to radiation therapy alone, but at the cost of increased side effects (Table 6.3).

A subsequent Intergroup trial took the concept of definitive concurrent chemoradiation with cisplatin and 5-FU a step further, by testing whether it was more effective to give a higher dose of radiation with concurrent chemotherapy—64.8 Gy versus the standard 50.4 Gy (15). Two hundred eighteen patients were randomized, of which 85% had squamous cell carcinoma and 15% had adenocarcinoma. There was no significant difference in survival between the arms: median survival was 13 months for the high-dose radiation and 18.1 months for the standard radiation; 2-year survival was 31% versus 40% (Table 6.3). Therefore, cisplatin and 5-FU in combination with 50.4 Gy of radiation was considered the standard of care.

The Study of Chemoradiotherapy in OesoPhageal cancer with Erbitux (SCOPE1) trial was a randomized study conducted at 36 centers in England to determine if patients who were selected to receive definitive chemoradiation would benefit from the addition of cetuximab to a regimen of cisplatin, capaecitabine, and radiation (16). Two hundred fifty-eight patients were recruited, but the trial

was stopped early for futility. The chemoradiation plus cetuximab group had a shorter median survival than those treated with chemoradiation alone (22.1 vs. 25.4 months, $P$ = .035), and more nonhematological toxicities. Therefore, cetuximab in combination with chemoradiation is not recommended for patients with esophageal cancer.

The NCCN guidelines note that numerous regimens and dosing schedules of chemotherapy have been used in combination with radiation as definitive therapy for patients with esophageal cancer. Some of the agents listed in various combinations include cisplatin and 5-FU/capecitabine, oxaliplatin and a fluoropyrimidine, a taxane and cisplatin, paclitaxel and carboplatin, irinotecan and cisplatin, a taxane with a fluoropyrimidine, or even triplet therapy. Very recent trials are also exploring the addition of targeted agents to chemoradiation.

## Summary

Nonsurgical therapy is best for bulky, inoperable disease, for patients who are not surgical candidates due to significant comorbidities, or for patients whose tumors are so proximal that the surgery required would be very extensive and extremely morbid with minimal chance of cure. For these patients who have a good performance status and desire aggressive treatment, concurrent chemoradiation is indicated (Figure 6.1). However, although survival is better with chemoradiation, the physician must remember that it is also significantly more toxic, and so radiation alone may be the best option for very frail patients. Our patient, M.W., is relatively young and relatively healthy. After a frank discussion about the substantial possibility of severe hematological and GI side effects, concurrent chemoradiation would be initiated. These patients have to be monitored closely for nutrition, fluid intake, and pain.

## Metastatic Esophageal Cancer

L.J. is a 66-year-old male veteran. He had been married for 36 years and his wife had prompted him to go to his primary care physician because he had been losing weight. His past medical history was significant for diabetes and he attributed his recent 62-pound weight loss over the past 7 months to his recent limitation of sweets from his diet. His wife reported to the physician that he looked relatively pale and his energy was decreasing. On review of symptoms, he reported epigastric pain and difficulty swallowing solid foods. He could ingest food, but had to take several drinks of water to accomplish this. He described the pain as dull and fairly constant. He denied any change in his bowel habits.

On examination, L.J. had conjunctival pallor, and his sclera were anicteric. Palpation of his neck revealed a Virchow's node. His lung examination revealed rales. His cardiac examination was unremarkable. He was tender in the epigastrum and there was a vaguely palpable mass. He did not have abdominal distention and no lower extremity edema.

A CBC revealed a hemoglobin of 10.1 mg/dL and a comprehensive metabolic panel demonstrated a mild transaminitis. CT scan of the chest, abdomen, and pelvis was ordered in addition to a GI referral for endoscopy. At the time of endoscopy, L.J. was found to have a circumferential narrowing at the GEJ with a friable and ulcerated mass. Biopsies of the mass were taken and revealed a moderately well-differentiated adenocarcinoma. The CT scan demonstrated a 6 × 7 cm mass at the GEJ, multiple low attenuation lesions in the liver ranging in size from 5 mm to 2.3 cm, diffuse adenopathy consistent with metastatic disease involving celiac, lesser curvature, posterior mediastinal, and a left supraclavicular node. There were scattered lung nodules bilaterally, all <5–8 mm in diameter. One of the liver nodules was biopsied and unfortunately was also positive for adenocarcinoma. The biopsy was tested for human epidermal growth factor receptor 2 (HER2)/neu with immunohistochemistry and the results were 3+ positive.

## Evidence-Based Case Discussion

Determination of treatment for a patient with metastatic esophageal cancer starts with a discussion between the physician and patient regarding goals of care. In order to make a reasonable decision for the best quality of life, the patient must understand that this stage of disease is incurable, and that chemotherapy is palliative in nature. If the patient has no symptoms to palliate, the best decision might be to elect no treatment. However, this patient has abdominal pain and dysphagia; so he has symptoms to palliate. It may be possible to relieve his dysphagia with placement of a stent, but because he has a reasonable performance status, palliative chemotherapy is also an option (Figure 6.1).

### Chemotherapy

The choices for chemotherapy typically include a combination of 2 to 3 drugs, and the most commonly used active agents are the platinums (cisplatin, carboplatin, and oxaliplatin); the fluoropyrimidines (5-FU and capecitabine); the taxanes (paclitaxel and docetaxel); irinotecan; and epirubicin (see Table 6.4). In 2008, the Randomized ECF for Advanced and Locally Advanced Esophagogastric Cancer 2 "REAL-2" trial conducted in the United Kingdom compared 4 triplet chemotherapy regimens: all regimens contained epirubicin, combined with either cisplatin and 5-FU (ECF), cisplatin and capecitabine (ECX), oxaliplatin and 5-FU (EOF), or oxaliplatin and capecitabine (EOX) (17). In the study, 1002 patients were enrolled and the endpoint

**Table 6.4**  Select Randomized Chemotherapy Trials for Metastatic Esophageal Cancer

| Author (Ref. No.) | No. of Patients | Regimen | Response Rate (%) | Median Survival (Months) | Survival (1 Yr, %) |
|---|---|---|---|---|---|
| Cunningham et al. (REAL-2) (17) | 1002 | Epirubicin/cisplatin/5-FU (ECF) | 40.7 | 9.9 | 37.7 |
| | | Epirubicin/cisplatin/capecitabine (ECX) | 46.4 | 9.9 | 40.8 |
| | | Epirubicin/oxaliplatin/5-FU (EOF) | 42.4 | 9.3 | 40.4 |
| | | Epirubicin/oxaliplatin/capecitabine (EOX) | 47.9 | 11.2 | 46.8 |
| Bang et al. (ToGA) (18) | 584 HER2+ patients | Cisplatin/5-FU or capecitabine | 35 | 11.1 | |
| | | Cisplatin/5-FU or capecitabine + Trastuzumab | 47 | 13.8 (P = .0046) | |
| Kang et al. (AVAGAST) (19) | 774 | Cisplatin/capecitabine | 37 | 10.1 | |
| | | Cisplatin/capecitabine + bevacizumab | 46 | 12.1 (P = .1002) | |
| Fuchs et al. (REGARD) (20) | 355 | Placebo | | 3.8 | 11.8 |
| | | Single-agent ramucirumab | | 5.2 (P = .047) | 17.6 |
| Hansjochen et al. (RAINBOW) (21) | 665 | Paclitaxel | | 7.4 | |
| | | Paclitaxel + ramucirumab | | 9.6 (P < .0001) | |

5-FU, 5-fluorouracil; HER2, human epidermal growth factor receptor 2; REAL-2, Randomized ECF for Advanced and Locally Advanced Esophagogastric Cancer 2.

was noninferiority in OS for triplet therapies comparing the newer agents, oxaliplatin and capecitabine, as opposed to the older agents, cisplatin and infusional 5-FU. Patients enrolled in the study had either metastatic or locally advanced cancers of the esophagus, GEJ, or stomach. At a minimum, 87% of patients in each arm had an Eastern Cooperative Oncology Group (ECOG) performance status of 0 or 1. Eighty-six percent to 90% of patients had adenocarcinomas. The median number of cycles of therapy in each group was 6. Regarding the primary endpoint, both capecitabine and oxaliplatin performed well with HRs for death of 0.86 and 0.92 compared to infusional 5-FU and cisplatin, respectively. The overall response rate in the EOX arm was 47.9% versus 40.7%, 46.4%, and 42.4% for the ECF, ECX, and EOF arms, respectively. PFS was 7 months in the EOX arm versus 6.2–6.7 months in the 3 comparator arms. The EOX arm was associated with a 11.2-month median survival compared with 9.9, 9.9, and 9.3 months in the ECF, ECX, and EOF arms, respectively. Cisplatin-containing regimens were associated with greater frequencies of hair loss and grade 3 or 4 leukopenia, whereas oxaliplatin-containing regimens were associated with a greater incidence of grade 3 or 4 peripheral neuropathy. The primary endpoint was achieved and capecitabine and oxaliplatin were proven noninferior to 5-FU and cisplatin, respectively. Since this trial, EOX has become a frequently used regimen for metastatic disease.

The NCCN guidelines list numerous possible chemotherapy combinations, involving cisplatin, carboplatin, oxaliplatin, 5-FU, capecitabine, paclitaxel, docetaxel, irinotecan, and epirubicin. The regimen is typically chosen by weighing its potential side effects and the patient's characteristics and medical history.

## Targeted Therapy

Recent studies have shown that approximately 20% of adenocarcinomas of the esophagus overexpress the HER2 receptor. This suggested the possibility of therapeutic utility for trastuzumab, which is a monoclonal antibody that binds to the HER2 receptor. Therefore, a phase III randomized open-labeled controlled study, called the Trastuzumab for Gastric Cancer (ToGA) trial, was conducted (18). In the ToGA study, 3665 patients were screened, and 810 had tumors that were HER2+, for an overall positivity rate of 22%, which included 20% of gastric cancers and 34% of GEJ cancers. HER2 receptor positivity was determined by immunohistochemistry (3+), or fluorescent in situ hybridization (FISH) (HER2:CEP17 ratio ≥2). Five hundred eighty-four patients were included in the primary analysis and were randomized to either the control arm (cisplatin 80 mg/m$^2$ on day 1 and either capecitabine 1000 mg/m$^2$ orally twice per day for 14 days of a 21-day cycle or fluorouracil 800 mg/m$^2$ by continuous infusion on days 1–5 of each cycle) or the experimental

arm (the same chemotherapy plus trastuzumab 8 mg/kg on day 1 of the first cycle, followed by 6 mg/kg every 3 weeks). Approximately 90% of patients in each treatment arm had good ECOG performance status, and 80–83% of patients had gastric cancer. The median OS was 13.8 months for those assigned to the trastuzumab plus chemotherapy arm, and 11.1 months for those assigned to chemotherapy alone (HR = 0.74). The rates of grade 3 or 4 toxicities including cardiac toxicities did not differ greatly between the treatment arms. Trastuzumab plus chemotherapy is the standard of care for patients with advanced HER2+ GEJ, and gastric cancers.

Bevacizumab is a monoclonal antibody that binds to the vascular endothelial growth factor receptor (VEGF-R). The Avastin in Gastric Cancer (AVAGAST) trial was a randomized, double-blind, placebo-controlled trial that compared outcomes of 774 patients treated with capecitabine and cisplatin plus bevacizumab versus the same chemotherapy alone (19). The study unfortunately did not meet its primary objective of demonstrating a significant increase in OS. Within the intent to treat population, the median OS was 10.1 months with chemotherapy and placebo, as compared to 12.1 months in the chemotherapy plus bevacizumab arm (HR = 0.87, $P$ = .1002). However, PFS significantly favored the bevacizumab-containing arm: 29.5 months in the placebo arm compared with 38.0 months in the treatment arm ($P$ = .0121). Bevacizumab was well tolerated overall.

A newer agent, ramucirumab, is a fully human monoclonal antibody directed against the VEGF receptor 2 (VEGF-R2). Ramucirumab was evaluated in 2 recent trials for previously treated metastatic gastric and GEJ cancers. The REGARD trial randomized 355 patients previously treated with fluoropyrimidine- or platinum-containing chemotherapy to receive ramucirumab monotherapy ($n$ = 238) or placebo ($n$ = 117). Median OS was 5.2 months in the ramucirumab group and 3.8 months with placebo group (HR = 0.78, 95% CI [0.60–0.998]; $P$ = .047). The major side effect was hypertension, but the drug was otherwise very well tolerated (20). Additionally, the RAINBOW trial examined ramucirumab plus paclitaxel versus paclitaxel alone in the treatment of 665 patients with metastatic GEJ and gastric adenocarcinoma following disease progression on first-line platinum- and fluoropyrimidine-containing combination therapy (21). In this study, the median OS with the combination was 9.6 months compared with 7.4 months with paclitaxel alone (HR = 0.8, 95% CI [0.68–0.96], $P$ = .017). Ramucirumab is now approved for metastatic GEJ adenocarcinoma after failure of platinum- or fluoropyrimidine-based first-line therapy.

## Summary

L.J.'s tumor was 3+ positive for HER2 receptor, he had a reasonable performance status, and he wished to pursue at least 1 regimen of palliative chemotherapy to try to relieve his discomfort and dysphagia. Therefore, we can elect to offer to treat him with cisplatin, 5-FU or capecitabine, and trastuzumab. We first need to address that he has an adequate means of maintaining nutrition, possibly a feeding tube or stent if he cannot swallow enough on his own, before initiating the chemotherapy.

## ACKNOWLEDGMENT

The authors would like to thank Dr. David Shepard for his significant contributions to the first edition of this chapter.

## REVIEW QUESTIONS

1. You have been treating a 50-year-old man for stage IV gastroesophageal junction adenocarcinoma with cisplatin and 5-fluorouracil. HER2 immunohistochemistry on the tumor was 2+ and fluorescent in situ hybridization was negative. After the third cycle of chemotherapy, a CT scan revealed progression of disease. His blood pressure is 160/90 mmHg. Pulse is 100. Hemoglobin is 10.8 g/dL and platelet count is 90,000/μL. Performance status is Eastern Cooperative Oncology Group 2. Which of the following would be a relative contraindication to using ramucirumab?

   (A) Hypertension
   (B) Thrombocytopenia
   (C) Anemia
   (D) Asthma

2. A 65-year-old man presented with dysphagia. His primary care physician ordered an upper endoscopy that revealed a mass at the distal esophagus and biopsy demonstrated adenocarcinoma. A CT scan showed multiple liver lesions, and these are $^{18}$F-fludeoxyglucose-avid on follow-up PET scan. You order a biopsy of one of the liver lesions to confirm metastatic disease. Which of the following tests should be added to the pathology assessment?

   (A) ERCC1 expression level
   (B) HER2 immunohistochemistry
   (C) Epidermal growth factor receptor expression
   (D) Vascular endothelial growth factor receptor assessment

3. A 42-year-old man was diagnosed with squamous cell carcinoma of the upper esophagus. Gastric biopsies during esophagogastroduodenoscopy (EGD) revealed the presence of *Helicobacter pylori* infection. He comes to you for further management accompanied by his wife and 3 children. History is positive for heavy alcohol abuse and smoking, as well as long standing GE reflux disease (GERD). Physical examination reveals an obese man (body mass index = 35). He inquires about risk factors that may have contributed to developing this cancer. Which of the following modifiable risk factors put him at increased risk for this malignancy?

   (A) Obesity
   (B) *Helicobacter pylori* infection
   (C) Smoking and alcohol use
   (D) Uncontrolled GERD

4. A 60-year-old woman with a history of stage II breast cancer treated with neoadjuvant adriamycin (450 mg/m² total dose) and cyclophosphamide followed by lumpectomy is now diagnosed with gastroesophageal junction adenocarcinoma metastatic to the lung. Immunohistochemistry for HER2 was 1+. Additional medical history is significant for diabetes with an estimated glomerular filtration rate of 40. She comes to your office with multiple clinical research reports, including findings from the landmark Randomized ECF for Advanced and Locally Advanced Esophagogastric Cancer 2 trial. After discussing the different options, you believe she can safely receive which of the following chemotherapy regimens?

   (A) Epirubicin, oxaliplatin, capecitabine
   (B) Epirubicin, cisplatin, 5-fluorouracil (5-FU)
   (C) Cisplatin + 5-FU
   (D) Capecitabine and oxaliplatin

5. You are seeing a 45-year-old woman with a heavy smoking history, who recently underwent an upper endoscopy in the emergency department after presenting with a food bolus impaction. A large fungating and partially obstructing mass was seen in the distal esophagus. Biopsy confirmed adenocarcinoma, and HER2 was 3+. Her case was reviewed by a thoracic surgeon, and the tumor was determined to be unresectable due to tumor invasion of local structures. PET scan did not show evidence of metastatic disease. Which regimen would be most appropriate for this patient?

   (A) Radiation plus herceptin
   (B) Radiation plus cisplatin and fluorouracil
   (C) Radiation plus epirubicin, cisplatin, fluorouracil, and herceptin
   (D) Epirubicin, oxaliplatin, fluorouracil

6. You are asked to give a second opinion regarding treatment options for a 50-year-old man who was recently found to have a large mass in the middle third of the esophagus. Biopsy was positive for

adenocarcinoma, and HER2 status was negative. CT and PET scans did not reveal any signs of metastatic disease. Endoscopic ultrasound was done, and the resultant staging was T3N1 disease. Which of the following treatment regimens do you recommend?

(A) Preoperative chemotherapy followed by surgery and then postoperative chemoradiation

(B) Preoperative chemoradiation followed by surgery and then postoperative chemotherapy

(C) Referral for surgical resection with perioperative chemotherapy

(D) Perform immunohistochemistry for HER2 on the tumor specimen

7.  A 40-year-old man presents to his physician with dysphagia that has been worsening over the past 2 months. He is undergoing endoscopy to establish a diagnosis, and an ulcerated tumor is noted. Unfortunately, an esophageal perforation occurs, and the patient is taken immediately to the surgical suite for esophagectomy. He recovers without sequelae, and the pathological staging of the tumor is T2N1 disease. Which of the following treatment options are most appropriate at this time for the patient?

(A) Observation

(B) Radiation therapy

(C) Chemotherapy with carboplatin and paclitaxel × 4 cycles

(D) Radiation plus concurrent fluoropyrimidine-based chemotherapy

## REFERENCES

1.  Hongo M, Nagasaki Y, Shoji T. Epidemiology of esophageal cancer: orient to occident. Effects of chronology, geography and ethnicity. *J Gastroenterol Hepatol.* 2009;24(5):729–735.

2.  Girling DJ, Bancewicz J, Clark PI, et al. Surgical resection with or without preoperative chemotherapy in oesophageal cancer: a randomized controlled trial. *Lancet.* 2002;359(9319):1727–1733.

3.  Walsh TN, Noonan N, Hollywood D, et al. A comparison of multimodal therapy and surgery for esophageal adenocarcinoma. *N Engl J Med.* 1996;335(7):462–467.

4.  Urba SG, Orringer MB, Turrisi A, et al. Randomized trial of preoperative chemoradiation versus surgery alone in patients with locoregional esophageal carcinoma. *J Clin Oncol.* 2001;19(2):305–313.

5.  Tepper J, Krasna MJ, Niedzwiecki D, et al. Phase III trial of trimodality therapy with cisplatin, fluorouracil, radiotherapy, and surgery compared with surgery alone for esophageal cancer: CALGB 9781. *J Clin Oncol.* 2008;26(7):1086–1092.

6.  Stahl M, Stuschke M, Lehmann N, et al. Chemoradiation with and without surgery in patients with locally advanced squamous cell carcinoma of the esophagus. *J Clin Oncol.* 2005;23(10):2310–2317.

7.  Gaast AV, van Hagen P, Hulshof M, et al. Effect of preoperative concurrent chemoradiotherapy on survival of patients with resectable esophageal or esophagogastric junction cancer: results from a multicenter randomized phase III study. *J Clin Oncol.* 2010;28(15s):[abstract] #4004.

8.  Gebski V, Burmeister B, Smithers BM, et al.; Australasian Gastro-Intestinal Trials Group. Survival benefits from neoadjuvant chemoradiotherapy or chemotherapy in oesophageal carcinoma: a meta-analysis. *Lancet Oncol.* 2007;8(3):226–234.

9.  Medical Research Council Oesophageal Cancer Working Party. Surgical resection with or without preoperative chemotherapy in oesophageal cancer: a randomized controlled trial. *Lancet.* 2002;359(9319):1727–1733.

10. Cunningham D, Allum WH, Stenning SP, et al. Perioperative chemotherapy versus surgery alone for resectable gastroesophageal cancer. *N Engl J Med.* 2006;355(1):11–20.

11. Kelsen DP, Ginsberg R, Pajak TF, et al. Chemotherapy followed by surgery compared with surgery alone for localized esophageal cancer. *N Engl J Med.* 1998;339(27):1979–1984.

12. Thirion PG, Michiels S, Le Maitre A, Tierney J, on behalf of the Meta-Analysis of Chemotherapy in Esophagus Cancer Collaborative Group. Individual patient data-based meta-analysis assessing pre-operative chemotherapy in resectable oesophageal carcinoma. *J Clin Oncol.* 2007;25(18S): (Abstract #4512).

13. Macdonald JS, Smalley SR, Benedetti J, et al. Chemoradiotherapy after surgery compared with surgery alone for adenocarcinoma of the stomach or gastroesophageal junction. *N Engl J Med.* 2001;345(10):725–730.

14. Herskovic A, Martz K, al-Sarraf M, et al. Combined chemotherapy and radiotherapy compared with radiotherapy alone in patients with cancer of the esophagus. *N Engl J Med.* 1992;326(24):1593–1598.

15. Minsky BD, Pajak TF, Ginsberg RJ, et al. INT 0123 (Radiation Therapy Oncology Group 94–05) phase III trial of combined-modality therapy for esophageal cancer: high-dose versus standard-dose radiation therapy. *J Clin Oncol.* 2002;20(5):1167–1174.

16. Crosby T, Hurt CN, Falk S, et al. Chemoradiotherapy with or without cetuximab in patients with oesophageal cancer (SCOPE1): a multicentre, phase 2/3 randomised trial. *Lancet Oncol.* 2013;14(7):627–637.

17. Cunningham D, Starling N, Rao S, et al.; Upper Gastrointestinal Clinical Studies Group of the National Cancer Research Institute of the United Kingdom. Capecitabine and oxaliplatin for advanced esophagogastric cancer. *N Engl J Med.* 2008;358(1):36–46.

18. Bang YJ, Van Cutsem E, Feyereislova A, et al.; ToGA Trial Investigators. Trastuzumab in combination with chemotherapy versus chemotherapy alone for treatment of HER2-positive advanced gastric or gastro-oesophageal junction cancer (ToGA): a phase 3, open-label, randomised controlled trial. *Lancet.* 2010;376(9742):687–697.

19. Kang AY, Ohtsu E, Van Cutsem E, et al. AVAGAST: A randomized, double-blind, placebo-controlled, phase III study of first-line capecitabine and cisplatin plus bevacizumab or placebo in patients with advanced gastric cancer (AGC). *J Clin Oncol.* 2010;28:[abstract] #4007.

20. Fuchs CS, Tomasek J, Yong CJ, et al. Ramucirumab monotherapy for previously treated advanced gastric or gastro-oesophageal junction adenocarcinoma (REGARD): an international, randomised, multicentre, placebo-controlled, phase 3 trial. *Lancet.* 2014;383(9911):31–39. doi: 10.1016/S0140–6736(13)61719–5.

21. Hansjochen W, Van Cutsem E, Oh SC, et al. RAINBOW: A global, phase III, randomized, double-blind study of ramucirumab plus paclitaxel versus placebo plus paclitaxel in the treatment of metastatic gastroesophageal junction (GEJ) and gastric adenocarcinoma following disease progression on first-line platinum- and fluoropyrimidine-containing combination therapy rainbow IMCL CP12–0922 (I4T-IE-JVBE). *J Clin Oncol.* 2014(Suppl 3; Abstract LBA7).

# 7

## *Gastric Cancer*

JOSH WILFONG AND MARK M. ZALUPSKI

## EPIDEMIOLOGY, NATURAL HISTORY, RISK FACTORS, AND PATHOLOGY

In 2013, an estimated 21,600 new cases of gastric cancer were diagnosed in the United States, with 10,990 deaths resulting from this malignancy. The incidence of gastric cancer showed wide geographical variation. Worldwide, gastric cancer represents the fourth most common cancer and the second most common cause of cancer death, whereas in the United States it accounts for only 1.3% of cancer diagnoses per year (1,2). High incidence rates of the disease are seen in China, Japan, Korea, and countries in Latin America and Eastern Europe. In contrast, low incidence rates are observed in Northern Africa, South and Southeast Asia, and North America. This regional variation is probably related to differences in epidemiological factors, but may also be attributable to differences in the molecular biology of the disease. Within the United States, this neoplasm has been in decline over the past 3 decades, with an overall decrease of 5.2 cases per 100,000 people from 1976 to 2010, corresponding to approximately 15,000 fewer cases. This observation is likely related to changes in dietary habits, improvement in food preparation and storage, and treatment of *Helicobacter pylori* infection. Mortality associated with the malignancy also has declined, with a decrease in deaths of 5.1 cases per 100,000 people, approximating 15,000 fewer deaths over that time period (1).

The National Cancer Institute (NCI) Surveillance, Epidemiology, and End Results (SEER) Cancer Statistics Review indicates that the median age of diagnosis of gastric cancer from 2006 to 2010 was 69 years, with 81% of the cases occurring after 55 years of age. Approximately 28% of the patients presented with localized disease, 34% with locally advanced disease involving regional lymph nodes, and 38% with distant metastasis. Survival correlated with stage, with 5-year survival rates of 63%, 28%, and 3% for localized, regional, and distant disease, respectively.

Gastric cancer is not a single disease. Its classification can be established based on the anatomical location of the primary tumor and/or the histological pattern displayed. On the basis of the anatomical location in the stomach, gastric carcinoma is subdivided into cardia or proximal stomach, often involving the gastroesophageal junction (GEJ), and noncardia or distal tumors located predominantly in the corpus or antral area. Despite the overall decrease of gastric cancer within Western populations, the proportion of tumors originating in the cardia has been increasing since 1975, which now represents the most common location (3). Distal tumors continue to predominate in Asia and South America.

When characterized by histology, gastric cancer is divided into intestinal or diffuse subtypes (4). Intestinal gastric cancer forms rudimentary glands and displays varying degrees of differentiation, from well to moderate to poorly differentiated tumors. This subtype arises in a background of intestinal metaplasia. In the other histological subtype, diffuse gastric cancer, malignant cells fail to form any recognizable structures resembling glands, with the classical appearance of signet ring cells, named due to intracellular mucin forcing the nucleus to the periphery. At the present time, both classifications are used simultaneously because the epidemiological factors, precursor lesions, phenotypic and clinical features correlate specifically with each subtype (Table 7.1). Therefore, a 3-category classification is widely used: GEJ/cardia, intestinal noncardia, and diffuse subtype.

Analytical epidemiology studies have identified multiple risk factors involved in the pathogenesis of this disease, reflecting the multifactorial nature of gastric cancer. The strength of each association varies depending on the subtype of gastric cancer analyzed. Traditional risk factors

**Table 7.1**  Summary of the Characteristics of Gastric Cancer Based on Tumor Subtype

|  | Cardiac GEJ | Noncardiac Intestinal | Noncardiac Diffuse |
|---|---|---|---|
| Epidemiology | Incidence increasing in Western countries | Incidence decreasing worldwide | Incidence stable |
| Biology | Possible link with HER2 | HNPCC-related | *CDH1* mutations<br>Loss of E-Cadherin |
| Clinical features | GERD<br>Obesity | *H. pylori* infection<br>Tobacco/alcohol<br>Salt intake<br>Low-fruit/vegetable diet | No clear relation to classical risk factors |
| Pathology |  | Stepwise progression model:<br>– Chronic gastritis<br>– Intestinal metaplasia<br>– Dysplasia | No stepwise progression<br>No precursor lesion<br>Signet ring cells<br>Interstitial mucin |
| HER2 status | 32% positive GEJ | 32% positive intestinal | 6% positive diffuse |

GC, gastric cancer; GEJ, gastroesophageal junction; GERD, gastroesophageal reflux disease; HER2, human epidermal growth factor receptor 2; HNPCC, hereditary nonpolyposis colorectal cancer.

for gastric carcinoma including high salt diet, presence of nitrates in cured foods, tobacco exposure, and *H. pylori* infection have been linked to the intestinal subtype. *H. pylori* infection leads to the development of chronic gastritis, resulting in genetic instability and progression through atrophy, intestinal metaplasia, dysplasia, and malignancy. Protective factors such as a diet rich in fruits and vegetables, refrigeration of food, and exposure to vitamin C and carotenoids have been related to decreased risk. It is noteworthy that the decrease in the incidence of gastric cancer observed during the last few decades is clearly attributable to interventions leading to the modifications of these risk factors, thus impacting the burden of intestinal gastric cancer. In contrast, relationships between diffuse gastric cancer and specific environmental factors have not been clearly identified, although *H. pylori* may also account for an increase in the risk of the diffuse subtype.

A genetic predisposition has been recognized in the development of the intestinal subtype, including deficiencies of mismatch repair proteins and a diagnosis of Lynch syndrome. Additionally, genetic factors have also been strongly associated with the development of early onset, diffuse gastric carcinoma. The presence of a germ-line truncating mutation in Cadherin-1 (*CDH1*), encoding for the protein E-Cadherin, leads to the autosomal dominant cancer genetic syndrome known as hereditary diffuse gastric cancer (HDGC), which is also associated with the development of lobular breast cancer. The diagnosis of HDGC confers by age 80 years an estimated cumulative risk of gastric carcinoma of 67% for men (95% confidence interval [CI], [39–99]) and 83% for women (95% CI [58–99]), as well as a cumulative risk of breast cancer in women of approximately 39% (95% CI [12–84]). Strikingly, immunohistochemical (IHC) evidence for the loss of E-Cadherin is also observed in approximately 50% of sporadically occurring gastric cancers, although these cases are typically associated with the presence of somatic missense mutations of *CDH1*.

Finally, risk factors for the development of GEJ tumors include alcohol, tobacco, past medical history of gastroesophageal reflux, and obesity. The incidence of GEJ tumors among young white individuals has increased in the past decade in Western countries, likely secondary to increases in obesity and reflux disease.

Gastric cancer spreads by local invasion, lymphatic extension, distant hematogenous metastasis, and peritoneal dissemination. Initially, the malignancy invades locally into, along, and through the gastric wall, further advancing into neighboring organs and anatomical structures. Intestinal type gastric carcinomas are commonly limited to a restricted area of the stomach. In contrast, diffuse carcinomas tend to more widely involve the stomach, the so-called linitis plastica, which often extends into the duodenum. Lymph node involvement correlates with size and depth of the primary tumor and follows an orderly fashion spreading into regional lymph node stations. This behavior influences the surgical principles underlying the extent of lymphadenectomy in those patients who are candidates for surgical resection. Venous invasion leads to the development of distant metastasis, most commonly located in the liver, lungs, and bone. Local invasion of the serosal surfaces precedes the development of peritoneal metastases. Not uncommonly, bilateral ovarian metastases are observed in premenopausal women diagnosed with gastric carcinoma, the so-called Krukenberg's tumor.

Generally, intestinal gastric cancer will develop distant metastasis via hematogenous dissemination. Diffuse tumors often present with extensive lymph node and peritoneal involvement. Tumors of the GEJ resemble the behavior of esophageal tumors: not infrequently, the esophagus

| Stage | Definition |
|-------|------------|
| 0 | Carcinoma in situ: intraepithelial tumor without invasion of the lamina propria |
| IA | Tumor invades lamina propria, muscularis mucosae, or submucosa without lymph node involvement or metastasis |
| IB | Tumor invades muscularis propria without lymph node involvement or metastasis; *or* tumor invades lamina propria, muscularis mucosae, or submucosa with metastasis in 1–2 regional lymph nodes |
| IIA | Tumor penetrates subserosal connective tissue without invasion of visceral peritoneum or adjacent structures and without lymph node involvement or metastasis; *or* tumor invades muscularis propria with metastasis in 1–2 regional lymph nodes; *or* tumor invades lamina propria, muscularis mucosae, or submucosa with metastasis in 3–6 regional lymph nodes |
| IIB | Tumor invades serosa (visceral peritoneum) without lymph node involvement or metastasis; *or* tumor penetrates subserosal connective tissue without invasion of visceral peritoneum or adjacent structures with metastasis in 1–2 regional lymph nodes; *or* tumor invades muscularis propria with metastasis in 3–6 regional lymph nodes; *or* tumor invades lamina propria, muscularis mucosae, or submucosa with metastasis in 7 or more regional lymph nodes |
| IIIA | Tumor invades serosa (visceral peritoneum) with metastasis in 1–2 regional lymph nodes; *or* tumor penetrates subserosal connective tissue without invasion of visceral peritoneum or adjacent structures with metastasis in 3–6 regional lymph nodes; *or* tumor invades muscularis propria with metastasis in 7 or more regional lymph nodes |
| IIIB | Tumor invades adjacent structures with metastasis in 0–2 regional lymph nodes; *or* tumor invades serosa (visceral peritoneum) with metastasis in 3–6 regional lymph nodes; *or* tumor penetrates subserosal connective tissue without invasion of visceral peritoneum or adjacent structures with metastasis in 7 or more regional lymph nodes |
| IIIC | Tumor invades adjacent structures with metastasis in 3 or more regional lymph nodes; *or* tumor invades serosa (visceral peritoneum) with metastasis in 7 or more regional lymph nodes |
| IV | Distant metastasis |

*Source:* American Joint Committee on Cancer (AJCC), *AJCC Cancer Staging Handbook, 7th edition.*

is involved with submucosal extension, and lymph node metastases may be located in the lower mediastinum (upward progression) or in the esophagogastric angles and other para-aortic structures (downward progression).

Molecular characterization of gastric cancer has further defined our understanding and is impacting the therapy of this disease. Thus far, the identification of over-expression of the oncoprotein human epidermal growth factor receptor 2 (HER2) has been most meaningful. The HER2 protein is a 185-kDa *trans*-membrane tyrosine kinase receptor that is a member of the family of the epidermal growth factor receptors (EGFR). HER2 is encoded by a gene located at chromosome 17q21. It has been shown to be overexpressed and/or amplified in 13–22% of gastric cancers (5). Overexpression may be determined using IHC with a monoclonal antibody (Herceptest) and amplification using fluorescent in situ hybridization (FISH), as assayed in breast cancer. The trastuzumab for gastric cancer (ToGA) trial analyzed a total of 1527 gastric cancers for HER2 overexpression using both IHC and FISH, with an observed frequency of 22%. These analyses showed a higher correlation between HER2 overexpression and the intestinal subtype (vs. the diffuse and mixed subtypes) and GEJ location (vs. a noncardiac origin). The role of HER2 as a prognostic factor in gastric cancer is debated, although a majority of studies suggest a negative prognostic effect for tumors overexpressing HER2. Important therapeutic implications for HER2-positive tumors are discussed in further detail in the metastatic disease section of this chapter. Molecular profiling has also revealed numerous

somatic gene mutations and pathway alterations in gastric cancer, with involvement of *p53, PTEN, PIK3CA, FGFR2, EGFR,* and *MET* (6). The clinical utility of these findings is undergoing prospective evaluation.

## STAGING

Gastric cancer is staged by using the tumor, node, metastases (TNM) classification, which is based on the extent of tumor and involvement of local and distant structures. The American Joint Committee on Cancer (AJCC) staging of gastric tumors is shown in Table 7.1.

## CASE SUMMARIES

### Resectable Gastric Cancer

S.C. is a 66-year-old man with a past medical history relevant for myocardial infarction secondary to coronary artery disease, hyperlipidemia, peripheral vascular disease with intermittent claudication, and sleep apnea. He has a 20-pack-year history of tobacco exposure and no history of alcohol use. S.C. presented with epigastric pain over a 3-month period and subsequently had 1 episode of gastrointestinal bleeding that required admission to a local hospital. During that admission a complete workup was performed, including an esophagogastroduodenoscopy (EGD) that revealed the presence of an ulcerated and friable mass in the gastric fundus as well as mild gastritis in the antrum. Biopsies demonstrated invasive adenocarcinoma. A CT scan of chest, abdomen, and pelvis showed thickening of the fundus and cardia of the stomach with adjacent pathologically enlarged lymph nodes. There was no evidence of distant metastatic disease. A combined PET-CT scan confirmed the presence of increased uptake in the posterior aspect of the fundus and in regional lymph nodes. Endoscopic ultrasound (EUS) examination revealed tumor in the gastric wall involving the muscularis propria, with enlarged lymph nodes in the vicinity (uT2 N1 Mx). S.C. was evaluated and was considered to be a candidate for total gastrectomy with Roux-en-Y esophagojejunostomy and placement of jejunostomy feeding tube. At this point S.C. was referred to the medical oncology clinic for evaluation.

## Evidence-Based Case Discussion

The staging workup for gastric cancer should include history and physical examination, blood count and differential, liver and renal function tests, upper endoscopy (EGD), CT of the abdomen and pelvis, and either x-ray or CT scan of the thorax. The role of EGD is crucial in the diagnosis of gastric cancer since it enables the visualization of the tumor as well as evaluation of its localization and extent. Moreover, EGD allows biopsy for diagnosis

of the tumor and simultaneously determines the presence of *H. pylori* infection or Barrett's esophagus. EUS is helpful in determining the depth of tumor invasion and the proximal and distal extent of the tumor, although it is less useful for this purpose in tumors located in the antrum. In women, pelvic CT or ultrasound (US) may help to rule out the presence of ovarian metastasis. PET-CT has been shown to be superior for preoperative staging when compared to CT scan or PET alone. PET-CT is especially useful to evaluate the presence of distant metastasis and to help accurately determine the nodal staging. The utility of laparoscopy, with or without cytology of peritoneal washings, is debated. Some institutions perform this routinely as an initial maneuver in all patients who are medically fit and candidates for surgical resection. Especially in those patients planned to be treated with neoadjuvant therapy, laparoscopy may be performed in order to exclude the presence of metastatic disease. The staging classification of gastric cancer is based on the data collected with these procedures depicted previously. In clinical settings, however, a frequently used classification is based on the potential for resection and evidence for extent of disease, dividing patients into 3 categories: resectable, unresectable, and metastatic (Figure 7.1).

An attempt at curative resection is often the initial treatment for gastric cancer. The major surgical issues

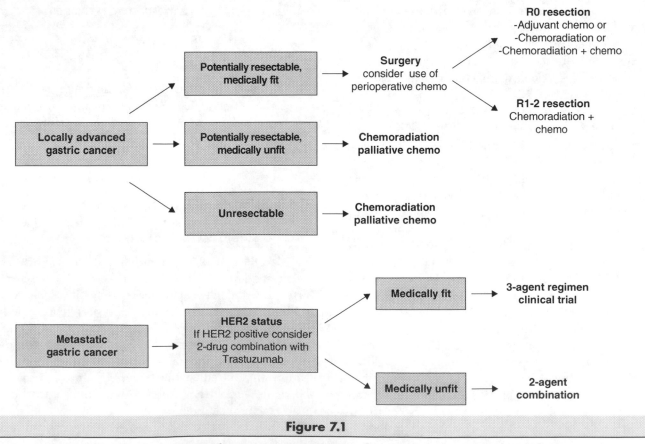

### Figure 7.1

Algorithm for the treatment of gastric cancer. HER2, human epidermal growth factor receptor 2.

include the extent of luminal resection and lymph node dissection. Regarding the extent of luminal resection, tumors located distally can be addressed either by a total gastrectomy or a distal subtotal gastrectomy. Several prospective studies have shown no difference in terms of survival between these 2 surgical approaches. However, quality of life is superior after subtotal gastrectomy. For those tumors located more proximally, factors such as an association with Barrett's esophagus, the exact location (i.e., within the GEJ vs. subcardial region) and the differentiation of the tumor (well/moderately vs. poorly differentiated) needs to be considered. Proximal subtotal gastrectomy is appropriate for well or moderately differentiated tumors that arise within the GEJ, but not for those associated with Barrett's esophagus or those located in the subcardial region. Poorly differentiated tumors, those associated with Barrett's esophagus, and those extending into any portion of the esophagus require total gastrectomy with some extent of esophagectomy and a Roux-en-Y reconstruction.

An area of controversy in the surgical treatment of gastric cancer is the extent of the lymph node dissection. This is classified into different categories, designated D0 to D3, as the extent of lymphadenectomy increases. A D1 dissection includes perigastric lymph nodes located in the lesser and greater curvatures and is a minimum standard surgical treatment. A classical D2 dissection includes nodes located along the hepatic, left gastric, celiac, and splenic arteries, including the splenic hilum, requiring a splenectomy for proximal tumors. A D2 dissection requires a high degree of expertise and should be performed only in those centers with sufficient experience. A D3 dissection involves removal of the portahepatic and periaortic nodes. These regions are considered metastatic locations, and therefore this extent of lymphadenectomy is not often performed. Studies have analyzed the effect of D1 versus D2 dissection on survival. Generally, it is believed that D2 dissections offer a small survival advantage over D1 dissections. In Asian countries, the standard of care includes the classical D2 dissection, whereas in Western countries the standard is a modified D2 dissection, excluding splenectomy or pancreatectomy and achieving the goal of removing at least 15 lymph nodes.

Characterization of failure patterns in patients following surgical treatment of gastric cancer identifies relapse in locoregional sites, peritoneal dissemination, and distant metastatic disease (primarily liver) (7). To decrease the likelihood of disease recurrence in resectable gastric cancer, various "adjuvant" strategies have been studied, including the use of perioperative chemotherapy, postoperative adjuvant chemotherapy, and postoperative adjuvant chemoradiation. To date, these different approaches have not been directly compared with one another.

The rationale for the use of perioperative chemotherapy (pre- and postoperative treatment) includes providing systemic therapy to all patients, earliest possible treatment of micrometastasis, downstaging to improve rates of complete resection, and avoidance of disruption in the delivery of adjuvant therapy following surgery due to postoperative complications that may delay or prevent its use. The UK Medical Research Council Adjuvant Gastric Infusional Chemotherapy (MAGIC) trial was a phase III randomized trial of 503 patients (3). This study demonstrated a significant survival benefit with up to 6 cycles of perioperative chemotherapy using a regimen that included epirubicin, cisplatin, and 5-fluorouracil (5-FU; ECF) as compared to surgery alone. Survival rates at 5 years were improved from 23% with surgery alone to 36% with surgery and chemotherapy ($P = .009$). The use of perioperative chemotherapy did not affect the rate of surgical resection (91.6% in the chemotherapy arm vs. 94.6% in the surgery arm). A significant downstaging effect was observed, however, in the perioperative arm with regard to tumor stage (T1–2 disease 52% in the chemotherapy arm vs. 37% in the surgery-only arm, $P = .002$) and nodal disease, described by an increase in the fraction of patients with N0–1 disease (84% in the chemotherapy arm vs. 70% in the surgical arm, $P = .01$). Regarding the extent of lymphadenectomy in this trial, approximately 40% of patients underwent some type of D2 dissection, 21% had D1 dissection, 20% had surgical resection of the primary without lymph node dissection, and 19% were not resected. These data reflect the quality of the surgery performed in patients enrolled in the MAGIC trial, and should be taken into account when comparing trials testing other modalities of adjuvant treatment.

Chemoradiation therapy was evaluated in the randomized Intergroup 0116 trial, a North American study that compared surgery alone to surgery followed by combined modality adjuvant treatment in 556 patients (8). Adjuvant therapy consisted of 1 cycle of 5-FU/leucovorin, followed by 5-FU chemotherapy concurrent with radiation to the gastric bed and regional lymph nodes, followed by 2 additional cycles of 5-FU chemotherapy. Five-year survival in the surgery-alone group was 41%, compared with 50% in the adjuvant treatment group (hazard ratio [HR] = 1.31; 95% CI [1.09–1.59]; $P = .005$). The majority of the patients included in this trial underwent D0 dissections, whereas 36% had D1 and only 10% had D2 dissections, raising the question of a possible compensatory effect of chemoradiotherapy in a suboptimally resected population.

More recently, the CALGB-80101 trial compared combination chemotherapy to single-agent treatment sandwiched around a course of chemoradiation as used in the Intergroup 0116 trial. In this phase III trial, 826 patients with stage IB–IVA resected gastric cancer were randomized to adjuvant chemotherapy with 5-FU/leucovorin (LV) or to combination chemotherapy with epirubicin, cisplatin, and 5-FU (ECF) before and after combined modality treatment. Results, currently available in abstract form only, demonstrate no difference in overall survival between the 2 chemotherapy regimens, with median survival reported as 37 and 38 months, respectively ($P = .80$).

The role of adjuvant chemoradiation and chemotherapy following adequate surgery (D2 lymph node dissection) was evaluated in the Adjuvant Chemoradiation Therapy in Stomach Cancer (ARTIST) trial, a phase III study randomizing 458 patients to postoperative therapy consisting of chemotherapy alone (6 cycles of capecitabine and cisplatin) or chemotherapy and chemoradiation (2 cycles capecitabine and cisplatin followed by concurrent capecitabine and radiation therapy with 2 subsequent cycles of capecitabine and cisplatin). The results of this trial showed similar disease-free survival (DFS) with the addition of radiation therapy compared with chemotherapy alone (3-year DFS of 78.2% and 74.2%, $P = .86$). In subgroup analysis, however, patients with node-positive disease treated with radiation and chemotherapy demonstrated a DFS benefit as compared to those treated with only chemotherapy (3-year DFS of 77.5% vs. 72.3%, $P = .03$). To confirm this finding, a prospective trial restricted to node-positive patients is currently in process (ARTIST II).

The benefit of postoperative chemotherapy alone was demonstrated in the Adjuvant Chemotherapy Trial of S-1 for Gastric Cancer (ACTS-GC) study, a Japanese trial in which postoperative patients with D2 nodal dissection were randomized to receive S-1 (a combination of the oral fluoropyrimidine tegafur with the dihydropyrimidine dehydrogenase inhibitors 5-chloro-2,4-dihydroxypyridine, and potassium oxonate) or observation (9). The investigators reported a significant improvement in 5-year survival from 61% with surgery alone to 71% with the addition of S-1 (HR = 0.66; 95% CI [0.54–0.82]). The utility of adjuvant chemotherapy with S-1 in non-Japanese populations is uncertain, however. Clinical trials performed with this agent in Western populations with advanced disease have shown less benefit, and the drug is not available in North America. A second, more recent Asian trial conducted in South Korea, China, and Taiwan investigated adjuvant combination chemotherapy in 1035 patients with stage II–IIIb gastric cancer who had undergone gastrectomy and D2 lymph node dissection (capecitabine and oxaliplatin adjuvant study in stomach cancer [CLASSIC] trial). Patients were randomized postoperatively to capecitabine plus oxaliplatin for 6 months versus observation. Three-year DFS was prolonged in the chemotherapy arm, with 74% of patients remaining disease free as compared to 59% in the observation arm ($P < .0001$). No difference in overall survival was seen at the 34-month analysis, but may be demonstrated with continued follow-up.

A recent meta-analysis in resected gastric cancer compared adjuvant chemotherapy to observation and demonstrated an overall survival benefit with chemotherapy (10). This study retrieved single-patient data from 17 randomized clinical trials that completed accrual before 2004,

thus not including the positive results from the ACTS-GC or CLASSIC trials. Adjuvant chemotherapy was associated with a statistically significant benefit in terms of overall survival (HR = 0.82; 95% CI [0.76–0.90]; $P = .001$) and DFS (HR = 0.82; 95% CI [0.75–0.90]; $P = .001$). The mortality hazard was reduced by 18%, with an absolute improvement in survival of 6% observed at 5 years, maintaining this improvement through 10 years. This finding, as well as results from the ACTS-GC and CLASSIC trials, support the use of adjuvant chemotherapy in resected gastric cancer.

There are ongoing phase III clinical trials further exploring multimodality therapies. For example, the CRITICS study is investigating the value of adding postoperative radiation therapy to chemotherapy as compared to chemotherapy alone. The trial, based in the Netherlands, has a targeted recruitment of 788 patients with stage IB–IVA gastric cancer. Randomization is to perioperative chemotherapy with 3 cycles of epirubicin, cisplatin, and capecitabine (ECX) before and after surgery, versus 3 cycles of neoadjuvant ECX followed by adjuvant radiation with concurrent cisplatin and capecitabine. It is anticipated that recent and current trials will inform future practice.

In summary, patients with localized and likely resectable gastric cancer should be offered multimodal therapy with curative intent. Surgical treatment should provide adequate gastric resection with at least D1 dissection and removal of >15 regional nodes. Sequencing of therapies is often center- and sometimes surgeon-specific. Resected patients with stage IB or greater cancer should be considered for postoperative adjuvant therapy. As T and/or N stage increases, we would favor incorporation of combined modality therapy, but chemotherapy alone is an acceptable strategy. Based on available data, single-agent fluoropyrimidine therapy ± platinum is a reasonable systemic treatment. Preoperative chemotherapy with a fluoropyrimidine and a platinum ± epirubicin might also be considered, with additional adjuvant treatment offered following resection, based on surgical and pathology findings.

## Locally Advanced Unresectable and Metastatic Gastric Cancer

D.K. is a 35-year-old man without significant past medical history who presented with chest pain. He was initially evaluated at the emergency department and underwent a complete cardiology workup, which was negative. Subsequently, with a diagnostic suspicion of dyspepsia, he was initiated on treatment with a proton pump inhibitor, without clinical response. In the following 2 weeks, he began to complain of pain in a band-like region across the upper abdomen, along with bloating and burping. He also noted the presence of fevers and night sweats. His primary care physician ordered an abdominal US that revealed the presence of multiple liver lesions. A CT scan of the chest, abdomen, and pelvis confirmed the presence of >30 low-attenuation liver lesions, an enhancing mass arising from the lesser curvature of the stomach, and multiple enlarged lymph nodes along the gastrohepatic ligament. A US-guided biopsy of one of the liver lesions was positive for undifferentiated carcinoma. An endoscopy was subsequently performed and visualized a large, fungating, ulcerated mass arising in the cardia and extending into the gastric body and the lesser curvature of the stomach. Biopsies were positive for anaplastic carcinoma. IHC staining for HER2/neu on the stomach lesion was negative. Laboratory studies demonstrated mildly decreased hemoglobin of 10.6 g/dL, a normal creatinine value of 0.7 mg/dL, and abnormal liver function tests relevant for aspartate transaminase (AST) of 42 IU/L, alanine transaminase (ALT) of 79 IU/L, and alkaline phosphatase (ALK) of 194 IU/L, with total bilirubin within the normal range. DK was referred to medical oncology with the diagnosis of stage IV gastric cancer. At the initial visit, the performance status of the patient was Eastern Cooperative Oncology Group (ECOG) 1 and his pain was well controlled with a regimen of long-acting morphine. Following discussion with the patient and family, it was decided to initiate chemotherapy with a regimen combining intravenous epirubicin and oxaliplatin and oral capecitabine.

## Evidence-Based Case Discussion

The standard treatment for patients diagnosed with locally advanced, unresectable, or metastatic gastric cancer is systemic chemotherapy administered with palliative intent. This approach is based on several meta-analyses performed to assess the value of chemotherapy on quality of life and overall survival, the 2 main therapeutic endpoints in this patient population. The most recent update of this series of meta-analyses from the Cochrane Collaboration published in 2010 shows a significant benefit in survival for chemotherapy versus best supportive care (BSC) (11 vs. 4.3 months; HR = 0.37; 95% CI [0.24–0.55]). Moreover, the average quality-adjusted survival was longer in the group of patients randomized to chemotherapy compared with the BSC group. Of note, between 10% and 24% of patients treated with chemotherapy were alive after 2 years. These results dictate that further phase III studies evaluating therapeutic interventions in advanced gastric cancer require a control chemotherapy arm (11).

Numerous drugs have demonstrated single-agent activity in gastric cancer including 5-FU and oral fluoropyrimidine agents (S-1 and capecitabine); topoisomerase inhibitors (irinotecan, etoposide); taxanes (paclitaxel, docetaxel); platinum analogs (cisplatin, oxaliplatin, carboplatin); anthracyclines (doxorubicin, epirubicin); and antibiotics (mitomycin-C). Although the majority of these drug agents show only modest single-agent activity, with response rates in the range of 20–30%, these data suggest

classes of drugs to be considered for combination therapy. Clinical trials in the advanced setting have addressed 2 important questions: (1) Is combination chemotherapy superior to single-agent therapy? and (2) Which drugs should be incorporated into combination chemotherapy regimens?

Several meta-analyses have provided the answer to the first question. The medical literature consistently demonstrates that combination chemotherapy is superior to single-agent treatment in terms of overall survival (HR = 0.82; 95% CI [0.74–0.90]), progression-free survival, and response rate, the latter 2 measures often correlating with improvement or maintenance of quality-of-life measures. Various combinations have shown significant activity, with relatively tolerable toxicity. Cisplatin and 5-FU (CF) often serve as a comparator or backbone in the majority of regimens studied. Other agents or classes of drugs combined with or added to this backbone include the anthracyclines, taxanes, and topoisomerase inhibitors. The most studied 3-drug regimens include ECF and docetaxel, cisplatin, and 5-FU (DCF). A total of 580 patients were randomized in a phase III clinical trial to receive ECF or mitomycin, cisplatin, and 5-FU (MCF) as first-line treatment in advanced disease. The overall response rate (42.4% and 44.1%, P = .692) and median survival (9.4 and 8.7 months, P – .315) were not statistically different between the 2 regimens (12). However, ECF was judged to be better tolerated, with activity similar to MCF. Despite ECF not having been compared to CF in a phase III trial, ECF was selected for further development and has become an accepted standard regimen. Conversely, the DCF regimen was compared with CF in a phase III clinical trial showing a statistically significant prolongation time to progression (5.6 vs. 3.7 months; P < .001) and survival (9.2 vs. 8.6 months; P = .02). The toxicity of the DCF combination is concerning, however, with 82% of the patients developing grade 3/4 neutropenia and 29% febrile neutropenia (13). This effect is attenuated when patients treated with DCF receive granocyte-colony stimulating factor (G-CSF) as secondary prophylaxis. Modification to the DCF regimen, with 5-FU administered as continuous infusion and dose reductions to docetaxel and cisplatin, has been shown to reduce toxicity while maintaining efficacy in a phase II trial (14).

Regarding the use of fluoropyrimidine analogs, 2 Japanese studies have shown noninferiority of the combination of cisplatin plus S-1 compared to cisplatin plus infusional 5-FU. Finally, an irinotecan-based regimen combining 5-FU and folinic acid was compared in a phase III trial to the CF regimen, with both treatments found to be equivalent in terms of time to progression and survival.

The REAL-2 study evaluated the substitution of oxaliplatin for cisplatin, and capecitabine for infusional 5-FU. This study, involving 1002 patients, had a 2 × 2 factorial design where patients were assigned to ECF, EOF (substituting oxaliplatin for cisplatin), ECX (substituting capecitabine for 5-FU), and EOX (substituting both oxaliplatin and capecitabine), and was sample sized for noninferiority assumptions. The results demonstrated that oxaliplatin was equivalent to cisplatin, as was capecitabine to infusional 5-FU. Of some interest, the EOX combination was superior to standard ECF. A second randomized phase III clinical trial addressed the equivalence of capecitabine and infusional 5-FU added to cisplatin with a similar noninferiority design. In this study, patients were randomized to receive CF or cisplatin plus capecitabine (CX), and the response rate was statistically superior for those patients receiving CX compared to CF (41% vs. 29%, $P$ = .03). However, no differences were seen for the primary end points of this trial, progression-free survival (5.6 vs. 5 months) or overall survival (10.5 vs. 9.3 months) (15). A meta-analysis combining 1318 patients treated with an oral fluoropyrimidine versus infusional 5-FU from these 2 studies observed that overall survival was superior for those receiving capecitabine (16).

The suitability of 3-drug combinations to treat advanced gastric cancer is dependent on the general health and functional status of the patient, and only patients with high performance status should be considered for such regimens. Although 2-drug regimens have shown lower response rates as compared to 3-drug combinations, many are quite active as described in phase II/III clinical trials in the first-line setting (Table 7.2).

Therefore, 2-drug regimens may also be considered in those patients not suitable for polychemotherapy based on lower performance status, comorbid conditions, advanced age, or previous intolerance to chemotherapy.

Targeted agents have been evaluated in advanced gastric cancer, with varying degrees of success. Following the discovery of the overexpression of HER2 in gastric cancer, a logical therapeutic consequence was the application of agents known to target this pathway. The ToGA trial was a phase III multicenter study conducted in 130 institutions worldwide evaluating the cisplatin–fluoropyrimidine doublet with or without trastuzumab in advanced, untreated, HER2 positive gastric cancer (17). A total of 584 patients were enrolled. Those receiving trastuzumab had improved survival as compared to controls (13.8 vs. 11.1 months; HR = 0.74; 95% CI [0.60–0.91]; $P$ = .0046). This trial led to the approval of trastuzumab for use in HER2+, metastatic gastric cancer. Tyrosine kinase inhibitors targeting HER2, including lapatinib, are currently undergoing evaluation in combination with chemotherapy in the first-line setting.

Epidermal growth factor receptor (EGFR) inhibition has not demonstrated a clinical benefit when added to first-line cytotoxic chemotherapy in metastatic disease. A phase III trial involving treatment with capecitabine and cisplatin with or without cetuximab failed to show a difference in progression-free survival or overall survival between the 2 groups, and patients receiving cetuximab experienced an increase in grade 3 and 4 toxicities (18).

Agents targeting the vascular endothelial growth factor (VEGF) pathway (bevacizumab, sorafenib, and ramucirumab) continue to be evaluated in the metastatic setting in first- and second-line therapy. The addition of bevacizumab to cytotoxic chemotherapy in the first-line setting was studied in the avastin in gastric cancer (AVAGAST) trial. The trial randomized 387 patients to cisplatin and capecitabine with bevacizumab or placebo. The results showed a statistically significant improvement in overall response rate (46% vs. 37.4%) and progression-free survival (6.7 vs. 5.3 months) favoring bevacizumab, but without an improvement in overall survival (19).

Ramucirumab, a vascular endothelial growth factor receptor 2 (VEGFR-2) antagonist, has shown efficacy in the second-line setting in 2 phase III studies. The first trial involved 355 patients with advanced gastric cancer who had progressed on first-line chemotherapy. Patients were randomized to ramucirumab (8 mg/kg every 2 weeks) or placebo. An improvement in median survival was noted in the ramucirumab arm, with patients surviving for 5.2 months compared to 3.8 months in those who received placebo ($P$ = .047). The major toxicity in treated patients was hypertension, with a severity of grade 3 or greater occurring in 8% of patients receiving ramucirumab. The second trial involved the combination of ramucirumab with paclitaxel as compared to paclitaxel monotherapy in 665 patients with advanced gastric cancer who had progressed within 4 months following first-line therapy with a platinum and fluoropyrimidine. An improvement in median survival was observed in the combination arm compared to single-agent paclitaxel, with median survival of 9.6 months and 7.4 months, respectively ($P$ = .0169). There was an improved response rate in the combination arm, 28% versus 16% ($P$ = .001) as well as an increase in grade 3 toxicities, with greater rates of neutropenia (40.7% vs. 18.8%), leukopenia (17.4% vs. 6.7%), hypertension

**Table 7.2** Activity of 2-Drug Combination Regimens in Gastric Cancer Based on Data Extracted From Phase II and III Clinical Trials

| Treatment | N | RR (%) |
| --- | --- | --- |
| 5-FU/leucovorin/oxaliplatin | 112 | 34 |
| 5-FU/leucovorin/cisplatin | 110 | 27 |
| 5-FU/leucovorin/irinotecan | 172 | 32 |
| 5-FU/doxorubicin | 49 | 27 |
| Docetaxel/cisplatin | 158 | 26 |
| Docetaxel/oxaliplatin | 71 | 38 |
| Docetaxel/capecitabine | 44 | 39 |
| Cisplatin/5-FU | 165 | 26 |
| Cisplatin/capecitabine | 160 | 41 |
| Cisplatin/S-1 | 153 | 54 |
| Cisplatin/paclitaxel | 41 | 51 |

FU, fluorouracil; RR, response rate.

(14.1% vs. 2.4%), and fatigue (7.0% vs. 4.0%). As a result of these trials, ramucirumab was approved by the Food and Drug Administration (FDA) in April 2014 for the treatment of gastric cancer following progression on first-line chemotherapy.

Irinotecan has also been evaluated in the second-line setting as a single agent and as part of combination therapy. One randomized phase II clinical trial compared single-agent irinotecan to BSC and observed a significant survival advantage for the treated group. Irinotecan when combined with fluorouracil and leucovorin (FOLFIRI) displayed activity and was shown to be tolerable in a single-arm phase II trial. Other single-arm phase II trials with 2-drug regimens such as irinotecan–capecitabine, irinotecan–docetaxel, docetaxel–capecitabine, and FOLFOX show very similar median progression-free (approximately 4 months) and overall survival times (approximately 9 months). This observation suggests that it is not the particular agent or combination but adequate patient selection and good performance status that are essential in decision making for treatment in the second-line setting.

In conclusion, while the incidence of gastric cancer is declining in Western countries, the mortality associated with this disease remains high. Surgery is the only curative treatment for this malignancy. Multimodality approaches that include the use of chemotherapy and radiation therapy are needed in those with resectable disease to increase the fraction of those cured with this malignancy. In the advanced disease setting, systemic therapy, typically chemotherapy combinations with or without targeted agents, is the best option to improve quality of life and extend survival. Treatment selection should be based on the performance status of the patient and goals of therapy. Finally, improvement in our knowledge of the molecular biology of gastric cancer has led to the use of new treatments for this disease. Further investigation and characterization of the molecular basis of this disease will expand options for therapy, with resultant improvements in outcome.

## REVIEW QUESTIONS

1. Which of the following statements about the incidence of gastric cancer is *true*?

   (A) The incidence of gastric cancer in the United States has increased since 1976
   (B) The frequency of gastric cancer occurring within the cardia has decreased since 1976
   (C) The incidence of gastric cancer is far greater in Japan, China, and Korea than in North America
   (D) The incidence of gastric cancer is distributed evenly throughout the world

2. Traditional risk factors for the development of gastric cancer include all of the following *except*:

   (A) *Helicobacter pylori* infection
   (B) Tobacco exposure
   (C) High-salt diet
   (D) Vitamin C exposure
   (E) Obesity

3. A 45-year-old woman presents after a recent diagnosis of metastatic gastric cancer involving the peritoneum and the liver. She reports being diagnosed with a T1N1 lobular adenocarcinoma of the breast 5 years ago and received breast conservation therapy with adjuvant chemotherapy. She also reports that her mother and maternal grandfather were diagnosed with gastric cancer prior to the age of 50 years. A mutation in which of the following genes is likely present?

   (A) *BRCA 2*
   (B) *E cadherin*
   (C) *BRCA 1*
   (D) *p53*
   (E) *PTEN*

4. A 65-year-old man presented to his primary care provider with 3 months of epigastric abdominal pain and weight loss. A CT scan of the abdomen and pelvis with oral and IV contrast reveals a mass within the body of the stomach with perigastric lymphadenopathy. An esophagogastroduodenoscopy with concurrent endoscopic ultrasound was performed revealing an ulcerative lesion within the body of the stomach with lymphadenopathy along the greater curvature of the stomach. A forceps biopsy of the stomach lesion and a fine needle aspiration of the lymph node both revealed adenocarcinoma. The case is presented at a multidisciplinary tumor board. The malignancy is felt to be surgically resectable and the patient is an appropriate surgical candidate. All of the following are appropriate first-line treatment options *except*:

   (A) Perioperative chemotherapy with epirubicin, cisplatin, and 5-fluorouracil (5-FU) and total gastrectomy and lymph node dissection
   (B) Total gastrectomy and lymph node dissection followed by postoperative chemoradiation using 5-FU
   (C) Total gastrectomy and a D2 lymph node dissection followed by adjuvant chemotherapy using capecitabine or 5-FU
   (D) Total gastrectomy and lymph node dissection followed by observation

*The following vignette applies to Questions 5 and 6*

A 62-year-old man with a history of obesity and GE reflux disease was recently diagnosed with metastatic gastric cancer following a 2-month history of epigastric pain and fatigue. He remains symptomatic from the disease and is not capable of working but spends <50% of time in bed. He wishes to pursue cancer-directed treatment.

5. Further diagnostic evaluation should include which of the following?

    (A) MRI of the brain
    (B) Immunohistochemical (IHC) staining for HER2-neu expression
    (C) Mutational analysis for epidermal growth factor receptor mutation
    (D) Bone scan
    (E) No further evaluation indicated at this time

6. For the aforementioned patient, treatment with all of the following regimens are reasonable *except:*

    (A) Cisplatin and 5-fluorouracil (5-FU)
    (B) Oxaliplatin and 5-FU
    (C) Docetaxel, cisplatin, and 5-FU
    (D) Irinotecan and 5-FU

7. A 68-year-old man with metastatic gastric cancer presents for evaluation regarding further treatment options after progression on first-line chemotherapy. Which of the following statements regarding second-line chemotherapy is *correct*?

    (A) The majority of therapy trials in this setting demonstrate median progression-free survivals of approximately 4 months and a median overall survival of approximately 9 months
    (B) Ramucirumab, alone or in combination with paclitaxel, is a reasonable palliative therapy
    (C) Irinotecan has shown clinical benefit as a single agent and in combination therapy
    (D) All of the above statements are correct

## REFERENCES

1. Surveillance, Epidemiology, and End Results (SEER) Program, (www.seer.cancer.gov) Research Data (1973–2011). 2013, Cancer statistics, National Cancer Institute.
2. Parkin DM. International variation. *Oncogene.* 2004;23(38): 6329–6340.
3. Blot WJ, Devesa SS, Kneller RW, Fraumeni JF Jr. Rising incidence of adenocarcinoma of the esophagus and gastric cardia. *JAMA.* 1991;265(10):1287–1289.
4. Shah, MA, Kelsen DP. Gastric cancer: a primer on the epidemiology and biology of the disease and an overview of the medical management of advanced disease. *J Natl Compr Canc Netw.* 2010 Apr;8(4):437–447.
5. Gravalos C, Jimeno A. HER2 in gastric cancer: a new prognostic factor and a novel therapeutic target. *Ann Oncol.* 2008;19(9): 1523–1529.
6. Nadauld LD, Ford JM. Molecular profiling of gastric cancer: toward personalized cancer medicine. *J Clin Oncol.* 2013;31(7): 838–839.
7. hang JS, Lim JS, Noh SH, et al. Patterns of regional recurrence after curative D2 resection for stage III (N3) gastric cancer: implications for postoperative radiotherapy. *Radiother Oncol.* 2012;104(3): 367–373.
8. Macdonald JS, Smalley SR, Benedetti J, et al. Chemoradiotherapy after surgery compared with surgery alone for adenocarcinoma of the stomach or gastroesophageal junction. *N Engl J Med.* 2001;345(10):725–730.
9. Sakuramoto S, Sasako M, Yamaguchi T, et al.; ACTS-GC Group. Adjuvant chemotherapy for gastric cancer with S-1, an oral fluoropyrimidine. *N Engl J Med.* 2007;357(18):1810–1820.
10. Paoletti X, Oba K, Burzykowski T, et al. Benefit of adjuvant chemotherapy for resectable gastric cancer: a meta-analysis. *JAMA.* 2010;303(17):1729–1737.
11. Wagner AD, Unverzagt S, Grothe W, et al. Chemotherapy for advanced gastric cancer. *Cochrane Database Syst Rev.* 2010;(3):CD004064.
12. Ross P, Nicolson M, Cunningham D, et al. Prospective randomized trial comparing mitomycin, cisplatin, and protracted venous-infusion fluorouracil (PVI 5-FU) With epirubicin, cisplatin, and PVI 5-FU in advanced esophagogastric cancer. *J Clin Oncol.* 2002;20(8):1996–2004.
13. Van Cutsem E, Moiseyenko VM, Tjulandin S, et al.; V325 Study Group. Phase III study of docetaxel and cisplatin plus fluorouracil compared with cisplatin and fluorouracil as first-line therapy for advanced gastric cancer: a report of the V325 Study Group. *J Clin Oncol.* 2006;24(31):4991–4997.
14. Chi Y, Ren JH, Yang L, et al. Phase II clinical study on the modified DCF regimen for treatment of advanced gastric carcinoma. *Chin Med J.* 2011;124(19):2997–3002.
15. Kang YK, Kang WK, Shin DB, et al. Capecitabine/cisplatin versus 5-fluorouracil/cisplatin as first-line therapy in patients with advanced gastric cancer: a randomised phase III noninferiority trial. *Ann Oncol.* 2009;20(4):666–673.
16. Okines AF, Norman AR, McCloud P, et al. Meta-analysis of the REAL-2 and ML17032 trials: evaluating capecitabine-based combination chemotherapy and infused 5-fluorouracil-based combination chemotherapy for the treatment of advanced oesophago-gastric cancer. *Ann Oncol.* 2009;20(9): 1529–1534.
17. Bang YT, Van Cutsem E, Feyereislova A, et al. Trastuzumab in combination with chemotherapy alone for treatment of HER-2 positive advanced gastric cancer or gastro-esophageal junction cancer (ToGA): a phase 3, open label, randomised controlled trial. *Lancet.* 2010; 9742(376):687–697.
18. Lordick F, Kang YK, Chung HC, et al. Capecitabine and cisplatin with or without cetuximab for patients with previously untreated advanced gastric cancer (EXPAND): a randomised, open-label phase 3 trial. *Lancet Oncol.* 2013;14(6):490–499.
19. Ohtsu A, Shah MA, Van cutsem E, et al. Bevacizumab in combination with chemotherapy as first-line therapy in advanced gastric cancer: a randomized, double-blind, placebo-controlled phase III study. *J Clin Oncol.* 2011;29(30):3968–3976.

# 8

# *Pancreatic Cancer*

YUE C. WANG, DONGXIN LIU, AHMED A. EID, AND AIHUA EDWARD YEN

## EPIDEMIOLOGY, RISK FACTORS, NATURAL HISTORY, AND PATHOLOGY

Pancreatic cancer is the second most common gastrointestinal malignancy with 12.2 cases per 100,000 population in the United States, and it is the fourth most common cause of cancer related deaths in men and women. In 2014, there were 46,420 estimated new cases diagnosed and 39,590 estimated deaths from pancreatic cancer (1). The incidence of pancreatic cancer increases with age, rising steeply from age 50 years and peaking around age 70 years. The disease is extremely unusual in patients younger than 30 years and rarely occurs before age 50 years. Men are 30% more likely to develop pancreatic cancer than women. There are racial and socioeconomic differences in the incidence of pancreatic cancer: The incidence is higher in African Americans than in whites or Asian American/ Pacific Islanders and also higher in those with lower socioeconomic status. Despite substantial international variation, geographical differences do not affect pancreatic cancer incidence in the United States.

The exact causes of pancreatic cancer are not well understood; however, there are several factors known to increase the risk. The most important risk factor for pancreatic cancer is age. People in the eighth decade of life experience a risk approximately 40 times that of those in the fourth decade. Cigarette smoking is another important risk factor for pancreatic cancer with a relative risk of at least 2. The risk increases proportionally with greater cigarette use and returns to baseline 5–10 years after smoking cessation. Diet also appears to be a risk factor: Diets rich in red or processed meat seem to be associated with the development of pancreatic cancer, whereas fruits and vegetables seem to have a protective effect. Obesity is fairly consistently linked with pancreatic cancer with 20% higher risk. Other possible risk factors for pancreatic cancer include coffee and alcohol consumption, use of aspirin and nonsteroidal anti-inflammatory drugs (NSAIDs), low 25-hydroxy-vitamin D, and *Helicobacter pylori* infection. However, these relationships are not consistent across studies. Several medical conditions, such as diabetes and chronic pancreatitis, have been shown to be associated with increased risk of pancreatic cancer. Genetic factors play an important role in the development of pancreatic cancer. An estimated 5–10% of pancreatic cancer cases result from a hereditary genetic predisposition. Mutations of *BRCA2/BRCA1* are perhaps the most studied, but other less common genetic syndromes that have been linked to pancreatic cancer include hereditary pancreatitis, hereditary nonpolyposis colon cancer (HNPCC), multiple endocrine neoplasia, familial melanoma with *p16* mutation, Peutz–Jeghers syndrome, Gardner syndrome, von Hippel–Lindau syndrome, and ataxia telangiectasia. Other noninherited genetic alterations have been implicated in pancreatic cancer development as well. More than 80% of resected pancreatic cancers harbor an activating point mutation of *KRAS*. Several tumor suppressor genes such as *CDKN2A*, *p53*, and *DPC4* are frequently inactivated in this cancer.

Pancreatic cancer is a highly lethal disease with a 6% 5-year survival rate when all stages are taken together. This fact is highlighted when looking at the discordance between its incidence and mortality. Its incidence rate is ranked twelveth, but it is the fourth leading cause of cancer death in the United States. The poor prognosis of pancreatic cancer is due, in part, to a delay in diagnosis and a low resection rate. Approximately 80% of patients have already developed local or distant metastasis at the time of diagnosis, prohibiting the chance of curable resection. Chemotherapy and radiation therapy offer only modest survival benefits for those patients. Even for those who undergo surgical resection, the 5-year survival is only

25–30% for node-negative disease and 10% for node-positive disease due to the fact that most of them will develop recurrence within 2 years.

The pancreas consists of exocrine and endocrine components, and pancreatic cancers can arise from either portion. More than 90% of pancreatic cancers are adenocarcinomas derived from ductal cells of the exocrine portion, of which two thirds occur in the head of the pancreas, and one third occurs in other parts of the pancreas such as the body or tail. A variety of other malignant and premalignant tumors may arise from the ductal epithelia of the pancreas. Malignant lesions include acinar cell carcinoma, cystadenocarcinoma, giant cell carcinoma, adenosquamous carcinoma, and carcinosarcoma among others. Pancreatic intraepithelial neoplasia as well as intraductal papillary mucinous neoplasms and mucinous cystic neoplasm are thought to be precursors of invasive ductal adenocarcinoma. Pancreaticoblastoma arises from multipotential cells that can differentiate into mesenchymal, endocrine, or acinar cells, and it occurs primarily in children. Other uncommon pancreatic tumors including small cell carcinoma, schwannoma, leiomyosarcoma, liposarcoma, and malignant fibrous histocytoma can also arise in the pancreas.

Pancreatic neuroendocrine tumors (PNETs) are rare. They arise from the islet cells of the pancreas. Functional endocrine tumors are named after the hormone or the peptide they secrete. Insulinomas are the most common, followed by gastrinomas, glucagonomas, VIPomas, and somatostatinomas in terms of frequency. Nonfunctional PNETs (NF-PNETs) are not associated with an excess production of any hormone or peptide. PNETs have metastatic potential but are relatively slow growing with better survival as compared to ductal adenocarcinoma of the exocrine pancreas.

## STAGING

Pancreatic cancer is staged by using tumor/node/metastasis (TNM) classification, which is based on the extent of tumor and involvement of local and distant structures. The 7th edition of the American Joint Committee on Cancer (AJCC) staging of endocrine and exocrine pancreatic tumors is shown as follows.

| AJCC 7th Edition Staging System for Pancreatic Cancer | |
| --- | --- |
| **Stage** | **Definition** |
| 0 | Carcinoma in situ (Tis) without regional lymph nodes (N0) or distant metastasis (M0) (Tis N0 M0) |
| IA | Tumor limited to the pancreas (≤2 cm) (T1) without regional lymph nodes (N0) or distant metastasis (M0) (T1 N0 M0) |
| IB | Tumor limited to the pancreas (>2 cm) (T2) without regional lymph nodes (N0) or distant metastasis (M0) (T2 N0 M0) |
| IIA | Tumor extends beyond the pancreas but without involvement of the celiac axis or the superior mesenteric artery (T3) and also without regional lymph nodes (N0) or distant metastasis (M0) (T3 N0 M0) |
| IIB | Tumor with T1–3 with regional lymph nodes metastasis (N1) but without distant metastasis (M0) (T1–3 N1 M0) |
| III | Tumor involves the celiac axis or the superior mesenteric artery (unresectable primary tumor) (T4) with or without regional lymph nodes metastasis (Tany) but without distant metastasis (T4 Nany M0) |
| IV | Tumor with distant metastasis (M1) (Tany Nany M1) |

AJCC, American Joint Committee on Cancer.

## CASE SUMMARIES

### Resectable Pancreatic Adenocarcinoma

G.S. is a 61-year-old woman with a 70-pack-year history of smoking who presented with constant dull abdominal pain for the last few months. Two weeks prior to presentation, she noticed dark tea-colored urine, clay-colored white stools, and yellowing of her eyes and skin. She also complained of progressive fatigue, loss of appetite, and unintentional weight loss of 30 lbs during the last several months. She denied fever, chills, emesis, shortness of breath, chest pain, or urinary symptoms. She denied regular alcohol consumption as well. Her past medical/surgical history was only significant for hypertension. Her physical examination was remarkable for icteric sclerae, jaundice, and periumbilical tenderness on deep palpation without rebound or guarding. Blood tests showed markedly elevated total and direct bilirubin (10.9 and 9.7 mg/dL, respectively) with a modest elevation of her alkaline phosphatase and transaminases. Complete blood count (CBC), basic metabolic panel (BMP), amylase, and lipase were within normal limits. A CT scan of the abdomen and pelvis revealed an ill-defined heterogeneous mass in the pancreatic head measuring approximately 2.5 × 2.6 × 2.7 cm with marked dilatation of the common bile duct as it narrowed to complete/near-complete occlusion at the level of the pancreatic head. Intrahepatic biliary ductal dilation was also observed. No arterial involvement, hepatic lesions, or abdominal lymphadenopathy was seen. The serum CA19–9 was elevated to 221.57 U/mL (reference range = 0–37 U/mL).

Because pancreatic adenocarcinoma was highly suspected, endoscopic ultrasonography (EUS) and EUS-guided fine-needle aspiration (FNA) biopsy were performed and revealed a T3 N0 M0 pancreatic adenocarcinoma (stage IIA). On the basis of a discussion in a multidisciplinary tumor board, G.S. was judged to be a good candidate for surgical resection. She underwent a complete (R0) resection and started adjuvant chemotherapy with gemcitabine 6 weeks after the surgery.

## Evidence-Based Case Discussion

G.S. represents a patient with early-stage, resectable pancreatic adenocarcinoma (stage IIA). While her history of cigarette use, abdominal pain, and weight loss are concerning for cancer, these features are nonspecific, which is often the case. CT scan and EUS helped to stage her cancer and the diagnosis was confirmed by EUS-guided biopsy. Because the cancer did not involve any vascular structures and there were no distant metastases, she was treated with surgical resection followed by an adjuvant therapy.

The diagnosis of pancreatic cancer is often made on the basis of history, imaging studies, and laboratory tests (Figure 8.1). There are no good screening tests for pancreatic cancer, and therefore, the possibility of an early diagnosis of pancreatic cancer is hampered by the nonspecificity and

subtle onset of symptoms. Pain is the most common presenting symptom, typically midepigastric in location with radiation to the back or right upper quadrant if bile duct obstruction is present. When the cancer is located in the head of the pancreas, obstructive jaundice is the most characteristic sign. Patients usually notice jaundice, pruritus, the darkening of urine, and lightening of the color of stools. Significant weight loss is another characteristic feature of pancreatic cancer. Other common presenting symptoms include fatigue, anorexia, nausea, vomiting, early satiety, constipation, and glucose intolerance. Migratory thrombophlebitis and venous thrombosis (Trousseau's sign) occur with high frequency in patients with pancreatic cancer and could be the first manifestation. Depression is found to be more common in patients with pancreatic cancer. Physical examination may reveal temporal wasting, jaundice, Virchow's node (left supraclavicular node), palpable gallbladder (Courvoisier's sign), hepatomegaly, or ascites.

Routine laboratory findings in pancreatic cancer are usually nonspecific such as elevated bilirubin; elevated alkaline phosphatase and transaminases levels; elevated

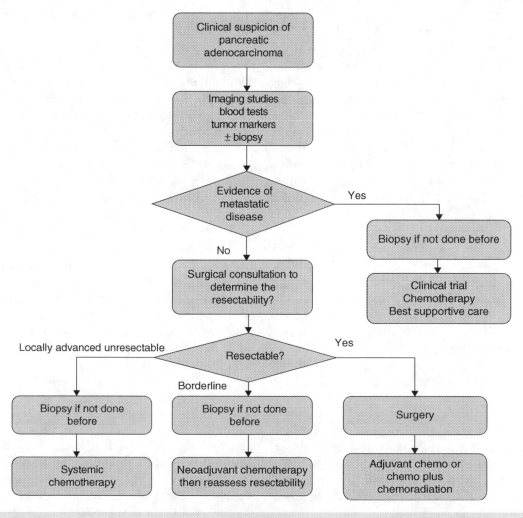

**Figure 8.1**

Algorithm of diagnosis and treatment for resectable pancreatic adenocarcinoma.

amylase and/or lipase; coagulopathy; thrombocytosis; and a low serum albumin level due to malnutrition. Several tumor markers such as CA19–9, CA125 or carcinoembryonic antigen (CEA) may be elevated in pancreatic cancer, but they all lack sensitivity and specificity. CA19–9 is the most extensively studied and clinically useful biomarker for pancreatic cancer. It has no role in screening asymptomatic populations due to its low positive predictive value and has a sensitivity and specificity of 79–81% and 82–90%, respectively, in symptomatic patients. The level of CA19–9 correlates with the tumor burden and is useful in disease monitoring and in assessing the adequacy of resection or chemotherapy. It is recommended to measure serum CA19–9 levels prior to surgery (if bilirubin level is normal), following surgery prior to adjuvant therapy, and for surveillance. It is noteworthy that CA19–9 should be interpreted with caution in patients with obstructive jaundice as it is falsely positive in such patients and can be falsely low in 10% of the population whose tumors are unable to synthesize this cancer antigen.

A number of imaging modalities are available to assist in the diagnosis and staging of pancreatic cancer. These include CT scanning, MRI, endoscopic retrograde cholangiopancreatography (ERCP), transcutaneous ultrasonography (TUS), EUS, and PET scanning. The abdominal CT scan is the mainstay modality for the diagnosis of pancreatic cancer as well as assessing resectability. Dual or triple phase thin-cut spiral CT has approximately 70% sensitivity for tumors <1.5 cm and almost 100% for tumors >1.5 cm. It also has 90% accuracy in the determination of resectability of pancreatic cancer. EUS is excellent for tumor staging and can detect the presence of portal vein invasion, hepatic lesions, and lymph node involvement. Concurrent EUS-guided FNA allows the simultaneous cytological confirmation of pancreatic adenocarcinoma. The role of MRI in pancreatic cancer has been less well studied than CT scanning, but is not superior to spiral CT scanning. PET scanning by itself does not appear to offer additional benefits over a high-quality CT scan, but PET scanning with simultaneous CT imaging may be more sensitive than conventional imaging. Pathological diagnosis can be achieved with EUS-guided or CT-guided biopsy; brush cytology; and forceps biopsy via ERCP, peritoneal cytology, or laparoscopy. If patients have suspected liver metastatic disease based on the initial imaging findings, they should undergo biopsy of liver lesions for confirmation.

Laparoscopy that allows for direct visualization of the liver and peritoneal surfaces with biopsy of any suspicious area can facilitate staging of pancreatic cancer. However, the invasiveness of the procedure and associated risks and complications should be taken into account. Routine staging laparoscopy is controversial and the yield of the procedure depends on surgeons and institutional factors.

Despite the advances in cancer therapy, the treatment of pancreatic cancer still remains challenging. To date,

radical surgical resection of pancreatic adenocarcinoma is the only treatment with survival benefit. Unfortunately, only 10–20% of patients present with resectable disease at the time of diagnosis. Patients with pancreatic adenocarcinoma can be classified into 4 groups: resectable, borderline resectable, locally advanced unresectable, and disseminated (Figure 8.1). In general, stage 0–IIA tumors are usually considered resectable. Some of the stage IIB tumors are also resectable if involved lymph nodes are contained within the resection area. Stage III and IV tumors are generally felt to be unresectable. Studies are underway to determine whether selected patients with locally advanced disease can benefit from neoadjuvant therapy; however, evidence supporting a survival benefit for this approach is limited. For patients with resectable disease, surgical resection followed by adjuvant therapy is the standard of care.

Curative resection options include pancreaticoduodenectomy (Whipple procedure), total pancreatectomy, or distal pancreatectomy depending on the anatomical location of the tumor. Each procedure is associated with its own set of perioperative complications and risks. If a tumor is located in the head of the pancreas, patients will most likely benefit from a Whipple procedure, which consists of removal of the distal half of the stomach (antrectomy); the gallbladder and its cystic duct (cholecystectomy); the common bile duct (choledochectomy); and the head of the pancreas, duodenum, proximal jejunum, and regional lymph nodes with surgical drainage of the distal pancreatic duct and biliary system, usually accomplished through anastomosis to the jejunum. Pancreaticoduodenectomy is considered, by any standard, a major surgical procedure with a significant mortality rate. The leading causes of postoperative mortality are sepsis, bleeding, and cardiovascular events. Many studies have shown that pancreaticoduodenectomy outcomes are significantly better overall if performed at high-volume hospitals than at low-volume centers. Operative mortality of pancreaticoduodenectomy is currently <6% in major surgical centers. Distal pancreatectomy is done for tumors located in the body and tail of the pancreas. Total pancreatectomy is the least commonly done procedure with the highest associated mortality. However, it still remains a viable option in the surgical treatment of pancreatic cancer.

Even with surgery, patients often have poor long-term survival due to early relapse. At least 80% of patients who undergo surgery will develop local or distant relapse within 2 years of surgery. The 5-year survival rate after surgical resection alone is <20%. In an attempt to reduce the incidence of relapse and death, postoperative adjuvant treatment in the form of systemic chemotherapy alone or chemoradiotherapy is commonly administered. Adjuvant therapy should only be considered for patients who have adequately recovered from surgery, and treatment should ideally be initiated within 4–8 weeks after surgery.

There is as yet no consensus regarding the standard of adjuvant therapy after resection of pancreatic cancer. Several multicenter randomized trials have studied the potential benefit of adjuvant therapy with either chemotherapy alone or chemoradiation, whereas very few clinical trials have addressed the benefit of adjuvant radiation alone. The approach is different in the United States and Europe due to inconsistent results and differing interpretations of these trials. Generally, chemotherapy alone is currently the most popular adjuvant therapy in Europe while postoperative chemoradiation is widely adopted in the United States.

The landmark U.S. trial, Gastrointestinal Tumor Study Group (GITSG) 9173, was the first multicenter randomized phase III trial that evaluated the role of postoperative chemoradiotherapy. Forty-three patients after surgical resection were randomized to observation or concomitant chemoradiotherapy (5-fluorouracil [5-FU]) followed by 2-year maintenance 5-FU. There was a significant survival advantage in patients receiving adjuvant chemoradiation compared to observation (median survival = 21 vs. 11 months, $P = .03$) (2). On the basis of the results from this trial, 5-FU-based chemoradiation became the standard of care in the United States for nearly 2 decades.

The survival benefit of adjuvant chemoradiotherapy demonstrated in GITSG 9173 was not replicated by European groups. In a similar phase III trial, European Organization for Research and Treatment of Cancer (EORTC) 40891, 114 patients with resected pancreatic head cancers or periampullary cancers were randomized to observation versus concurrent chemoradiation (3). There was only a trend toward improved survival with chemoradiotherapy in patients with cancer of the pancreatic head (at 2 years, 34% vs. 26%, $P = .099$). Long-term follow-up results from this trial demonstrated no progression-free survival (PFS) or overall survival (OS) benefit of chemoradiotherapy in the adjuvant setting for resected pancreatic adenocarcinoma. The study, however, was criticized for its design and statistical analyses, which minimized its influence in the United States.

European Study Group for Pancreatic Cancer (ESPAC) 1 was the largest reported multicenter phase III trial evaluating the role of adjuvant chemotherapy or chemoradiotherapy in patients with resected pancreatic adenocarcinoma. A total of 541 patients with pancreatic adenocarcinoma undergoing resection were randomized to 1 of 4 arms including concurrent chemoradiotherapy alone (radiation plus FU), chemotherapy alone (FU), and concurrent chemoradiotherapy followed by chemotherapy or observation. Patients who received chemotherapy had a statistically significant survival benefit over patients who did not receive chemotherapy (median survival = 20.1 vs. 15.5 months; HR for death = 0.71; 95% confidence interval [CI] [0.55–0.92]; $P = .009$), while patients in the chemoradiotherapy arm showed worse median survival compared with those who did not receive chemoradiotherapy (median

survival = 15.9 vs. 17.9 months; HR for death = 1.28; 95% CI [0.99–1.66]; $P = .05$) (4). This study concluded that adjuvant chemotherapy has a significant survival benefit in patients with resected pancreatic cancer, whereas adjuvant chemoradiotherapy has a deleterious effect on survival. However, the design and interpretation of this study were complicated, and were subject to criticism.

A subsequent European trial CONKO (Charité Onkologie) 001 randomized 369 patients with early-stage pancreatic cancer to adjuvant gemcitabine for 6 months versus observation after completing surgical resection. There was a statistically significant improvement in disease-free survival (DFS) (13 vs. 7 months; 95% CI [6.1–7.8]; $P < .001$) with adjuvant gemcitabine. However, the improvement in OS was very modest and was not statistically significant (2-month improvement with gemcitabine, 22.8 vs. 20.2 months; $P = .06$) (5). Based on the results from EORTC, ESPAC 1, and CONKO 001 trials, chemotherapy alone is presently recommended after surgical resection, and adjuvant chemoradiotherapy has been essentially abandoned at most European centers.

Unlike in Europe, where chemoradiation fell out of favor as the standard adjuvant treatment for pancreatic cancer, it continued to be widely used and studied in the United States. The Radiation Therapy Oncology Group (RTOG) 9704 is the most recent American phase III study evaluating adjuvant chemoradiotherapy since the landmark GITSG trial was completed. The trial was conducted to evaluate adjuvant therapy of resected pancreatic adenocarcinoma with concurrent FU-based chemoradiation in combination with either gemcitabine or 5-FU. Chemotherapy with either FU or gemcitabine was administered for 3 weeks prior to standard chemoradiation therapy, and similarly for 12 weeks after. Chemoradiation was identical for all patients and administered with a continuous infusion of FU. Five-year analysis of the trial showed no difference in OS between the 2 arms, though patients with pancreatic head adenocarcinoma showed a trend of improved survival with gemcitabine (20.5 vs. 16.9 months; hazard ratio [HR] = 0.82; 95% CI [0.65–1.03]; $P = .09$). Gemcitabine was found to have higher grade 4 hematologic toxicity without a difference in the incidence of febrile neutropenia or infection as compared to FU (14% vs. 1%, $P < .001$) (6).

Similar to the outcome of RTOG 9704, the results of a multicenter randomized European phase III trial, ESPAC-3, found no survival advantage of gemcitabine in the adjuvant chemotherapy setting as compared to FU. A total of 1088 patients with resected pancreatic adenocarcinoma received either bolus FU or gemcitabine. The median survival was 23 months with FU and 23.6 months with gemcitabine (HR = .94; 95% CI [0.81–1.08]; $P = .39$). There were no significant differences in either PFS or global quality-of-life scores between the 2 treatment groups. However, there were more treatment-related serious adverse events in the group of patients who received FU plus folinic acid (14%) compared to those who received gemcitabine (14% vs. 7.5%, $P < .001$) (7).

Although no definitive standard has been established for the adjuvant treatment of resected pancreatic cancer, the acceptable options include systemic chemotherapy alone with gemcitabine or 5-FU, or combined modality concurrent chemoradiotherapy plus additional chemotherapy. When chemotherapy alone is used as adjuvant treatment, gemcitabine is preferred over 5-FU due to its favorable toxicity profile.

## Metastatic (Unresectable) Pancreatic Cancer

P.Y. is a 67-year-old man who came to his primary care physician (PCP) with a complaint of left arm swelling for 3 days. Notably, he had been diagnosed with a right lower extremity deep vein thrombosis (DVT) and pulmonary embolism (PE) 2 months previously, and he was anticoagulated with warfarin. His international normalized ratio (INR) was monitored by his PCP regularly and the level was very stable in the therapeutic range. His other past medical history was limited to treatment for hypertension. He had a 40-pack-year history of smoking and quit after he was diagnosed with PE and DVT. He did not have a family history of cancer.

Further review of systems revealed that for the last 3 months, P.Y. had experienced vague abdominal discomfort with decreased appetite and >10 lbs of unintentional weight loss. His physical examination was remarkable for left arm and right leg swelling and mild abdominal tenderness in the periumbilical area. A venous Doppler ultrasound of the left upper extremity revealed an acute thrombus in the left axillary vein. His anticoagulation was switched from warfarin to enoxaparin.

Trousseau's syndrome was suspected and additional imaging tests were ordered. An abdominal CT scan showed a 3-cm mass in the pancreatic head with evidence of multiple hepatic lesions ranging in size from 1 to 2 cm. Laboratory analysis revealed markedly elevated CA19–9 and CEA levels. Other routine laboratory tests were within normal limits except for a slightly elevated total bilirubin, transaminases, and alkaline phosphatase. A core biopsy of a liver lesion revealed moderately differentiated adenocarcinoma consistent with metastasis from pancreatic carcinoma.

Because of the presence of hepatic metastases, his disease was unresectable and he was referred to the medical oncology clinic, and the patient agreed to initiate palliative chemotherapy.

### Evidence-Based Case Discussion

P.Y. represents a patient with unresectable stage IV pancreatic adenocarcinoma who presented with venous thromboembolism (VTE). More than 50% of patients with pancreatic adenocarcinoma have metastatic disease at the time of diagnosis because of relatively nonspecific symptoms, the lack of an effective screening modality, and the aggressive biology of this cancer. Patients who present with unexplained VTE should undergo a workup for an occult malignancy. Thromboembolic disease associated with malignancy including DVT, PE, and thrombophlebitis migrans, is one of the common complications of pancreatic cancer with an incidence ranging from 17% to 57%, which is one of the highest among all forms of cancer. Anticoagulation with low-molecular-weight heparin rather than vitamin K antagonists is recommended in this setting because of evidence of decreased risk of recurrent clots. There is some evidence that prophylactic anticoagulation reduces the incidence of thromboembolic events and is associated with improved response to chemotherapy and improved OS. Treatment of the underlying cause is also indicated, and the patient was started on palliative chemotherapy.

Despite advancement in the understanding of the molecular biology and pathogenesis of pancreatic cancer, the prognosis of patients with advanced disease remains poor. Progress is hampered in part by the limited sensitivity of pancreatic cancer to current chemotherapy and radiation therapy. The median survival for patients with untreated metastatic disease is about 2–3 months, and 6 months for patients who are treated. Thus, while the efficacy of treatment is modest, supportive care is an extremely important element in the care of these patients.

Symptomatic relief of patients with advanced pancreatic cancer requires consideration of specific palliative techniques in addition to those offered to cancer patients in general. With obstructive jaundice or gastric outlet obstruction, surgical bypass or endoscopic stent placement should be considered. Advanced pancreatic cancer can be especially painful since the tumor commonly invades neural and perineural tissues. Therefore, the pain associated with advanced pancreatic cancer is a major debilitating symptom and needs to be treated aggressively with a combination of long- and short-acting narcotics. In cases of refractory pain, celiac plexus neurolysis is recommended. Nutritional support is required for all patients with pancreatic cancer. Pancreatic enzyme supplements can help ameliorate malabsorption and provide good relief for patients with bloating, diarrhea, or gas after meals. Megestrol acetate, dronabinol, or steroids can help stimulate appetite in some patients. Nutritional supplements are also highly recommended.

Before offering chemotherapy, it is important to determine if the patient is a suitable candidate for chemotherapy (Figure 8.2). Considerations should include performance status (PS); adequate hematological, renal, and hepatic function; nutritional status; and the potential toxicity of the proposed therapy. Patients who are debilitated with poor PS are generally not candidates for chemotherapy

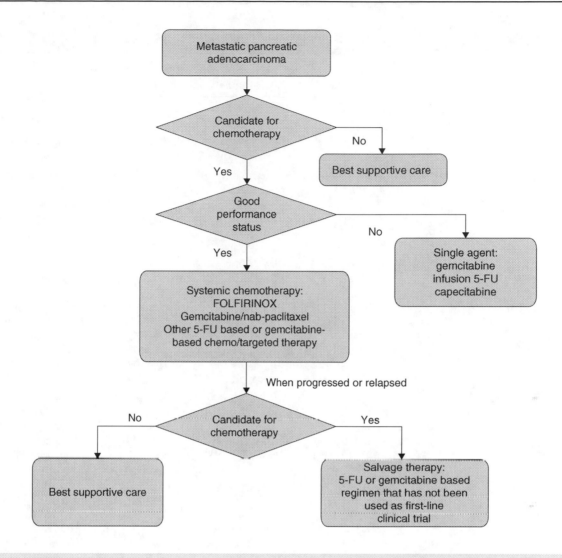

**Figure 8.2**

Algorithm of diagnosis and treatment for metastatic pancreatic adenocarcinoma. 5-FU, 5-fluorouracil; FOLFIRINOX, fluorouracil, leucovorin, irinotecan, and oxaliplatin.

since the likelihood of deriving benefit from chemotherapy is extremely low. For these patients, best supportive care should be the treatment option. However, for patients with good performance status who desire therapy, chemotherapy may be offered in addition to supportive management, or, whenever possible, they should be encouraged to participate in clinical trials. Major phase III clinical trials of front-line chemotherapy for advanced pancreatic cancer including metastatic pancreatic cancer are summarized in the following sections, and outlined in Table 8.1.

## Single-Agent Chemotherapy

Gemcitabine, a pyrimidine antimetabolite inhibiting DNA synthesis, was initially established as first-line treatment for advanced pancreatic adenocarcinoma, following the results of a pivotal trial published in 1997. The study randomized 126 patients with advanced pancreatic cancer to receive either gemcitabine or 5-FU. The patients with gemcitabine showed modest survival advantage (5.6 vs. 4.4 months, $P = .0025$), improved 1-year survival rate (18% vs. 2%) and response rate (24% vs. 5%) over those with 5-FU (8).

Further studies were conducted to determine if fixed-dose rate of gemcitabine improved clinic outcome as compared to standard dose. In the phase III E6201 trial, fixed-dose rate gemcitabine showed no significant difference in response rate compared with standard-dose gemcitabine, and there was only a small trend toward survival improvement with fixed-dose rate regimen (6.2 vs. 4.9 months, $P = .05$) (9). Other monotherapy in pancreatic cancer treatment include capecitabine and continuous infusion 5-FU. Any of these 3 single-agent regimens (gemcitabine, capecitabine, or 5-FU) can be considered for patients with advanced pancreatic adenocarcinoma and poor PS.

**Table 8.1**   Summary of Major Phase III Clinical Trials of Front-Line Chemotherapy for Advanced Pancreatic Adenocarcinoma

| Chemotherapy Regimen | N | Response Rate (%) | PFS (Months) | Median OS (Months) | Reference |
|---|---|---|---|---|---|
| Gem vs. 5-FU | 126 | 23.8 vs. 4.8[a] (P = .0022) | n/a | 5.65 vs. 4.41 (P = .0025) | Burris et al., *JCO* 1997 (8) |
| Gem/5-FU vs. gem | 327 | 6.9 vs. 5.6[b] | 3.4 vs. 2.2 (P = .022) | 6.7 vs. 5.4 (NS) | Berlin et al., *JCO* 2002 (ECOG 2297) |
| IRINOGEM vs. gem | 360 | 16.1 vs. 4.4 (P < .001) | 3.5 vs. 3.0 (NS) | 6.3 vs. 6.6 (NS) | Rocha Lima et al., *JCO* 2004 |
| Gem/pemetrexed vs. gem | 565 | 14.8 vs. 7.1 (P = .004) | 3.9 vs. 3.3 (NS) | 6.2 vs. 6.3 (NS) | Oet, *Ann Onc* 2005 |
| GemOX vs. gem | 326 | 27 vs. 17 (P = .04) 38.2 vs. 26.9[a] (P = .03) | 5.8 vs. 3.7 (P = .04) | 9 vs. 7 (NS) | Louvet et al., *JCO* 2005 (GERCOR/GISCAD) |
| GemCis vs. gem | 195 | 10.2 vs. 8.2[b] | 5.3 vs. 3.1 (P = .053) | 7.5 vs. 6.0 (NS) | Heinemann et al., *JCO* 2006 |
| IRINOGEM vs. gem | 145 | 15 vs. 10 (NS) | 2.8 vs. 2.9 (NS) | 6.4 vs. 6.5 (NS) | Stathopoulos et al., *Br J Cancer* 2006 |
| GemCap vs. gem | 319 | 32 vs. 30[b] | 4.3 vs. 3.9 (NS) | 8.4 vs. 7.2 (NS) 10.1 vs. 7.4 (P = .014) for KPS 90–100 | Herrmann et al., *JCO* 2007 |
| GemOX vs. gem FDR vs. gem | 832 | 9 vs. 10 vs. 6 (NS) | 2.7 vs. 3.5 vs. 2.7 (NS) | 5.7 vs. 6.2 vs. 4.9 (NS) | Poplin et al., *JCO* 2009 (ECOG 6201) (9) |
| GemCap vs. gem | 533 | 19.1 vs. 12.4 (P = .034) | 5.3 vs. 3.8 (P = .004) | 7.1 vs. 6.2 (P = .08) | Cunninghams et al., *JCO* 2009 |
| GemCis vs. gem | 400 | 10.1 vs. 12.9 (NS) | 3.9 vs. 3.8 (NS) | 8.3 vs. 7.2 (NS) | Colucci et al., *JCO* 2010 (GIp) |
| FOLFIRINOX vs. gem | 342 | 31.6 vs. 9.0 (P < .001) | 6.4 vs. 3.3 (P < .0001) | 11.1 vs. 6.8 (P < .0001) | Conroy et al., *JCO* 2010 (ACCORD 11 ) |
| Gem/nab-paclitaxel vs. gem | 861 | 23 vs. 7 (P = 1.1 x 10–10) | 5.5 vs. 3.7 (P = .000024) | 8.5 vs. 6.7 (P = .000015) | Von Hoff et al., *NEJM* 2013 (MPACT) |
| Gem/erlotinib vs. gem | 569 | 8.6 vs. 8.0[b] | 3.75 vs. 3.55 (P = .004) | 6.4 vs. 5.9 (P = .025) | Moore et al., *JCO* 2007 (15) |
| Gem/cetuximab vs. gem | 766 | n/a | 3.5 vs. 3.0 (P = .058) | 5.8 vs. 5.9 (NS) | Philip et al., *JCO* 2007 (SWOG S0202) (16) |
| Gem/erlotinib/bevacizumab vs. gem | 607 | 13.5 vs. 8.6 (P = .057) | 4.6 vs. 3.6 (P = .0002) | 7.1 vs. 6.0 (NS) | Van Cutsem et al., *JCO* 2009 |
| Gem/bevacizumab vs. gem | 602 | 13 vs. 10[b] | 3.8 vs. 2.9 (P = .07) | 5.8 vs. 6.1 (NS) | Kindler et al., *JCO* 2010 (CALGB 80303) (17) |

FDR, fixed dose rate; GERCOR, Groupe Cooperateur Multidisciplinaire en Oncologie; 5-FU, 5-fluorouracil; ECOG, Eastern Cooperative Oncology Group; FOLFIRINOX, fluorouracil, leucovorin, irinotecan, and oxaliplatin; Gem, gemcitabine; GemOX, gemcitabine–oxaliplatin; GISCAD, Gruppo italiano per lo studio dei carcinomi dell' apparato digerente; GemCis, gemcitabine and cisplatin; GemCap, gemcitabine and capecitabine; IRINOGEM, irinotecan and gemcitabine; KPS, Karnofsky performance status; NS, not significant; OS, overall survival; PFS, progression-free survival.
[a]Clinical response; all others refer to tumor response.
[b]*P* value not reported.

## Combination Chemotherapy

Since the approval of gemcitabine by the FDA in 1997 for the management of advanced pancreatic cancer, studies of several combination therapies with cytotoxic agents including FU, capecitabine, oxaliplatin, irinotecan, and pemetrexed have demonstrated no survival benefit compared with gemcitabine alone. A modest survival benefit was observed for the combination gemcitabine plus erlotinib at the expense of increased side effects and high cost of treatment (see Targeted Therapy in this chapter for detailed discussion).

A milestone phase III trial (Actions Concertées dans les Cancers Colo-Rectaux et Digestifs [ACCORD] 11) published in 2009 compared the safety and efficacy of multidrug combination FOLFIRINOX (fluorouracil, leucovorin, irinotecan, and oxaliplatin) with gemcitabine alone in metastatic pancreatic cancer. A total of 342 chemotherapy-naive patients with metastatic pancreatic cancer were randomized and all had Eastern Cooperative Oncology Group (ECOG) PS 0 or 1. The objective response rate (ORR), PFS, and median OS (mOS) were significantly higher with FOLFIRINOX as compared with gemcitabine (ORR = 31.6% vs. 9.4%; PFS = 6.4 vs. 3.3 months, $P < .001$; mOS = 11.1 vs. 6.8 months, $P < .0001$). FOLFIRINOX, however, also produced significantly higher grade 3 or 4 toxicity, including grade 3 or 4 neutropenia (46% vs. 21%), febrile neutropenia (5.4% vs. 1.2%), thrombocytopenia (9.1% vs. 3.6%), sensory neuropathy (9% vs. 0%), and diarrhea (12.7% vs. 1.8%). Despite significantly greater toxicities, patients on FOLFIRINOX experienced a better quality of life than those on gemcitabine alone (10). On the basis of this trial, FOLFIRINOX has been established as a standard front-line therapy for patients with metastatic pancreatic cancer who have excellent PS.

Nab-paclitaxel, an albumin-bound form of paclitaxel has synergic effect with gemcitabine in preclinical models of pancreatic cancer. Previous phase I/II trials demonstrated that the combination of gemcitabine and nab-paclitaxel in advanced pancreatic cancer patients was tolerated and efficacious with a 48% response rate and OS of 12.2 months (11). The safety and efficacy of this combination regimen were further investigated by a multicenter phase III trial Metastatic Pancreatic Adenocarcinoma Clinical Trial (MPACT) that randomized 861 patients with metastatic pancreatic cancer to receive either nab-paclitaxel plus gemcitabine or gemcitabine alone. All patients were treatment naive and had Karnofsky performance status (KPS) ≥70%. The doublet regimen (nab-paclitaxel/gemcitabine) showed significant superiority to single-agent gemcitabine with improved survival (8.5 vs. 6.7 months; $P = .000015$), PFS (5.5 vs. 3.7 months; $P = .000024$), and ORR (23% vs. 7%, $P = 1.1 \times 10^{-10}$). Combination therapy was associated with more grade 3 or 4 adverse events compared with gemcitabine alone including neutropenia (38% vs. 27%), febrile neutropenia (3% vs. 1%), fatigue (17% vs. 7%), peripheral neuropathy (17% vs. 1%), and diarrhea (6% vs. 1%) (12). Based on these results, nab-paclitaxel combined with gemcitabine was approved by the FDA in late 2013 for treatment of patients with metastatic pancreatic cancer who have a good PS.

As shown in Table 8.1, cisplatin combined with gemcitabine did not prolong the survival of patients with metastatic pancreatic cancer compared with gemcitabine alone. However, patients who have a family history of pancreatic cancer or who are carriers of a *BRCA1* or *BRCA2* mutation may uniquely benefit from a platinum-based regimen (13,14).

## Targeted Therapy

Targeted agents offer the promise of being able to tailor therapy to specific cancers and reduce the toxicity of traditional chemotherapy. In pancreatic cancer, targeting the angiogenesis and growth factor pathways has been tested in several clinical trials (Table 8.1). A Canadian phase III study that randomized 569 patients with metastatic or locally advanced pancreatic cancer to receive either gemcitabine with erlotinib or gemcitabine alone showed a small but statically significant survival benefit favoring the combination arm (6.4 vs. 5.9 months; HR = 0.81; 95% CI [0.67–0.97]; $P = .025$). The 1-year survival rate was 24% and 17%, respectively. There was a slight increase in the incidence of grade 3/4 rash and diarrhea with erlotinib (15). On the basis of the results from this trial, gemcitabine combined with erlotinib can be considered an acceptable treatment option for advanced pancreatic cancer. However, the modest survival benefit might be offset by increased toxicity and high cost of treatment.

In contrast, phase III trials of similar design comparing combinations of cetuximab or bevacizumab plus gemcitabine versus gemcitabine alone failed to demonstrate statistically significant improvement in OS (16,17). Trials in which other targeted agents administered in combination with gemcitabine including sorafenib, sunitinib, aflibercept, axitinib, lapatinib, and trastuzumab were similarly negative, failing to demonstrate a survival benefit for the combination.

## Salvage Therapy

For patients who progress or relapse after first-line therapy, those with excellent PS and organ reserve may be candidates for clinical trial or, in the absence of clinical trial availability, may be offered single-agent or combination therapy using potentially active drugs not employed in first-line therapy (e.g., fluoropyrimidine-based therapy for patients who received gemcitabine-based first-line therapy; gemcitabine-based therapy for patients who received fluoropyrimidine-based first-line therapy). Of note, the CONKO-003 phase III trial compared 5-FU/leucovorin/oxaliplatin to 5-FU/leucovorin as a salvage therapy among patients who failed gemcitabine-based first-line treatment and demonstrated that addition of oxaliplatin to 5-FU/leucovorin improved PFS (13 vs. 9 weeks; $P = .012$) and OS (20 vs. 13 weeks; $P = .014$) (18,19).

## Borderline Resectable Disease and Treatment Consideration

Efforts have been made to determine whether an aggressive approach of neoadjuvant therapy followed by surgical resection is effective in borderline resectable pancreatic adenocarcinoma. There is no uniformly accepted set of criteria to define patients with "borderline resectability" and this often varies between or even within institutions. The most common cited definitions include those proposed by the MD Anderson Cancer Center (MDACC) group and the Americas Hepato-Pancreato-Biliary Association/Society for Surgery of the Alimentary Tract/Society of Surgical Oncology (AHPBA/SSAT/SSO). The National Comprehensive Cancer Network (NCCN) adapted the criteria from AHPBA/SSAT/SSO and considered borderline resectable tumors to have the following characteristics listed in Table 8.2 (20). Although lacking high level of evidence, many clinicians prefer neoadjuvant therapy for borderline resectable pancreatic adenocarcinoma given the increased risk of positive margins at initial surgery. The use of neo-adjuvant therapy in borderline resectable disease is highly debatable and the best regimen is unknown at present. Modern chemotherapy regimens such as FOLFIRINOX that offer improved response rates and survival benefit are currently being investigated for neoadjuvant use.

## Locally Advanced Unresectable Disease and Treatment Options

Like the term "borderline resectable," standard criteria for locally advanced unresectable pancreatic adenocarcinoma does not exist. Most experts differentiate borderline resectable tumor from unresectable tumor on the basis of radiographic evidence of limited *superior mesenteric artery* (SMA) involvement (tumor–SMA interface <180° by radiographic prediction) that would allow resection of tumor without reconstruction of the artery (21). While localized unresectable pancreatic cancer and metastatic cancer are staged differently, the standard recommendation for both of these is palliative chemotherapy. The mono- or combination systemic therapy discussed in metastatic setting can be employed for locally advanced unresectable disease. Chemoradiation has been used in the management of unresectable locoregional pancreatic cancer in the past although no strong evidence is available. A recent international phase III study Locally Advanced Pancreatic Cancer (LAP) 07 has shown that chemoradiation did not improve OS or PFS as compared to chemotherapy alone among patients with LAP controlled after induction chemotherapy (22). Occasionally, up-front palliative chemoradiation is considered if patients experience severe pain or have local obstructive symptoms. There is no standard radio

**Table 8.2** Characteristics of Locally Advanced Resectable Pancreatic Adenocarcinoma

No distant metastasis

Venous involvement of the SMV or PV with distortion or narrowing of the vein or occlusion of the vein with suitable vessel proximal and distal, allowing for safe resection and replacement.

Gastroduodenal artery encasement up to the hepatic artery with either short-segment encasement or direct abutment of the hepatic artery, without extension to the celiac axis.

Tumor abutment of the SMA not to exceed >180° of the circumference of the vessel wall.

PV, pulmonary vein; SMA, superior mesenteric artery.
*Source*: National Comprehensive Cancer Network (NCCN) adapted from Americas Hepato-Pancreato-Biliary Association/Society for Surgery of the Alimentary Tract/Society of Surgical Oncology (AHPBA/SSAT/SSO).

sensitizer in this setting. 5-FU, gemcitabine, and capecitabine have been assessed and appear to be effective.

## Metastatic Pancreatic Neuroendocrine (Islet) Carcinoma

R.G. is a 56-year-old man who presented to his PCP complaining of constant and worsening midepigastric pain of several months' duration having previously experienced midepigastric abdominal pain with nausea and bloating for 2 years. Over the previous 12 months, he lost 20 lbs unintentionally. An over-the-counter proton pump inhibitor (PPI) initially improved his symptoms but failed to provide long-term relief. His review of systems was negative except for the gastrointestinal complaints as described. He denied fatigue, vomiting, diarrhea, flushing, shortness of breath, or chest pain. His physical examination was remarkable only for the mild tenderness at the midepigastric area.

A CT of the abdomen and pelvis revealed a 3-cm hypodense mass in the area of the pancreatic head and multiple diffuse liver lesions. Serum measurements of CA19–9, CEA, and alpha-fetoprotein (AFP) were within normal limits as were other laboratory tests including: CBC, metabolic panel, and coagulation profile. However, a serum chromogranin A level was found to be markedly elevated. A CT-guided biopsy of the liver mass was performed, and showed a well-differentiated neuroendocrine carcinoma. Immunohistochemical stains were positive for cytokeratin as well as neuroendocrine markers chromogranin A and synaptophysin.

The case was discussed at the Multidisciplinary Tumor Board, and hepatic artery chemoembolization to the hepatic metastases was recommended. R.G. underwent the procedure and tolerated it well without major complications. After the procedure, he was subsequently treated with octreotide.

## Evidence-Based Case Discussion

This patient presented with a metastatic NF-PNET with nonspecific symptoms of abdominal pain of several years' duration and unintentional weight loss. More than 50% of patients with PNET have metastatic disease at presentation, and nearly all of these have evidence of liver metastases. The diagnosis for this case was made by imaging study (CT scanning), laboratory tests (elevated chromogranin A level) and definitive pathology via biopsy (Figure 8.3). Because the patient was symptomatic and had significant tumor burden in the liver, he required treatment intervention. He was not a surgical candidate due to the bilobar distribution of his liver metastases. As he had hepatic dominant disease, he underwent nonsurgical intervention with hepatic artery embolization in order to reduce the tumor burden in the liver. Octereotide long-acting release (LAR) was also administered for subsequent disease control.

PNETs arise from the exocrine component of the pancreas and constitute <5% of pancreatic neoplasms. The prognosis and OS of patients with these tumors are much better than those for patients with pancreatic adenocarcinomas. The majority of PNETs is sporadic, but may be associated with genetic syndromes such as multiple endocrine neoplasm-1 (MEN-1), von Hippel-Lindau (VHL) disease, neurofibromatosis, and tuberous sclerosis.

PNETs are divided into 2 groups clinically: functional PNETs (F-PNETs) and NF-PNETs. F-PNETs secrete biologically active peptides causing endocrine tumor syndromes. The relatively common tumor syndromes are insulinoma with secretion of insulin, gastrinoma (Zollinger–Ellison syndrome) with secretion of gastrin, glucagonoma with secretion of glucagon, VIPoma with secretion of vasoactive intestinal polypeptide (VIP), and somatostatinoma with secretion of somatostatin. NF-PETs are not associated with a specific hormonal syndrome either because no peptide or hormone is secreted or the substance secreted does not cause specific symptoms. NF-PNETs are more frequent than F-PNETs, and also have worse survival rates than F-PNETs.

In 2000, the World Health Organization (WHO) introduced a histological classification system for gastroenteropancreatic neuroendocrine tumors (GEP-PNETs) including PNETs, in which tumor location, extension, proliferative capacity, and angio-/perineural invasion are assessed. This grading system discriminates well-differentiated endocrine tumors with benign features from well-differentiated and poorly differentiated endocrine carcinomas. Well-differentiated endocrine carcinomas demonstrate slow growth, low proliferative index, and late spread with metastasis. In contrast, poorly differentiated endocrine carcinomas have high Ki67 proliferation and mitotic rate and rapid progression with lymph node and other distant metastases (to liver, bone, lung, etc.). Table 8.3 demonstrates the WHO 2010 definitions of well-differentiated and poorly differentiated PNETs. All PNETs are staged using the same AJCC TNM staging system as mentioned earlier.

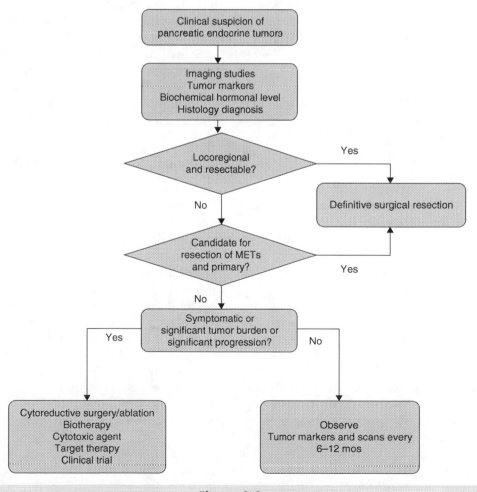

**Figure 8.3**

Algorithm of diagnosis and treatment for pancreatic endocrine tumor.

**Table 8.3** Classification of PNETs

| Differentiation | History Grade | Gastroenteropancreatic NETs |
| --- | --- | --- |
| Well-differentiated PNET | Low grade (G1) | <2 mitoses/10 HPF and/or <3% Ki67 |
| Well-differentiated PNET | Intermediate grade (G2) | 2–20 mitoses/10 HPF and/or 3–20% Ki67 |
| Poorly differentiated PNET | High grade (G3) | >20 mitoses/10 HFP and/or >20% Ki67 |

HFP, high-powered fields; NETs, neuroendocrine tumors; PNETs, pancreatic neuroendocrine tumors.

The diagnostic assessment for PNET should include localization of the primary tumor, nodal status, metastatic disease, presence of functional syndrome, histological classification of the tumor, and the familial genetic background (Figure 8.3). Imaging studies are essential for the management of patients with PNETs. Conventional imaging techniques such as CT, MRI, and ultrasound (US) are still the most commonly used modalities. For identifying patients with liver metastases, high-resolution spiral CT and MRI are much more sensitive than US. EUS/FNA is useful for tissue diagnosis to distinguish PNETs from adenocarcinoma and also to localize tumors not imaged with conventional studies. EUS is more effective at localizing intrapancreatic PNETs, and can identify tumors in approximately 90% of cases, particularly when the tumor is small and frequently missed by conventional studies. Functional imaging studies play an important role in the diagnosis of PNETs. Most PNETs express high levels of somatostatin receptors that have high affinity for the somatostatin analogs such as octreotide. Radiolabeled octreotide scanning (octreoscan) has been proved sensitive and specific for localizing both primary PNETs and metastases. Standard [18]F-fludeoxyglucose (FDG)-PET scanning is not useful because of the low metabolic activity of most PNETs.

In addition to the specific hormone released by a functional PNET, other tumor markers have been used for initial diagnosis and treatment response, most notably the serum chromogranin A that is elevated in 88–100% of PNETs.

Surgery is the only treatment modality with the potential to cure patients with PNETs. Even for PNETs with liver or lung metastases, they should be evaluated for metastectomy or radical resection whenever possible (Figure 8.3). When curative surgery is not feasible, tumor debulking may also render medical therapy more effective by decreasing the secretion of bioactive substances. Most of the PNETs present at an advanced stage; therefore, nonsurgical treatments play a crucial role in controlling symptoms, improving quality of life, and prolonging survival. Nonsurgical treatment approaches include biotherapies with somatostatin analogs and interferons (IFNs), systemic chemotherapy, and targeted therapy. For patients with hepatic dominant diseases, nonsurgical regional hepatic therapy such as hepatic artery embolization, radiofrequency ablation, cryoablation, and radioembolization can

be considered as treatment options. Liver transplantation should be considered in only highly selective patients.

Radiation therapy can be considered as a palliative modality for locally advanced disease or symptomatic metastasis such as bone metastasis. The utilization of radiolabeled octreotide in the treatment of PNETs has been tested, but it remains in the research area and has not been approved by the FDA. Depending on the secreted hormone, symptom management for F-PNETs may significantly improve quality of life. PPI and H2-receptor antagonists are useful in the symptomatic management of gastrinomas. Diazoxide, an insulin-release inhibitor, and glucagon are useful for treatment of insulinoma in conjunction with frequent high-carbohydrate meals. Patients with glucagonoma syndrome are treated symptomatically with insulin.

Somatostatin analogs are the mainstay of treatment for palliating symptoms by decreasing the secretion of peptides and inhibiting tumor growth. Even in patients presenting with metastatic PNET, excellent survival can still be achieved by using a multimodality approach.

## Biotherapy With Somatostatin Analogs and IFNs

Somatostatin is an endogenous inhibitor of various hormones secreted from the endocrine system including insulin, glucagon, and gastrin. However, it has limited clinical use due to its short half-life (<3 minutes). Somatostatin analogs such as octreotide, lanreotide, and pasireotide have been developed and used as the first-line medical therapy for well-differentiated NETs including PNETs. Octreotide was the first available somatostatin analog, and was introduced into clinical practice in 1983 for treatment of neuroendocrine tumors (NETs). The development of a LAR formulation, which is administered monthly, eliminates the need for daily injection. The result of a double-blind, placebo-controlled randomized phase III study (PROMID) treating well-differentiated metastatic midgut NETs with either octreotide LAR or placebo demonstrated that octreotide LAR significantly improved time to tumor progression compared with placebo in patients with functionally active and inactive metastatic midgut NETs (14.3 vs. 6.0 months; HR = 0.34; $P$ = .000072). After 6 months of treatment, stable disease was observed in 66.7% of patients in the octreotide LAR group and 37.2%

of patients in the placebo group. Moreover, the survival benefit of octreotide was independent of tumor functionality, chromogranin A level, PS, or age (23). A follow-up data analysis of long-term survival from the PROMID study demonstrated octreotide LAR extended OS in the subgroup of patients with metastatic midgut NETs that had a low hepatic tumor load (≤10%) but not in those who had a high hepatic tumor load (>10%) (24). The response to octreotide may depend on the cell type. For example, insulinomas are marginally responsive to octreotide, while gastrinomas and VIPomas often respond.

IFN therapy is generally recommended as a second-line approach in treatment of PNETs. IFN-α can inhibit tumor growth by inhibiting proliferation and hormone synthesis as well as by stimulating T cells and natural killer (NK) cell function. As a single agent, IFN-α can produce approximately 40% biochemical response and approximately 10% of objective tumor response (25), but with a less favorable toxicity profile than the somatostatin analogs.

## Cytotoxic Chemotherapy

Systemic chemotherapy has been tested in the treatment of patients with PNETs including 5-FU, capecitabine, dacarbazine, doxorubicin, streptozocin, and temozolomide. Streptozocin is a broad-spectrum antibiotic isolated from *Streptomyces achromogenes* and was the first agent shown to have significant benefit as monotherapy for PNETs (26). A phase II study conducted in 1973 demonstrated a biochemical and a measurable disease (tumor size) response of 64% and 50%, respectively, for patients with metastatic islet cell carcinoma treated with streptozocin (27). Combination of chemotherapeutic agents seems more effective than monotherapy. A trial conducted by ECOG involving 84 patients with PNETs demonstrated a higher response rate (63% vs. 36%) as well as a better complete response rate (33% vs. 12%) in streptozocin/5-FU group as compared to that observed in the streptozocin-only group (28). A streptozocin–doxorubicin combination significantly improved OS compared with streptozocin/5-FU (2.2 vs. 1.4 years; P = .004) (29). For poorly differentiated PNETs, chemotherapy with cisplatin and etoposide is recommended.

## Targeted Therapy

The expression of several signaling pathways has been shown to be enhanced in PNETs including vascular endothelial growth factor (VEGF), platelet-derived growth factor (PDGF), and insulin-like growth factor (IGF-1). Accordingly, agents that inhibit the activity of various tyrosine kinases and mammalian target of rapamycin (mTOR) have been assessed for activity against PNETs. In a recent phase III trial, 171 patients with advanced, well-differentiated PNETs (all with documented disease progression) were randomized to treatment with either

sunitinib, a multitargeted TKI (tyrosine kinase inhibitor), or to placebo. The ORR and median PFS were 9.3% and 11.4 months, respectively, in the sunitinib group versus 0% and 5.5 months, respectively, in the placebo group (HR for progression of death = 0.42; 95% CI [0.26–66]; P < .001). The most common grade 3/4 side effects of sunitinib included diarrhea (97%), abdominal pain (7%), neutropenia (12%), hand–foot syndrome (7%), and hypoglycemia (7%) (30). Another therapeutic target is mTOR, a threonine kinase that regulates downstream signaling pathways. In a phase III study, 410 patients with advanced, low- or intermediate-grade, progressive PNETs were randomized to treatment with either everolimus (an mTOR inhibitor) or placebo. Similar to the results of the sunitinib phase III trial, treatment with everolimus was associated with an improved PFS of 11.0 months as compared to 4.6 months in the placebo group (HR for disease progression or death from any cause for everolimus = 0.35; 95% CI [0.27–0.45]; P < .001). The most common side effects (all grades) of everolimus were stomatitis (64%), rash (49%), diarrhea (34%), fatigue (31%), and infections (23%) (31). In both trials, the data on OS have not matured yet. Based on the positive results, sunitinib and everolimus were FDA approved in 2011 for the treatment of PNETs.

## REVIEW QUESTIONS

1. A 62-year-old female presented to the emergency department with 1-month history of worsening back pain. Review of systems revealed an unintentional weight loss of 7 kg in 2 months. The physical examination showed some epigastric tenderness and decreased breath sounds in left lower lung, otherwise no abnormalities. A CT scan demonstrated a 2.4-cm mass in the body of the pancreas and multiple 1–3 cm liver lesions in different lobes, consistent with metastases. An upper endoscopy with endoscopic ultrasound-directed biopsy of the pancreases mass was positive for adenocarcinoma. CA19–9 was elevated (89 U/mL). Hydrocodone/acetaminophen (10–325 mg) every 4–6 hours PRN was started for pain control. She has an Eastern Cooperative Oncology Group performance status of 1. The patient asks you about treatment advice. Which of the following would you recommend?

   (A) Gemcitabine-alone chemotherapy
   (B) Combination therapy of 5-fluorouracil (5-FU)/leucovorin plus irinotecan and oxaliplatin (FOLFIRINOX)
   (C) Gemcitabine-based chemotherapy followed by concurrent chemoradiotherapy
   (D) No therapy and referral to hospice

2. The aforementioned patient was started with appropriate first-line chemotherapy. Except for 1 episode

of grade 4 neutropenia without fever and grade 2 diarrhea, she tolerated therapy relatively well. After 6 cycles of treatment, a restaging CT scan showed the pancreatic tumor had increased in size from 2.4 cm to 3.1 cm, and 2 new liver metastases. The CA 19–9 rose to 115 U/mL from 89 U/mL. She still has intermittent back and right upper quadrant pain, which is relieved by hydrocodone/acetaminophen (10 mg/325 mg) PRN. Her performance status is 1. The patient would like to continue treatment and asks you about the options. What is your recommendation?

(A) Fluorouracil/oxaliplatin combination chemotherapy
(B) Clinical trial or gemcitabine/nab-paclitaxel chemotherapy
(C) Chemoradiation therapy for the primary tumor
(D) No other choices of systemic chemotherapy and referral to hospice

3. A 52-year-old previously healthy male was incidentally found to have a 1.5-cm mass in the pancreatic head in a CT scan. He has no symptoms. Physical examination was unremarkable. CA19–9 was normal at 43 U/mL. A CT of the chest, abdomen, and pelvis with pancreatic protocol confirmed the pancreatic mass, and there were no enlarged lymph nodes, vascular involvement, or distant metastasis. He was referred to surgery and underwent pancreaticoduodenectomy. The surgery was uneventful. The final pathology demonstrated pancreatic adenocarcinoma, stage IA (pT1N0); margins free. He is now in your clinic 6 weeks after surgery and has recovered well. His performance status is 1. He asks you about further treatment plans. Which of the following would be the best choice?

(A) Surveillance
(B) Adjuvant 5-fluorouracil concurrently with radiotherapy
(C) Concurrent chemoradiation followed by systemic chemotherapy
(D) Radiation alone

4. The aforementioned patient wants to avoid radiotherapy. What would you recommend?

(A) 5-Fluorouracil/leucovorin
(B) Gemcitabine
(C) Erlotinib
(D) Bevacizumab

5. A 55-year-old female with diabetes presented with a 4-month-history of epigastric pain. Physical examination demonstrated epigastric tenderness on palpation. A CT scan showed 4.5 × 5.2 cm mass in the pancreatic neck/proximal body, which encases the common bile duct, proximal superior mesenteric artery (>180°)

and superior mesenteric vein. The pancreatic duct is dilated to 6 mm and the common bile duct is dilated to 10 mm. An endoscopic ultrasound confirmed the pancreatic mass and biopsy was positive for adenocarcinoma. CA 19–9 was 51 U/mL. Her pain is improved with morphine sulfate. She has excellent performance status. What would be the next appropriate step?

(A) Pancreatoduodenectomy
(B) Up-front concurrent chemoradiation
(C) Chemotherapy such as FOLFIRINOX or gemcitabine/nab-paclitaxel
(D) Radiotherapy

6. A 65-year-old male with a past medical history of pancreatic cancer presented to the emergency room for a 3-day history of intractable abdominal pain, nausea, vomiting, and anorexia. He had been diagnosed with locally advanced pancreatic adenocarcinoma (stage III cT4N1M0) 2 years ago and was deemed unresectable. He was initially treated with FOLFIRINOX and had a partial response after 6 cycles of treatment. Irinotecan was discontinued after cycle 6 due to diarrhea. He continued with FOLFOX and received the last treatment 10 days ago. On physical examination, he appears chronically ill and cachectic; epigastric tenderness is present on palpation; his abdomen is soft but moderately distended. A CT scan shows stable dimensions of the primary tumor size, but also the presence of new moderate ascites. No colonic obstruction or perforation is seen. A diagnostic paracentesis is performed, and the fluid cytology is positive for malignant cells. He was treated supportively with IV fluid, antiemetics, and narcotics but the symptoms persisted. An esophagogastroduodenoscopy was done showing a large amount of gastric residual debris with partial duodenal obstruction. His Eastern Cooperative Oncology Group performance status is 3. Which of the following should be considered to improve patient's quality of life?

(A) Enteral stent placement
(B) Gastrojejunostomy (duodenal bypass)
(C) Celiac plexus neurolysis
(D) A and C

7. A 68-year-old female was incidentally found to have 3 liver masses in both lobes with a maximum diameter of 2 cm on a CT scan for evaluation of a possible kidney stone. A repeat CT scan with liver protocol confirmed the finding and also reveals a 3.2-cm mass in the pancreatic body. Routine laboratory tests including liver function tests were normal. A US-guided fine needle aspiration and biopsy of the liver mass demonstrated a well-differentiated metastatic neuroendocrine tumor with 2 mitoses per 10 high-powered fields

and 3% Ki67. Her performance status was 0 and she had no symptoms such as diarrhea or flushing; her initial pain symptoms resolved spontaneously. Which of the following would you recommend?

(A) Interventional radiology referral for liver chemoembolization
(B) Everolimus
(C) Streptozocin and doxorubicin
(D) Obtain a baseline chromogranin A level, then observe and repeat imaging in a few months

8. A 51-year-old male presented with right upper quadrant pain and left hip pain for 2 months. A CT scan showed 4-cm mass in the pancreatic body; innumerable hepatic lesions in both lobes, the largest one measures 8 × 6.5 cm; prominent round sclerotic lesions are seen through the visualized bony spine and pelvis, including the bilateral iliac bones, femurs, and sacrum, measuring between 1 and 2 cm. A fine needle aspiration and biopsy of the liver mass revealed a low-grade neuroendocrine tumor with 6 mitotic counts per 10 high-powered fields and 6% Ki67. His performance status was 0–1. Which of the following would be the best course of action?

(A) Everolimus
(B) FOLFIRINOX
(C) Gemcitabine
(D) Observe and repeat image in 3 months

9. In the preceding case, if the fine needle aspiration and biopsy of the liver mass instead revealed a high-grade neuroendocrine tumor with 25 mitoses per 10 high-powered fields and 30% Ki67, and the patient has a good performance status, which of the following would you recommend?

(A) Everolimus
(B) Sunitinib
(C) Cisplatin/etoposide
(D) FOLFIRINOX

## REFERENCES

1. Siegel R, Ma J, Zou Z, Jemal A. Cancer statistics, 2014. *CA Cancer J Clin.* 2014;64(1):9–29.
2. Kalser MH, Ellenberg SS. Pancreatic cancer. Adjuvant combined radiation and chemotherapy following curative resection. *Arch Surg.* 1985;120(8):899–903.
3. Klinkenbijl JH, Jeekel J, Sahmoud T, et al. Adjuvant radiotherapy and 5-fluorouracil after curative resection of cancer of the pancreas and periampullary region: phase III trial of the EORTC gastrointestinal tract cancer cooperative group. *Ann Surg.* 1999;230(6):776–782.
4. Neoptolemos JP, Stocken DD, Friess H, et al. A randomized trial of chemoradiotherapy and chemotherapy after resection of pancreatic cancer. *N Engl J Med.* 2004;350(12):1200–1210.
5. Oettle H, Post S, Neuhaus P, et al. Adjuvant chemotherapy with gemcitabine vs observation in patients undergoing curative-intent resection of pancreatic cancer: a randomized controlled trial. *JAMA.* 2007;297(3):267–277.
6. Regine WF, Winter KA, Abrams RA, et al. Fluorouracil vs gemcitabine chemotherapy before and after fluorouracil-based chemoradiation following resection of pancreatic adenocarcinoma: a randomized controlled trial. *JAMA.* 2008;299(9):1019–1026.
7. Neoptolemos JP, Stocken DD, Bassi C, et al. Adjuvant chemotherapy with fluorouracil plus folinic acid vs gemcitabine following pancreatic cancer resection: a randomized controlled trial. *JAMA.* 2010;304(10):1073–1081.
8. Burris HA III, Moore MJ, Andersen J, et al. Improvements in survival and clinical benefit with gemcitabine as first-line therapy for patients with advanced pancreas cancer: a randomized trial. *J Clin Oncol.* 1997;15(6):2403–2413.
9. Poplin E, Feng Y, Berlin J, et al. Phase III, randomized study of gemcitabine and oxaliplatin versus gemcitabine (fixed-dose rate infusion) compared with gemcitabine (30-minute infusion) in patients with pancreatic carcinoma E6201: a trial of the Eastern Cooperative Oncology Group. *J Clin Oncol.* 2009;27(23):3778–3785.
10. Conroy T, Desseigne F, Ychou M, et al. FOLFIRINOX versus gemcitabine for metastatic pancreatic cancer. *N Engl J Med.* 2011;364(19):1817–1825.
11. Von Hoff DD, Ramanathan RK, Borad MJ, et al. Gemcitabine plus nab-paclitaxel is an active regimen in patients with advanced pancreatic cancer: a phase I/II trial. *J Clin Oncol.* 2011; 29(34):4548–4554.
12. Von Hoff DD, Ervin T, Arena FP, et al. Increased survival in pancreatic cancer with nab-paclitaxel plus gemcitabine. *N Engl J Med.* 2013; 369(18):1691–1703.
13. Oliver GR, Sugar E, Laheru D, et al. Family history of cancer and sensitivity to platinum chemotherapy in pancreatic adenocarcinoma [abstract]. *Gastrointestinal Cancer Symposium* 2010:180.
14. Lowery MA, Kelsen DP, Stadler ZK, et al. An emerging entity: pancreatic adenocarcinoma associated with a known *BRCA* mutation: clinical descriptors, treatment implications and future directions. *Oncologist.* 2011;16(10):1397–1402.
15. Moore MJ, Goldstein D, Hamm J, et al. National Cancer Institute of Canada Clinical Trials Group. Erlotinib plus gemcitabine compared with gemcitabine alone in patients with advanced pancreatic cancer: a phase III trial of the National Cancer Institute of Canada Clinical Trials Group. *J Clin Oncol.* 2007;25(15): 1960–1966.
16. Philip PA, Benedetti J, Fenoglio-Preiser C, et al. Phase III study of gemcitabine plus cetuximab versus gemcitabine in patients with locally advanced or metastatic pancreatic adenocarcinoma: SWOG S0205 study. *J Clin Oncol.* 2007;25(18S):LBA 4509 (abstract)
17. Kindler HL, Niedzwiecki D, Hollis D, et al. Gemcitabine plus bevacizumab compared with gemcitabine plus placebo in patients with advanced pancreatic cancer: phase III trial of the Cancer and Leukemia Group B (CALGB 80303). *J Clin Oncol.* 2010;28(22):3617–3622.
18. Pelzer U, Kubica K, Stieler J, et al. A randomized trial in patients with gemcitabine refractory pancreatic cancer. Final results of the CONKO 003 study. *J Clin Oncol.* 2008;26(May 20 suppl):4508.
19. Saif MW. New developments in the treatment of pancreatic cancer. Highlights from the "44th ASCO Annual Meeting." Chicago, IL, USA. May 30–June 3, 2008. *JOP.* 2008;9(4):391–397.
20. Tempero, MA, Malafa, MP, Behrman SW et al. Pancreatic adenocarcinoma, NCCN clinical practice guidelines in oncology. version 1.2014, http://www.nccn.org/professionals/physician_gls/f_guidelines.asp#pancreatic.
21. Katz MH, Marsh R, Herman JM et al. Borderline resectable pancreatic cancer: need for standardization and methods for optimal clinical trial design. *Ann Surg Oncol.* 2013;20(8):2787–2795.
22. Hammel P, Huguet F, Van Laethem J-L et al. Comparison of chemoradiotherapy (CRT) and chemotherapy (CT) in patients with a locally advanced pancreatic cancer (LAPC) controlled after

4 months of gemcitabine with or without erlotinib: final results of the international phase III LAP 07 study. 2013 ASCO meeting. *J Clin Oncol.* 2013;31(suppl;abstr LAB4003).

23. Rinke A, Müller HH, Schade-Brittinger C, et al.. Placebo-controlled, double-blind, prospective, randomized study on the effect of octreotide LAR in the control of tumor growth in patients with metastatic neuroendocrine midgut tumors: a report from the PROMID Study Group. *J Clin Oncol.* 2009;27(28):4656–4663.

24. Arnold R, Wittenberg M, Rinke A et al. Placebo controlled, double blind, prospective, randomized study on the effect of octreotide LAR in the control of tumor growth in patients with metastatic neuroendocrine midgut tumors (PROMID): results on long-term survival. 2013 ASCO meeting. *J Clin Oncol.* 31, 2013 (suppl;abstr 4030).

25. Dirix LY, Vermeulen PB, Fierens H, et al. Long-term results of continuous treatment with recombinant interferon-alpha in patients with metastatic carcinoid tumors——an antiangiogenic effect? *Anticancer Drugs.* 1996;7(2):175–181.

26. Murray-Lyon IM, Eddleston AL, Williams R, et al. Treatment of multiple-hormone-producing malignant islet-cell tumour with streptozotocin. *Lancet.* 1968;2(7574):895–898.

27. Broder LE, Carter SK. Pancreatic islet cell carcinoma. II. Results of therapy with streptozotocin in 52 patients. *Ann Intern Med.* 1973;79(1):108–118.

28. Moertel CG, Hanley JA, Johson LA. Streptozocin alone compared with streptozocin plus fluorouracil in the treatment of advanced islet-cell carcinoma. *N Engl J Med.* 1980;303:1189–1194.

29. Moertel CG, Lefkopoulo M, Lipsitz S, et al. Streptozocine-doxorubicin, streptozocin-fluorouracil or chlorozotocin in the treatment of advanced islet-cell carcinoma. *N Engl J Med.* 1992;326(8):519–523.

30. Raymond E, Dahan L, Raoul JL, et al. Sunitinib malate for the treatment of pancreatic neuroendocrine tumors. *N Engl J Med.* 2011;364:501–513.

31. Yao JC, Shah M, Tetshide I, et al. Everolimus for advanced pancreatic neuroendocrine tumors. *N Engl J Med.* 2011;364(6):514–523.

# 9

# *Neuroendocrine Cancer*

DANIEL DA GRACA, MARIELA BLUM, GARRETT R. LYNCH, AND JUN ZHANG

## EPIDEMIOLOGY, RISK FACTORS, NATURAL HISTORY, AND PATHOLOGY—GENERAL

The incidence of neuroendocrine tumors (NETs) is increasing. An analysis of the Surveillance, Epidemiology, and End Results (SEER) database demonstrated a 4.8-fold increase in incidence of NETs during the past 3 decades. In the United States, the annual age-adjusted incidence rose from 1.09 to 5.25 per 100,000 people between 1973 and 2004. This increase is likely due to the improvement in classification of these tumors, and the widespread use of endoscopy for cancer screening (1). The risk of developing NETs is higher in African American individuals (overall NET incidence of 6.50) compared to whites. NETs comprise a diverse group of neoplasms that share morphological and cellular features, biological behavior, and functional abilities. NETs originate in tissues derived from neuroectoderm and endoderm. These tumors can develop from various endocrine glands, such as the pituitary, the parathyroid, or the neuroendocrine portions of the adrenal glands, as well as in endocrine islets within the thyroid or pancreas. They can also develop from endocrine cells found dispersed among the exocrine cells of the digestive and respiratory tracts. NETs can occur in virtually all tissues and organs, but are more frequently located in the digestive tract. Most NETs have endocrine function and secrete peptides and neuroamines that cause clinical syndromes; however, some are clinically silent or nonfunctional until late presentation when mass effects result. Diagnosis of NETs is complex and often requires sophisticated laboratory and scanning techniques (2).

Unlike many other cancers, a unified classification system for NETs does not exist. These tumors share certain features, including their microscopic appearance and immunohistochemistry characteristics, as well as their biology and functions. Given their diversity, a variety of different nomenclature systems have been developed based on organ or embryonic site of origin for use in grading and staging of NETs (3). However, these classification schemas became outdated since it has been observed that patient prognosis is highly dependent on the biological behavior of the tumor and its histological differentiation, rather than its site of origin.

Histologically, NETs are classified based on tumor differentiation (well or poorly differentiated) and tumor grade (grades 1–3), with differentiation being linked to tumor grade. Grading relies mostly on proliferative rate, which can be assessed by the number of mitoses per unit area of tumor or percentage of neoplastic cells immune labeling for the proliferation index Ki67. Low-grade NETs are considered indolent, whereas high-grade tumors behave very aggressively. Intermediate-grade tumors tend to be less predictable, but often follow a moderately aggressive course (3). Well-differentiated NETs are either low or intermediate grade, whereas poorly differentiated NETs are always considered high grade. The pathological diagnosis of NETs is based on morphological and immunohistochemical (IHC) features including positive IHC staining for neuroendocrine markers, which include chromogranin, synaptophysin, and neuron-specific enolase (NSE).

Functionality also should be considered when referring to NETs. Functionality is based on the presence of excess hormone secretion that causes different clinical symptoms. This is particularly important in pancreatic tumors, where such tumors are designated according to their primary hormone production and related clinical syndrome (e.g., insulinomas, gastrinomas, Verner–Morrison syndrome [VIPomas], polypeptideomas, glucagonomas, somatostatinomas, and nonfunctioning islet cell tumors). The current recommended practice is to describe NETs according to their location of primary origin (e.g., pancreas, duodenum, small intestine, etc.), their grade, differentiation, and reference to the resultant hormone secretion or symptoms.

## WELL-DIFFERENTIATED NEUROENDOCRINE TUMORS

### Epidemiology, Risk Factors, Natural History, and Pathology

Oberndofer first coined the term carcinoid (or "Karzinoid") in 1907 to describe all NETs. He chose the term "carcinoid" for these tumors because they grew so slowly that he considered them to be "cancer-like" rather than truly cancerous. In 1929, he reported that some such tumors in the pancreas were not as indolent as previously thought. He used the term neuroendocrine tumors to distinguish these from what most authorities call carcinoids. Today the term carcinoid has been retained and is used synonymously with the term well-differentiated NET, as well as for the low-grade carcinoma associated with the classic carcinoid syndrome.

Carcinoid tumors are the most common endocrine tumors of the gut, with the small bowel being the most common site, followed by the appendix. Carcinoids, however, may also occur in the bronchus, pancreas, rectum, ovary, lung, and thymus. Approximately 2500 new cases of carcinoid tumor are diagnosed annually in the United States. These tumors grow slowly and are often clinically silent for many years before metastasizing. The most common sites for metastases in order of frequency are regional lymph nodes, liver, lung, and bone. Carcinoid tumors may secrete various hormones and vasoactive peptides including adrenocorticotropic hormone, antidiuretic hormone, gastrin, pancreatic polypeptide (PP), somatostatin, serotonin, histamine, and tachykinins. Carcinoid syndrome occurs in <10% of patients with carcinoid tumors. It is related to the secretion of serotonin, histamine, or tachykinins into the systemic circulation resulting in classic symptoms of episodic cutaneous flushing, abdominal cramps, and diarrhea. For gut-derived carcinoid tumors, carcinoid syndrome most commonly occurs in the setting of hepatic metastases that provide access to the systemic circulation. However, hepatic metastases are not necessary for carcinoid syndrome in non-gut-derived carcinoid tumors.

The major clinical manifestations of carcinoid syndrome include the following:

- Cutaneous flushing (90%)
- Gastrointestinal hypermotility with diarrhea (70%)
- Abdominal pain (40%)
- Heart disease (right sided) (37%)
- Severe sweating (15%)
- Bronchial constriction/wheezing (17%)
- Myopathy (7%)
- Pellagra, dermatitis (5%)

Two of these clinical manifestations deserve further comment. Carcinoid heart disease is reported in approximately 50% of all patients with malignant carcinoid syndrome and is severe in approximately 25% of cases. Carcinoid heart disease occurs primarily on the right side of the heart but may involve the left side to a lesser degree. It is caused by serotonin-induced fibrosis of the tricuspid and pulmonary valves, and by fibrous deposits in the endocardium. The tricuspid valve is most commonly affected. These deposits are thought to be responsible for the thickening of the endocardium of the cardiac chambers and papillary muscles. Thickening and deformation of the valve cusps and chordae tendineae can be seen and may result in heart failure, valvular dysfunction, or combined functional lesions.

Another condition that can develop with carcinoid tumors is pellagra. Pellagra is caused by niacin deficiency (vitamin B3) characterized by diarrhea, dermatitis, dementia, and death. It can develop through several mechanisms, but it develops primarily via the action of functioning tumor cells in diverting tryptophan toward serotonin production and thereby away from the niacin production pathway. Anorexia and diarrhea, frequently present in the carcinoid syndrome, reduce the availability of exogenous niacin by decreasing the amount ingested and absorbed. The decreased availability of endogenous and exogenous niacin eventually results in the depressed tissue niacin levels responsible for the development of pellagra.

The occurrence and severity of the carcinoid syndrome are directly related to elevation of serotonin or its metabolites and tumor size. The patient often has a long history of vague abdominal symptoms, a series of visits to his or her primary care practitioner, and referral to a gastroenterologist. Many individuals with carcinoid tumors are initially misdiagnosed with irritable bowel syndrome.

The diagnosis includes a strong clinical suspicion in patients who present with flushing, diarrhea, wheezing, myopathy, or right-sided heart disease. Appropriate biochemical confirmation and imaging studies are often needed to assess disease burden and evaluate primary location.

In clinical practice, the following constitute the best markers for diagnosis and follow-up of carcinoid tumors: chromogranin A, 24-hour urine 5-hydroxyindoleacetic-acid (5-HIAA), gastrin, serotonin, pancreastatin, and NSE.

Commonly used standard imaging techniques include CT (triple-phase studies are required when CT is used in the evaluation of liver metastases), MRI, and octreotide scan. The majority of carcinoid tumors possess high-affinity receptors for somatostatin, and an octreotide scan (radiolabeled somatostatin receptor scintigraphy [SRS]) can be used in diagnosis.

### Staging

Historically, no formal TNM-based staging systems existed for NETs for any anatomical site. In 2010, the

American Joint Committee on Cancer (AJCC) 7th edition for the first time applied TNM-staging system to NETs of all different anatomic sites (4). To exemplify the AJCC staging system, the following table outlines the system for NETs of the colon or rectum.

### AJCC Staging for NETs of the Colon or Rectum

| Stage | Description |
|---|---|
| I | Primary tumor <2 cm in greatest dimension (T1) with invasion of lamina propria or submucosa with no regional lymph node (N0) or distant metastases (M0) |
| IIA | Tumor invades muscularis propria or >2 cm with invasion of lamina propria or submucosa (T2) with no regional lymph node (N0) or distant metastases (M0) |
| IIB | Tumor invades through the muscularis propria into the subserosa or into nonperitonealized pericolic or perirectal tissues (T3) with no regional lymph node (N0) or distant metastases (M0) |
| IIIA | Tumor directly invades peritoneum or other adjacent organs (T4) without lymph node (N0) or distant metastases (M0) |
| IIIB | Any T with regional lymph node metastases (N1); no distant metastases (M0) |
| IV | Any T, any N, with distant metastases (M1) |

AJCC, American Joint Committee on Cancer; NETs, neuroendocrine tumors.

## CASE SUMMARY

### Well-Differentiated NETs

A.C. is a 58-year-old man with a history of gastroesophageal reflux disease (GERD) who had been well until 2 years ago when he developed loose stools. He was treated initially for reflux and his symptoms were attributed to a long-term history of proton pump inhibitors use. Two months prior to evaluation, he became increasingly fatigued. He noticed a metallic taste in his mouth, flushing in his face, sweats, and worsening diarrhea (small-volume stools up to 20 times a day). He also experienced a 33-pound weight loss over a 2-month period. The patient presented to his primary care physician, who admitted him to the hospital with dehydration and malnutrition.

He underwent esophagogastroduodenoscopy (EGD) and colonoscopy, which revealed only telangiectasia. He underwent further evaluation with CT of the chest, abdomen, and pelvis, which revealed numerous poorly defined enhancing lesions throughout the liver, with the largest lesion measuring 12 x 15 cm. Oncology was consulted, and at that time, he denied any dizziness, lightheadedness, fever, or chills. He reported some dysphagia without odynophagia. He denied any nausea, vomiting, or abdominal pain, but had lost 38 pounds in a 4-week period.

His past medical history was positive for GERD, hypertension, hypercholesterolemia, and colonic polyps, and his family history was significant for leukemia. Previous surgical procedures included cholecystectomy and incisional hernia repair. His Eastern Cooperative Oncology Group (ECOG) performance status was 1. He rarely drank alcoholic beverages and denied any illicit drug use. He had smoked cigarettes for 20 years, but stopped 10 years ago. His medications included atenolol, ranitidine, amlodipine, and multivitamin. He has had prior allergic reactions to penicillin and iodine.

On physical examination, he appeared ill. His weight was 193 pounds, and he was afebrile. His blood pressure was 102/71 mm Hg and his pulse was 70 beats per minute. He had no lymphadenopathy. The lung and cardiac examinations were normal. His abdomen was soft with normal bowel sounds and no tenderness or hepatosplenomegaly. Skin and neurologic examinations were normal.

Laboratory test results for hemoglobin and comprehensive metabolic panel were normal, but serum chromogranin A was elevated at 4900 ng/mL (normal value <225 ng/mL) as well as urine 5-HIAA at 361 mg/24 hr (normal value <6 mg/24 hr). Other selective tumor marker results included normal serum levels of neuron-specific enolase, insulin growth factor 1, and gastrin. An octreotide scan was performed, which showed octreotide uptake in the liver, as well as the terminal ileum.

Cytologic examination of a specimen obtained via a CT-guided fine needle aspiration (FNA) biopsy of one of the liver lesions showed metastatic low-grade NET with Ki67 index <3%.

### Evidence-Based Case Discussion

Diarrhea is a common symptom, with multiple causes making determination of its etiology sometimes difficult. Common causes of chronic diarrhea include irritable bowel syndrome, inflammatory bowel disease, malabsorption syndromes, chronic infections, and neoplasm. Irritable bowel syndrome, in particular, should be a diagnosis of exclusion; and patients should initially undergo assessment for "alarm symptoms," such as weight loss, nocturnal diarrhea, rectal bleeding, or anemia. Upper gastrointestinal endoscopy with small bowel biopsy and colonoscopy are indicated and will assist in the diagnosis of the previously mentioned conditions. Our patient's characteristic symptoms of flushing and diarrhea raised the concern for a NET, and biomarker data accompanied by imaging and pathology confirmed the presence of a metastatic low-grade NET with a likely primary in the terminal ileum.

Depending on the results obtained from imaging studies, carcinoid tumors are classified as being locoregional or metastatic disease.

## Therapy for Localized Disease

For localized disease, surgical resection should be performed (5).

*Stomach*: For hypergastrinemic patients (types 1 and 2) with tumor of 2 cm or less, endoscopic resection or observation are recommended. For patients with normal gastrin level (type 3), radical resection should be considered.

*Appendix*: For appendiceal tumors of 2 cm or less, simple appendectomy is recommended, and no further follow-up is required. If the tumor is >2 cm in diameter, CT or MRI of the abdomen/pelvis is recommended. If no distant disease is found, right hemicolectomy with lymph node resection should be performed.

*Small bowel*: For tumors 2 cm or less, segmental resection with operative search for other sites is recommended. If the tumor is >2 cm in size or multifocal, hemicolectomy is advised. If primary is not discovered, mesenteric resection to minimize bowel obstruction should be considered.

*Colon*: For colonic tumors, hemicolectomy with appropriate lymph node resection is recommended.

*Rectal*: For lesions 2 cm or less, transanal or endoscopic resection and regular follow-up is recommended. For tumors >2 cm, abdominoperineal resection or lower anterior resection should be considered.

Figure 9.1 shows an algorithm of the management of well-differentiated NETs.

## Therapy for Unresectable and/or Metastatic Disease

For metastatic disease or unresectable carcinoid tumors in symptomatic patients, somatostatin analogs are indicated for symptom control (5). In the United States, octreotide is the only somatostatin analog approved for the management of carcinoid syndrome. Octreotide comes in 2 forms: immediate release and long-acting release (LAR). When there is a need for immediate symptom control, a subcutaneous rescue injection of short-acting octreotide (100–500 µg every 8–12 hours) should be administered. For long-term treatment, octreotide LAR 20–30 mg IM every 4 weeks should be used. Octreotide LAR is also recommended to control tumor growth in patients with significant tumor burden. This is based on the result of the PROMID study, a placebo-controlled, double-blind phase III trial of 85 treatment naive patients with well-differentiated metastatic midgut NET (42 and 43 patients were randomly assigned to receive octreotide LAR and placebo, respectively), which showed that octreotide LAR significantly lengthened the time to tumor

progression compared with placebo: 14.3 months for octreotide LAR group versus 6 months for placebo group (6). An update of the PROMID study on long-term survival was recently reported. The median overall survival (OS) was not significantly different between 2 treatment arms: OS was not reached in octreotide LAR arm versus 84 months in placebo arm (hazard ratio [HR] = 0.85, 95% confidence interval [CI] [0.46–1.56], $P = .59$). However, this result might have been confounded by patients in the placebo group receiving octreotide LAR after disease progression (7).

Whether symptomatic or not, resection of liver metastases should be considered if feasible. In cases where liver metastases are unresectable, local ablative radiofrequency therapy, cryotherapy, or microwave therapy should be considered. Hepatic regional therapy (arterial embolization, chemoembolization, or radioembolization) or cytoreductive surgery are also available options. If none of these options can be offered, systemic therapy with cytotoxic agents such as interferon, temozolamide, dacarbazine, 5-fluorouracil (5-FU), and capecitabine can be used in patients with progressive metastases. Figure 9.1 provides an algorithm of the management of metastatic disease.

A number of investigational therapies have shown preliminary evidence of activity in patients with advanced carcinoid tumors. These include inhibitors of the vascular endothelial growth factor receptor (VEGFR) pathway (bevacizumab, sunitinib, and sorafenib), as well as inhibitors of mammalian target of rapamycin (mTOR inhibitors). A phase III study (RADIANT-2) comparing octreotide LAR with or without everolimus in patients with advanced carcinoid tumors, and carcinoid syndrome showed improved median progression-free survival in patients treated with octreotide plus everolimus (16.4 vs. 11.3 months, $P = .026$) (8).

## Surveillance

Patients with carcinoid tumors should be reevaluated 3–12 months after resection, and annually thereafter by performing a complete patient history and physical examination as well as CT or MRI imaging studies. Serum chromogranin A and urinary 5-HIAA in 24-hour samples may be used as tumor markers. Octreotide scan is not routinely needed.

For A.C., treatment with octreotide LAR was initiated, and within 2 months, the patient's overall condition improved. He gained approximately 10 lbs and his diarrhea resolved. After 6 months, the patient was back to his baseline weight and was completely asymptomatic. Previously elevated levels of serum chromogranin A and urinary 5-HIAA both declined to near normal. Even though excellent control of the patient's symptoms was achieved with the use of octreotide, surgical resection of

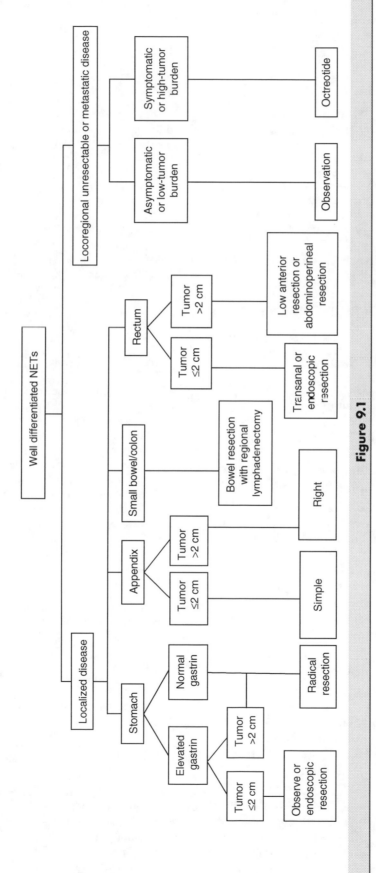

**Figure 9.1**

Therapeutic algorithm of the management of well-differentiated NETs. NETs, neuroendocrine tumors.

**Table 9.1**  Clinical Syndromes Associated With PNETs

| Tumor (Secreted Product) | Clinical Presentation |
|---|---|
| Gastrinoma (gastrin) | Zollinger–Ellison syndrome (ZES) |
| Insulinoma (insulin) | Whipple's triad |
| Glucagonoma (glucagon) | Glucagonoma syndrome |
| Vasoactive intestinal peptidoma | Verner–Morrison syndrome |
| Somatostatinoma (somatostatin) | Somatostatinoma syndrome |
| Well-differentiated NF-PNETs | Mass effect (jaundice, hemorrhage) |
| Poorly differentiated | Mass effect/syndromes reported |

NF-PNETs, neurofibromatosis-pancreatic neuroendocrine tumors.
*Source:* From Ref. (9). Ehehalt F, Saeger HD, Schmidt CM, et al. Neuroendocrine tumors of the pancreas. *Oncologist.* 2009;14(5):456–467.

the hepatic metastases, which has been shown to prolong survival, should be considered.

## PANCREATIC NEUROENDOCRINE TUMORS (INTERMEDIATE GRADE)

### Epidemiology, Risk Factors, Natural History, and Pathology

The adult endocrine pancreas contains "micro-organs" called islets of Langerhans. The average human islet consists of approximately 3000 cells producing insulin (β-cells, 54%), glucagon (α-cells, 34%), somatostatin (δ-cells, 10%), vasoactive intestinal polypeptide (VIP) (δ2 cells), PP cells, and substance P/serotonin (enterochromaffin cells). Pancreatic neuroendocrine tumors (PNETs), or islet cell tumors, are assumed to originate in these islets of Langerhans. In theory, each pancreatic endocrine cell type could give rise to a PNET (9).

PNETs are rare neoplasms. Although the peak incidence is between ages 40 and 60 years, a significant number of patients diagnosed with islet cell tumors are under the age of 35 years. PNETs are classified as functional or nonfunctional. Recent clinical studies suggest that majority (40–90%) of pancreatic NETs are nonfunctioning (10,11). Clinical presentations of PNETs are summarized in Table 9.1.

The pathogenesis of PNETs is poorly understood. The majority of PNETs are sporadic, but PNETs may also be associated with genetic syndromes such as multiple endocrine neoplasia (MEN-1), von Hippel-Lindau (VHL) disease, neurofibromatosis 1 (NF-1), and tuberous sclerosis (TSC) (Table 9.2).

In 2000, the WHO introduced a histological classification system for PNETs. This system was intended to allow benign tumors to be distinguished from malignant tumors. For the WHO classification system, tumor localization, extension, proliferative capacity, and vascular and perineural invasion are assessed (9) (Table 9.3).

**Table 9.2**  Hereditary Syndromes Associated With PNETs

| Genetic Syndrome | Gene Abnormality | Associated NET Type |
|---|---|---|
| MEN 1 | Menin 11q13 | Gastrinoma, insulinoma, thymic |
| MEN 2 | RET | Medullary thyroid carcinoma (CMT) and pheochromocytoma |
| Neurofibromatosis type I | Hamartin 17q11 | Duodenal somatostatinoma |
| VHL disease | pVHL 3q25 | NFNET |
| Tuberous sclerosis | Tuberin | Rarely NFNET, insulinoma, and gastrinoma |
| Familial carotid paraganglioma | 11q | |

MEN, multiple endocrine neoplasia; NET, neuroendocrine tumor; NFNET, nonfunctioning neuroendocrine tumor; PNETs, pancreatic neuroendocrine tumors; VHL, von Hippel-Lindau.
*Source:* From Ref. (9). Ehehalt F, Saeger HD, Schmidt CM, et al. Neuroendocrine tumors of the pancreas. *Oncologist.* 2009;14(5):456–467.

**Table 9.3**  WHO Classification of PNETs

1. Well-differentiated endocrine tumor (WDET)
    1.1. Benign behavior. Confined to the pancreas, <2 cm in diameter, <2 mitosis per 10 HPF, <2% Ki67 positive cells, no angioinvasion or perineural invasion
    1.2. Uncertain behavior. Confined to the pancreas and 1 or more of the following features: >2 cm in diameter, >2 mitosis per 10 HPF, >2% Ki67 positive cells, angioinvasion, perineural invasion
2. Well-differentiated endocrine carcinoma (WDEC)
    2.1. Low-grade malignant
    2.2. Gross local invasion and/or metastases
3. Poorly differentiated endocrine carcinoma (PDEC)
    3.1. High-grade malignant
    3.2. >10 mitoses per HPF

HPF, high-power field; PNET, pancreatic neuroendocrine tumors.
*Source:* From Ref. (9). Ehehalt F, Saeger HD, Schmidt CM, et al. Neuroendocrine tumors of the pancreas. *Oncologist.* 2009;14(5):456–467.

### Staging

Because PNETs do not arise in the luminal gut, separate TNM staging systems are used for PNETs (4).

**AJCC Staging of Pancreatic NETs**

| Stage | Description |
|---|---|
| IA | Tumor limited to the pancreas, ≤2 cm in greatest dimension (T1) without regional lymph node (N0) or distant metastases (M0) |
| IB | Tumor limited to the pancreas, >2 cm in greatest dimension (T2) without regional lymph node (N0) or distant metastases (M0) |

*(continued)*

| Stage | Description |
|-------|-------------|

**AJCC Staging of Pancreatic NETs (continued)**

| Stage | Description |
|-------|-------------|
| IIA | Tumor extends beyond the pancreas, but without involvement of celiac axis or the superior mesenteric artery (T3) without regional lymph node (N0) or distant metastases (M0) |
| IIB | T1, T2, or T3 tumor with regional lymph node metastases (N1); no distant metastases (M0) |
| III | Tumor involves the celiac axis or the superior mesenteric artery (T4; unresectable), any N, without distant metastases (M0) |
| IV | Any T, any N, with distant metastases (M1) |

AJCC, American Joint Committee on Cancer; NETs, neuroendocrine tumors.

## CASE SUMMARY

### Pancreatic Neuroendocrine Tumors

R.B. is a 33-year-old woman who was referred to the outpatient cancer center for further evaluation and therapy of a PNET. The patient had been well until 2 weeks prior to this visit when she developed jaundice and dark urine. She had been having intermittent abdominal pain, nausea, and postprandial diarrhea for 2 months. She presented to the emergency department of an outside hospital where she was found to have elevated liver enzymes. Her total bilirubin was 8.4 mg/dL, direct bilirubin 4.0 mg/dL, alkaline phosphatase 99 IU/L, aspartate aminotransferase (AST) 539 IU/L, and alanine aminotransferase (ALT) 539 IU/L. An ultrasound of the abdomen was performed that showed liver masses with bile duct dilatation. CT of the abdomen confirmed multiple liver masses, bile duct dilatation, and a pancreatic mass with retroperitoneal lymphadenopathy. Two days later, she underwent endoscopic retrograde cholangiopancreatography (ERCP) with fine needle aspiration (FNA) of the pancreatic mass, as well as stent placement in the common bile duct. The ERCP visualized a pancreatic mass involving the head of the pancreas that appeared highly vascular. There was vascular involvement of the splenic and portal vessels. Cytology from the aspirate revealed an NET based on immunohistochemistry that was positive for synaptophysin, S-100, and chromogranin. Ki67 was positive in 50% of the cells and there were 6 mitoses per 10 HPF. Six days later, a colonoscopy was performed, which was normal. A diagnostic laparoscopy with liver biopsy was performed 2 days later. The cytology report from the liver biopsy confirmed a neuroendocrine carcinoma (NECA). The patient presented to the CancerCenter for further recommendation.

On examination, the patient appeared well. Her vital signs were normal. Her abdomen was soft with no tenderness, hepatomegaly, splenomegaly, or palpable masses. The remainder of the examination was normal. Basic laboratory test results, including a complete blood count, electrolytes, glucose, total protein, globulin, albumin, and calcium, as well as tests of coagulation and renal and hepatic function, were normal. Other specific markers were as follows: chromogranin A and neuron-specific enolase were elevated at 970 ng/mL (normal <225 ng/mL) and 58 ng/mL (normal <15 ng/mL), respectively. Serum VIP, gastrin, and urinary 5-HIAA were within the normal range.

### Evidence-Based Case Discussion

R.B. presented with a pancreatic mass and liver metastases. The biopsy was consistent with an NET with 6 mitoses per 10 HPF, a feature consistent with an intermediate-grade NET. Her tumor was nonfunctional, but had she presented with symptoms characteristic of a functional PNET, the diagnostic evaluation described in the next section would have been performed.

### Diagnostic Evaluation of Functional PNETs

The classic description of an *insulinoma* is the Whipple's triad, which includes symptoms of hypoglycemia, a measured low blood glucose concentration, and resolution after the ingestion of glucose. Ninety percent of these tumors are benign. The major symptoms caused by insulinomas are those of hypoglycemia, which include the adrenergic symptoms of nervousness, sweating, palpitation, and diaphoresis.

The gold standard test for diagnoses is a positive 72-hour fasting blood glucose and insulin levels. This test excludes all differential diagnoses of hypoglycemia. Patients with insulinoma have elevated levels of C-peptide. An insulin level >3 µU/mL (and often found to be >6 µU/mL) when blood glucose is <45 mg/dL and an insulin to glucose ratio is 0.3 or greater is diagnostic, reflecting the inappropriate secretion of insulin at the time of hypoglycemia.

Preoperative localization of tumors over 0.5 cm can be achieved with abdominal ultrasound, endoscopic ultrasound, CT, or MRI. SRS is positive in 60% of all benign insulinomas. Percutaneous selective arterial calcium stimulation and portal venous sampling are used when other localization studies fail to identify the tumor.

Although most insulinomas are benign, malignancy might be found in tumors >2 cm. It is important to document any possible site of metastases by CT scan or MRI since this may change the treatment strategy.

*Gastrinomas* are NETs that produce gastrin. The chronic effects from hypergastrinemia result in a marked gastric acid hypersecretion that ultimately causes severe peptic ulcer disease. They are often accompanied by refractory diarrhea and GERD (Zollinger–Ellison syndrome). Fifty to 60% of gastrinomas are malignant.

Diagnosis of a gastrinoma requires measuring fasting gastrin levels (basal level, stimulated level, and gastric acidity). Gastrin levels (basal and stimulated) should be measured after the patient is off proton pump inhibitor therapy for at least 1 week. If the fasting serum gastrin level (FSG) is elevated <10-fold and the gastric pH is <2, then a basal acid output (BAO) measurement should be performed. In patients with Zollinger–Ellison syndrome, serum parathormone, fasting calcium, and prolactin levels should be assessed to rule out MEN-1 (9).

Tumor localization involves upper gastrointestinal endoscopy, CT scan, SRS, or PET Octreotide. If these tests fail to localize the gastrinoma, endoscopic ultrasonography and selective angiography with secretin stimulation and hepatic venous sampling should be considered.

Surgical exploration for gastrinoma should include investigation of the pancreas with intraoperative ultrasonography, duodenal transillumination, and duodenotomy. Laparoscopic approaches are typically not feasible.

*Glucagonomas* are generally large tumors associated with liver metastases. They are characterized by glucose intolerance, weight loss, and a pathognomonic rash called migratory necrolytic erythema. This rash has a characteristic annular pattern of erythema with central crusting and bullae. The diagnosis of glucagonoma requires the demonstration of increased plasma glucagon levels (usually 500–1000 pg/mL, whereas normal is <50 pg/mL) in the presence of symptoms (3).

*VIPomas* are PNETs that secrete VIP that leads to large-volume diarrhea, hypokalemia, and achlorhydria. The diagnosis requires the demonstration of an elevated VIP plasma level.

*Somatostatinomas* are PNETs that can occur in the duodenum or pancreas. Most cases reported in the literature are PNETs containing somatostatin by immunohistochemistry, without a specific somatostatinoma syndrome, which is a classic clinical pentad of diabetes mellitus, cholelithiasis, weight loss, steatorrhea and diarrhea, and hypochlorhydria and achlorhydria.

The diagnosis is made by the presence of a PNET with the appropriated elevated somatostatin hormone assay result (3). For functioning and nonfunctioning tumors, global neuroendocrine parameters such as chromogranin A and neuron-specific enolase should be assessed. SRS, octreotide scan, or other radionucleotide PET should be performed to evaluate octreotide receptor status and localization. Additional imaging modalities include contrast-enhanced ultrasound (CEUS), CT scan, and MRI (9).

## Treatment for Localized Disease

Surgical resection is the optimal treatment for localized PNETs. Any hormone-related symptoms should be addressed prior to resection. For gastrinomas, gastrin hypersecretion may be treated with histamine H2 receptor antagonists or proton pump inhibitors. For insulinomas, stabilization of glucose levels with diet or diazoxide (200–600 mg/d) is advised. Treatment of electrolyte imbalance with intravenous fluid and octreotide (if octreotide scan results are positive) may be useful in patients with VIPoma or glucagonoma.

For insulinomas <2 cm, laparoscopic enucleation is the preferred procedure. Central or distal partial pancreatectomy may be required in certain cases (9). If laparoscopic enucleation is not possible due to the size of tumor or invasion, then pancreaticoduodenectomy or distal pancreatectomy with lymphadenectomy and removal of resectable liver metastases is recommended.

In nonresectable cases, palliative tumor debulking may be justified to achieve hypoglycemic control and may prolong survival. Other procedures such as radiofrequency ablation (RFA), cryotherapy, or transarterial chemoembolization (TACE) for liver metastases can also be considered.

The treatment approach for gastrinomas usually depends on the results of preoperative localization studies. In patients with occult gastrinoma (i.e., no primary tumor or metastases seen on imaging), observation is recommended. Alternatively, if the tumors are identified at surgery, duodenectomy with removal of periduodenal lymph nodes can be performed. Gastrinomas in the head of the pancreas, but not adjacent to the pancreatic duct, should be resected via duodenectomy. Gastrinomas that are deeper or invasive in proximity to the main pancreatic duct should be managed by pancreaticoduodenectomy with periduodenal node dissection. Because most tumors are located in the "gastrinoma triangle" (pancreatic head, duodenum, and surrounding lymph nodes), a distal pancreatectomy allows for removal of the extremely rare distally located gastrinomas. Because primary lymph node gastrinomas have been reported, lymphadenectomy should always be performed, even in the absence of a pancreatic or duodenal primary (12).

Most glucagonomas are malignant, calcified, and located in the tail of the pancreas with regional node involvement. The recommended treatment includes either excision of the tumor with peripancreatic nodal dissection or distal pancreatectomy with resection of lymph nodes and splenectomy.

As with nonfunctioning tumors, depending on the size, location, and invasiveness of the tumor, recommended options for VIPomas are excision, distal pancreatectomy, and resection of peripancreatic lymph nodes and spleen. Pancreaticoduodenectomy with dissection of peripancreatic nodes are recommended for tumors in the head of the pancreas.

Long-acting somatostatin analogs (e.g., octreotide, lanreotide) are generally successful in the initial management of patients with glucagonomas, VIPomas, and in some patients with somatostatinomas (13).

See Figure 8.3 in Chapter 8 for an algorithm for the management of PNETs.

## Management of Locoregional Unresectable Disease and/or Metastatic PNETs

PNETs demonstrate a highly variable growth pattern, with most insulinomas being benign (>85%), whereas >50% of the other symptomatic PNETs and the nonfunctioning

PNETs demonstrate liver metastases (14). Surgical excision of both the primary tumor and metastases should be considered if possible. Observation is recommended for patients with unresectable disease who have low tumor burden and are asymptomatic.

For patients with symptomatic or significant disease progression, there are a few treatment options. The results of 2 phase III trials have demonstrated the effects of inhibitors of multiple tyrosine kinases associated with platelet-derived growth factor receptor (PDGFR), stem cell factor (c-kit), and VEGFR, and inhibitors of the mTOR. A randomized double-blinded trial of sunitinib (an oral multi-targeted tyrosine kinase inhibitor) versus placebo as salvage therapy in advanced, well-differentiated PNET after documented progression (86 patients in the sunitinib group and 85 patients in the placebo group) showed a median progression-free survival of 11.4 months in the sunitinib arm versus 5.5 months for the patients who received placebo. The objective response rate was 9.3% in the sunitinib arm and 0% in the placebo arm (15). Equally promising phase III results have also been reported with the mTOR inhibitor everolimus. Four hundred ten patients with advanced-, low-, or intermediate-grade PNET with recent radiographic progression were randomized to receive oral everolimus (207 patients) or placebo (203 patients) both in conjunction with best supportive care. The median progression-free survival in the everolimus group was 11.0 months as compared with 4.6 months in the control group (the HR for disease progression or death from any cause with everolimus was 0.35, 95% CI [0.27–0.45], $P < .001$). At 18 months' follow-up, the proportion of patients who were alive and free of progression was 34% (CI [26–43]) in the everolimus group versus 9% (CI [4–16]) in the placebo group (16).

For symptomatic or significant disease progression, patients with a positive octreotide scan or elevated biomarkers can be treated with short-acting octreotide of 150–250 mcg subcutaneously 3 times a day. If a symptomatic response occurs, then an initial monthly dose of 20–30 mg octreotide LAR I.M. is recommended. In addition to the improvement of symptoms, recent study demonstrated that somatostatin analogs improve progression-free survival in patients with nonfunctioning PNETs. The CLARINET study is a large phase III trial evaluating the antiproliferative effects of lanreotide in 204 patients with advanced well or moderately differentiated, nonfunctioning gastroenteropancreatic NETs. Forty-five percent of patients recruited in this study had primary pancreatic NETs, an important subgroup of patients not included in the PROMID study. The patients were randomized to receive either 120 mg lanreotide Autogel ($n$ = 101) or placebo ($n$ = 103) every 4 weeks for 96 weeks or until progressive disease (PD) or death. At a time point of 2 years following initiation of treatment, median progression-free survival was not reached in lanreotide arm compared to 18 months in placebo arm (HR = 0.47; 95% CI [0.30–0.73], $P$ = .0002) (17).

Systemic chemotherapy should also be considered in rapidly progressing disease (see Figure 8.3 in Chapter 8: Pancreatic Cancer). A number of chemotherapy agents alone or in combination, such as doxorubicin, streptozocin, 5-fluorouracil [5-FU], temozolamide, and dacarbazine, have established antitumor effects in PNETs. A retrospective analysis of 84 patients with either locally advanced or metastatic disease who received streptozocin, 5-FU, and doxorubicin showed that this regimen was associated with an overall response rate of 39% and median survival duration of 37 months (18). In patients with poorly differentiated PNETs, the chemotherapy regimen used for small-cell lung cancer (SCLC) such as cisplatin and etoposide or its analogs is recommended (13). Recently, a number of newer chemotherapeutic agents with some efficacy in malignant PNETs have been described. Temozolamide-based regimens represent an alternative to streptozocin-based therapy in patients with advanced PNETs. Temozolamide has been commonly administered as a single agent or in combination with capecitabine (13).

For patients with incurable liver metastases and dominant metastases, treatment options include hepatic regional therapies such as arterial embolization, radioembolization, chemoembolization, and local ablative therapy (RFA, cryotherapy, microwave), which may provide cytoreductive therapy of the liver metastases (14).

In the case of R.B., as described previously, she was initiated on chemotherapy with adriamycin, streptozocin, and 5-FU, which resulted in a sustained progression-free interval.

## ADRENOCORTICAL CARCINOMA

### Epidemiology, Risk Factors, Natural History, and Pathology

Adrenocortical carcinomas (ACCs) are rare malignancies (incidence of 1–2 per million population) with a heterogeneous presentation and a variable but generally poor prognosis (19). There is a bimodal age distribution with an initial peak in childhood and a second higher peak in the fourth or fifth decade of life. Women are more affected than men; the female-to-male ratio is approximately 1.5:1.

The majority of cases are sporadic; nevertheless, cases of adrenal carcinoma have been seen in association with several hereditary syndromes including the Li–Fraumeni syndrome, Beckwith–Wiedmann syndrome, and MEN1. The molecular pathogenesis of ACC is still poorly understood. However, inactivating mutations at the 17p13 locus, including the $p53$ tumor suppressor gene, and alterations of the 11p15 locus, leading to IGF-II overexpression are frequently observed (19).

Approximately 60% of patients present with signs and symptoms of adrenal steroid hormone excess, usually in the form of rapidly progressing Cushing's syndrome, with or without virilization. Signs and symptoms of Cushing's syndrome are caused by hypercortisolism and include weight gain with centripetal obesity, rounded face (moon face), increased fat deposition around the neck (buffalo hump), relatively proximal muscle wasting, psychiatric disturbances, hyperglycemia, and hypokalemia. Androgen-secreting ACCs in women may induce hirsutism, deepening voice, male pattern baldness, and oligo/amenorrhea. In men, estrogen-secreting tumors may induce gynecomastia and testicular atrophy. Aldosterone-producing ACCs present with hypertension and marked hypokalemia. Nonfunctioning or hormone-inactive ACCs, usually present with abdominal discomfort, including nausea, vomiting, abdominal fullness, or back pain caused by the mass effect of a large tumor.

## Staging

| AJCC Staging of Adrenocortical Carcinoma | |
| --- | --- |
| Stage | Description |
| I | Tumor <5 cm in greatest dimension without invasion (T1) without regional lymph node (N0) or distant metastases (M0) |
| II | Tumor >5 cm in greatest dimension without invasion (T2) without regional lymph node (N0) or distant metastases (M0) |
| III | T1 or T2 tumor with regional lymph node metastases (N1) *or* tumor extends beyond adrenal invading fat (T3) without regional lymph node (N0); no distant metastases (M0) |
| IV | T3 or T4 tumor with regional lymph node metastases (N1) *or* T4 tumor without regional lymph node metastases; no distant metastases (M0) OR any T, any N, with distant metastases (M1) |

AJCC, American Joint Committee on Cancer.

## CASE SUMMARY

### Metastatic ACC

G.H. is a 32-year-old woman who was referred to the cancer center because of an adrenal mass. She had been in her usual state of health until 2 months prior to her evaluation when she began to experience back pain and generalized swelling. Her back pain was most noticeable in her cervical and lumbar areas. She reported increased irritability, facial hair, and easy bruising. She also became more anxious over the previous 3 months and noticed an elevation in her blood pressure. The patient presented to her primary care physician who believed her symptoms were related to polycystic ovarian syndrome. She underwent a dexamethasone suppression test, which revealed an elevated cortisol level. The urinary free cortisol was also found to be elevated. Subsequently, an ultrasound of the abdomen revealed a 5.3 x 1.5 cm mass in the superior margin of the right kidney, which was suspected to be of adrenal origin. This was followed by an MRI, which confirmed the mass to be located in the adrenal gland. One week prior to her cancer center referral, she was admitted to the hospital with hypokalemia and hypertension. Her potassium was replaced and blood pressure medications were adjusted. On the basis of her evaluation to date, she was diagnosed with Cushing's syndrome secondary to an adrenocortical mass concerning for malignancy.

At her cancer center visit, G.H. reported anxiety and episodes of flushing. She had gained approximately 12 pounds in the last month. She had difficulty sleeping for the last 2 months and she had recently noticed a numbness and tingling sensation in her upper extremities. Her medications were metoprolol, potassium chloride, alprazolam, and zolpidem. She did not drink alcohol, smoke, or use illicit drugs. Her father had prostate cancer, and 1 grandmother had a history of cervical carcinoma.

On physical examination, the patient was overweight with a moon face with increased facial hair. Her blood pressure was elevated at 157/99 mmHg with a normal pulse rate. Her body mass index (BMI) was 32. There was an unusual distribution of her body fat, particularly noticeable at the top of her back. Her lungs were clear to auscultation and her heart was regular without murmur. The abdomen was soft, with no tenderness, hepatomegaly, splenomegaly, or palpable masses. The remainder of the examination was normal. Her cortisol level was elevated to 50.4 µg/dL (reference range = 4.3–22 µg/dL), but her adrenocorticotropic hormone (ACTH), free metanephrine, aldosterone, and renin levels were within the normal range. Dehydroepiandrosterone and testosterone levels were also elevated at 626 mcg/dL (31–228 mcg/dL) and 314 ng/dL (14–76 ng/dL), respectively. Other laboratory test results were normal, including complete blood cell count, electrolytes, glucose, total protein, globulin, albumin, and calcium. Renal and hepatic functions were also normal.

Review of CT scans of the abdomen and pelvis confirmed the presence of a large heterogeneous mass with central calcification arising from the superior portion of the right adrenal gland, and also showed multiple scattered ring-enhanced lesions in the liver and numerous pulmonary nodules in lung bases consistent with metastases. A small lytic lesion was identified in the costochondral junction suggestive of bone metastasis in her eighth rib. An MRI of the cervical, thoracic, and lumbosacral spine was requested due to the patient's symptoms of numbness and tingling in the upper extremities. It revealed a severe compression fracture of C6 with retropulsion, and an epidural tumor causing mild C6 cord compression. Epidural metastases from C5 to C7, as well as S4 and S5 epidural disease was noted in addition to multiple other bone metastases. G.H. underwent an FNA of the right adrenal mass. Pathological examination showed adrenal carcinoma.

## Evidence-Based Case Discussion

G.H. is a patient with ACC with metastases to liver, lung, and bone.

## Diagnosis and Evaluation

In the evaluation of adrenal masses, screening should be performed to exclude a pheochromocytoma. Pheochromocytomas are NETs derived from adrenal chromaffin cells, which produce, store, metabolize, and secrete catecholamines or their metabolites. About 10% of these tumors are malignant, and 90% arise in the adrenal medulla, while extra-adrenal pheochromocytomas usually occur within the para-aortic sympathetic chain. Pheochromocytomas may occur sporadically or as a part of a hereditary syndrome (such as MEN 2A, MEN 2B, NF-1, VHL, and Osler–Weber–Rendu syndrome). The main signs and symptoms of catecholamine excess include hypertension, palpitation, headache, sweating, and pallor. According to the degree of catecholamine excess, patients can present with myocardial infarction, arrhythmia, stroke, or other signs of ischemic events resulting in serious morbidity and mortality. Because imaging often cannot reliably differentiate between ACC and pheochromocytoma, screening should include a 24-hour urinary estimation of catecholamines (epinephrine, norepinephrine, and dopamine) and its metabolites, including metanephrines and normetanephrines. In addition, plasma metanephrines and catecholamines can be assayed in order to establish the diagnosis in most patients. For functional ACCs, a thorough hormonal workup is needed to identify the type of hormone with abnormal level as a biomarker for disease monitoring after surgical treatment and subsequent detection of tumor recurrence (see Table 9.4) (19).

Evaluation with CT or MRI using an adrenal protocol is recommended for initial tumor localization, and morphological evaluation. According to the National Institute of Health consensus conference, tumors >6 cm are highly suspicious for malignancy. On unenhanced CT scan, the Hounsfield Unit (HU) number is typically higher in carcinomas than in adenomas and a threshold value of 10 HU has been proposed as a means of distinguishing benign from malignant adrenal tumors (20). Adrenal lesions with an attenuation value >10 HU in unenhanced CT scan, or an enhancement washout of <50% and a delayed attenuation of >35 HU (on 10–15 min delayed enhanced CT) are suspicious for malignancy. Because the lung and liver are the most common sites of metastatic spread, thoracic and abdominal scans are integral to the staging workup of ACCs.

Because histological analysis of an adrenal mass may be unreliable, fine or core tissue needle aspiration biopsies

**Table 9.4** Hormonal Workup and Imaging in Patients With Suspected or Proven ACC[a]

| | |
|---|---|
| Glucocorticoid excess (minimum 3 of 4 tests) | Dexamethasone suppression test (1 mg, 23:00 hr) |
| | Excretion of free urinary cortisol (24-hr urine) |
| | Basal cortisol (serum) |
| | Basal ACTH (plasma) |
| Sexual steroids and steroid precursors | DHEA-S (serum) |
| | 17-OH-progesterone (serum) |
| | Androstendione (serum) |
| | Testosterone (serum) |
| | 17 B-estradiol (serum, only in men and postmenopausal women) |
| Mineral corticoid excess | Potassium (serum) |
| | Aldosterone-to-renin ratio (only in patients with arterial hypertension and/or hypokalemia) |
| Exclusion of a pheochromocytoma (1 of 2 tests) | Catecholamine excretion (24-hr urine) |
| | Meta- and normetanephrines (plasma) |
| Imaging | CT or MRI of abdomen and thorax |
| | Bone scintigraphy (when suspecting skeletal metastases) |
| | FDG-PET (optional) |

ACTH, adrenocorticotropic hormone; DHEA, dehydroepiandrosterone; FDG, $^{18}$F-fludeoxyglucose.

[a]As per recommendations of the Adrenocortical Carcinoma (ACC) Working Group of the European Network of the Study of Adrenal Tumors (ENSAT), May 2005.

*Source*: From Ref. (19). Allolio B, Fassnacht M. Clinical review: adrenocortical carcinoma: clinical update. *J Clin Endocrinol Metab.* 2006;91(6):2027–2037.

(percutaneous) are generally not recommended except in possible metastatic deposits. Laparoscopic excision of the tumors is the preferred method of removal of benign adrenal tumors. When tumors are thought to be malignant, an open or laparoscopic-assisted operation should be done since these malignant tumors are prone to rupture. If pheochromocytoma is suspected, patients should receive a preoperative blocking agent in order to counteract the significant release of catecholamines on target tissues due to anesthesia and surgical manipulation of the tumor. Nuclear atypia, atypical and frequent mitoses (>5 per 50 HPF), vascular and capsular invasion, and necrosis are suggestive of malignancy. Several studies have demonstrated the value of Ki67 staining in differentiating benign from malignant lesions. In addition, Ki67 expression may be of prognostic relevance, as high expression (>10%) has been associated with poor survival (19).

## Therapy for Localized and Advanced ACC

ACCs are rare; therefore, clinical series are small, and only limited prospective evaluation of treatment strategies exists.

In stages I through III, complete tumor removal by a specialized surgeon offers the best chance of cure. Surgical resection is often extensive with en bloc resection of the invaded organs and lymph nodes. At present, there is a consensus that open adrenalectomy remains the operation of choice for ACC with invasion to adjacent organs, enlarged regional lymph nodes, and tumors >10–12 cm in size (19).

Owing to its rarity, there are no published randomized prospective trials for adjuvant therapy. The majority of retrospective trials of adjuvant therapy have included the use of mitotane, an oral adrenocorticolytic agent. Mitotane exerts a specific cytotoxic effect on adrenocortical cells, producing focal degeneration of the fascicular, and particularly the reticular zone, whereas changes in the zona glomerulosa are minimal. The main side effects of mitotane are weakness, fatigue, dizziness, loss of appetite, nausea, vomiting, and diarrhea. The largest study thus far retrospectively analyzed 177 patients who underwent tumor resection and subsequent treatment in Italy and Germany. In the Italian cohort, 47 of the 102 patients received adjuvant mitotane at doses ranging from 1 to 5 g daily, whereas none of the 75 German patients received adjuvant mitotane. Recurrence-free survival was significantly prolonged in the mitotane group as compared with the 2 control groups (median recurrence-free survival was 42 months as compared with 10 months in control group 1 and 25 months in control group 2). HRs for recurrence were 2.91 (95% CI [1.77–4.78]; $P < .001$) and 1.97 (95% CI [1.21–3.20]; $P = .005$), suggesting that adjuvant mitotane may be an effective postoperative strategy (21). For patients on adjuvant mitotane, 13% required temporary discontinuation or dose reduction. Due to the adrenolytic effects of mitotane, replacement doses of corticosteroids (hydrocortisone or prednisone) should be prescribed in order to prevent adrenal insufficiency.

For patients with high-grade adrenal carcinoma suspected of having residual disease due to invasion and incomplete resection, the National Comprehensive Cancer Network (NCCN) recommends adjuvant mitotane or radiation therapy to the adrenal tumor bed. Follow-up with imaging and biomarkers every 3–6 months in functional tumors is also recommended. Figure 9.2 demonstrates an algorithm for the management of patients with localized ACC.

G.H. presented with stage IV ACC with metastases to the liver, lungs, and bones. In advanced stages, such as this case, the treatment is often palliative (see Figure 9.2 for treatment algorithm).

Treatment strategies include treatment of endocrine excess syndromes in functional adrenal carcinomas, the use of mitotane or several multiagent chemotherapy regimens and/or radiation for low-grade tumors, or palliative chemotherapy or radiation for high-grade tumors. The role of tumor debulking in the presence of metastatic disease is debatable. Incomplete resection of the primary tumor or metastatic disease not amenable to surgery is associated with a particularly poor prognosis (19). In most studies, the overall survival is <12 months.

Several studies have evaluated the combination of mitotane with cytotoxic agents, including cisplatin and etoposide. In a large prospective phase II trial, the combination of cisplatin, etoposide, and doxorubicin with mitotane 4 g daily yielded an overall response rate of 49% (by WHO criteria). Median time to tumor progression and overall survival of the entire cohort were 9.1 versus 28.5 months, respectively (18.2 and 47.7 months, respectively, in the patient subset attaining a disease response) (22). Another study reported an objective response rate of 36% with the combination of mitotane plus streptozocin. The overall 2-year and 5-year survival rates were 70% and 32.5%, respectively (23). In the First International Randomized Trial in Locally Advanced and Metastatic Adrenocortical Carcinoma Treatment (FIRM-ACT), 304 patients with advanced ACC were randomly assigned to receive etoposide, doxorubicin, cisplatin, and mitotane, or streptozocin and mitotane. There was no significant difference in overall survival (14.8 vs. 12 months, HR = 0.79, 95% CI [0.61–1.02], $P = .07$) with the crossover design. However, for those who did not cross over to the other arm, the overall survival for the 4-drug regimen and 2-drug regimen was 17.1 and 4.7 months, respectively. The rates of serious adverse events were not significantly different between 2 treatment groups (24). Currently, the first-line chemotherapy treatment for advanced metastatic ACC includes the combination of cisplatin, adriamycin, etoposide, and mitotane, while second-line therapy is mitotane plus streptozocin. Given potential toxicity of combined chemotherapy, single-agent mitotane may still be considered as an option.

For most bone and brain metastases, radiation therapy is the treatment of choice. In the case of G.H., palliative radiation was initiated for the epidural metastases from C6 to C7 in order to relieve the mild cord compression. Mitotane was given concurrently. Subsequently, she received a chemotherapy combination of cisplatin, adriamycin, etoposide, and mitotane with few reported side effects.

## POORLY DIFFERENTIATED (HIGH-GRADE) EXTRAPULMONARY NEUROENDOCRINE CARCINOMAS

### Epidemiology, Risk Factors, Natural History, and Pathology

The terms poorly differentiated (PD) and high-grade NECA are used interchangeably. The classic small cell carcinoma occurs in the lung, but extrapulmonary poorly differentiated NECAs can originate in the skin (Merkel cell), larynx, gastrointestinal tract (including pancreas),

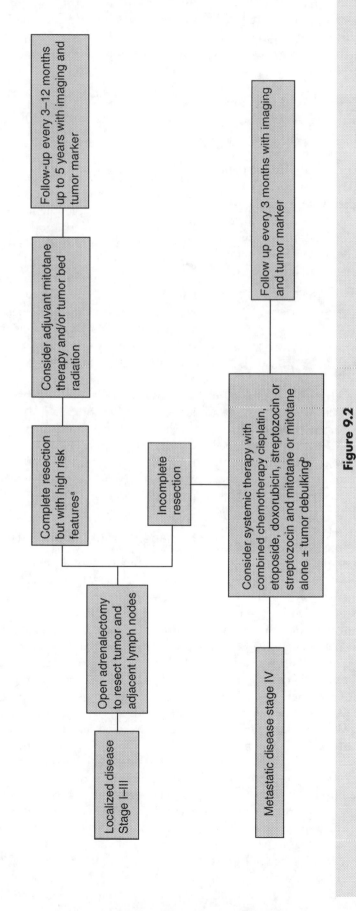

**Figure 9.2**

Management algorithm for adrenal cortical carcinoma.

<sup>a</sup>High risk local recurrence features: positive margins, rupture of capsule, larger size, and high grade. <sup>b</sup>If >90% of tumor and metastases can be removed.

bladder, cervix, and prostate. NECAs are characterized by a high mitotic rate (>10–20 mitoses per 10 HPFs) and extensive necrosis (25). They can present with paraneoplastic syndrome such as syndrome of inappropriate antidiuretic hormone (SIADH) secretion, ectopic ACTH secretion, and so on.

Extrapulmonary PD NECAs are exceedingly rare and they confer a poor prognosis with median survival durations in patients with localized, regional, and distant disease of 34, 14, and 5 months, respectively.

Particularly, 1–2% of prostate cancer has mainly small cell carcinoma in histology. Their clinical characteristics and presentations are different from those of the typical prostate adenocarcinoma. Possible signs for these kinds of prostate malignancies include inappropriate level of prostate-specific antigen (PSA), atypical metastatic sites such as brain, lung, or liver, or poor response to hormonal therapy. In such cases, initial biopsy specimen needs to be reexamined for small cell and/or neuroendocrine features.

## CASE SUMMARY

### High-Grade/Poorly Differentiated NETs

M.M. is a 32-year-old man who was seen in consultation by oncology during inpatient hospitalization because of a high-grade NET. The patient had been well until approximately 3 weeks before this evaluation when he developed abdominal pain, heartburn, cramping, nausea, vomiting, and constipation. The pain was most noticeable after eating. He had been vomiting for 2 weeks and reported a weight loss of 30 pounds over the same time period. He presented to the emergency department with the previously mentioned symptoms and the gastroenterology service was consulted. CT scan of the abdomen, obtained on the day of admission, showed a large mass in the gastrohepatic area that abutted the stomach and the esophagus, as well as multiple large liver lesions. An upper gastrointestinal endoscopy showed a large, lobular mass in the body of the stomach. Biopsies were taken and the pathology was consistent with a poorly differentiated NECA with 20 mitosis per 10 HPFs.

He did not have any medical and surgical history in the past. He had lost approximately 40 pounds of body weight during the previous month, which he attributed to emesis. He exercised regularly, drank alcohol, and smoked socially, but denied any illicit drug use. There was no history of cancer in the family.

On physical examination, the patient appeared well and his vital signs were normal. His BMI was 25. The abdomen was soft, with tenderness in the epigastric area. There was no distention, hepatomegaly, splenomegaly, lymphadenopathy, or palpable masses. The remainder of the examination was also normal. Other laboratory test results, including complete blood cell count, glucose, total protein, globulin, albumin, and calcium, as well as tests of coagulation, renal, and hepatic function were normal. Immunohistochemistry examination of the pathology specimen was positive for synaptophysin, chromogranin, CK7, CAM 5.2, CK5/6. Morphological and immunophenotypic features were consistent with a high-grade NET.

## Evidence-Based Case Discussion

### Management of Limited Disease

Similar to small cell lung carcinoma, poorly differentiated NECAs tend to metastasize even in patients with apparently localized tumors. Surgery alone is rarely curative. Given their aggressive behavior, surgical resection followed by adjuvant chemotherapy (4 or 6 cycles of cisplatin or carboplatin and etoposide), with or without radiation, is recommended. Based on the treatment for limited stage SCLC, a course of definitive chemotherapy with 4–6 cycles of cisplatin or carboplatin and etoposide with radiation can be considered in patients with localized extrapulmonary involvement, particularly when surgical resection is difficult. Concurrent chemotherapy with radiation is more efficacious as reported in clinical trials for limited stage SCLC, but at the expense of increased toxicity (25).

Data on extrapulmonary PD NECAs suggest a lower incidence of central nervous system metastases as compared to SCLC. Therefore, routine prophylactic cranial irradiation is not recommended in this population, but it may be considered for patients with poorly differentiated NECAs of the head and neck or unknown primary (25).

### Management of Extensive Disease

The combination of cisplatin and etoposide has been studied in metastatic PD NECAs of the gastrointestinal tract. Moertel reported a response rate of 67% in patients with poorly differentiated NECA with a response duration of 8 months and a median survival of 19 months (26). Mitry also studied this combination in PD NECAs of the gastrointestinal tract and reported a response rate of 42% with a response duration of 9 months and a median survival of 15 months (27). On the basis of these studies, cisplatin in combination with etoposide is recommended as first-line therapy for metastatic PD NECAs. The length of treatment remains unclear and whether treatment beyond 4 cycles is associated with a survival benefit is debatable.

There are no data for second-line chemotherapy regimens. Retreatment with a platinum and etoposide regimen can be considered in patients who initially responded, but then relapsed >3–6 months after termination of first-line chemotherapy. Other agents with activity in second-line treatment for SCLC include irinotecan, paclitaxel, docetaxel, vinorelbine, and gemcitabine.

In the case of M.M., a CT scan showed complete remission following 6 cycles of cisplatin and etoposide, after which he was placed on surveillance with imaging and physical examinations.

## REVIEW QUESTIONS

1. A 62-year-old man presented with abdominal pain. A CT scan showed 2 liver lesions and a 15-cm left adrenal mass invading pancreas, left kidney, spleen, and descending colon. Biopsy revealed adrenocortical carcinoma. He has good performance status and would like to explore his systemic treatment options. Which of the following regimen would you least likely consider in the first-line setting?

   (A) Mitotane
   (B) Streptozocin and mitotane
   (C) Cisplatin and paclitaxel
   (D) Cisplatin, etoposide, doxorubicin, and mitotane

2. A 66-year-old man was told to have "low blood sugar" during a routine preoperative evaluation for hernia repair. Patient mentions that he has been having episodes of feeling dizzy, shaky, and nervous since about 6 months ago. He noticed he would get better after eating some snacks or drinking a glass of orange juice. His astute internist suspects his patient has an insulinoma. Which of the following tests would be helpful in making this diagnosis?

   (A) Chromogranin
   (B) Glucagon and glucose
   (C) Insulin and glucose
   (D) Insulin

3. A 50-year-old woman was referred to you due to a recent diagnosis of pancreatic neuroendocrine tumor (NET). You ordered a CT scan, which showed a pancreatic mass as well as multiple liver lesions highly suggestive of metastases. The patient is an accountant and has spent the last 2 days reading materials of NET on the Internet. She prefers no intravenous treatment. Which of the following medications would you recommend?

   (A) Everolimus
   (B) Temsirolimus
   (C) Sorafenib
   (D) Temodar

4. A 45-year-old man with a history of peptic ulcer disease presented to his gastroenterologist with persistent abdominal pain. He underwent an esophagogastroduodenoscopy, which showed a 2.5-cm gastric lesion. Biopsy was taken from this lesion. The pathology was consistent with well-differentiated neuroendocrine tumor. The patient has normal gastrin level. A staging CT showed no other suspicious lesions. What is the next step in management?

   (A) Start octreotide
   (B) Observe
   (C) Perform endoscopic resection
   (D) Perform radical resection of tumor with regional lymphadenectomy

5. A 33-year-man presented with intermittent palpitation, flushing, headache, and hypertension. Workup showed a 3-cm right adrenal mass. He was very anxious and would like to have it resected as soon as possible. He was referred to a general surgeon. What preoperative evaluation would be most relevant for this patient given his symptoms?

   (A) Complete blood count and liver function test
   (B) Transthoracic echocardiogram
   (C) Plasma metanephrine
   (D) Chromogranin and 5-HIAA

6. A 30-year-old man with no significant medical history, presented to the emergency department with sudden onset of right lower quadrant abdominal pain with related nausea and vomiting for 8 hours. On physical examination, his temperature was 98.3°F, blood pressure was 120/78 mmHg, pulse was 100/min; his abdomen was soft, tenderness to palpation to the right lower quadrant with positive rebound. White blood cell count was 15.3 × 109 L with left shift. CT abdomen and pelvis suggested acute appendicitis. The patient underwent laparoscopic appendectomy. Pathology confirmed acute appendicitis. In addition, a 2.1 × 1.5 cm tumor was found at the tip of the appendix. The tumor cells were positive for CK20, carcinoembryonic antigen, chromogranin, and neuron-specific enolase, Ki67 was <3%, consistent with low-grade carcinoid tumor. What is the next step in management?

   (A) Re-exploration and right hemicolectomy
   (B) Observation
   (C) Octreotide long-acting release
   (D) Everolimus

7. A 48-year-old man with history of hypertension presented to his primary care physician's office with right upper quadrant pain and intermittent diarrhea for the past 3 months. He also complains of episodes of flushing and recent unintentional weight loss of 10 lbs in the past 3 months. His esophagogastroduodenoscopy and colonoscopy were normal. However, a CT abdomen and pelvis showed multiple liver lesions involving both lobes of the liver, size ranging from 3 to

6 cm in diameter. The patient underwent ultrasound-guided core biopsy of a liver lesion. The pathology was consistent with low-grade neuroendocrine tumor. Clinically, the patient has an Eastern Cooperative Oncology Group performance status of 0. What treatment would you recommend for this patient?

(A) Cisplatin plus etoposide
(B) Everolimus
(C) Observation
(D) Octreotide long-acting release (LAR)

8. RET proto-oncogene mutation is associated with which of the following neuroendocrine tumor type:

(A) MEN1
(B) MEN2
(C) Medullary thyroid carcinoma
(D) B and C
(E) All of the above

9. A 68-year-old man with hypothyroidism and benign prostatic hypertrophy presented to his urologist with gross hematuria, dysuria, and tenesmus for 1 month. A cystoscopy showed normal urethra and bladder and a large prostate causing the narrowing of the bladder neck. His prostate-specific antigen was 8. CT abdomen and pelvis showed a markedly enlarged prostate gland with a hypodense lesion measuring 8.9 × 7.2 × 5.3 cm, extending to the base of the bladder and lateral pelvic wall. Core biopsy of the prostate mass showed high-grade carcinoma, consistent with small cell carcinoma of the prostate. Which one of the following treatments would you recommend for him?

(A) Cisplatin/etoposide
(B) External beam radiation therapy of the prostate
(C) Prostatectomy
(D) Leuprorelin

10. Which of the following germ-line mutation is associated with MEN1 syndrome?

(A) von Hippel–Lindau, 3q25
(B) Hamartin, 17q11
(C) Menin, 11q13
(D) RET

## REFERENCES

1. Yao JC, Hassan M, Phan A, et al. One hundred years after "carcinoid": epidemiology of and prognostic factors for neuroendocrine tumors in 35,825 cases in the United States. *J Clin Oncol.* 2008;26(18):3063–3072.
2. Vinik A, O'Dorisio T, Woltering E, et al. *Neuroendocrine Tumors: A Comprehensive Guide to Diagnosis and Management.* Inglewood, CA: Inter Science Institute; 2009.
3. Klimstra DS, Modlin IR, Coppola D, et al. The pathologic classification of neuroendocrine tumors: a review of nomenclature, grading, and staging systems. *Pancreas.* 2010;39(6):707–712.
4. Edge SB, Byrd DR, Compton CC, et al. *AJCC Cancer Staging Handbook: From the AJCC Cancer Staging Manual.* New York, NY: Springer; 2010.
5. Anthony LB, Strosberg JR, Klimstra DS, et al. The NANETS consensus guidelines for the diagnosis and management of gastrointestinal neuroendocrine tumors (NETS): well-differentiated NETS of the distal colon and rectum. *Pancreas.* 2010;39(6): 767–774.
6. Rinke A, Müller H, Schade-Brittinger C, et al. Placebo-controlled, double-blind, prospective, randomized study on the effect of octreotide LAR in the control of tumor growth in patients with metastatic neuroendocrine midgut tumors: a report from the PROMID Study Group. *J Clin Oncol.* 2009;27(28):4656–4663.
7. Arnold R, Wittenberg M, Rinke A, et al. Placebo controlled, double blind, prospective, randomized study on the effect of octreotide LAR in the control of tumor growth in patients with metastatic neuroendocrine midgut tumors (PROMID): results on long-term survival (abstract). *J Clin Oncol.* 2013;31(suppl; abstr 4030).
8. Pavel ME, Hainsworth JD, Baudin E, et al. RADIANT-2 Study Group. Everolimus plus octreotide long-acting repeatable for the treatment of advanced neuroendocrine tumours associated with carcinoid syndrome (RADIANT-2): a randomised, placebo-controlled, phase 3 study. *Lancet.* 2011;378(9808):2005–2012.
9. Ehehalt F, Saeger HD, Schmidt CM, et al. Neuroendocrine tumors of the pancreas. *Oncologist.* 2009;14(5):456–467.
10. Zerbi A, Falconi M, Rindi G, et al. AISP-Network Study Group. Clinicopathological features of pancreatic endocrine tumors: a prospective multicenter study in Italy of 297 sporadic cases. *Am J Gastroenterol.* 2010;105(6):1421–1429.
11. Halfdanarson TR, Rabe KG, Rubin J, et al. Pancreatic neuroendocrine tumors (PNETs): incidence, prognosis and recent trend toward improved survival. *Ann Oncol.* 2008;19(10): 1727–1733.
12. Jensen RT, Niederle B, Mitry E, et al. Gastrinoma (duodenal and pancreatic). *Neuroendocrinology.* 2006;84(3):173–182.
13. Kulke MH, Anthony LB, Bushnell DL, et al. NANETS treatment guidelines: well-differentiated neuroendocrine tumors of the stomach and pancreas. *Pancreas.* 2010;39(6):735–752.
14. Metz DC, Jensen RT. Gastrointestinal neuroendocrine tumors: pancreatic endocrine tumors. *Gastroenterology.* 2008;135(5): 1469–1492.
15. Raymond E, Dahan L, Raoil J-L, et al. Sunitinib maleate for the treatment of pancreatic neuroendocrine tumors. *N Engl J Med.* 2011;364:501–573.
16. Yao JC, Shah MH, Ito T, et al. Everolimus for advanced pancreatic neuroendocrine tumors. *N Engl J Med.* 2011;364:514–523.
17. Caplin ME, Pavel M, Ćwikła JB et al.; CLARINET Investigators. Lanreotide in metastatic enteropancreatic neuroendocrine tumors. *N Engl J Med.* 2014;371(3):224–233.
18. Kouvaraki MA, Ajani JA, Hoff P, et al. Fluorouracil, doxorubicin, and streptozocin in the treatment of patients with locally advanced and metastatic pancreatic endocrine carcinomas. *J Clin Oncol.* 2004;22(23):4762–4771.
19. Allolio B, Fassnacht M. Clinical review: adrenocortical carcinoma: clinical update. *J Clin Endocrinol Metab.* 2006;91(6): 2027–2037.
20. Caoili EM, Korobkin M, Francis IR, et al. Adrenal masses: characterization with combined unenhanced and delayed enhanced CT. *Radiology.* 2002;222(3):629–633.
21. Terzolo M, Angeli A, Fassnacht M, et al. Adjuvant mitotane treatment for adrenocortical carcinoma. *N Engl J Med.* 2007;356(23):2372–2380.
22. Berruti A, Terzolo M, Sperone P, et al. Etoposide, doxorubicin and cisplatin plus mitotane in the treatment of advanced

adrenocortical carcinoma: a large prospective phase II trial. *Endocr Relat Cancer.* 2005;12(3):657–666.

23. Khan TS, Imam H, Juhlin C, et al. Streptozocin and o,p'DDD in the treatment of adrenocortical cancer patients: long-term survival in its adjuvant use. *Ann Oncol.* 2000;11(10):1281–1287.

24. Fassnacht M, Terzolo M, Allolio B, et al. Combination chemotherapy in advanced adrenocortical carcinoma. *N Engl J Med* 2012;366(23):2189–2197.

25. Strosberg JR, Coppola D, Klimstra DS, et al. The NANETS consensus guidelines for the diagnosis and management of poorly differentiated (high-grade) extrapulmonary neuroendocrine carcinomas. *Pancreas.* 2010;39(6):799–800.

26. Moertel CG, Kvols LK, O'Connell MJ, et al. Treatment of neuroendocrine carcinomas with combined etoposide and cisplatin. Evidence of major therapeutic activity in the anaplastic variants of these neoplasms. *Cancer.* 1991;68(2):227–232.

27. Mitry E, Baudin E, Ducreux M, et al. Treatment of poorly differentiated neuroendocrine tumours with etoposide and cisplatin. *Br J Cancer.* 1999;81(8):1351–1355.

# 10

# Hepatobiliary Cancers

GHANA KANG, AHMED AWAIS, PAUL ZHANG, AND YVONNE SADA

## BILIARY TRACT CARCINOMAS

### Epidemiology, Risk Factors, Natural History, and Pathology

Biliary tract cancers (BTCs) include cholangiocarcinoma (CC) and gallbladder cancer (GBC), which are malignant tumors arising from the epithelial lining of the bile duct and gallbladder, respectively. These tumors comprise 3% of all gastrointestinal malignancies. There are approximately 9000 new cases per year in the United States (1), with almost twice as many cases of GBC than CC. High-incidence areas of BTC worldwide include Thailand, China, India, and Chile. The incidence of BTC peaks in the sixth and seventh decades of life. A significantly higher proportion of GBC cases occur in women, whereas CC affects men and women equally.

Risk factors for CC include a history of primary sclerosing cholangitis (PSC), congenital biliary cysts, hepatolithiasis, liver flukes (*Clonorchis sinensis* and *Opisthorchis viverrini*), Thorotrast dye, dietary nitrosamines, and chemical agents such as dioxin and asbestos. Recently, an association between CC and hepatitis C infection has been established. The association of primary sclerosing cholangitis (PSC) with CC is as high as 40%. The most common risk factor for GBC is gallstones, which are identified in 65–90% of GBC cases. Other risk factors for GBC include porcelain gallbladder, anomalous pancreaticobiliary duct junction, obesity, various chemicals, *Salmonella typhi*, and *Helicobacter pylori*. These risk factors cause chronic inflammation of the biliary epithelium, resulting in dysplasia, carcinoma in situ, and eventually invasive carcinoma. Genetic defects involving *k-ras* and *p53* have been described in a significant number of cases of BTC (2).

More than 90% of BTCs are adenocarcinomas. Anatomically, CC can be divided into intrahepatic cholangiocarcinoma (ICC), extrahepatic cholangiocarcinoma (ECC), and hilar (i.e., Klatskin tumor) types. Hilar CC occurs at the bifurcation of the common hepatic duct. ICC occurs in the liver and can present a diagnostic challenge due to difficulty in differentiating ICC from hepatocellular carcinoma (HCC) by imaging. ECC originates in the bile duct along the hepatoduodenal ligament. The distribution of these tumors is 10% ICC, 20% ECC, and 70% hilar. Hilar CC and ECC often present with painless jaundice due to biliary obstruction. Other symptoms may include pruritus, weight loss, dark urine, pale stools, and fever. In contrast, ICC usually presents with dull, right upper quadrant pain without evidence of biliary obstruction. The incidence of ICC has been rising, while the incidence of ECC seems to be declining. Most cases of GBC arise in the fundus of the gallbladder and are often diagnosed incidentally during surgical exploration for cholelithiasis. Frequently, GBC cases are diagnosed in advanced stages and present with many of the symptoms described previously.

BTCs are curable, if caught early, with surgical resection; however, only 10–20% of patients present in an early stage. Even after surgical resection, the recurrence rate can be as high as 50%. The average 5-year survival for BTC is 5% for GBC and 10–20% for CC. The majority of patients with unresectable disease die within 6–12 months of diagnosis.

### Staging

The Cancer Staging System of the American Joint Committee on Cancer (AJCC) is the standard staging system. ICC, ECC, and GBC have independent staging criteria. The extrahepatic bile duct tumors are further subclassified into perihilar (proximal) and distal groups. However, for clinical practice, all patients with BTC may be divided into 3 distinct groups: localized (resectable), locally advanced (unresectable), or metastatic disease. Staging studies include advanced imaging and sometimes laparoscopy to evaluate for peritoneal metastases.

## AJCC 7th Edition Staging System for Perihilar (Proximal) Bile Duct Tumors

| Stage | Definition |
|-------|------------|
| I | Tumor confined to bile duct histologically |
| II | Tumor invades beyond bile duct wall to adjacent adipose tissue or liver parenchyma |
| IIIA | Tumor invades unilateral branches of portal vein (PV) or hepatic artery (HA) |
| IIIB | Regional lymph node metastasis |
| IVA | Tumor invades main PV or its branches bilaterally; or the common HA; or the second-order biliary radicals bilaterally; or unilateral second-order biliary radicals with contralateral PV or HA involvement |
| IVB | Distant metastasis (includes distant lymph nodes) |

AJCC, American Joint Committee on Cancer.

## AJCC 7th Edition Staging System for Distal Bile Duct Tumors

| Stage | Definition |
|-------|------------|
| IA | Tumor confined to bile duct histologically |
| IB | Tumor invades beyond bile duct wall |
| IIA | Tumor invades duodenum, pancreas, gallbladder, or other adjacent organs and does not involve the celiac or superior mesenteric artery |
| IIB | Any regional nodal involvement |
| III | Tumor involves celiac axis or superior mesenteric artery |
| IV | Distant metastasis |

AJCC, American Joint Committee on Cancer.

## AJCC 7th Edition Staging System for Intrahepatic Bile Duct Tumors

| Stage | Definition |
|-------|------------|
| I | Solitary tumor, without vascular invasion |
| II | Multiple tumors or solitary tumor with vascular invasion |
| III | Tumor perforating the visceral peritoneum or involving the local extrahepatic structures by direct invasion |
| IVA | Tumor with periductal invasion; or regional lymph node metastasis present |
| IVB | Distant metastasis present |

AJCC, American Joint Committee on Cancer.

# CASE SUMMARIES

## Locally Advanced/Unresectable BTC

R.T. is a 67-year-old male with no significant past medical history who presented with a 5-day history of jaundice, dark urine, and pale stools. His wife confirmed a 10-pound weight loss over the last month. Examination revealed icteric sclera and tenderness to deep palpation in the right upper quadrant of the abdomen. Laboratory tests revealed a total and direct bilirubin level of 7.1 and 5.8 mg/dL, respectively. Alkaline phosphatase was elevated at 273 U/L. Alanine aminotransferase (ALT) and aspartate aminotransferase (AST) were within normal limits. An abdominal ultrasound revealed a suspicious mass in the hilar region of the liver and no gallstones. An MRI scan of the abdomen was performed to better characterize the lesion. MRI revealed intrahepatic bile duct dilatation and a 3.5 × 4.0 × 3.7 cm T2 hyperintense mass at the confluence of the bile ducts that was suspicious for hilar CC. The mass partially infiltrated hepatic segments 4 and 5 and also invaded the porta hepatis, HA, and PV. No extrahepatic biliary ductal dilatation was noted. No other abnormalities were noted in the liver or pancreas, and no regional lymphadenopathy was seen. The carbohydrate antigen 19–9 (CA 19–9) was 500 U/mL, and the carcinoembryonic antigen (CEA) was 0.5 U/mL.

R.T. was admitted to the hospital for further workup. An endoscopic retrograde cholangiopancreatography (ERCP) revealed a hilar stricture with dilation of the left and right hepatic ducts. Brushings and cytology were obtained, and a stent was placed to relieve the obstruction. An endoscopic ultrasound (EUS) confirmed the locally invasive mass and no regional lymphadenopathy. EUS-guided biopsy of the mass revealed a cytokeratin (CK) 7 positive and CK 20 negative adenocarcinoma. The cytology from brushings was negative. A chest CT was negative for metastatic disease. According to the AJCC, this tumor was a stage IVA (T4 N0 M0).

## Evidence-Based Case Discussion

The differential diagnosis for a patient with jaundice and biliary obstruction includes cholelithiasis, benign biliary strictures, PSC, pancreatic tumors, and hepatobiliary malignancies. However, painless jaundice and weight loss are highly suggestive of a hepatobiliary tumor. R.T. initially had an ultrasound to assess the biliary tree. An ultrasound is very sensitive for detection of biliary tract dilatation or other obvious biliary pathology, but MRI or CT scan is required to better characterize the extent of the tumor and to identify regional or distant metastases. The relationship of the tumor to the surrounding structures, including the vasculature, is extremely important when assessing resectability. An early surgical opinion should be obtained, since surgery represents the only chance for cure. In general, stages III and IV disease are not amenable to surgery. Four factors affect tumor resection: (a) the extent of the tumor within the biliary tree; (b) vascular invasion; (c) hepatic lobar atrophy; and (d) metastatic disease. The extensive invasion of this patient's tumor into the porta hepatis, HA, and PV made this an unresectable tumor. Neoadjuvant therapy is not considered a standard approach for the treatment of patients with CC. Photodynamic therapy and orthotopic liver transplant have been used in some studies with encouraging results; however, they are not yet the standard of care. Unresectable disease carries a poor prognosis, and the only remaining option is palliative chemoradiation or chemotherapy alone.

Stent placement to relieve biliary obstruction before initiation of chemotherapy or radiation is an important intervention. The median survival for unresectable CC is approximately 6 months with biliary drainage and 3 months without drainage. Bacterial cholangitis or liver failure is a potentially fatal complication. For patients who are expected to live longer and who wish to avoid repeated procedures, surgical bypass may be considered.

Both CEA and CA 19–9 are often checked in patients with suspected biliary tumors, although neither is specific nor sensitive for CC. In patients with biliary obstruction alone, serum CA 19–9 may be elevated, so serum CA 19–9 should be reevaluated after stent placement and when the bilirubin has normalized. In a recent study, serum CA 19–9 combined with abdominal ultrasound, CT scan, or MRI had a sensitivity of 90–100% for detecting CC (3). When CEA and CA 19–9 are evaluated together, the accuracy is greater than that when either is used alone. The sensitivity of brush cytology for diagnosing CC is also quite low due to the desmoplastic reaction associated with the tumor. In a large prospective study, the sensitivity of cytology varied from 9% to 24%, and the specificity varied from 61% to 100% (3).

Treatment decisions for locally advanced BTC can be challenging. The 3 most common scenarios for locally advanced BTC are residual disease after surgery, unresectable disease at diagnosis, or local recurrence in the surgical bed. Currently, there is no standard treatment for locally advanced BTC. No randomized trials have demonstrated a therapeutic benefit for chemoradiation therapy in locally advanced BTC. However, radiation with or without chemotherapy may provide palliation of symptomatic disease and has resulted in improvement of median survival in a small number of patients (4). A retrospective analysis of 28 patients with localized, nonmetastatic extrahepatic bile duct cancer showed a significantly increased median survival in patients who received external beam radiation therapy (EBRT) after transtumoral dilatation and intubation of the bile duct compared with those patients who underwent surgical decompression alone (12.2 vs. 2.2 months, respectively; $P = 0.05$). A similar study reported an increase in median survival with the use of EBRT after surgical decompression compared with surgical decompression alone (16 vs. 3 months, respectively). A study at the Mayo Clinic reported a median survival of 18.5 months, and 1- and 5-year survival rates of 69% and 7%, respectively, in 14

patients with unresectable ECC who were treated with intraoperative radiation therapy (IORT) and EBRT. In most studies, the use of BT or IORT and EBRT in patients with unresectable ECC resulted in a median survival of 12–14 months and a 1-year survival rate of 50–70%. Long-term survival is possible in approximately 10–20% of highly selected patients. A retrospective study at the MD Anderson Cancer Center showed that adjuvant chemoradiation after resection did not prolong survival, and adjuvant chemotherapy was actually associated with decreased overall survival (OS) (5).

Patients with known distant metastases should not be subjected to local treatment unless symptomatic relief is required. In such cases, local radiation may help relieve biliary obstruction. Radiosensitizing chemotherapy can also be used. The most extensively studied agent is 5-fluorouracil (5-FU). Capecitabine is fairly well tolerated and may be substituted if needed. Gemcitabine can be administered concurrently with radiation, but may be associated with an increased risk of toxicity.

Chemotherapy alone has been used for locally advanced disease when radiation is not an option. A detailed review of chemotherapy is presented in the section on metastatic disease.

R.T. received oral capecitabine (850 mg/m$^2$/d) concurrently with 5 weeks of EBRT and tolerated therapy well. A repeated CT scan 6 weeks after completion of treatment showed stable disease, and serum CA 19–9 decreased to 100 U/mL. He is followed every 3 months with a history and physical examination, liver function tests, and serum CA 19–9 levels.

BTC treatment requires a multidisciplinary approach that should also focus on supportive care. Pain control with narcotics, antiemetics, bowel regimens, and appetite stimulants are essential components of the treatment plan.

Figure 10.1 depicts the general approach to management of CC.

## Metastatic BTC

J.V. is a 77-year-old Hispanic woman with a long-standing history of gallstones who presented with 1 month of abdominal pain and 1 week of jaundice, decreased appetite, and 15-pound weight loss. She complained of fatigue and a low energy level, but continued to work and perform all her household chores. In the last few days, she also noticed itching of her skin. Examination revealed icteric sclera and tenderness on palpation in the right upper quadrant of the abdomen. On deep palpation, a firm mass was felt in the same region. Laboratory tests revealed a total and direct bilirubin of 10.1 mg/dL and 8.8 mg/dL, respectively. Alkaline phosphatase was elevated at 373 U/L. ALT and AST were mildly elevated at 75 U/L and 94 U/L, respectively. CA 19–9 and CEA levels

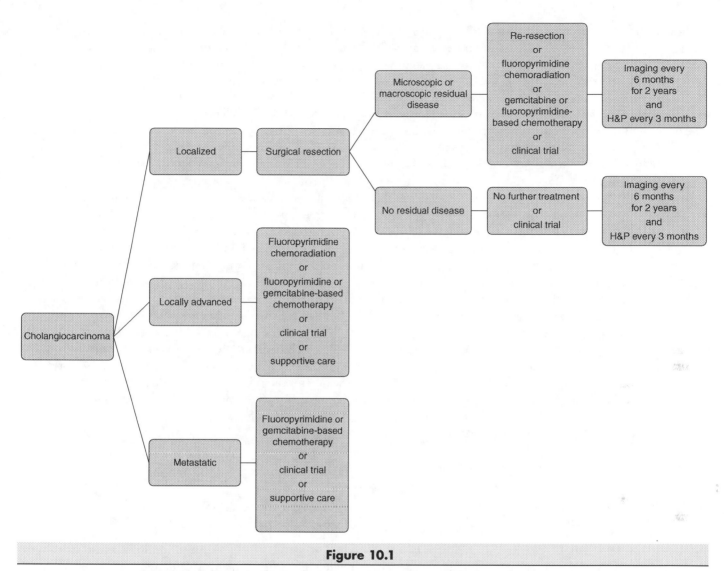

**Figure 10.1**

Treatment algorithm for cholangiocarcinoma. H&P, history and physical examination.

were normal. Hematopoietic and kidney functions were well preserved.

Abdominal ultrasound showed a suspicious mass in the gallbladder, with small gallstones, but no evidence of cholecystitis. CT of the abdomen showed a 4.6 × 5.5 × 4.2 cm heterogeneously enhancing, centrally necrotic mass occupying the gallbladder fossa, causing compression of the common bile duct and also associated with intra- and extrahepatic biliary dilatation. An irregular, peripherally enhancing, centrally low-attenuating mass was also visualized in the left lobe of the liver, measuring 4.8 × 7.5 × 8.7 cm. Numerous smaller, peripherally enhancing, low attenuation lesions were seen throughout the liver. Necrotic 1.8-cm para-aortic lymph nodes were identified, as well as a 2-cm necrotic porta hepatis lymph node. A percutaneous CT-guided biopsy of the gallbladder mass was performed. The pathology was consistent with adenocarcinoma of the gallbladder. A metal stent was placed in the common bile duct to relieve the obstruction. The metastases to the liver

and lymph nodes resulted in a T3 N1 M1 (stage IV) disease classification.

## Evidence-Based Case Discussion

J.V. has advanced GBC with Eastern Cooperative Oncology Group (ECOG) performance status of 1 and was performing daily household chores. Jaundice as a presenting sign in GBC indicates a poor prognosis, and 50% of these tumors are unresectable. The presence of metastases to the lymph nodes and liver does not favor a local treatment modality such as surgery or radiation. In these situations, palliative chemotherapy would be the only option. J.V.'s ECOG performance status is crucial to determining the treatment approach, since patients with poor performance status are not good candidates for chemotherapy and should receive supportive care.

GBC, like CC, is a rare tumor, and most of the evidence for treatment is derived from small retrospective studies or phase II trials of advanced BTC. The survival benefit of chemotherapy over best supportive care (6.0 months for treated patients vs. 2.5 months untreated) was demonstrated approximately 2 decades ago in a study that used 5-FU and etoposide in patients with advanced pancreaticobiliary malignancies. Quality of life was also improved with chemotherapy. Historically, 5-FU alone had a response rate of 10%. When combined with other agents such as oxaliplatin and cisplatin, the response rate increased between 25% and 55%, with a median survival of 6–12 months. Capecitabine showed similar results to 5-FU when used in combination with platinum compounds. Later, gemcitabine was found to be active in biliary tract neoplasms and was successful in various combinations, with median survivals of 9–12 months. A recent meta-analysis of 104 trials, including 2810 patients with advanced BTCs (both locally advanced and metastatic), demonstrated an average response rate of 22.8% to various chemotherapy regimens (6). The median times to progression and OS were 4.1 and 8.2 months, respectively. Gemcitabine as a single agent was found to be superior to the fluoropyrimidines. Doublet chemotherapy demonstrated superior response rates (28% vs. 15.3%) and a trend toward increased OS (9.3 vs. 7.5 months) compared to single agents. Three or more drug combinations added no extra benefit over 2-drug regimens. Gemcitabine and platinum (cisplatin and oxaliplatin)-based doublets demonstrated the best response rates, with some as high as 50%. There was a trend toward a longer time to progression with the gemcitabine–platinum doublet compared to the fluoropyrimidine–platinum combination (5.5 vs. 3.7 months).

There are only 2 phase III trials conducted to date studying chemotherapy for advanced BTC. The first trial compared 5-FU, etoposide, and leucovorin (FELV) to epirubicin, cisplatin, and 5-FU (ECF). However, due to poor recruitment, it was underpowered to detect any difference in OS. The median OS was 9.02 versus 12.03 months for ECF and FELV, respectively, and this was not statistically significant. The overall response rates and nonhematologic toxicities were very similar in both groups. The other phase III trial (ABC-02) recruited 410 patients from 37 centers in the United Kingdom. Half of the patients were assigned to gemcitabine as a single agent, and the other half received a gemcitabine–cisplatin combination (1). The tumor control rate was 81.4% for the combination versus 71.8% for the single agent. Progression-free survival (PFS) and median OS were 8 and 11.7 months, respectively, for the gemcitabine–cisplatin combination. PFS and OS were 5 and 8.1 months, respectively, for single-agent gemcitabine. There was a nonsignificant increase in the incidence of neutropenia in the gemcitabine–cisplatin group; however, infections were similar in the 2 groups.

Therefore, in patients with good performance status, the combination of cisplatin and gemcitabine is the chemotherapy of choice. Other commonly used combinations include gemcitabine–oxaliplatin, gemcitabine–capecitabine, and capecitabine–oxaliplatin; however, none has been compared head to head. Single-agent 5-FU, capecitabine, or gemcitabine can be offered in patients who have borderline ECOG performance status of 1–2, that is, those who are able to carry out daily life activities with some difficulty, as long as the patient can tolerate treatment. Chemotherapy is generally continued until there is evidence of disease progression. There is no approved second-line treatment regimen, but the aforementioned chemotherapy drugs may be used if they were not used as part of the first-line treatment.

There are currently several trials investigating the role of targeted therapies, such as erlotinib, cetuximab, or bevacizumab. Although encouraging data are emerging, randomized trials are needed to determine the efficacy of targeted agents in patients with BTCs.

J.V. in the clinical vignette was started on gemcitabine–cisplatin chemotherapy, which was well tolerated except for some nausea and mucositis. A CT scan performed 8 weeks after the initiation of treatment showed no evidence of progression. She was maintained on the same treatment and continues to follow up in the clinic.

## HEPATOCELLULAR CARCINOMA

### Epidemiology, Risk Factors, Natural History, and Pathology

HCC ranks as the fifth most common cause of cancer-related mortality in the world and is responsible for up to 1 million deaths worldwide (7). The prevalence of HCC parallels the distributions of hepatitis B virus (HBV) and hepatitis C virus (HCV) infections, and the incidence of HCC has been on the rise worldwide due to HBV and HCV epidemics (8). Significant improvements in the management of cirrhosis complications have led to increased survival of patients who carry these viruses. High-incidence areas for HCC include mainland China, Taiwan, Hong Kong, and sub-Saharan Africa (9).

Most patients with HCC have underlying liver disease, which further complicates the diagnosis and management of HCC. HCC can be distinguished from other tumor types where the organ function is well preserved despite malignant transformation. HCC generally has a progressive course and poor overall prognosis. Surgical resection and ablation of a localized tumor are the only curative options, and less than one third of the patients present at this early stage. Overall, the 5-year survival for HCC is approximately 5%.

HCC arises from the liver epithelium, and the morphology can vary from well differentiated to very poorly differentiated. Tumors arise in the context of chronic hepatocyte injury, which results in inflammation and increased hepatocyte turnover. Dysplastic changes and subsequent fibrosis can predispose the patient to develop HCC. In fact, patients with HCC often have underlying fibrotic nodules and hyperplasia that make the diagnostic process more complex. However, up to 10% of patients with HCC have no underlying liver disease. These tumors arise in young people (fibrolamellar variant) and sometimes in the elderly (de novo HCC).

Risk factors for HCC include HBV and HCV infection (80% of all cases) and other causes of cirrhosis such as alcoholism, adult fatty liver disease, hemochromatosis, alpha-1 antitrypsin deficiency, primary biliary cirrhosis, autoimmune hepatitis, and carcinogens such as aflatoxin and Thorotrast. The HBV genome may become integrated into the hepatocyte DNA, leading to mutations and malignant transformation without cirrhosis. Male sex and advanced age are also risk factors. Because HCC is largely a preventable disease, surveillance guidelines now incorporate both alpha-fetoprotein (AFP) and ultrasound to screen high-risk populations (9).

## Staging

Many staging systems have been used for HCC, including the Tumor, Lymph Nodes, Metastasis (TNM); Okuda; and Cancer of the Liver Italian Program classifications. The AJCC TNM staging system was recently revised and is the only system that has been validated in patients treated with either surgical resection or transplantation. However, this system does not include liver function. Because underlying liver function affects prognosis, Child-Pugh score can also be used in treatment planning. The Barcelona Clinic Liver Cancer (BCLC) system (Figure 10.2) has been chosen as the best staging system by the American Association for the Study of Liver Diseases (AASLD) (8). The BCLC incorporates tumor stage, liver function, physical condition of the patient, and cancer-related symptoms; all of these factors appear to impact the prognosis and the treatment approach.

**AJCC 7th Edition TNM Staging System for Hepatocellular Carcinoma**

| Stage | Definition |
|---|---|
| I | Solitary tumor without vascular invasion |
| II | Solitary tumor with vascular invasion or multiple tumors but none >5 cm |
| IIIA | Multiple tumors >5 cm |
| IIIB | Single tumor or multiple tumors of any size involving a major branch of the portal vein or hepatic vein |
| IIIC | Tumor/tumors with direct invasion of adjacent organs other than the gallbladder or with perforation of visceral peritoneum |
| IVA | Regional nodal metastasis |
| IVB | Distant metastasis |

AJCC, American Joint Committee on Cancer.

## CASE SUMMARIES

### Locally Advanced HCC

S.R. is a 53-year-old woman with a history of alcoholic cirrhosis and portal hypertension who presented with mild abdominal distension. She denied any history of hepatic encephalopathy, but did have a bleeding esophageal varix a few months ago. On examination, she had mild ascites. Labs revealed a platelet count of 105,000/µL, albumin of 3 g/dL, prothrombin time prolonged 4 s beyond normal, and a bilirubin of 1.5 mg/dL. A CT of the abdomen showed an irregular mass measuring 6.6 × 4.3 cm in the lateral segment of the left hepatic lobe. Another mass measuring 5.5 × 2.8 cm was identified in the left hepatic lobe. Both lesions showed arterial enhancement and rapid washout in the venous and delayed phases. The liver had a nodular contour consistent with cirrhosis. Prominent esophageal, gastric, and periportal venous collaterals were seen, as well as signs of portal hypertension such as an enlarged PV and splenomegaly. No significant intra-abdominal lymphadenopathy was noted. A CT of the chest did not show any metastases. AFP was 500 ng/mL. The ECOG performance status was 0.

### Evidence-Based Case Discussion

S.R. was diagnosed with HCC based on the size of the tumor and the classic findings on imaging of arterial enhancement and washout. Due to multiple tumors >5 cm in diameter, her cancer was stage IIIA according to the TNM classification. Thus, she was not a candidate for surgical resection or transplant. Her cirrhosis was Child-Pugh class B, so her cancer was classified as BCLC stage B. She was referred to interventional radiology for transarterial chemoembolization (TACE).

TACE is a combination of targeted chemotherapy (chemotherapeutic agents delivered via hepatic arterial infusion through a catheter directly into the HCC) and arterial embolization (selective obstruction of blood flow to the tumor using gelatin sponge particles). The rationale behind this approach is the fact that the HA is the major source of blood supply to the tumor. Antineoplastic agents can include doxorubicin, mitomycin, and cisplatin. Clinical trials have demonstrated TACE response rates from 16% to 60% (10). The OS benefits of TACE over best-supportive care have been shown in phase III clinical trials (11); however, meta-analyses of several phase III trials by different groups generated conflicting results (10,12). The improvement in survival in patients undergoing TACE ranges from 20% to 60% at 2 years and 20% to 50% at 3 years in prospective trials. Some studies have also documented the success of TACE as an effective bridge to potentially curative treatments such as surgery or liver transplant. Contraindications for TACE are advanced (Child-Pugh Class C) cirrhosis, PV thrombosis, hepatic

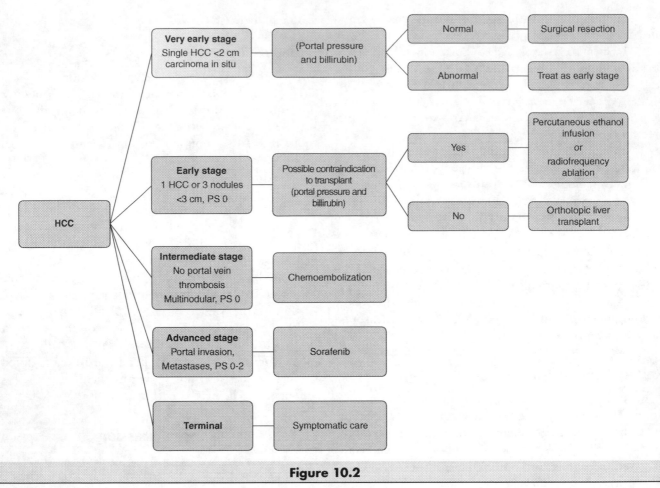

**Figure 10.2**

The BCLC Scale system and treatment algorithm. BCLC, Barcelona Clinic Liver Cancer Scale; HCC, hepatocellular carcinoma; PS, performance status.

encephalopathy, and biliary obstruction. Performing TACE in such cases may cause hepatic failure. S.R. had no contraindications and was prepared for the procedure with vigorous intravenous hydration and prophylactic antibiotics. The first TACE was uncomplicated; however, the second TACE 4 weeks later was followed by a low-grade fever and abdominal pain. This "postembolization syndrome" occurs in up to 50% of patients and is due to acute hepatic ischemia and tumor necrosis. Characterized by fevers, abdominal pain, and ileus, the syndrome is generally self-limited and can be treated with IV hydration and no oral intake. Major complications from TACE include PV thrombosis, hepatic abscess, HA dissection or thrombosis, and liver failure. S.R. recovered within 2 days and was discharged in stable condition. A CT scan post-TACE showed necrosis of 80% of the tumor, and a repeat AFP level decreased to 200 ng/mL. S.R. continues to be monitored with serial scans.

Recently, several small studies and 2 larger randomized-controlled trials have evaluated TACE with sorafenib (13,14). Tumor cells that survive after TACE upregulate hypoxia-inducible factor and vascular endothelial growth factor (VEGF), which promote angiogenesis. Sorafenib inhibits the activity of VEGF receptors and other proangiogenic signaling pathways. Thus, sorafenib administered during and after TACE treatment may counteract hypoxia-induced angiogenesis and potentially yield synergistic efficacy in decreasing tumor burden. Studies have suggested that the combination of TACE and sorafenib is feasible and has a manageable side effect profile. However, whether sorafenib combined with TACE yields additive or synergistic efficacy compared to TACE alone still remains unclear. One randomized phase III study demonstrated no added benefit of TACE with sorafenib versus placebo (14). However, in this study, sorafenib was administered >9 weeks after TACE in 60% of patients, which may have been after the hypoxia-inducible factor and VEGF surge occurred. In contrast, the randomized phase II SPACE trial showed that TACE in combination with sorafenib exhibited a trend for increased time to progression compared to TACE alone (hazard ratio [HR] = 0.79, P = .07) (13). According to National Comprehensive Cancer Network (NCCN) guidelines, sorafenib may be considered after local arterial therapy if liver function returns to baseline, and local therapies cannot be performed for residual cancer. Other randomized phase III trials are ongoing to further investigate combination approaches.

Transarterial radioembolization (TARE) is another liver-directed therapy that has been evaluated mostly in patients with large, infiltrating, or multifocal disease. Yttrium-90 (Y-90) microspheres emit high doses of beta radiation (100–1000 Gy) that penetrate 2.5–11 mm, which limits radiation exposure to normal liver surrounding the tumor. The microspheres are deposited into the hepatic vasculature. TARE can be performed in patients who have PV thrombosis and preserved synthetic liver function. Sangro et al. recently reported long-term survival outcomes after TARE, stratified by BCLC stages. The median OS was 12.8 months, which varied significantly by disease stage (BCLC A, 24.4 months; BCLC B, 16.9 months; and BCLC C, 10 months) (15). A prospective phase II trial showed that the median time to progression after TARE was 11 months and the median OS was 15 months. There was a nonsignificant trend in OS favoring patients without PV thrombosis compared to patients with PV thrombosis (18 vs. 13 months) (16).

In recent years, early stages of HCC have been increasingly recognized due to efficient screening guidelines and better imaging techniques. HCC in the early stage can be treated with surgical resection and demonstrates a 5-year survival up to 70% (17). Hepatic resection is a potentially curative option in patients with adequate liver function, those with a solitary mass, no evidence of major vascular invasion and adequate future liver remnant. Interestingly, the size of the tumor may not limit surgical consideration. In some centers, hepatic vein catheterization is performed to assess the hepatic vein pressure gradient prior to surgical planning. Only those patients with a hepatic venous pressure gradient <10 mmHg and a normal bilirubin level are cleared for surgery. This policy is in accordance with the most recent 2010 AASLD practice guidelines (17). There is currently no role for pre- or post-resection therapy; however, in clinical practice, neoadjuvant local techniques are sometimes used to shrink the tumor so that it may become surgically resectable. Also, PV embolization may be carried out preoperatively in an attempt to induce hypertrophy of the residual liver segments after surgical resection. This is especially beneficial for those with chronic liver disease who are being considered for major liver resection. The Sorafenib as Adjuvant Treatment in the Prevention of Recurrence of Hepatocellular Carcinoma (STORM) trial investigated the effect of adjuvant sorafenib after surgery, but did not meet the primary end point of improving recurrence-free survival.

Liver transplant is indicated for patients with underlying portal hypertension and cirrhosis. On the basis of the Milan criteria, any patient with a solitary tumor <5 cm in diameter, or up to 3 lesions, each <3 cm in diameter, without evidence of vascular invasion or extrahepatic spread, may be eligible for transplantation (18). Patients with HCC within these criteria have posttransplant survival rates of 70% at 5 years. There is level II evidence to support the use of preoperative therapy if the waiting list for transplant exceeds 6 months. This approach helps minimize the risk of progression during the waiting time.

Radiofrequency ablation or percutaneous ethanol injection is the local technique that can be used with curative intent if the patient is not a transplant candidate because the disease burden falls outside the Milan criteria or the patient has other comorbidities. The local control and OS rates for these procedures are very similar to surgical resection (7,17). Even after successful surgery, the risk of recurrence remains up to 50% at 5 years. Therefore, the NCCN guidelines recommend patients be followed with serial imaging every 3–6 months.

## Metastatic HCC

F.S. is a 50-year-old white man with a long-standing history of chronic HCV infection and liver cirrhosis who was admitted to the hospital with abdominal pain and a 20-pound weight loss over the last 3 months. He also noted decreased appetite and fatigue. He had been treated for HCV infection a few years ago. He denied any history of encephalopathy, varices, or ascites. Abdominal examination revealed mild tenderness to palpation in the right upper quadrant. No jaundice or ascites was appreciated. Laboratory testing revealed an albumin of 3.6 g/dL, bilirubin of 1.9 mg/dL, and a prothrombin time within normal limits. A complete blood count and liver chemistry were also within normal limits. A CT scan of the abdomen with contrast was performed and showed several heterogeneous lesions with areas of necrosis in the liver measuring 2–6 cm in diameter. The lesions showed arterial enhancement and early venous washout, and there was concern for PV invasion. Multiple retroperitoneal lymph nodes were enlarged, suggesting metastatic disease. Serum AFP was 800 ng/mL. His ECOG performance status was 1.

### Evidence-Based Case Discussion

F.S. was diagnosed with HCC based on the size of the tumor and the classic findings seen on imaging of arterial enhancement followed by washout of contrast in the venous-delayed phases. The tumor was classified as stage IV according to the TNM classification. The Child-Pugh score was class A with a good performance status. Thus, the BCLC stage was C, advanced disease.

In this case, tissue biopsy is not required to diagnose HCC. As per the NCCN guidelines, presence of a tumor >1 cm with 2 classic enhancements on 1 imaging study (usually CT or MRI with contrast) in a patient with cirrhosis is diagnostic of HCC. A tumor with no or 1 classic enhancements requires a second type of contrast-enhanced scan. If there are no classic findings in imaging, biopsy is indicated to establish the diagnosis. Once the diagnosis was confirmed in this case, CT of the chest was performed to complete the staging and was negative.

Four main factors determine prognosis in HCC: (a) stage, (b) tumor aggressiveness, (c) liver function, and (d) performance status of the patient. The BCLC system uses all of these factors to determine stage, recommended treatment, and prognosis (17).

The most appropriate treatment for F.S. is systemic therapy due to his advanced disease. Historically, many different treatment strategies have been used in such advanced cases, including systemic doxorubicin, interferon, tamoxifen, and radiation therapy, but none has demonstrated a survival benefit (9). The median survival in untreated patients is usually <6 months. The landmark study that significantly impacted clinical practice was the Study of Heart and Renal Protection (SHARP) trial (19). This was a multicenter, double-blinded, phase III clinical study that proved the efficacy of sorafenib, a multikinase inhibitor that targets vascular endothelial growth factor receptor 2 (VEGFR2), platelet-derived growth factor receptor (PDGFR), Raf-1, B-Raf, c-Kit, other tyrosine kinases, and serine threonine kinases. This trial enrolled 602 patients with advanced HCC who were not candidates for local treatment or had progressed after failing local treatment. All patients had an ECOG of ≤ 2, and 97% were classified as Child-Pugh Class A. All had adequate renal and hematopoietic function, and were randomized to either sorafenib (400 mg) twice a day or placebo. Overall median survival was significantly longer in the sorafenib group than the placebo group (10.7 vs. 7.9 months). A 31% reduction in the risk of death was noted. The disease control rate was also significantly higher in the sorafenib group than the placebo group (43% vs. 32%). The 2 most relevant adverse effects of sorafenib were diarrhea and hand–foot syndrome, both of which occurred in 8% of patients.

The other major phase III trial that evaluated sorafenib in HCC patients was the Asia-Pacific study, a randomized, double-blind, placebo-controlled study (20). Compared with the SHARP trial, this trial was smaller, randomizing a total of 226 patients with advanced HCC to receive either oral sorafenib (400 mg twice daily) or placebo. All patients were Child-Pugh Class A. The median OS was significantly longer in the sorafenib group compared with the placebo group (6.5 vs. 4.2 months). Median time to progression was also improved with sorafenib (2.8 vs. 1.4 months). Sorafenib did not produce a significant response rate. The safety profile of sorafenib was similar to that reported in the SHARP trial. As a result, the NCCN and AASLD guidelines now recommend sorafenib as the first-line treatment for advanced disease (extrahepatic spread or portal invasion) not amenable to other modalities in patients with well-preserved liver function (i.e., Child-Pugh Class A).

F.S. was started on sorafenib, which he tolerated well except for mild diarrhea. A dynamic CT scan was repeated 12 weeks after initiation of treatment and showed no change in the size of the liver mass; however, increased necrosis throughout the tumor was observed. Such necrosis is typically seen in patients who respond to sorafenib, and this patient continues to have stable disease after 1 year on sorafenib.

Sorafenib is not recommended in patients who are Child-Pugh Class C, and data on the use of sorafenib in Child-Pugh Class B are limited. The Global Investigation of therapeutic DEcisions in hepatocellular carcinoma and Of its treatment with sorafeNib (GIDEON) study is a global, prospective study evaluating the safety of sorafenib in real-life practice. In the second interim analysis of the GIDEON cohort, 74% of patients received the full 800-mg sorafenib dose, but median duration of therapy was shorter in patients with Child-Pugh B cirrhosis. Adverse effects were similar across Child-Pugh, BCLC, and initial dosing subgroups (21).

Bevacizumab has been studied both as monotherapy and in combination with other agents. Most trials have been small phase II trials with variable results, and larger randomized trials are needed to determine the role of bevacizumab in the treatment of advanced HCC (22). Fibroblast growth factor (FGF) is another key driver of angiogenesis in HCC. Brivanib is an oral tyrosine kinase inhibitor that inhibits VEGF and FGF signaling. The BRISK-FL study examined the role of first-line brivanib compared to sorafenib in advanced HCC. The BRISK-PS study investigated the use of second-line brivanib compared to placebo after progression on sorafenib (23,24).

## REVIEW QUESTIONS

1. A 47-year-old Asian man with a history of hepatitis B infection and Child-Pugh class B cirrhosis presented for his 6-month surveillance for hepatocellular carcinoma. Ultrasonography revealed a new solitary 2.5-cm lesion in the right lobe of the liver. Triphasic contrast-enhanced CT showed arterial enhancement of the lesion without venous washout. The serum level of alpha-fetoprotein was 20 ng/mL. Which of the following is the most appropriate next step?

   (A) Six-month follow-up with ultrasound
   (B) Three-month follow-up with CT
   (C) Treat the lesion with radiofrequency ablation
   (D) Dynamic MRI
   (E) Orthotropic liver transplantation

2. A 58-year-old man with primary biliary cirrhosis and Child-Pugh class A cirrhosis was referred for evaluation. The serum level of alpha-fetoprotein (AFP) was 5 mg/mL and the results of recent abdominal ultrasonography were negative. Six months later, the serum AFP was stable at 7 ng/mL, but ultrasonography showed a new 6-cm mass in the right lobe of the liver

and a 3-cm nodule in the left lobe. CT demonstrated arterial phase enhancement of the mass, with washout in the portal and venous phases but no portal vein thrombosis or other evidence of extrahepatic disease. The patient was living independently and working full time. The most appropriate management for him is:

(A) Surgical resection
(B) Radiofrequency ablation
(C) Comfort care
(D) Transarterial chemoembolization
(E) Orthotropic liver transplantation

3. A 55-year-old man with hepatitis C infection and liver cirrhosis presented with a large infiltrative hepatocellular carcinoma (HCC) in the right lobe of the liver and right portal vein thrombosis. He had ascites, which required 3 large volume paracentesis during the past 2 months. He was capable of only limited self care and was confined to the bed >50% of the day. On physical examination, he was malnourished and in a wheelchair. He was slow in his thinking but oriented to self, place, and time. He had spider angiomas, moderate ascites, and asterixis. Labs: Na = 129, K = 3.5, Cl = 100, $CO_2$ = 16, BUN = 40, creatinine = 1.6, glucose = 80, albumin = 2.7, total bilirubin = 3.1, ALT = 20, AST = 130, Alk Phos = 250, INR = 1.8, WBC = 12,000, Hgb = 8.5, Hct = 26, Plt = 87,000, and AFP = 400,000. The most appropriate management for his HCC at this time is:

(A) Sorafenib
(B) Liver transplantation
(C) Transarterial chemoembolization
(D) Surgical resection
(E) Supportive measures

4. A 45-year-old obese white man with fatty liver disease and liver cirrhosis was referred to an oncologist after a biopsy showed hepatocellular cancer. Abdominal CT revealed multifocal infiltrative hepatocellular carcinoma involving the left and right hepatic lobes with retroperitoneal lymphadenopathy. He complained of fatigue, but was still very active. He was able to work and perform household chores. On physical examination, he was fully oriented, in no acute distress. His abdomen was obese without ascites. Labs: Na = 137, K = 4.2, Cl = 105, $CO_2$ = 22, BUN = 17, creatinine = 1.0, glucose = 120, albumin = 3.5, total bilirubin = 1.0, PT = 12 s, INR = 1.1, ALT = 40, AST = 78, Alk Phos = 142, WBC = 8000, Hgb = 11.3, Plt = 130,000, and AFP = 20 ng/mL. Which of the following is the most appropriate next step?

(A) Liver transplantation
(B) Transarterial chemoembolization
(C) Sorafenib
(D) Supportive measures
(E) Portal vein embolization and surgical resection

5. A 52-year-old Japanese man with a past medical history of hepatitis B infection and Child-Pugh class A cirrhosis presented for his 6-month surveillance for hepatocellular carcinoma (HCC). Ultrasonography showed a new solitary 2-cm lesion in the left lobe of the liver. Triphasic contrast-enhanced CT and MRI both showed arterial enhancement of the lesion without venous washout. Transcutaneous biopsy of the liver mass was consistent with HCC. There was no portal vein thrombosis or other evidence of extrahepatic disease. He was very fit and ran 2 miles every day. On physical examination, he was found to be alert and fully oriented, with no evidence of ascites. Labs: Na = 140, K = 4.1, Cl = 105, $CO_2$ = 24, BUN = 15, creatinine = 0.80, glucose = 98, albumin = 3.7, total bilirubin = 1.0, PT = 11 s, INR = 1.0, ALT = 71, AST = 81, Alk Phos = 142, WBC = 8000, Hgb = 12.5, Plt = 160,000. Which of the following is the most appropriate next step?

(A) Liver transplantation
(B) Surgical resection
(C) Transarterial chemoembolization
(D) Sorafenib

6. A 53-year-old white man received a screening abdominal ultrasound due to a history of hepatitis C virus and Child-Pugh class B cirrhosis. The ultrasound showed 2 lesions measuring 2.4 cm and 1 cm in the right and left hepatic lobes, respectively, with moderate ascites. Triphasic contrast-enhanced CT revealed arterial enhancement of both lesions with venous washout, without portal vein thrombosis or other evidence of extrahepatic disease. He had mild fatigue when performing housework. Esophagogastroduodenoscopy showed grade I esophageal varices. The serum level of alpha-fetoprotein was 15 ng/mL. Labs: Na = 139, K = 4.2, Cl = 107, $CO_2$ = 21, BUN = 19, creatinine = 0.9, glucose = 110, albumin = 3.0, total bilirubin = 2.1, PT = 12 s, INR = 1.1, ALT = 51, AST = 78, Alk Phos = 157, WBC = 4300, Hgb = 11.3, and Plt = 115,000. Which of the following is the most appropriate next step?

(A) Liver transplantation
(B) Surgical resection
(C) Transarterial chemoembolization
(D) Sorafenib

7. A 30-year-old Hispanic woman with a past medical history of primary sclerosing cholangitis presented to the emergency department with 3 days of abdominal pain, nausea, vomiting, and subjective fever. She had been otherwise healthy and active prior to this illness. Labs: Na = 140, K = 4.0, Cl = 106, $CO_2$ = 26, BUN = 4, creatinine = 0.7, glucose = 121, total protein = 6.1, albumin = 3.0, ALT = 217, AST = 100, Alk Phos = 498, and total bilirubin = 3.9 (direct bilirubin = 3.6). CT

scan of the abdomen showed mild intrahepatic ductal dilatation, a 4.3-cm hypodense mass surrounding the proximal extrahepatic common bile duct, inseparable from the pancreatic head and second portion of the duodenum, and multiple subcentimeter mesenteric and retroperitoneal lymph nodes. Endoscopic retrograde cholangiopancreatography revealed a beading appearance of the intra- and extrahepatic bile ducts. The suspicious lesion was biopsied and showed cholangiocarcinoma. Which of the following is the most appropriate treatment for her cancer?

(A) Concurrent chemoradiation with capecitabine
(B) Systemic chemotherapy with cisplatin and gemcitabine
(C) Systemic chemotherapy with 5-fluorouracil/ leucovorin
(D) Systemic chemotherapy with gemcitabine
(E) Supportive care

## REFERENCES

1. Valle J, Wasan H, Palmer DH, et al. Cisplatin plus gemcitabine versus gemcitabine for biliary tract cancer. *N Engl J Med.* 2010;362(14):1273–1281.
2. Wistuba II, Gazdar AF. Gallbladder cancer: lessons from a rare tumour. *Nat Rev Cancer.* 2004;4(9):695–706.
3. Aljiffry M, Walsh MJ, Molinari M. Advances in diagnosis, treatment and palliation of cholangiocarcinoma: 1990–2009. *World J Gastroenterol.* 2009;15(34):4240–4262.
4. Macdonald OK, Crane CH. Palliative and postoperative radiotherapy in biliary tract cancer. *Surg Oncol Clin N Am.* 2002;11(4):941–954.
5. Glazer ES, Liu P, Abdalla EK, et al. Neither neo-adjuvant nor adjuvant therapy increases survival after biliary tract cancer resection with wide negative margins. *Gastrointest Surg.* 2012;16:1666–1671.
6. Eckel F, Schmid RM. Chemotherapy in advanced biliary tract carcinoma: a pooled analysis of clinical trials. *Br J Cancer.* 2007;96(6):896–902.
7. Verslype C, Van Cutsem E, Dicato M, et al. The management of hepatocellular carcinoma. Current expert opinion and recommendations derived from the 10th World Congress on Gastrointestinal Cancer, Barcelona, 2008. *Ann Oncol.* 2009;20(suppl 7):vii1–vii6.
8. El-Serag HB, Marrero JA, Rudolph L, et al. Diagnosis and treatment of hepatocellular carcinoma. *Gastroenterology.* 2008;134(6):1752–1763.
9. Bartlett DL, Di Bisceglie AM, Dawson LA. Cancer of the liver. In: Pine JW, Jacobs AE, eds. *DeVita, Hellman, and Rosenberg's Cancer: Principles & Practice of Oncology.* 8th ed. Philadelphia, PA: Lippincott Williams & Wilkins; 2008:1129–1155.
10. Llovet JM, Bruix J. Systematic review of randomized trials for unresectable hepatocellular carcinoma: chemoembolization improves survival. *Hepatology.* 2003;37(2):429–442.
11. Llovet JM, Real MI, Montaña X, et al. Arterial embolisation or chemoembolisation versus symptomatic treatment in patients with unresectable hepatocellular carcinoma: a randomized control trial. *Lancet.* 2002;359(9319):1734–1739.
12. Geschwind JF, Ramsey DE, Choti MA, et al. Chemoembolization of hepatocellular carcinoma: results of a metaanalysis. *Am J Clin Oncol.* 2003;26(4):344–349.
13. Leicioni R, Llovet JM, Han G, et al. Sorafenib or placebo in combination with transarterial chemoembolization (TACE) with doxorubicin-eluting beads (DEBDOX) for intermediate-stage hepatocellular carcinoma (HCC): phase II, randomized, double-blind SPACE trial. *J Clin Oncol.* 2012;30(suppl 4_sabstr LBA154).
14. Kudo M, Imanaka K, Chida N, et al. Phase III study of sorafenib after transarterial chemoembolisation in Japanese and Korean patients with unresectable hepatocellular carcinoma. *Eur J Cancer.* 2011;47(14):2017–2027.
15. Sangro B, Carpanese L, Cianni R, et al. Survival after Yttrium-90 resin microsphere radioembolization of hepatocellular carcinoma across Barcelona clinic liver cancer stages: a European evaluation. *Hepatology.* 2011;54(3):868–878.
16. Mazzaferro V, Sposito C, Bhoori S, et al. Yttrium-90 radioembolization for intermediate-advanced hepatocellular carcinoma: a phase 2 study. *Hepatology.* 2013;57(5):1826–1837.
17. Bruix J, Sherman M. Management of hepatocellular carcinoma: an update. *Hepatology.* 2011;53(3):1020–1022.
18. Mazzaferro V, Regalia E, Doci R, et al. Liver transplantation for the treatment of small hepatocellular carcinomas in patients with cirrhosis. *New Engl J Med.* 1996;334(11):728–729.
19. Llovet JM, Ricci S, Mazzaferro V, et al. Sorafenib in advanced hepatocellular carcinoma. *New Engl J Med.* 2008;359(4):378–390.
20. Cheng AL, Kang YK, Chen Z, et al. Efficacy and safety of sorafenib in patients in the Asia-Pacific region with advanced hepatocellular carcinoma: a phase III randomised, double-blind, placebo-controlled trial. *Lancet Oncol.* 2009;10(1):25–34.
21. Lencioni R, Kudo M, Ye S-L, et al. GIDEON (Global Investigation of therapeutic DEcisions in hepatocellular carcinoma and Of its treatment with sorafeNib): second interim analysis. *Int J Clin Pract.* 2014;68(5):609–617.
22. Fang, P, Hu, J, Cheng Z, et al. Efficacy and safety of bevacizumab for the treatment of advanced hepatocellular carcinoma: a systematic review of phase II trials. *PLoS ONE.* 2012;7(12):e49717.
23. Llovet JM, Decaens T, Raoul J-L, et al. Brivanib in patients with advanced hepatocellular carcinoma who were intolerant to sorafenib or for whom sorafenib failed: results from the randomized phase III BRISK PS study. *J Clin Oncol.* 2013;31(28):3509–3516.
24. Johnson PJ, Quin S, Park JW, et al. Brivanib versus sorafenib as first-line therapy in patients with unresectable, advanced hepatocellular carcinoma: results from the randomized phase III BRISK-FL study. *J Clin Oncol.* 2013;31(28):3517–3524.

# 11

# *Colorectal Cancer*

JASMINE KAMBOJ, YVONNE SADA, AND BENJAMIN L. MUSHER

## EPIDEMIOLOGY, RISK FACTORS, NATURAL HISTORY, AND PATHOLOGY

As the most common gastrointestinal cancer and the third leading cause of cancer-related mortality in the United States, colorectal cancer (CRC) is expected to account for 136,830 new cases and 50,310 deaths in 2014. Although the overall incidence of CRC has been slowly declining, presumably due to the excision of premalignant adenomatous polyps during routine screening of appropriate individuals, emerging data suggest a rising incidence among patients younger than 50 years. Advances in treatment continue to improve 5-year survival rates for both early- and late-stage CRC; however, outcomes among minority populations, in particular African Americans, remain significantly worse because of less access to medical care and perhaps more aggressive tumor biology.

The pathogenesis of CRC involves a well-described evolution from normal colonic epithelium, to adenoma, and ultimately to frank carcinoma. Because this transformation generally requires 10 years, experts recommend colonoscopy every 5–10 years for people at "average risk" for CRC. Two distinct processes have been implicated in this adenoma–carcinoma sequence: chromosomal instability and microsatellite instability (MSI). Chromosomal instability, which accounts for the majority (80–85%) of cases, occurs when inactivating mutations in genes that regulate DNA replication alter chromosome copy number or function, leading to loss of function of tumor suppressor genes. Loss of function of the adenomatous polyposis coli (APC) tumor suppressor gene initiates the process, and the accumulation of additional mutations leads to carcinogenesis. While tumorigenesis typically requires 2 somatic "hits" (1 to each allele of the *APC* gene), carriers of an *APC* germ-line mutation require only 1 somatic mutation to initiate the adenoma–carcinoma sequence. Thus, in contrast to the 5–10-year adenoma–carcinoma sequence observed in average-risk patients, carriers of *APC* germ-line mutations develop thousands of adenomatous polyps at a young age (familial adenomatous polyposis [FAP]) and are at high risk for CRC by late adolescence.

MSI, which accounts for the remaining 15–20% of CRCs, occurs when mutation or epigenetic silencing of 1 or more of the DNA mismatch repair (MMR) enzymes MLH1, MSH2, MSH6, and PMS2 causes slippage within short repetitive DNA sequences (microsatellites). Epigenetic hypermethylation of the MLH1 promoter, which silences MLH1 expression in tumor tissue only, accounts for 80% of microsatellite unstable CRC. The remaining 20% of MSI-related tumors (accounting for 3–4% of all CRC cases) arise in individuals who harbor either a germ-line mutation in 1 of the 4 aforementioned *MMR* genes or a deletion in the *EpCAM* gene, which induces silencing of MSH2 by promoter hypermethylation. Starting at a relatively young age, carriers of a germ-line MMR enzyme mutation are at high risk of colorectal, as well as gastric, small bowel, hepatobiliary, genitourinary, gynecologic, and brain tumors—a syndrome known as hereditary non-polyposis colon cancer, or Lynch syndrome. Although carriers of germ-line APC or MMR mutations hold the highest known lifetime risk of CRC, other high-risk populations include those with inflammatory bowel disease, family history of CRC without an identifiable germ-line mutation, or a personal history of adenomatous polyps or colon cancer. More frequent screening should be offered to any individual deemed at higher than average risk for developing CRC.

Because only a minority of CRCs can be attributed to known genetic syndromes, epidemiologists and scientists have hypothesized that environmental exposures may alter an individual's risk of developing CRC. Smoking, diabetes, obesity, red meat consumption, and high-fat diet may increase the risk of developing CRC, whereas high-fiber diet, hormone replacement therapy, active lifestyle, and anti-inflammatory drug use (nonsteroidal anti-inflammatory drugs [NSAIDs] and aspirin) have been identified as protective factors. The precise impact of these factors on CRC risk and how they should influence CRC screening have, however, not yet been identified.

Colon cancer and rectal cancer share histopathological, molecular, and genetic features, but due to anatomical considerations, their clinical behaviors differ. Although large or perforated colonic tumors may spread locally to involve adjacent organs or peritoneum, colon cancer more commonly metastasizes by lymphovascular invasion. Because colonic vasculature drains into the portal venous system, the liver is the most common site of metastases, followed by the lungs, remote lymph nodes, bones, and rarely the central nervous system. Compared to colon cancer, rectal cancer has a greater propensity for local spread and recurrence, due to the absence of a rectal serosa and the rectum's proximity to other pelvic structures. As a result, measures to improve local control, namely, total mesorectal excision (TME) and neoadjuvant chemoradiotherapy, have been incorporated into standard therapy for rectal cancer. Rectal cancer also metastasizes remotely, but due to the rectum's dual portal and systemic venous drainage, it commonly bypasses the liver directly and spreads directly to the lungs.

CRC may be diagnosed during routine screening or may present with tumor-related symptoms. Symptoms of early disease include anemia-induced fatigue, gross blood per rectum, crampy abdominal pain, change in stool caliber, or tenesmus. Advanced CRC can present with focal symptoms related to the primary tumor and/or metastases, but may also present with generalized weakness, fatigue, and weight loss.

## Colorectal Cancer Staging

| Stage | Description |
|-------|-------------|
| I | Primary tumor invades no deeper than muscularis propria (T1 or T2), no lymph nodes (N0) or metastases |
| IIA | Primary tumor invades pericolorectal tissue (T3), no lymph nodes (N0) or metastases |
| IIB | Primary tumor invades visceral peritoneum surface (T4a), no lymph nodes (N0) or metastases |
| IIC | Primary tumor invades other organs (T4b), no lymph nodes (N0) or metastases |
| IIIA | Primary tumor invades no deeper than muscularis propria (T1 or T2), ≤2–3 regional lymph node involvement (N1a, N1b), no metastases |
|  | Primary tumor invades only submucosa (T1), 4–6 regional lymph nodes involved (N2a), no metastases |

## CASE SUMMARIES

### Unresectable Metastatic CRC

L.L. is a 57-year-old woman who presented with a 2-month history of abdominal pain, thin caliber stools, and weight loss. Laboratory evaluation was significant for a hemoglobin of 6.5 g/dL and ferritin of 3 µg/L, consistent with iron deficiency anemia. A CT scan revealed circumferential thickening of the sigmoid colon and numerous bilateral liver masses, the largest of which measured 10.7 × 7.7 cm. Colonoscopy showed a nonobstructing, circumferential sigmoid mass, and pathology revealed poorly differentiated adenocarcinoma. No *KRAS* mutation was identified. The serum carcinoembryonic antigen (CEA) was 155 ng/mL. Aside from having well-controlled diabetes and hypertension, L.L. was healthy and extremely functional. She had no family history of cancer.

The patient initially received 4 cycles of FOLFOX (5-fluorouracil [5-FU], leucovorin [LV], and oxaliplatin) with bevacizumab (BV), the latter of which caused mild hypertension requiring initiation of amlodipine. Restaging CT scans showed a 40% decrease in the size of the liver masses, and the CEA now measured 2 ng/mL. After 2 more cycles of FOLFOX, she developed grade II neuropathy; so oxaliplatin was discontinued. After 12 additional cycles of 5-FU/LV/BV (10 months total of systemic chemotherapy), the CEA rose to 11 ng/mL, and CT scans showed new bilateral pulmonary nodules. Oxaliplatin was reintroduced due to an absence of persistent neuropathy, and CT imaging after 4 more cycles showed response. Almost 16 months into her treatment, her disease progressed again, and FOLFIRI (5-FU, LV, and irinotecan) with BV was initiated. After initial stabilization of her disease, a CT scan 6 months into starting FOLFIRI/BV showed progression. Her performance status remained excellent, so further treatment options were considered.

### Evidence-Based Case Discussion

L.L. has stage IV colon cancer in the context of unresectable liver metastases. Due to her excellent Eastern Cooperative Oncology Group (ECOG) performance status and her *KRAS* wild-type (WT) tumor, she is an appropriate candidate for any of the available systemic therapies for metastatic CRC (mCRC), including monoclonal antibodies targeting the epidermal growth factor receptor (EGFR). This case illustrates the armamentarium that has become available to clinicians treating mCRC, the sequential approach to using these agents, the factors that guide clinical decision making, and the management of treatment-related toxicity.

### Determining the Goals of Therapy

Treatment of mCRC should be guided by the primary goal of care: palliation or long-term survival. Until relatively recently, mCRC was considered uniformly fatal and therefore treated exclusively with palliative intent. With the emergence of aggressive multidisciplinary management, consisting of novel surgical and ablative techniques combined with modern chemoimmunotherapy, a growing number of patients with mCRC are being treated with curative intent (see the section titled Potentially Resectable or Resectable Metastatic CRC). However, most patients with mCRC present with widespread disease and are therefore not candidates for curative therapy. While the primary goal of therapy in such cases is palliation—controlling tumor growth, alleviating tumor-related symptoms, prolonging life, and maintaining quality of life (QOL)—the possibility of long-term survival should be entertained during the course of treatment in case a dramatic clinical response occurs and/or new local therapies emerge. Owing to the number and distribution of her metastases, L.L. has unresectable disease, and her oncologist should explain unambiguously during the initial visit that the primary goal of therapy is palliation.

## Addressing the Primary Tumor in CRC With Unresectable Metastases

On evaluating the patient with unresectable mCRC, the oncologist must decide whether the primary colorectal tumor requires intervention after carefully assessing the patient's symptomatology, tumor burden, prognosis, comorbidities, and performance status. Symptoms related to the primary colorectal tumor include obstruction, perforation, and bleeding. Patients with clinical perforation and/or heavy bleeding should generally undergo surgical resection, while those with obstruction can be treated with resection, diversion, or stent placement depending on operative risk, overall tumor burden, anatomical location, and available expertise. If symptoms related to the primary tumor are mild or absent, the question of whether to address the primary tumor is more complicated. Prior to the advent of effective chemotherapy for mCRC, the risk of developing bowel obstruction or clinically significant gastrointestinal bleeding during the course of systemic treatment was unacceptably high. Primary tumor resection (PTR) to prevent local complications therefore became common practice. As more effective chemotherapy for mCRC emerged, it made less sense to expose patients to the risks of major abdominal surgery, which, even without major complications, could postpone the initiation of systemic therapy by several weeks. To illustrate the safety of foregoing PTR in the context of mCRC, investigators at Memorial Sloan Kettering retrospectively reviewed the cases of 233 mCRC patients who had received combination chemotherapy without initial PTR. Over the course of treatment, 89% did not experience any primary tumor complication requiring intervention. Four percent required nonoperative palliation with stent placement or radiation,

and only 7% required emergent surgery for obstruction or perforation (1). These data indicate that, with modern chemotherapy and palliative interventions, the vast majority of mCRC patients with relatively asymptomatic primary tumors may safely forego PTR at diagnosis.

Newer data, however, suggest that selected patients who do not require urgent intervention at diagnosis may benefit from upfront PTR. From an analysis of 16,029 patients with stage IV disease identified from the Search Results Surveillance, Epidemiology, and End Results (SEER) Registry, Sada et al. showed that, although PTR became less frequently performed between 1998 and 2008, it was associated with an improved 1- and 3-year survival (2). Similarly, a retrospective analysis of 810 patients with unresectable mCRC enrolled in 4 prospective randomized controlled trials (RCTs) comparing various chemotherapy regimens reported that the hazard ratio (HR) for death in the 478 patients who had undergone PTR was 0.63, 95% confidence interval (CI) [0.53–0.75] (3). Due to potential selection bias, neither of these studies proves that patients with unresectable mCRC benefit from upfront PTR, but 2 ongoing RCTs (Dutch CAIRO4 and German SYNCHRONOUS) are addressing this very issue. For the time being, clinicians must make a recommendation after weighing the risks and benefits of upfront PTR versus upfront chemotherapy, conferring with an experienced surgical oncologist, and discussing available options with the patient.

L.L. had thin caliber stools but was not frankly obstructed; so urgent surgical intervention was not required. Due to the lack of randomized data supporting routine upfront PTR and the presence of large burden liver metastases, the treating oncologist recommended starting chemotherapy as soon as possible. L.L. was prescribed an aggressive bowel regimen and was reminded to call if she developed obstipation, worsening abdominal pain, or uncontrolled vomiting.

## Systemic Chemotherapy for mCRC

### 5-FU and LV

The median survival of mCRC with best supportive care (BSC) alone is approximately 6 months, but advances in chemotherapy (CTX), starting with the approval of 5-FU in 1957, have significantly improved outcomes. As a single agent, 5-FU yields an objective response rate of 15% and a median survival of 10–14 months. Adding LV, a reduced form of folic acid that stabilizes the binding of 5-FU to thymidylate synthase, improves the response rate to 25% but does not significantly change median survival.

Numerous studies have addressed the optimal administration of 5-FU—bolus, infusional, or oral. The original regimen, devised at the Mayo Clinic, consists of bolus 5-FU (b5-FU) daily for 5 days, repeated every 4 weeks. The Roswell Park regimen, which consists of weekly b5-FU for 6 weeks followed by a 2-week break, causes less myelosuppression and mucositis than its predecessor. The newest regimen, devised by de Gramont et al. (LV5-FU2), combines b5-FU, LV, and infusional 5-FU (i5-FU) (4). Having undergone several permutations to date, LV5-FU2 is most commonly administered as biweekly b5-FU 400 mg/m², LV 400 mg/m², and i5-FU 2400 mg/m² over 46 hours. Compared to the Mayo Clinic regimen, LV5-FU2 yields a higher response rate (32% vs. 14%), significantly longer progression-free survival (PFS; 28 vs. 22 weeks), and less myelosuppression, mucositis, and diarrhea. On the basis of its favorable efficacy and toxicity profile, the LV5-FU2 has become the standard for intravenous administration of 5-FU. Capecitabine, an oral pro-drug of 5-FU, has also proven to be as effective and more tolerable than b5-FU and therefore serves as a reasonable alternative to LV5-FU2 for patients who prefer an oral regimen. Aside from myelosuppression and mucositis, capecitabine can cause hand–foot syndrome (HFS), which is generally manageable with supportive care and dose adjustment.

## Irinotecan

5-FU remained the only available chemotherapeutic agent for CRC until the late 1990s, when the Food and Drug Administration (FDA) approved irinotecan for second-line therapy, based on randomized data showing that irinotecan improved survival and QOL over BSC in patients with 5-FU-refractory mCRC. Irinotecan was subsequently approved for CTX-naive mCRC after the combination of irinotecan and 5-FU demonstrated superior response rate (49% vs. 31%, P < .001), PFS (6.7 vs. 4.4 months, P < .001), and overall survival (OS; 17.4 vs. 14.1 months, P = .031) over 5-FU alone in patients with untreated mCRC (5). Because both irinotecan and 5-FU can cause nausea and diarrhea, gastrointestinal toxicity can be compounded when the agents are used simultaneously. During the chemotherapy consent process, patients need to be warned about CTX-induced diarrhea and taught how to manage it aggressively with antidiarrheal medications.

In order to maximize benefits while minimizing toxicity, clinical trials have tested various regimens that combine 5-FU and irinotecan. For example, the BICC-C trial compared LV5-FU2 plus biweekly irinotecan (FOLFIRI); b5-FU plus irinotecan (modified irinotecan, b5-FU, and LV [IFL]); and capecitabine plus Irinotecan (CapeIRI) (6). FOLFIRI yielded the best PFS and OS (7.6 and 23.1 months, respectively), while CapeIRI clearly caused the most gastrointestinal toxicity, with 25% of patients in this arm stopping treatment due to intolerable side effects. On the basis of the results from BICC-C and other published data, FOLFIRI (biweekly irinotecan 180 mg/m² plus LV5-FU2) remains the standard regimen for combining irinotecan and 5-FU. Although subsequent trials have shown that CapeIRI may be more tolerable than the BICC-C data

indicate, this regimen is not included in commonly referenced guidelines, such as the National Comprehensive Cancer Network (NCCN), and should therefore be used with extreme caution or avoided altogether.

## Oxaliplatin

A third-generation antineoplastic platinum derivative, oxaliplatin forms platinum–DNA adducts that appear to be more cytotoxic than those formed by cisplatin and carboplatin. Oxaliplatin has demonstrated cytotoxic synergy with 5-FU in cancer cell lines and carries a different side-effect profile than its predecessors, causing considerably less nausea, ototoxicity, and nephrotoxicity than cisplatin; less myelosuppression than carboplatin; and more neurotoxicity than either. As opposed to irinotecan, which has proven antineoplastic activity when used alone or in combination with 5-FU, oxaliplatin has only demonstrated benefit when combined with 5-FU. In 2002, the FDA approved oxaliplatin plus 5-FU/LV for mCRC refractory to 5-FU/LV and irinotecan. Two years later, oxaliplatin was approved in the first-line setting based on randomized data showing that FOLFOX (oxaliplatin 85 mg/m² plus LV5-FU2) yielded a significantly better response rate (50% vs. 21.9%) and PFS (9 vs. 6 months) than LV5-FU2 in patients with untreated mCRC (7). Although FOLFOX was well tolerated, it caused more neutropenia, mucositis, diarrhea, and neuropathy than 5-FU/LV alone.

The question of whether intravenous 5-FU and capecitabine can be used interchangeably with oxaliplatin was addressed by NO16966—a noninferiority trial comparing CAPEOX (capecitabine 1000 mg/m² twice daily on days 1–14 and oxaliplatin 130 mg/m² on day 1 of a 21-day cycle) to FOLFOX in patients with untreated mCRC (8). Initially, NO16966 included only 2 arms. However, the trial was amended to a 2 × 2 factorial design (CAPEOX vs. FOLFOX and BV vs. placebo) after a phase III trial showing improved survival from adding BV to chemotherapy was reported. NO16966 met its goal of noninferiority, with CAPEOX and FOLFOX yielding similar PFS (8 months) and OS (20 months).

Given that CAPEOX and FOLFOX appear to be equally effective, clinicians must help patients choose between these regimens based on other factors. CAPEOX offers patients the convenience of taking pills rather than wearing an infusion pump and receiving intravenous oxaliplatin every 3 weeks instead of every 2 weeks. On the other hand, it requires strict adherence to an oral medication schedule, raises the possibility of unpredictable drug levels due to variable gut absorption and interaction with other oral medications, and causes more HFS and diarrhea than i5-FU. FOLFOX does not require adherence to an oral regimen and is not affected by gut absorption, but it requires a 46-hour outpatient infusion and more frequent visits to an infusion suite. Because a Port-a-cath is required for i5-FU, patients are exposed to additional risk, primarily infection and thrombosis. FOLFOX causes less gastrointestinal toxicity and HFS than CAPEOX, but more neutropenia.

Distinguishing between the 2 neuropathic syndromes associated with oxaliplatin is crucial to proper oncological care. The first syndrome is an acute neurosensory complex that appears during or immediately after infusion and is characterized by cold-induced digital sensitivity and pharyngeal dysaesthesias. Although bothersome to patients, these symptoms are innocuous, transient, and reversible, generally disappearing by 1 week after oxaliplatin administration. Oncologists should warn their patients about the high likelihood of cold sensitivity and advise them to wear gloves in cold weather, to avoid holding cold objects, and to drink room temperature beverages until cold-induced symptoms subside. The second syndrome—an insidious, cumulative, and potentially debilitating "stocking and glove" peripheral sensory neuropathy (PSN)—develops with prolonged exposure to oxaliplatin. Unlike the acute syndrome, which can occur during or immediately following any oxaliplatin infusion, signs of true PSN tend to appear after 3–4 months of therapy. Clinicians must be particularly sensitive to the onset of true PSN so that oxaliplatin can be appropriately dose reduced or discontinued. Although oxaliplatin should be used cautiously in patients with preexisting neuropathy, diabetic patients without baseline neuropathy do not appear to be at higher risk for developing oxaliplatin-induced neurotoxicity and should therefore not be denied oxaliplatin based on diabetes alone.

Because PSN can significantly affect QOL and may necessitate oxaliplatin discontinuation before loss of treatment effect, various strategies to decrease oxaliplatin-induced neurotoxicity have been evaluated. OPTIMOX1 tested the hypothesis that using oxaliplatin on a "stop-and-go" basis would optimize duration of benefit by limiting cumulative toxicity (9). Patients were randomized to FOLFOX until progression or intolerance (control arm) or FOLFOX for 6 cycles, followed by 12 cycles of "maintenance" 5-FU, and reintroduction of FOLFOX for 6 more cycles ("stop-and-go" approach). All outcome measures (response rate, PFS, and OS) were similar between the 2 arms. However, because only 40% of patients in the experimental arm were reintroduced to FOLFOX and because 70% of these patients had a response or stable disease, the "stop-and-go" approach may have demonstrated improved survival with stricter protocol adherence. In fact, subsequent analysis confirmed that reintroducing oxaliplatin had a statistically significant impact on OS (HR = 0.56, $P$ = .009). Not surprisingly, patients receiving 5-FU alone ("stop-and-go" arm) experienced less grade 3 neurotoxicity. Taking the "stop-and-go" strategy 1 step further, OPTIMOX2 discontinued CTX altogether after an initial induction phase of FOLFOX. The control arm

in this study was similar to the experimental arm from OPTIMOX 1 (FOLFOX for 6 cycles followed by maintenance 5-FU until disease progression), but the experimental arm included a complete CTX "holiday" (FOLFOX for 6 cycles followed by observation until disease progression). Duration of disease control was superior (13 vs. 9 months, $P$ = .046) and median OS was numerically, but not statistically, superior (23.8 vs. 19.5 months, $P$ = NS) in the maintenance 5-FU arm (10).

Because oxaliplatin's metabolite oxalate may induce nerve damage by affecting permeability of $Ca^{2+}$-dependent neuronal voltage-gated $Na^+$ channels, 3 randomized trials have examined whether administering oxalate chelators, namely calcium and magnesium, can reduce the incidence and intensity of oxaliplatin-related neurotoxicity. While data from the CONcePT and N04C7 trials (both of which were stopped early after an unplanned and ultimately unsubstantiated interim analysis of CONcePT showed a lower response rate in the group receiving Ca/Mg) suggested that routine infusions of Mg and Ca before and after oxaliplatin mitigated oxaliplatin-infused neurotoxicity, the subsequent phase III N08CB/Alliance study, revealed no benefit whatsoever.

How can we synthesize the data from the various trials addressing oxaliplatin-induced neurotoxicity? First, based on OPTIMOX1, a "stop-and-go" approach (stopping oxaliplatin after 6 cycles and continuing 5-FU/LV alone until progression) may reduce the cumulative toxicity of oxaliplatin while maintaining, or even augmenting, its efficacy. Many experts and official guidelines therefore advocate stopping oxaliplatin after an initial induction phase and maintaining patients on 5-FU/LV (with a targeted agent if included previously) until documented progression, at which time oxaliplatin can be reintroduced. Based on the OPTIMOX2 data, discontinuing CTX altogether after an initial induction phase may be detrimental and therefore cannot be *routinely* recommended. A population of patients with indolent and/or exquisitely chemosensitive disease who may benefit from CTX "holidays" likely exists; however, this cohort has not been clearly defined. Finally, due to conflicting data regarding their neuroprotective benefit, Ca/Mg infusions cannot be recommended for prevention of PSN in patients receiving oxaliplatin.

## FOLFOX or FOLFIRI as First-Line Treatment in mCRC: Does Order Matter?

FOLFIRI and FOLFOX induce similar response rates and PFS in untreated mCRC, and each regimen is active in mCRC refractory to the other. To assess whether the precise order affects OS, Tournigand et al. randomized 220 patients to FOLFOX followed by FOLFIRI upon progression or vice versa (11). Both arms yielded similar median OS (21 months), time to first progression (8 months), and response rate (55%). Because these approaches appear to be equally effective, oncologists and patients must choose an initial regimen based on convenience and potential toxicity. Patients who suffer from preexisting neuropathy, who rely on fine motor skills professionally or vocationally, or who cannot avoid cold exposure may prefer FOLFIRI. On the other hand, patients who are particularly concerned about gastrointestinal toxicity or who prefer capecitabine over an infusion pump may opt for an oxaliplatin-containing regimen.

## 5-FU, LV, Oxaliplatin, and Irinotecan (FOLFOXIRI)

One approach to maximize benefit from available cytotoxic agents is to use them sequentially; another is to combine them into 1 regimen. An Italian study randomized 244 patients to FOLFOXIRI (biweekly irinotecan 165 mg/m$^2$, oxaliplatin 85 mg/m$^2$, LV 200 mg/m$^2$, and i5-FU 3200 mg/m$^2$ over 48 hours) or standard FOLFIRI. FOLFOXIRI yielded a significantly higher response rate (66% vs. 41%, $P$ = .0002), longer PFS (9.8 vs. 6.9 months, $P$ = .0006), and longer median OS (22 vs. 16.7 months, $P$ = .032) than FOLFIRI, and more patients receiving FOLFOXIRI underwent R0 resection of metastases. Not surprisingly, FOLFOXIRI caused more neurotoxicity and neutropenia (12). Thus, while FOLFOXIRI remains a first-line option for mCRC, especially in patients who have borderline resectable metastatic disease, it is more toxic and does not clearly provide a survival advantage over sequential FOLFOX and FOLFIRI.

## Vascular Endothelial Growth Factor Inhibitors

On the basis of laboratory evidence that tumors require a vascular supply to proliferate and clinical evidence that higher serum vascular endothelial growth factor (VEGF) correlates with worse prognosis in mCRC, BV, a humanized monoclonal antibody that binds VEGF, was the first biological agent tested in mCRC. In 2004, Hurwitz et al. published the results of a pivotal trial that randomized 813 patients to IFL plus BV 5 mg/kg or IFL plus placebo (13). The experimental arm demonstrated superior median OS (20.3 vs. 15.6 months, $P$ < .001) and PFS (10.6 vs. 6.2 months, $P$ < .001) but more grade 3 hypertension (11% vs. 2.3%). With BV's role in untreated mCRC having been established, ECOG 3200 randomized patients with FOLFIRI-refractory disease to FOLFOX/BV or FOLFOX. The combination arm yielded superior response rate, PFS, and OS (12.9 vs. 10.8 months), thereby establishing a role for BV in previously treated, BV-naive mCRC (14). NO16966, the first randomized trial to add BV to oxaliplatin-containing CTX in untreated mCRC showed that BV improved PFS over placebo when combined with CAPEOX or FOLFOX (9.4 vs. 8.0 months). Although BV did not, with statistical significance, improve OS over placebo (21.3 vs. 19.9 months, $P$ = .077), only 29% of

patients in the BV arm were treated with BV/CTX until disease progression (15), introducing the possibility of an underestimation of survival with this strategy. Finally, the AVEX study, which randomized patients aged 70 years or older with untreated mCRC to capecitabine or capecitabine/BV, showed a superior median PFS in the combination arm (9.1 vs. 5.1 months, $P$ < .0001) (16). Interestingly, the PFS of patients receiving capecitabine/BV in AVEX approximates that seen in most clinical trials combining 5-FU with oxaliplatin or irinotecan.

While these 4 trials support the use of BV as part of first- or second-line CTX for BV-naive patients, the phase III TML 18147 trial randomized patients with mCRC who had progressed up to 3 months after discontinuing first-line BV/CTX to second-line CTX with or without BV. The addition of BV yielded a modest but statistically significant improvement in both PFS and OS (11.2 vs. 9.8 months, $P$ = .0062) with little added toxicity (17). Adding aflibercept—a recombinant fusion protein that binds VEGF-A, VEGF-B, and placental growth factor—to second-line FOLFOX yielded a similar survival benefit (1.4 months) in the VELOUR study, which randomized patients with mCRC who had progressed on first-line FOLFIRI-based CTX to FOLFOX or FOLFOX/aflibercept. Although adding aflibercept improved the overall response rate by 9% ($P$ < .001), it also increased grade 3/4 diarrhea, stomatitis, and fatigue (by 19%, 15%, and 13%, respectively). In a preplanned subgroup analysis of the 30% of patients who had received BV with first-line CTX, the additions of aflibercept significantly improved PFS but not OS (18). Based on these data, either BV or aflibercept may be added to second-line chemotherapy in appropriate patients, including those who have progressed on a BV-containing regimen previously. To date, no study has directly compared BV with aflibercept. Nevertheless, the improvement in both OS and PFS in the BV arm of TML (vs. unproven OS benefit of afliberceptin the VELOUR subgroup previously treated with BV), the higher incidence of severe gastrointestinal toxicity seen with aflibercept in VELOUR, and the established familiarity with BV in clinical practice, make BV a more favorable option for continuing VEGF inhibition beyond progression.

Side effects attributed to VEGF inhibitors (VEGFIs) stem from their mechanism of action and therefore differ from those of traditional cytotoxic chemotherapy. Hypertension, proteinuria, arteriovenous thrombosis, and bleeding are attributed to their effects on normal vasculature, whereas gastrointestinal perforation and wound dehiscence are attributed to their effects on tissue regeneration. Because major complications tend to occur in patients with identifiable risk factors, a thorough history and physical examination to select appropriate candidates for anti-VEGF therapy is imperative. Blood pressure should be within normal range before starting a VEGFI, with the understanding that antihypertensive therapy may require intensification during treatment. VEGFIs may exacerbate preexisting proteinuria, but patients with healthy kidneys at baseline are not likely to develop clinically significant high-grade proteinuria from them. Following urinalysis closely during therapy, while reasonable, is of relatively low value in patients without baseline proteinuria.

Although VEGFIs have been used safely in patients with occult or bleeding, they should be used cautiously in patients with mild gross bleeding and should not be given to patients with heavy bleeding or untreated brain metastases. Patients with active deep venous thrombosis may safely receive VEGFIs as long as they are receiving effective, stable anticoagulation. Arterial thrombosis, however, poses a bigger concern, because adverse consequences are potentially much more serious. VEGFIs should therefore not be given to patients with recent stroke or myocardial infarction, ongoing symptomatic vascular disease, or uncontrolled risk factors for vascular disease. Finally, because VEGFIs have been shown to increase the incidence of wound dehiscence and gastrointestinal perforation, patients should not receive a VEGFI within 6 weeks of a major abdominal surgery.

## EGFR Inhibitors

Cetuximab (Cmab) and panitumumab (Pmab), monoclonal antibodies that compete with epidermal growth factor by binding to the extracellular domain of the EGFR, inhibit signaling through pathways that contribute to proliferation and survival of colon cancer cells. Because skin, the gastrointestinal tract, and the nephron highly express EGFR, rash, diarrhea, and hypomagnesemia are common side effects of EGFR inhibitors. As opposed to Pmab, which is fully humanized, Cmab is chimeric and can therefore cause infusion reactions.

In 2007, the first 2 randomized trials using EGFR inhibitors were published. NCIC CO.17 demonstrated a small, but statistically significant, survival benefit of Cmab over BSC alone in patients with chemotherapy-refractory mCRC (median OS = 6.1 vs. 4.6 months, $P$ = .01) (19). As had been the case with nearly every study testing EGFR inhibitors regardless of the underlying malignancy, the appearance of a rash during anti-EGFR therapy strongly correlated with treatment response. In the second trial, which included a similar design and patient population, Pmab (6 mg/kg every 2 weeks) demonstrated superior PFS but similar OS compared to BSC (20). Although both trials met their end points of *statistical* significance, implying that EGFR inhibitors do, in fact, exert some degree of antineoplastic activity, widespread use of these costly agents for a modest *clinical* benefit remained difficult to justify. Investigators therefore began searching for biomarkers that could help select those patients most likely to benefit from anti-EGFR therapy.

The *KRAS* story beautifully illustrates how advances in molecular biology can translate into meaningful improvements in clinical care. The *KRAS* oncogene encodes an intracellular GTPase located downstream from EGFR that, when mutated, becomes constitutively active and leads to unregulated cell signaling and proliferation. *KRAS* is mutated in approximately 40% of CRCs, in the form of single amino acid substitutions at codons 12 or 13, and concordance between metastatic and primary tumors nears 100%. Because an activating *KRAS* mutation would likely nullify any potential benefit of EGFR blockade, *KRAS* biomarker analysis was undertaken for clinical trials involving EGFR inhibitors, starting with NCIC CO.17. Using banked tumor from nearly 70% of the patients enrolled in CO.17, Karapetis et al. identified *KRAS* mutations in 42% of these specimens and reassessed benefit from EGFR inhibitors based on *KRAS* mutational status (21). Their findings were unequivocal. In the cohort of patients with *KRAS* WT tumors, Cmab yielded a survival benefit over BSC much greater than that reported for the unselected population (OS = 9.5 vs. 4.8 months, $P$ < .001; PFS = 3.7 vs. 1.9 months, $P$ < .001). Cmab provided no survival benefit over BSC in patients with *KRAS* mutated (MT) tumors, and the response rate was only 1% (vs. 13% in the *KRAS* WT group). While *KRAS* mutational status was highly predictive of treatment effect, it was not prognostic, in that it did not affect survival in the BSC group.

Having demonstrated the single-agent activity of EGFR inhibitors, investigators then combined EGFR inhibitors with standard chemotherapy. The BOND trial randomized patients previously treated with irinotecan-containing regimens to Cmab/irinotecan or Cmab alone. The combination of irinotecan/Cmab yielded a significantly higher response rate (23% vs. 11%) and time to progression (4.1 vs. 1.5 months), but no difference in OS (22). In addition to showing that adding chemotherapy to Cmab is more effective than Cmab alone, BOND proved the important principle that biological agents can resensitize tumor cells to a cytotoxic agent previously deemed ineffective. In the CRYSTAL trial, the first trial using Cmab with frontline therapy, patients were randomized to FOLFIRI/Cmab or FOLFIRI alone. While the addition of Cmab did not improve OS, PFS, or RR in patients with *KRAS* MT tumors, an analysis of the *KRAS* WT subgroup revealed that response rate, PFS, and OS were all significantly higher with FOLFIRI/Cmab compared to FOLFIRI alone (RR = 57% vs. 40%, $P$ < .0001; PFS = 9.9 vs. 8.4 months, $P$ = .001; OS = 23.5 vs. 20.0 months, $P$ = .009) (23). Because the only trial to date that has not shown benefit from adding Cmab to CTX in *KRAS* WT mCRC was the COIN trial, in which the majority of patients received capecitabine rather than i5-FU, questions have been raised about whether an EGFR inhibitor should be added to a regimen containing capecitabine (24).

Data from the trials combining Pmab with CTX closely resemble those reported with Cmab. In patients refractory to oxaliplatin-based CTX and naive to EGFR inhibitors, FOLFIRI/Pmab was compared to FOLFIRI alone. Adding Pmab significantly increased response rate (35% vs. 10%, P < .0001) and PFS (5.9 vs. 3.9 months, P = .004) in KRAS WT patients but provided no benefit in KRAS MT patients (25). Similar findings were observed when Pmab was added to frontline CTX in the PRIME study, which randomized patients with untreated mCRC to FOLFOX/Pmab or FOLFOX. Preplanned analysis of the KRAS WT group showed improved PFS and a strong trend toward improved OS with the addition of Pmab to chemotherapy (PFS = 9.6 vs. 8 months, P = .02; OS = 23.9 vs. 19.7 months, P = .07) (26). Interestingly, adding Pmab to CTX appeared to *worsen* PFS and OS of patients with KRAS MT tumors.

Because many patients with KRAS WT tumors still do not benefit from EGFR inhibitors, investigators have continued searching for biomarkers to help clinicians more accurately predict which patients should receive Cmab or Pmab. Preliminary data suggested that the proto-oncogene BRAF, which lies directly downstream from KRAS, may predict lack of benefit from Pmab. However, a review of subsequent data, including an extensive molecular analysis of specimens collected during the CRYSTAL trial, showed that BRAF mutations are strongly *prognostic* for a poorer outcome in patients with mCRC (mOS), and they do not appear to *predict* resistance to EGFR inhibition (23). Additional studies have shown that tumors harboring mutations in exons 3 and 4 of KRAS and exons 2, 3, and 4 of NRAS appear to confer resistance to EGFR inhibitors. In the PRIME study, the subgroup of patients whose tumors expressed KRAS WT but lacked exon 2, 3, and 4 mutations in NRAS demonstrated an increase in OS from 4.2 to 7.4 months when they received CTX plus EGFR inhibition (28.3 months with FOLFOX/Pmab vs. 20.9 months with FOLFOX, P = .02) (27).

## Combining Targeted Agents in mCRC

After initial phase II data strongly suggested benefit from combining VEGF and EGFR inhibitors, 2 subsequent phase III trials yielded disconcerting results. In CAIRO2, patients were randomized to CAPEOX/BV/Cmab (CBC) or CAPEOX/BV (CB). In the unrestricted population, CBC was associated with shorter PFS and a trend toward worse OS. When outcomes were compared according to KRAS status, KRAS WT patients did not benefit from combining biologics and, more disturbingly, KRAS MT patients receiving CBC patients were actively harmed when compared to those receiving CB alone (PFS = 8.1 vs. 12.5 months, P = .003; OS = 17.2 vs. 24.9 months, P = .03) (28). These findings could not easily be attributed to toxicity, because grade 3–4 nondermatologic toxicity was nearly identical between the treatment arms. The PACCE trial, which randomized patients to chemotherapy plus BV

or chemotherapy/BV/Pmab also showed worse PFS and OS with combined VEGF/EGFR inhibition, regardless of KRAS status.

Several important conclusions regarding EGFR inhibition can be drawn from the KRAS story. First KRAS is mutated frequently (40–50% of CRC cases) and serves as an excellent negative predictive biomarker, that is, it reliably identifies patients who will *not* benefit from EGFR inhibition. KRAS mutational analysis of paraffin-embedded tumor tissue is therefore recommended for all patients with mCRC. Although limiting the administration of EGFR inhibitors to patients whose tumors lack KRAS or NRAS mutations in exons 2, 3, or 4 appears to further increase the yield of EGFR inhibition, we must continue to search for additional predictive biomarkers. Second, EGFR inhibitors improve response rates, PFS, and OS in patients with RAS WT tumors, whether used alone or combined with chemotherapy. Cmab and Pmab appear to be equally effective and should therefore be regarded as interchangeable. Rash is clearly associated with benefit and should, if possible, be managed with supportive care (topical and/or oral antibiotics, sunscreen, and moisturizers) and dose reduction rather than drug discontinuation. Third, although the optimal time to start EGFR inhibitors (frontline or later in the treatment course) is not well-established pending randomized data, their single-agent activity in chemorefractory disease and their potential to resensitize tumor cells to cytotoxic agents makes them particularly attractive for mCRC that has progressed on prior therapy. Fourth, combining EGFR and VEGFIs, while making biological sense, has been shown to worsen outcomes. Toxicity does not seem to account for this antagonistic effect, and various hypotheses, including stimulation of escape pathways and alteration of chemotherapy metabolism, have been proposed. For the time being, such combinations should be avoided outside of research protocols.

### Regorafenib

Because mutations in the BRAF oncogene are associated with significantly poorer survival in mCRC, the international phase III CORRECT trial was conducted to assess the efficacy of the multi-kinase inhibitor regorafenib (29). A total of 760 patients with mCRC who had progressed after receiving all standard chemotherapy options were randomized in a 2:1 ratio to receive regorafenib 160 mg daily orally or placebo for days 1–21 of a 28-day cycle. CORRECT met its end point for OS (6.4 months with regorafenib vs. 5.0 months with placebo, P = .005), but at a cost of more toxicity in the experimental arm. The most common grade 3 or 4 adverse events (AEs) attributed to regorafenib were HFS, fatigue, diarrhea, hypertension, and rash. Based on its modest but statistically significant OS benefit and the absence of other available options, the FDA granted approval for regorafenib in chemotherapy-refractory mCRC.

## Summary

Compared to 15 years ago, presently patients with mCRC have numerous treatment options, from single-agent 5-FU to combination chemoimmunotherapy. Because no formula exists to dictate which regimen best suits an individual patient, clinicians can only make recommendations after considering goals of care, underlying age and comorbidity, side-effect profiles, matters of convenience, and patient preference. Figure 11.1 shows a treatment algorithm for managing unresectable metastatic colon cancer. FOLFOX, CAPEOX, and FOLFIRI are all standard frontline combination regimens. If FOLFOX or CAPEOX is chosen, strong consideration should be given to an OPTIMOX-like strategy. If a patient is not a candidate for intensive therapy, single-agent 5-FU (preferably LV5-FU2) or capecitabine can be used. In the absence of contraindications to VEGF therapy, BV may be added, as it has been shown to improve PFS and OS in the first-line setting and when continued during second-line therapy. Patients with *KRAS* WT tumors are eligible for EGFR inhibitors, which

may be used alone or with cytotoxic chemotherapy. EGFR inhibitors have demonstrated survival benefit in untreated mCRC and chemotherapy-refractory mCRC, but their optimal place in the treatment algorithm has not been well defined. Combining VEGF and EGFR inhibitors may worsen outcomes and should be avoided. Regorafenib is an option for those who have progressed on other therapies, but its survival benefit is modest and its toxicity can be problematic in this heavily treated population. Finally, although the prognosis of mCRC has improved considerably over the last few decades, the vast majority of patients ultimately succumb to their disease. Improving accrual to clinical trials during all stages of therapy should therefore remain a high priority.

Because of her excellent performance status and a *KRAS* WT tumor, L.L. was deemed eligible for further treatment. Based on the BOND data, she received irinotecan/Cmab rather than Cmab alone. After her first cycle, she developed a grade 2 acneiform rash that responded nicely to oral minocycline. She is now 10 months into

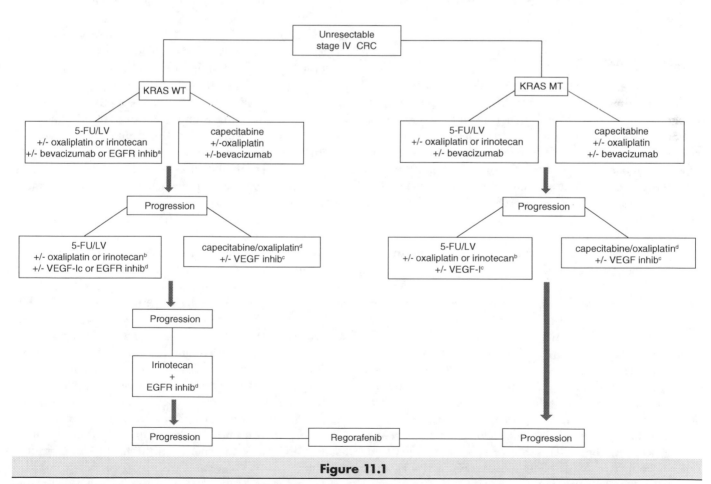

**Figure 11.1**

Treatment algorithm for unresectable stage IV colon cancer. [a]Cetuximab or panitumumab. [b]Whichever was not used previously. [c]Bevacizumab or aflibercept. [d]If not used previously. CRC, colorectal cancer; EGFR, epidermal growth factor receptor; 5-FU, 5-fluorouracil; LV, leucovorin; MT, mutated; VEGF-I, vascular endothelial growth factor inhibitor; WT, wild type.

irinotecan/Cmab, with CT scans and CEA indicating ongoing response.

## Potentially Resectable or Resectable Metastatic CRC

A.K. is a 51-year-old otherwise healthy male attorney who presented with rectal bleeding and constipation. Colonoscopy with biopsy showed a circumferential, partially obstructing adenocarcinoma, but the scope was successfully advanced to the cecum. Staging CT scans showed 2 masses in the right hepatic lobe measuring 1.3 and 1.1 cm and a cystic lesion in the left hepatic lobe measuring 1.2 cm. PET or CT showed marked [18]F-fludeoxyglucose (FDG) uptake in the colon mass and 2 right hepatic lobe lesions, but no uptake in the left hepatic lobe or lungs. A left hemicolectomy was performed, and pathological evaluation revealed a T3 N1 adenocarcinoma containing a codon 12 *KRAS* mutation. Intraoperative biopsy of a right liver mass showed adenocarcinoma. A preoperative CEA was 48 ng/mL and a postoperative CEA was 49 ng/mL. The patient recovered quickly from surgery and was referred to medical oncology to discuss prognosis and further treatment.

## Evidence-Based Case Discussion

A.K. has biopsy-proven stage IV colon cancer (T3 N2 M1) with radiographic evidence of 2 right hepatic metastases and a left hepatic lobe cyst. Although his prognosis is worse than that of patients with nonmetastatic colon cancer, the presence of limited metastases rather than widespread disease raises the possibility of long-term survival with aggressive multidisciplinary management. The treatment approach for A.K. therefore differs significantly from that of the previous patient.

In the 1990s, reports of long-term survival after R0 resection of primary colon cancer and its known sites of metastasis began to emerge. Excitement about potentially curative therapy for mCRC was, however, tempered by the following: (a) criteria for resectability were stringent (low burden disease confined to 1 liver lobe), thereby precluding surgery in the vast majority of patients; and (b) even though 5-year survival rates as high as 50% were reported, 75% of patients relapsed within a few years after surgery, making the actual cure rate very low. As more extensive metastasectomy proved to be safe, and as novel interventions such as radiofrequency ablation (RFA) and portal vein embolization (PVE) were devised to supplement surgical resection, the criteria for resectability liberalized, and the cohort of patients eligible for aggressive therapy expanded. On the other hand, it became clear that intensifying local therapy of known metastases without simultaneously eradicating micrometastatic disease would not further improve treatment outcomes.

Based on the high relapse rate with surgery alone, investigators hypothesized that a multidisciplinary approach of intensive local therapy combined with systemic chemotherapy would improve survival outcomes. Three randomized trials have addressed the issue of supplementing R0 resection of stage IV CRC with chemotherapy. Two European trials randomized patients who had undergone resection of gross disease to observation or 6 cycles of b5-FU/LV. Both trials closed prematurely due to slow accrual, so neither had power to demonstrate differences in disease-free survival (DFS) or OS. However, a pooled analysis demonstrated a trend toward improved survival with adjuvant chemotherapy over surgery alone (PFS = 27.9 vs. 18.8 months, P = .058; OS = 62.2 vs. 47.3 months, P = .095) (30). The third trial, EORTC 40983, randomized 364 patients with 4 or fewer resectable liver masses and no extrahepatic disease to metastasectomy alone or metastasectomy with perioperative chemotherapy (3 months of FOLFOX before and after surgery) (31). Because 7% of patients receiving FOLFOX progressed before surgery, more patients in the perioperative chemotherapy arm did not undergo surgery (12% vs. 4%). However, the rates of potentially curative resection were nearly identical (83% vs. 84%), and fewer patients in the perioperative chemotherapy arm underwent nontherapeutic laparotomy (5% vs. 11%). Postoperative morbidity was slightly higher in the chemotherapy arm, but postoperative mortality was 1% in both groups. In the intention-to-treat population, there was a trend toward improved median PFS in the perioperative chemotherapy arm (20 vs. 12.5 months, P = .068) and no difference in OS. Importantly, the subjects enrolled in European Organization for Research and Treatment of Cancer (EORTC) represented a biologically favorable population of stage IV colon cancer patients in that most (65%) presented with metachronous liver metastases and the vast majority (78%) had only 1 or 2 metastases.

Other nonrandomized studies have used perioperative FOLFIRI rather than FOLFOX or have added VEGF or EGFR inhibitors to chemotherapy. Although all regimens approved for mCRC appear to be effective in the setting of resectable oligometastatic disease, more aggressive regimens, possibly with the exception of FOLFOXIRI, have not been shown to be more effective than FOLFOX. Regardless of the regimen chosen, the risk of hepatotoxicity and postoperative complication seems to increase significantly with >3 months of preoperative combination chemotherapy. Based on retrospective data, BV can be safely added to preoperative chemotherapy, provided that the last dose is not given within 6 weeks of surgery.

Figure 11.2 outlines the algorithm for treating oligometastatic CRC. First, an experienced surgical oncologist must determine whether the patient is an appropriate candidate for aggressive resection, based on the predicted volume of healthy remnant liver following surgery, the ability to preserve vascular and biliary structures, and the overall health of the patient. Second, the surgical and medical oncologist

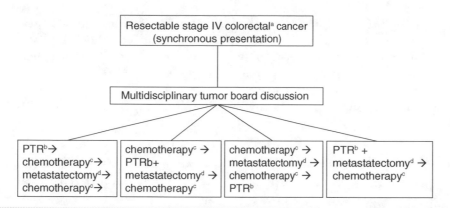

**Figure 11.2**

Treatment algorithm for resectable stage IV colon cancer (synchronous presentation). [a]Local therapy for a rectal primary may also include neoadjuvant chemoradiation. [b]Primary tumor resection. [c]Chemotherapy before liver resection should be limited to 3 months if possible to minimize risk of postoperative complications; total duration of chemotherapy should be up to 6 months. [d]Other modalities that can be incorporated into local therapy targeting metastases include radiofrequency ablation, stereotactic radiosurgery, portal vein embolization, and staged liver resection. PTR, primary tumor resection.

must decide how to incorporate chemotherapy into the treatment plan. While administering chemotherapy before and after R0 resection of gross disease is safe and effective, the optimal timing and duration have not been established. Neoadjuvant chemotherapy offers the potential advantages of (a) downsizing borderline resectable metastases to render them resectable; (b) testing the tumor's biology to spare patients with occult, widespread, aggressive disease from surgery that is unlikely to provide long-term benefit; (c) assessing the chemosensitivity of a tumor, which guides postoperative chemotherapy; and (d) serving as a "stress test" to select out those patients who are not medically fit enough to tolerate surgery. The primary disadvantage of neoadjuvant chemotherapy is the potential for toxicity severe enough to delay, complicate, or even preclude surgical resection.

Aside from cases of metachronous mCRC diagnosed after a lengthy disease-free interval, patients with oligometastatic colon cancer are, with increasing frequency, being treated with perioperative or postoperative chemotherapy. The precise sequencing of chemotherapy, PTR, and metastasectomy depends on various factors, including the urgency for PTR at presentation, the metastatic tumor burden, and the patient's overall health. Due to the complex decision-making process and meticulous coordination of care that such an aggressive approach demands, cases of newly diagnosed oligometastatic CRC should be presented in a multidisciplinary tumor board. More complex approaches incorporating RFA, stereotactic radiosurgery, hepatic arterial infusion, and staged resection following PVE (to induce hypertrophy of the future liver remnant) are increasingly being employed, but no single strategy has proven to be most effective.

A multidisciplinary tumor board recommended that A.K. undergo neoadjuvant chemotherapy prior to liver resection. He received FOLFOX/BV for 5 cycles, followed by an additional cycle of FOLFOX alone to provide at least 6 weeks between the last dose of BV and surgery.

Aside from some transient cold sensitivity following each dose of oxaliplatin, A.K. tolerated treatment well, continuing to work full-time and maintaining a normal diet and active lifestyle. Serum CEA fell from 49 to 3.8 ng/mL, and restaging CT scans showed that both right hepatic lobe lesions had decreased to <1 cm and that the left hepatic lobe lesion, which still appeared to be a cyst, was stable. Approximately 4 weeks after the completion of chemotherapy, he underwent right hepatectomy. Pathological evaluation confirmed R0 resection of 2 metastases, but no other foci of carcinoma. He recovered well from surgery and completed 3 more months of chemotherapy. Due to the onset of PSN after postoperative cycle #4, he received LV5-FU2 alone for the last 2 cycles. He remains without evidence of recurrence 2 years into surveillance.

## Stage III Colon Cancer: Adjuvant Chemotherapy

A.M. is a 76-year-old woman who, upon screening colonoscopy, was found to have an adenocarcinoma of the ascending colon. Staging CT scans showed no evidence of distant metastases. A right hemicolectomy was performed, and pathological evaluation revealed a moderately differentiated adenocarcinoma with metastasis to 6 of 20 resected lymph nodes. Her postoperative course was complicated by delayed wound healing, but she quickly regained bowel function and was discharged to her daughter's house on postoperative day 10.

During her initial consultation with medical oncology, A.M. had no major complaints. She was eating a full diet, having normal daily stools, and performing daily activities without compromise. She had multiple comorbidities, including obesity, atrial fibrillation, diabetes with mild sensory neuropathy, and hypertension. She denied any family history of colon cancer. She appeared well, and her wound was closed completely without surrounding erythema or drainage. Having been told by the surgeon that she would "need" adjuvant chemotherapy to reduce her risk of cancer recurrence, the patient and her family, although wanting to maximize her chance for cure, were concerned about the potential toxicity of chemotherapy in light of her recent wound infection and her underlying comorbidities.

## Evidence-Based Case Discussion

A.M. is an elderly patient who presents for consideration of adjuvant chemotherapy following resection of stage III colon cancer. Despite a complicated postoperative course, she has recovered completely and maintains an excellent performance status. This case raises the various issues that a medical oncologist needs to address during an initial consultation for stage III colon cancer. The oncologist should explain to A.M. that, although definitive therapy has been administered, her risk for recurrence without further treatment is 40–60% due to possible microscopic disease outside the surgical field at the time of resection. Although assays to detect circulating tumor cells exist, none has yet proven sensitive enough to guide decisions regarding adjuvant therapy. As a result, administration of adjuvant therapy is largely "empiric," that is, it is administered under the *assumption* that micrometastatic disease is both present and sensitive to cytotoxic chemotherapy. If the patient chooses to proceed with chemotherapy, the oncologist must review the various options and discuss timing, logistics, and potential side effects. Keeping this discussion in mind, we will review the data supporting the use of adjuvant therapy for resected colon cancer.

## 5-FU/LV as Adjuvant Therapy

Hoping to increase the cure rate of resected colon cancer by eradicating micrometastatic disease, investigators started to conduct RCTs comparing postoperative chemotherapy to observation in the 1980s. Due to the exceedingly high cure rate for resected stage I disease (90% or greater), they focused on stage III and, to lesser degree, stage II disease. Intergroup 0035—which randomized 929 patients with resected stage III colon cancer to 5-FU/levimasole for 1 year, levimasole alone for 1 year, or observation—was the first large phase III trial to demonstrate a survival benefit for adjuvant chemotherapy (32). At 3.5 years, 5-FU/levimasole yielded superior recurrence-free survival (RFS) and OS over observation alone (RFS 63% vs. 47%, *P* < .0001; estimated OS 71% vs. 55%, *P* < .0001). In 2 subsequent trials, 5-FU/LV was shown to be superior to 5-FU/levimasole, thereby establishing LV as the preferred 5-FU modulator. Finally, when a pooled analysis of >1500 patients with resected stage II or III colon cancer demonstrated that 6 months of 5-FU/LV conferred a survival advantage similar to that previously shown with 12 months of 5-FU/LV and that the benefit of chemotherapy at 3 years was

largely confined to stage III patients (event-free survival = 62% vs. 44%; OS = 76% vs. 64%), 6 months of 5-FU/LV became the standard backbone regimen for adjuvant chemotherapy (33).

## Combination 5-FU-Based Adjuvant Chemotherapy

Having already been approved for use in mCRC, irinotecan and oxaliplatin were logical choices to add to 5-FU/LV in the adjuvant setting. PETACC-3 randomized 3278 patients with resected stage II and III colon cancer to LV5-FU2 or FOLFIRI. There was no difference in 5-year DFS or median OS between the 2 arms, and FOLFIRI was associated with more grade 3 or 4 hematological and gastrointestinal toxicity (34). Two smaller randomized trials—CALGB 89803 and ACCORD—also failed to demonstrate a survival advantage of adding irinotecan to 5-FU/LV. Thus, while FOLFIRI has been shown to be superior to 5-FU/LV and equivalent to FOLFOX in mCRC, there are no available randomized data to support its use in the adjuvant setting.

On the other hand, 2 practice-changing trials—MOSAIC and NSABP C-07—demonstrated a statistically significant survival benefit of adding oxaliplatin to 5-FU/LV. The MOSAIC trial randomized 2246 patients with stage II (40%) or III (60%) colon cancer to 6 months of LV5-FU2 or FOLFOX (35). In the intention-to-treat population, FOLFOX yielded a modest but statistically significant OS benefit at 6 years (78.5% vs. 76%; HR = 0.84, *P* = .046). Among the 1247 patients with stage III disease, FOLFOX yielded a more pronounced OS benefit (72.9% vs. 68.7%; HR = 0.80; *P* = .023), as well as superior 5-year DFS (66.4% vs. 58.9%; HR = 0.78, *P* = .005). FOLFOX was not statistically superior to 5-FU/LV among the 899 patients with stage II disease, but subgroup analysis showed that FOLFOX improved DFS in the patients with high-risk stage II disease (82.3% vs. 74.6%; HR = 0.72; *P* not reported). Importantly, 24% of patients receiving FOLFOX had some degree of PSN by the end of treatment. Although the prevalence declined over time, 15% of patients examined 2 years after completion of FOLFOX complained of residual PSN (11.9%, 2.8%, and 0.7% with grade 1, 2, 3 PSN, respectively). Nearly identical results were reported from NSABP C-07, which randomized nearly 2500 patients to 5-FU/LV (Roswell Park regimen) with or without oxaliplatin. Three-year DFS and OS were superior in the FOLFOX arm, and PSN was still present in 10% of these patients 2 years after completion of adjuvant therapy.

Although adding oxaliplatin to 5-FU/LV clearly saves lives when applied to large populations, its potential benefit is modest in any 1 individual, and its potential long-term neurotoxicity is concerning. In fact, the likelihood that adjuvant FOLFOX will cause chronic PSN (10–12%) is 2–3 times greater than its absolute improvement in OS over 5-FU/LV alone in stage III disease (4–5%). In order to identify in *real time* those patients who will benefit from adjuvant chemotherapy and spare those who will not benefit from its potential toxicity, investigators continue to devise measures to "personalize therapy." Translational researchers are currently testing ultrasensitive peripheral blood assays to detect residual microscopic disease and designing tumor assays to quantify a patient's risk for recurrence and the potential benefit of adjuvant chemotherapy. Meanwhile, clinical researchers continue to devise strategies to prevent or counteract toxicity from available drugs such as oxaliplatin.

One such strategy is the basis for International Duration Evaluation of Adjuvant Chemotherapy (IDEA), an international effort to address the unacceptably high rate of chronic PSN in patients receiving adjuvant FOLFOX. Published data suggest that 3 months of adjuvant 5-FU/LV may confer benefit equivalent to that of 6 months (36). Furthermore, because PSN typically appears 4–5 months into oxaliplatin therapy, it stands to reason that reducing oxaliplatin exposure by a few months may reduce the likelihood of neurotoxicity. Five ongoing phase III trials (4 in Europe and 1 in North America) are therefore randomizing patients with resected stage III colon cancer to 3 or 6 months of FOLFOX. The North American trial, CALGB 80702, is randomizing 2500 patients in a 2 × 2 fashion to (a) 3 or 6 months of FOLFOX and (b) 3 years of celecoxib or placebo with a primary end point of showing equivalent DFS between 3 and 6 months of FOLFOX and superior DFS of celecoxib over placebo. The IDEA investigators will pool the data from all 5 trials ($n = 20,000$) to show equivalent DFS between 3 and 6 months of adjuvant FOLFOX.

The results of IDEA's analysis will be much anticipated, and clinicians are strongly encouraged to enroll patients in any of the participating trials. For the time being, without any commercially available biomarkers that can predict which individual patients will benefit from FOLFOX over 5-FU/LV alone and without any definitive data to show that a shorter duration of FOLFOX is equivalent to the standard 6 months, clinicians should carefully weigh the risks and benefits of adding oxaliplatin to 5-FU/LV and reevaluate the risk–benefit ratio of continuing oxaliplatin during FOLFOX therapy if PSN arises.

The addition of adjuvant chemotherapy demands special attention in the elderly. While data consistently show that administering adjuvant 5-FU to fit elderly patients after resection of stage III colon cancer confers a survival benefit similar to that seen in younger patients, the benefit of adding oxaliplatin to 5-FU in the adjuvant setting is not as clear. On the one hand, subgroup analyses from MOSAIC and NSABP C-07 have demonstrated that adding oxaliplatin to 5-FU improves DFS only in patients younger than 70 years; however, SEER-Medicare data strongly suggest that adding oxaliplatin to 5-FU does, in fact, benefit elderly patients, at least those between 70 and

75. 5-FU (or capecitabine) should therefore be offered to all fit elderly patients with stage III colon cancer, but a clinician must carefully account for each patient's functional status, comorbidities, social support, and understanding of the risk–benefit balance before making a formal recommendation regarding oxaliplatin.

## Capecitabine as Adjuvant Therapy

An appropriate substitute for 5-FU/LV in mCRC, capecitabine has also been rigorously tested in the adjuvant setting. In the X-ACT trial, Twelves et al. randomized 1987 patients with resected stage III colon cancer to 6 months of 5-FU/LV (Mayo Clinic regimen) or capecitabine 1250 mg/m$^2$ twice daily for days 1–14 every 21 days. Not only did the study meet its end point of noninferior DFS, capecitabine proved superior to 5-FU/LV for DFS (HR = 0.87; $P < .001$ for equivalence and $P = .05$ for superiority) and approached superiority for OS (HR = 0.84, $P < .001$ for equivalence and $P = .07$ for superiority) (37). Compared to 5-FU/LV, capecitabine caused less nausea, vomiting, diarrhea, stomatitis, alopecia, and neutropenia but more HFS and hyperbilirubinemia. Approximately, 50% of patients receiving capecitabine required dose reduction. Building on the results from MOSAIC and NSABP C-07, investigators set out to demonstrate superiority of CAPEOX over 5-FU/LV in the adjuvant setting. In the multicenter phase III trial NO16968, which randomized 1886 patients with resected stage III colon cancer to CAPEOX or b5-FU/LV, CAPEOX yielded statistically superior DFS and OS at 7 years (DFS = 63% vs. 56%; OS = 73% vs. 67%) (38).

## Targeted Agents as Adjuvant Therapy

Although targeted agents have proven beneficial in mCRC, clinical trials with VEGF and EGFR inhibitors in the adjuvant setting have yielded disappointing results. NSABP C-08 randomized 2672 patients with resected stage II or III colon cancer to 6 months of FOLFOX or 6 months of FOLFOX/BV followed by 6 months of maintenance BV. Adding BV to FOLFOX did not improve DFS at the predefined landmark of 3 years, and the primary end point for benefit was therefore not met; however, DFS was clearly superior with FOLFOX/BV until the 15-month landmark, declining thereafter (39). BV therefore appears to have exerted a "static effect" on micrometastatic disease, delaying recurrence with active VEGF inhibition but losing its effect once discontinued. While some investigators advocate designing a clinical trial with longer BV maintenance, others are concerned that indefinite continuation of BV would be required to control micrometastatic disease. The latter scenario would not only prove costly, it could also uncover cumulative or delayed toxicity of VEGF inhibition not previously described. The AVANT study (FOLFOX or CAPEOX ± BV) also showed no benefit of adding BV to 5-FU-based therapy, and the outcome of 2 ongoing trials—E5202 (FOLFOX vs. FOLFOX/BV in high-risk stage II disease) and QUASAR2 (capecitabine vs. capecitabine/BV in stage II/III disease)—have not yet been reported.

Perhaps more surprisingly, EGFR inhibitors also failed to improve outcomes when combined with adjuvant chemotherapy. Intergroup N0147, a randomized trial comparing FOLFOX and FOLFOX/Cmab in patients with resected, *KRAS* WT stage III colon cancer, was prematurely closed after interim analysis showed similar 3-year DFS and a trend toward worse 3-year OS. PETACC-8, a similarly designed trial in Europe also showed no benefit of Cmab in the adjuvant setting. In light of these reported data, BV, Cmab, and Pmab should not be administered to patients with resected nonmetastatic colon cancer outside of a research protocol.

### Surveillance

Stage III colon cancer patients, regardless of whether they receive adjuvant chemotherapy, should undergo surveillance for 5 years. Guidelines such as those published by NCCN include serial history and physical examination, serum CEA testing, and CT imaging to detect recurrent disease and colonoscopy to screen for second malignancies or premalignant polyps. While there are no published randomized data to define an optimal schedule for surveillance, large retrospective studies have demonstrated the benefit of intensive surveillance in stages I–III colon cancer, with the rationale that earlier detection of metastatic recurrence may facilitate earlier initiation of systemic therapy and, more importantly, R0 resection of oligometastatic disease. Clinicians should therefore personalize the schedule for surveillance based on an individual's risk of recurrence and whether aggressive treatment would be pursued if, in fact, recurrent disease was uncovered. As long as the endoscopist visualized the entire colon during the preoperative colonoscopy, the next colonoscopy can be performed 1 year later. If the entire colon was not visualized during initial endoscopy (due to obstruction, for example), colonoscopy should be performed 3–6 months after the completion of adjuvant therapy. If no advanced adenoma (polyp > 1 cm in size and/or containing villous histology or high-grade dysplasia) is seen on the first postoperative colonoscopy, colonoscopy should be repeated 3 years later, then every 5 years if there are still no advanced adenomas. Finally, with emerging data that strongly link an active lifestyle and healthy diet to lower recurrence rates of CRC, patients should be encouraged to adopt a low-fat, high-fiber diet and to engage in regular exercise. To date, no other measures are universally recommended to reduce risk of colon cancer recurrence. However, emerging data suggest that daily aspirin may improve OS in patients with resected PIK3CA mutated CRC.

### Summary

Figure 11.3 summarizes the current options for the treatment of patients with resected nonmetastatic colon cancer that include 6 months of 5-FU-based chemotherapy. FOLFOX or CAPEOX are the most aggressive options, significantly decreasing absolute recurrence rates by as much as 20% and improving OS compared to observation alone. However, it is important to remember (a) that most of the survival benefit conferred by combination chemotherapy is from the 5-FU component (absolute benefit = 15%), with an additional 5% derived from addition of oxaliplatin; and (b) that the risk of chronic PSN from FOLFOX is up to 15%. Therefore, patients who have pre-existing neuropathy or who are not deemed fit enough to tolerate oxaliplatin, should be offered 5-FU/LV or capecitabine, and patients who are deemed fit for combination chemotherapy should be offered FOLFOX or CAPEOX. Those receiving oxaliplatin should be followed closely for neurological symptoms, with careful attention to distinguish between the acute neurosensory complex and true PSN. At the first sign of PSN, strong consideration should be given to reducing or discontinuing oxaliplatin, given its relatively small marginal benefit over 5-FU alone and the possibility that all 12 doses may not be needed to confer benefit. In the case of oxaliplatin discontinuation, 5-FU (or capecitabine) should be continued to complete 6 total months of adjuvant therapy. Targeted agents currently have no role in the adjuvant setting outside of a clinical protocol.

Although A.M. is elderly and has multiple comorbidities, her performance status is excellent, and her chance of disease recurrence is appreciable, making her an appropriate candidate for adjuvant chemotherapy. After laying out the rationale for adjuvant chemotherapy, discussing the various chemotherapeutic options, and expressing concern over exacerbating her preexisting neuropathy with oxaliplatin, we recommended single-agent 5-FU therapy. Because the patient did not want a Port-a-cath or infusional pump, she chose capecitabine, which was started at 1000 mg/m$^2$ twice daily for 14 days of a 21-day cycle. Because she tolerated her first 2 cycles extremely well, her dose was increased to 1250 mg/m$^2$ twice daily, and she continued full-dose capecitabine to complete 6 months of adjuvant therapy. Five years of posttreatment surveillance revealed no evidence of recurrence.

### Stage II Colon Cancer: Adjuvant Chemotherapy

L.G. is a 38-year-old otherwise healthy woman without any family history of cancer who presented to the emergency department with rectal bleeding. Colonoscopy with biopsy revealed a circumferential, nonobstructing adenocarcinoma in the ascending colon. CT scans showed a right colon mass, but no evidence of regional adenopathy or distant metastases. She underwent right hemicolectomy and

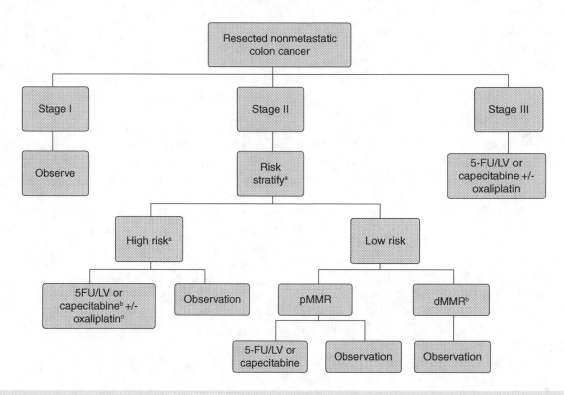

**Figure 11.3**

Treatment algorithm for resected nonmetastatic colon cancer. [a]High-risk features include T4 disease, poor differentiation (except if dMMR [deficient in mismatch repair]), tumor perforation/obstruction, microscopic lymphovascular, and/or perineural invasion, or <12 lymph nodes identified in resected specimen. [b]Patients with stage II dMMR tumors carry a better prognosis and do not appear to benefit from adjuvant 5-FU. [c]Adding oxaliplatin to 5-FU/LV has not been proven to improve survival in high-risk stage II colon cancer. dMMR, deficient in mismatch repair; 5-FU, 5-fluorouracil; LV, leucovorin; pMMR, proficient in mismatch repair.

had no postoperative complications. Pathological evaluation revealed a moderately differentiated adenocarcinoma invading pericolonic adipose tissue. None of the isolated 17 lymph nodes contained carcinoma, and there was no microscopic evidence of lymphovascular or perineural invasion. The tumor expressed MLH1, MSH2, MSH6, and PMS2 by immunohistochemistry (IHC), and molecular analysis demonstrated microsatellite stability. She was referred to medical oncology for an opinion regarding adjuvant therapy.

## Evidence-Based Case Discussion

L.G. presents with a resected stage IIA (T3 N0) adenocarcinoma that shows no high-risk histopathological or molecular features. Although her chance for tumor recurrence is relatively low (15–20%), she wants to know if adjuvant chemotherapy will further lower her risk for recurrence. This case highlights the controversy surrounding adjuvant chemotherapy in stage II colon cancer, the importance of risk stratification using established factors, and the need for more informative prognostic and predictive biomarkers.

## Adjuvant Chemotherapy in Stage II Colon Cancer

Many of the early adjuvant trials comparing chemotherapy to observation included a substantial number of patients with stage II disease. Although subgroup analyses of these trials consistently demonstrated a 15–20% lower relative risk for recurrence for stage II patients receiving chemotherapy, attaining statistical significance was difficult due to insufficient sample size and a low absolute risk for recurrence. To generate more statistical power, the IMPACT B2 investigators accumulated clinical data from 5 randomized trials comparing adjuvant 5-FU/LV to observation. Pooled analysis of the 1025 patients with stage II colon cancer demonstrated a strong trend toward superior 5-year event-free survival and OS with chemotherapy (EFS = 76% vs. 73%, $P = .061$; OS = 82% vs. 80%, $P = .057$) (40). The only large phase III trial to enroll primarily subjects with stage II disease was QUASAR, which randomized 3239 patients with resected CRC (91% of whom had stage II disease) to adjuvant 5-FU/LV or observation. Consistent with previously reported data from subgroup and pooled analyses, chemotherapy was associated with a 22% relative reduction of recurrence risk

($P$ = .001) and a 3.6% absolute improvement in OS (41). As for the benefit of adding oxaliplatin, subgroup analysis of the 1000 stage II patients in the MOSAIC trial showed no survival advantage of FOLFOX over LV5-FU2.

## Risk Stratification in Stage II Colon Cancer

Adjuvant 5-FU clearly improves survival when applied to large enough groups of patients with stage II colon cancer, but its absolute benefit of 2–4% makes an *individual's* chance of deriving benefit low. Working under the assumption that stage II patients with a worse prognosis are more likely to benefit from adjuvant therapy, investigators have identified various clinical and pathological features that increase risk for relapse, including bowel obstruction or perforation, invasion of adjacent structures (T4 lesion), poor differentiation, lymphovascular invasion, and inadequate (<12) lymph node dissection. Subgroup analyses of the major trials randomizing patients to 5-FU or observation have suggested that patients with stage II colon cancer meeting 1 or more of these criteria derive benefit from adjuvant therapy greater than the 2–4% reported for unselected stage II patients. Furthermore, analysis of "high-risk" stage II patients in the MOSAIC trial showed an improvement in DFS (HR = 0.72) conferred by FOLFOX over LV5-FU2 similar to that seen in stage III patients (HR = 0.78) (35). We must, however, keep in mind that these data were generated from post hoc subgroup analyses encompassing small numbers of patients and that the relative contribution of any single risk factor cannot possibly be quantified. In short, while it is fairly clear that these so-called high-risk features are *prognostic*, their *predictive* role has not been firmly established.

More recently, MSI has emerged as an important risk factor. After pooling data from 1027 patients with stage II and III colon cancer enrolled in 6 randomized trials comparing adjuvant 5-FU to observation, Sargent et al. published compelling data regarding the prognostic and predictive power of MSI. First, they reported that MSI was associated with improved DFS (HR = 0.51, $P$ = .009) and OS (HR = 0.51, $P$ = .004) in patients undergoing observation. Second, they showed that patients with stage III, microsatellite stable (MSS) tumors plainly benefit from adjuvant chemotherapy (HR = 0.64, $P$ = .001), whereas patients with stage III microsatellite unstable (MSI-H) tumors may not (HR = 1.01). Finally, they conclusively demonstrated inferior OS in patients with stage II, MSI-H tumors who received chemotherapy compared to those who did not (HR = 2.95, $P$ = .04) (42). These data therefore establish MSI as a positive *prognostic* factor as well as a negative *predictor* of benefit from adjuvant 5-FU, in stage II (and possibly stage III) patients.

Given the validation and widespread use of Oncotype Dx for breast cancer, translational scientists have also developed and tested similar assays for colon cancer.

By analyzing 761 candidate genes from 1851 resection specimens collected during large adjuvant therapy trials, Gray et al. identified 7 genes as being most predictive of recurrence and 6 genes as most predictive of treatment benefit. The final assay, a multigene reverse transcription-polymerase chain reaction (RT-PCR) that produces a recurrence (prognostic) score and a treatment benefit (predictive) score, was applied to specimens acquired from the QUASAR trial (43). Although the recurrence score successfully divided patients into low, intermediate, and high risk for recurrence, the differences were not particularly impressive (12%, 18%, and 22%, respectively), and the treatment score did not predict differential benefit from adjuvant chemotherapy. In other words, while the absolute risk of recurrence and therefore the absolute benefit from chemotherapy changed modestly with the recurrence score, HRs associated with chemotherapy stayed constant across the recurrence score continuum, thereby negating any true *predictive* power.

## Summary

The role of adjuvant chemotherapy for resected stage II colon cancer remains highly controversial. Studies have consistently shown a discernible treatment effect across large groups of patients, but an absolute benefit of <5% makes the number needed to treat (NNT) to prevent one from cancer recurrence uncomfortably high (>20). While a cohort of patients who stands to benefit more than others must exist, this population has not yet been identified despite much clinical investigation. Clinicopathological features, while proven to be prognostic, have not proven to predict benefit from chemotherapy. MSI is a strong positive prognostic factor and predicts lack of benefit, even harm, from adjuvant 5-FU in stage II disease. However, no predictive effect for patients receiving a fluoropyrimidine plus oxaliplatin has been established. Finally, the Oncotype Dx multigene assay provides limited prognostic but no predictive information.

In light of these inconclusive data, ASCO guidelines do not support the *routine* use of adjuvant chemotherapy in stage II colon cancer. As such, the oncologist and patient can only arrive at an appropriate, informed decision after engaging in a detailed conversation. The physician should delineate the known risk factors for cancer recurrence, acknowledging their aforementioned limitations; assess the patient's overall health status and life expectancy; explain the potential benefit of chemotherapy in layman's terms (using absolute benefit and NNT instead of relative benefit or HRs); and review the potential side effects of treatment. If the patient decides to proceed with adjuvant therapy, the clinician must recommend a specific treatment (see Figure 11.3). When considering a fluoropyrimidine-only regimen, the clinician should test the resected tumor for MMR expression (IHC) or MSI (PCR). LV5-FU2 and capecitabine are reasonable options for low-risk, MSS disease. However, patients with low-risk, MSI-H tumors should not receive adjuvant therapy due to their excellent prognosis and the potential harm of exposing them to 5-FU. Adding oxaliplatin is reasonable for high-risk disease, but it is important to remember that the data supporting this practice were derived from MOSAIC subgroup analysis, which showed improved DFS but not OS of FOLFOX over LV5-FU2. Finally, clinicians should encourage their patients to enroll in clinical trials and to donate tumor and blood to research tissue banks.

Because L.G.'s tumor expressed all 4 MMR enzymes and did not manifest any high-risk clinicopathological features, we explained that her risk of recurrence was approximately 15% and that adjuvant 5-FU/LV or capecitabine could reduce her recurrence risk by 3–4%. She chose not to undergo adjuvant therapy and therefore proceeded with surveillance alone.

## Rectal Cancer

G.F. is a 72-year-old white man who presented with a 5-month history of low caliber stools, intermittent rectal bleeding, tenesmus, and weight loss. Colonoscopy with biopsy revealed a friable, circumferential rectal adenocarcinoma, extending proximally from the anal verge to about 12 cm. CT imaging of the chest, abdomen, and pelvis showed an irregular rectal mass without perirectal adenopathy or distant metastases. Rectal endoscopic ultrasound (EUS) showed tumor invasion through the muscularis propria into the subserosa, but no lymphadenopathy (uT3N0). Because G.F. is otherwise healthy with an excellent performance status, he would like to receive the most aggressive treatment warranted to cure his cancer.

### Evidence-Based Case Discussion

Because they share cell of origin and pathogenesis, rectal cancer and colon cancer respond to identical chemotherapy regimens and are therefore treated similarly when metastatic. However, due to anatomical considerations, treatment of nonmetastatic rectal cancer differs from that of colon cancer. First, because of the rectum's proximity to pelvic structures, rectal cancer carries a high risk for local recurrence while maintaining its potential to metastasize remotely. Thus, lowering the risk for local recurrence, which is particularly morbid and extremely difficult to manage, has become an important focus of rectal cancer therapy. Second, because low-lying rectal tumors approximate or involve the anal sphincter and genitourinary nerves, surgical resection may require permanent colostomy and/or compromise of sexual and urinary function. With these considerations in mind, we briefly review the management of localized rectal cancer.

Surgery remains the mainstay of treatment for nonmetastatic rectal cancer. Although patients with superficial

tumors (T1 and some T2 tumors without nodal involvement) can be treated with local transanal excision, the majority of patients (those with T3 or T4 or node-positive tumors) will require more extensive resection. In these circumstances, the distance of the tumor from the anal verge will determine the type of procedure performed. Because the anal sphincter muscle fibers are located within 3-cm proximal of the dentate line, distal rectal tumors (<5 cm from the anal verge) frequently require abdominoperineal resection (APR), which leaves the patient with a permanent colostomy. Mid- to high-rectal tumors can generally be removed by low anterior resection (LAR), which spares the anal sphincter. Tumors that are low but not clearly low enough to require an APR may be downsized with neoadjuvant therapy (see the following sections), thereby facilitating resection by LAR instead. Regardless of whether APR or LAR is employed, TME—removal of the tumor, lymph nodes, rectal mesentery, and autonomic nerves en bloc by sharp dissection—increases the likelihood of negative margins and improves local control.

### Neoadjuvant Chemoradiation

Surgical resection alone for stage II or III rectal cancer yields an unacceptably high rate of local and distant relapse. Therefore, in contrast to colon cancer, both radiation and chemotherapy have been incorporated into the treatment algorithm for stages II–III rectal cancer. Although postoperative radiation has been shown to improve local control but not OS, concurrent 5-FU-based chemoradiation (CRT) improves both local control and OS over radiation alone, with i5-FU proving to be less toxic and possibly more effective than b5-FU. As a result, standard CRT for rectal cancer includes 5–6 weeks of radiation (5040 cGy over 5 weeks in 180-cGy fractions) with concurrent i5-FU 200–250 mg/m$^2$/d or capecitabine 800–850 mg/m$^2$ twice daily (44).

Administering preoperative rather than postoperative CRT offers the potential advantages of (a) downsizing tumors and facilitating sphincter preservation in some patients who would otherwise require APR; (b) expanding the number of patients who receive adjuvant therapy (because slow postoperative recovery may delay or preclude further therapy); and (c) reducing postoperative complications. To address the question of how best to sequence CRT in relation to surgery, Sauer et al. randomized 421 patients with stage II or III rectal cancer to preoperative or postoperative CRT. All patients underwent TME and received 4 additional cycles of adjuvant b5-FU. Although preoperative CRT did not improve OS when compared to postoperative CRT, it improved local control, caused significantly less grade 3 or 4 toxicity (both acute and chronic), and facilitated more frequent delivery of full-dose chemotherapy and radiation. The rate of sphincter-preserving surgery did not differ between the 2 groups; however, restricting analysis to the 194 patients determined before randomization to require APR revealed that patients receiving preoperative CRT had higher rates of sphincter-preserving surgery (45). This trial established the standard of care for clinical stage II or III rectal cancer: neoadjuvant CRT followed by TME and adjuvant 5-FU-based chemotherapy. Since all patients in this trial received both chemotherapy and CRT, the individual contribution of each modality could not be assessed; both are therefore included in standard therapy. With the publication of the MOSAIC and X-ACT trials, options for *adjuvant* chemotherapy have been expanded to include FOLFOX, capecitabine, or CAPEOX. However, 2 randomized phase III trials—ACCORD 12 and STAR-01—have shown that administering oxaliplatin *concurrently* with 5-FU-based CRT increased toxicity without improving pathological complete response (46).

Neoadjuvant full-dose chemotherapy without radiation is an emerging, but still experimental, paradigm to treat locally advanced rectal cancer for the following reasons: (a) locally advanced rectal cancer carries a substantial risk for distant relapse; in fact, the vast majority of recurrences after appropriate therapy of locally advanced rectal cancer are distant; (b) the current treatment strategy defers full-dose systemic chemotherapy by at least 4 months after diagnosis; (c) newer combination chemotherapy regimens have been shown to shrink primary rectal tumors at rates similar

to those seen with CRT; and (d) radiation can cause long-term toxicity and generally requires placement of temporary ostomy after TME. With single-arm studies having shown that chemotherapy alone yields rates of clinical response, pathological response, and R0 resection comparable to those seen with CRT, the ongoing N1048 trial is randomizing patients with T1–2N1 or T3N0–1 rectal cancer located ≥5 cm from the anal verge to standard neoadjuvant chemoradiation or neoadjuvant FOLFOX with "selective" chemoradiation (in the event of no clinical response to chemotherapy). Pending results of this study, standard therapy for locally advanced rectal cancer remains neoadjuvant chemo RT followed by resection and adjuvant chemotherapy.

## Summary

Evaluation of tissue-proven, nonmetastatic rectal cancer should include rigid proctoscopy by an experienced colorectal surgeon for precise tumor localization, as well as EUS or pelvic MRI for local staging. Patients with clinical stage I tumors should undergo surgical resection, followed by adjuvant therapy only if the pathological stage is higher than that expected. Because neoadjuvant CRT improves local control, facilitates higher rates of sphincter preservation, and causes less toxicity than adjuvant CRT, patients with clinical stage II or III tumors (see Figure 11.4) should

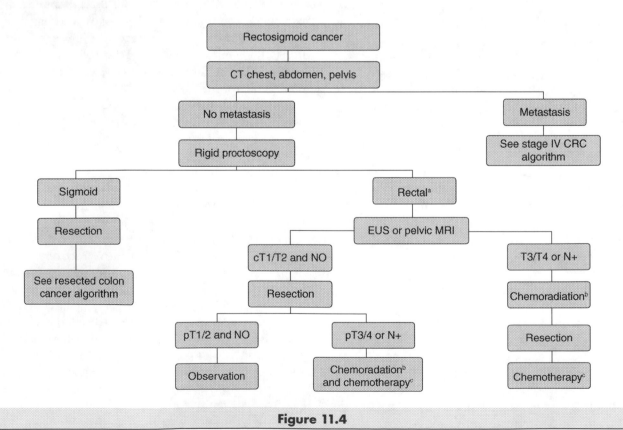

**Figure 11.4**

Treatment algorithm for rectal cancer. [a]Less than or equal to 12 cm from the anal verge. [b]Radiation administered concurrently with capecitabine or 5-FU by continuous infusion. [c]Capecitabine or 5-FU/LV or CAPEOX or FOLFOX for 4 months. CRC, colorectal cancer.

undergo neoadjuvant chemoradiation (using CIFU [continuous infusion 5-FU] or capecitabine), surgical resection, and 4 months of adjuvant chemotherapy (LV5-FU2, capecitabine, FOLFOX, or CAPEOX). Surveillance is similar to that of resected colon cancer. G.F. received neoadjuvant chemoradiotherapy (5040 cGy concurrently with capecitabine). Aside from mild radiation dermatitis, he tolerated treatment well. Six weeks after the completion of CRT, an experienced colorectal surgeon performed an APR (due to the tumor's proximity to the anal verge). Pathological evaluation revealed ypT2N0 adenocarcinoma with evidence of treatment-related tumor necrosis. After an additional 4 months of FOLFOX chemotherapy, surveillance was initiated.

## REVIEW QUESTIONS

1. An otherwise healthy 64-year-old woman is diagnosed with a sigmoid carcinoma after presenting with rectal bleeding. CT imaging shows diffuse bulky liver metastases. A *KRAS* mutation is detected in the sigmoid biopsy specimen. Her bilirubin is 2.2, and there is no radiographic evidence of biliary obstruction. Which is a reasonable option for this patient?

   (A) Proceed with resection of her primary tumor followed by staged resection of her liver metastases
   (B) Liver biopsy to confirm the presence of a *KRAS* mutation in her liver metastases
   (C) Start FOLFIRI/cetuximab chemotherapy
   (D) Start FOLFOX chemotherapy
   (E) Start FOLFIRI/BV chemotherapy

2. A 65-year-old woman undergoes screening colonoscopy, which reveals a nonobstructing mass in the descending colon. Biopsy shows well-differentiated carcinoma, and staging CT imaging of the chest, abdomen, and pelvis demonstrates a single 5-cm lesion in the right lobe of liver. The patient is otherwise healthy and is asymptomatic. Which of the following is the best treatment plan?

   (A) Palliative chemotherapy alone
   (B) Resection of the primary tumor and liver metastasis followed by observation
   (C) Chemotherapy for 6 months followed by consideration for resection of the primary tumor and liver metastasis
   (D) Chemotherapy for 3 months followed by consideration for resection of the liver metastasis, 3 more months of chemotherapy, then resection of the primary tumor
   (E) Resection of the primary mass followed by 6 months of chemotherapy, then resection of the liver metastasis

3. A 63-year-old man with hypertension, recent stroke, type II diabetes, and diabetic neuropathy is diagnosed with unresectable, *KRAS* wild-type colon cancer. Despite his comorbidities, he is highly functional (performance status = 0). Which would be the most appropriate regimen for him?

   (A) FOLFOX/BV
   (B) FOLFIRI/BV
   (C) FOLFOX/cetuximab
   (D) FOLFIRI/cetuximab

4. A 56-year-old woman with stage IV colon cancer characterized by metastases to lungs, liver, and retroperitoneal lymph nodes, has an excellent partial response to 6 cycles of FOLFOX. However, she has developed grade 2 neuropathy, and is unable to open jars while she is working in the kitchen. As her oncologist, what would you recommend as the next step in her disease management?

   (A) Ask her to tolerate the chemotherapy because she has shown a good response to treatment
   (B) Reduce the doses of 5-fluorouracil (5-FU) and oxaliplatin by 50% to reduce the risk of progressive neuropathy
   (C) Omit the oxaliplatin for now, but consider adding back later if her disease progresses on 15-FU/leucovorin and her neuropathy has improved
   (D) Start a chemotherapy holiday
   (E) Add calcium/magnesium 30 minutes before and after oxaliplatin infusions

5. Having recently undergone a left hemicolectomy for colon cancer, a 54-year-old man with well-controlled diabetes comes to your office for an evaluation. The patient appears well, and pathological evaluation of the resected tumor reveals T3N1 disease. Preoperative CT scans showed no evidence of distant metastasis. Molecular analysis shows the absence of a *KRAS* mutation. What do you recommend?

   (A) Observation
   (B) FOLFOX + cetuximab for 6 months
   (C) FOLFOX + BV for 6 months
   (D) FOLFIRI for 6 months
   (E) FOLFOX for 6 months

6. A 40-year-old man comes to your office regarding his recently resected colon cancer. The pathology report notes a T3N0 tumor (all 14 resected nodes are negative for metastasis) without evidence of perforation, lymphovascular invasion, or perineural invasion. Additional immunohistochemical analysis reveals absent MSH2 staining. He is otherwise healthy and has no baseline neuropathy. What do you recommend?

   (A) Observation
   (B) Single-agent 5-fluorouracil

(C) Capecitabine
(D) FOLFOX
(E) B or C

7. A 64-year-old woman presents with rectal bleeding and decreased stool caliber. Flexible sigmoidoscopy reveals a circumferential but nonobstructing rectosigmoid mass, and biopsy shows moderately differentiated adenocarcinoma. CT imaging of the chest, abdomen, and pelvis shows rectal thickening without evidence of distant metastasis. What other diagnostic testing do you recommend?

(A) Rigid proctoscopy by a colorectal surgeon
(B) MRI of the pelvis or endoscopic ultrasound
(C) PET/CT
(D) All of the above
(E) A and B

8. Further staging evaluation of the patient in Question 7 reveals a clinical T3N1 tumor located 6 cm from the anal verge. What treatment do you recommend?

(A) Surgical resection followed by adjuvant chemotherapy
(B) Chemotherapy followed by surgical resection
(C) Surgical resection followed by adjuvant chemoradiation and chemotherapy
(D) Neoadjuvant radiation with concurrent capecitabine, followed by surgery and adjuvant chemotherapy
(E) Neoadjuvant radiation with concurrent capecitabine and oxaliplatin, followed by surgery and adjuvant chemotherapy

9. A 66-year-old man presents with constipation and mild rectal bleeding. A CT scan shows a large distal rectal mass and multiple bilateral liver metastases without evidence of large bowel obstruction. Colonoscopy shows a circumferential, near-obstructing rectal mass 4 cm from the anal verge, and a pediatric scope is required to traverse the lesion. Biopsy is positive for poorly differentiated adenocarcinoma. What is the best treatment plan for this patient?

(A) An abdominoperineal resection followed by chemotherapy
(B) Full-course chemoradiation followed by chemotherapy
(C) Endoscopic placement of a rectal stent followed by chemotherapy
(D) Surgical diversion followed by chemotherapy

10. A 24-year-old man presents to the emergency department with shortness of breath and lightheadedness. He is found to have a microcytic anemia, and colonoscopy shows innumerable polyps as well as a large friable sigmoid cancer. His family history is strongly positive for colorectal cancer. Which of the following germ-line mutations likely explain his syndrome?

(A) MUTYH
(B) MSH2
(C) STK11
(D) APC

11. A 62-year-old man has just completed 6 months of adjuvant chemotherapy for stage III proficient in mismatch repair colon cancer. His last colonoscopy was before surgery and was incomplete due to obstruction. He has no prior history of cancer and no family history of cancer. What do you recommend?

(A) History and physical exam with carcinoembryonic antigen every 3–6 months and annual CT for 5 years
(B) A low fat, high-fiber diet and active lifestyle
(C) PET/CT
(D) All of the above
(E) A and B

12. Which of the following is the recommended endoscopic surveillance for the patient in Question 11?

(A) Colonoscopy now, then again in 1 year if no advanced adenoma or cancer, then every 3 years if no advanced adenoma or cancer
(B) Colonoscopy now, then again in 3 years if no advanced adenoma or cancer, then every 5 years if no advanced adenoma or cancer
(C) Colonoscopy 1 year after the initial colonoscopy, then yearly later if no advanced adenoma or cancer
(D) Colonoscopy 1 year after the initial colonoscopy, then every 3 years if no advanced adenoma or cancer

## REFERENCES

1. Poultsides GA, Servais EL, Saltz LB, et al. Outcome of primary tumor in patients with synchronous stage IV colorectal cancer receiving combination chemotherapy without surgery as initial treatment. *J Clin Oncol.* 2009;27(20):3379–3384.
2. Sada Y, Duan Z, El-Serag, et al. Utilization and outcomes of primary tumor surgery for stage IV colon cancer in the United States: a population-based study. *J Clin Oncol.* 2012(suppl);abstr 3542.
3. Ferrand F, Malka D, Bourredjem A, et al. Impact of primary tumour resection on survival of patients with colorectal cancer and synchronous metastases treated by chemotherapy: results from the multicenter, randomised trial Fédération Francophone de Cancérologie Digestive 9601. *Eur J Cancer.* 2013;49(1): 90–97.
4. de Gramont A, Bosset JF, Milan C, et al. Randomized trial comparing monthly low-dose leucovorin and fluorouracil bolus with bimonthly high-dose leucovorin and fluorouracil bolus plus continuous infusion for advanced colorectal cancer: a French intergroup study. *J Clin Oncol.* 1997;15(2):808–815.

5. Douillard JY, Cunningham D, Roth AD, et al. Irinotecan combined with fluorouracil compared with fluorouracil alone as first-line treatment for metastatic colorectal cancer: a multicentre randomised trial. *Lancet*. 2000;355(9209):1041–1047.

6. Fuchs CS, Marshall J, Mitchell E, et al. Randomized, controlled trial of irinotecan plus infusional, bolus, or oral fluoropyrimidines in first-line treatment of metastatic colorectal cancer: results from the BICC-C Study. *J Clin Oncol*. 2007;25(30):4779–4786.

7. de Gramont A, Figer A, Seymour M, et al. Leucovorin and fluorouracil with or without oxaliplatin as first-line treatment in advanced colorectal cancer. *J Clin Oncol*. 2000;18(16):2938–2947.

8. Cassidy J, Clarke S, Díaz-Rubio E, et al. Randomized phase III study of capecitabine plus oxaliplatin compared with fluorouracil/folinic acid plus oxaliplatin as first-line therapy for metastatic colorectal cancer. *J Clin Oncol*. 2008;26(12):2006–2012.

9. Tournigand C, Cervantes A, Figer A, et al. OPTIMOX1: a randomized study of FOLFOX4 or FOLFOX7 with oxaliplatin in a stop-and-Go fashion in advanced colorectal cancer—a GERCOR study. *J Clin Oncol*. 2006;24(3):394–400.

10. Chibaudel B, Maindrault-Goebel F, Lledo G, et al. Can chemotherapy be discontinued in unresectable metastatic colorectal cancer? The GERCOR OPTIMOX2 Study. *J Clin Oncol*. 2009;27(34):5727–5733.

11. Tournigand C, André T, Achille E, et al. FOLFIRI followed by FOLFOX6 or the reverse sequence in advanced colorectal cancer: a randomized GERCOR study. *J Clin Oncol*. 2004;22(2):229–237.

12. Falcone A, Ricci S, Brunetti I, et al.; Gruppo Oncologico Nord Ovest. Phase III trial of infusional fluorouracil, leucovorin, oxaliplatin, and irinotecan (FOLFOXIRI) compared with infusional fluorouracil, leucovorin, and irinotecan (FOLFIRI) as first-line treatment for metastatic colorectal cancer: the Gruppo Oncologico Nord Ovest. *J Clin Oncol*. 2007;25(13):1670–1676.

13. Hurwitz H, Fehrenbacher L, Novotny W, et al. Bevacizumab plus irinotecan, fluorouracil, and leucovorin for metastatic colorectal cancer. *N Engl J Med*. 2004;350(23):2335–2342.

14. Giantonio BJ, Catalano PJ, Meropol NJ, et al.; Eastern Cooperative Oncology Group Study E3200. Bevacizumab in combination with oxaliplatin, fluorouracil, and leucovorin (FOLFOX4) for previously treated metastatic colorectal cancer: results from the Eastern Cooperative Oncology Group Study E3200. *J Clin Oncol*. 2007;25(12):1539–1544.

15. Saltz LB, Clarke S, Díaz-Rubio E, et al. Bevacizumab in combination with oxaliplatin-based chemotherapy as first-line therapy in metastatic colorectal cancer: a randomized phase III study. *J Clin Oncol*. 2008;26(12):2013–2019.

16. Cunningham D, Lang I, Marcuello E, et al.; AVEX study investigators. Bevacizumab plus capecitabine versus capecitabine alone in elderly patients with previously untreated metastatic colorectal cancer (AVEX): an open-label, randomised phase 3 trial. *Lancet Oncol*. 2013;14(11):1077–1085.

17. Bennouna J, Sastre J, Arnold D, et al.; ML18147 Study Investigators. Continuation of bevacizumab after first progression in metastatic colorectal cancer (ML18147): a randomised phase 3 trial. *Lancet Oncol*. 2013;14(1):29–37.

18. Van Cutsem E, Tabernero J, Lakomy R, et al. Addition of aflibercept to fluorouracil, leucovorin, and irinotecan improves survival in a phase III randomized trial in patients with metastatic colorectal cancer previously treated with an oxaliplatin-based regimen. *J Clin Oncol*. 2012;30(28):3499–3506.

19. Jonker DJ, O'Callaghan CJ, Karapetis CS, et al. Cetuximab for the treatment of colorectal cancer. *N Engl J Med*. 2007;357(20):2040–2048.

20. Van Cutsem E, Peeters M, Siena S, et al. Open-label phase III trial of panitumumab plus best supportive care compared with best supportive care alone in patients with chemotherapy-refractory metastatic colorectal cancer. *J Clin Oncol*. 2007;25(13):1658–1664.

21. Karapetis CS, Khambata-Ford S, Jonker DJ, et al. K-ras mutations and benefit from cetuximab in advanced colorectal cancer. *N Engl J Med*. 2008;359(17):1757–1765.

22. Cunningham D, Humblet Y, Siena S, et al. Cetuximab monotherapy and cetuximab plus irinotecan in irinotecan-refractory metastatic colorectal cancer. *N Engl J Med*. 2004;351(4):337–345.

23. Van Cutsem E, Köhne CH, Láng I, et al. Cetuximab plus irinotecan, fluorouracil, and leucovorin as first-line treatment for metastatic colorectal cancer: updated analysis of overall survival according to tumor KRAS and BRAF mutation status. *J Clin Oncol*. 2011;29(15):2011–2019.

24. Maughan TS, Adams RA, Smith CG, et al.; MRC COIN Trial Investigators. Addition of cetuximab to oxaliplatin-based first-line combination chemotherapy for treatment of advanced colorectal cancer: results of the randomised phase 3 MRC COIN trial. *Lancet*. 2011;377(9783):2103–2114.

25. Peeters M, Price TJ, Cervantes A, et al. Randomized phase III study of panitumumab with fluorouracil, leucovorin, and irinotecan (FOLFIRI) compared with FOLFIRI alone as second-line treatment in patients with metastatic colorectal cancer. *J Clin Oncol*. 2010;28(31):4706–4713.

26. Douillard JY, Siena S, Cassidy J, et al. Randomized, phase III trial of panitumumab with infusional fluorouracil, leucovorin, and oxaliplatin (FOLFOX4) versus FOLFOX4 alone as first-line treatment in patients with previously untreated metastatic colorectal cancer: the PRIME study. *J Clin Oncol*. 2010;28(31):4697–4705.

27. Douillard JY, Oliner KS, Siena S, et al. Panitumumab-FOLFOX4 treatment and RAS mutations in colorectal cancer. *N Engl J Med*. 2013;369(11):1023–1034.

28. Tol J, Koopman M, Cats A, et al. Chemotherapy, bevacizumab, and cetuximab in metastatic colorectal cancer. *N Engl J Med*. 2009;360(6):563–572.

29. Grothey A, Van Cutsem E, Sobrero A, et al.; CORRECT Study Group. Regorafenib monotherapy for previously treated metastatic colorectal cancer (CORRECT): an international, multicentre, randomised, placebo-controlled, phase 3 trial. *Lancet*. 2013;381(9863):303–312.

30. Mitry E, Fields AL, Bleiberg H, et al. Adjuvant chemotherapy after potentially curative resection of metastases from colorectal cancer: a pooled analysis of two randomized trials. *J Clin Oncol*. 2008;26(30):4906–4911.

31. Nordlinger B, Sorbye H, Glimelius B, et al.; EORTC Gastro-Intestinal Tract Cancer Group; Cancer Research UK; Arbeitsgruppe Lebermetastasen und -tumoren in der Chirurgischen Arbeitsgemeinschaft Onkologie (ALM-CAO); Australasian Gastro-Intestinal Trials Group (AGITG); Fédération Francophone de Cancérologie Digestive (FFCD). Perioperative chemotherapy with FOLFOX4 and surgery versus surgery alone for resectable liver metastases from colorectal cancer (EORTC Intergroup trial 40983): a randomised controlled trial. *Lancet*. 2008;371(9617):1007–1016.

32. Moertel CG, Fleming TR, Macdonald JS, et al. Levamisole and fluorouracil for adjuvant therapy of resected colon carcinoma. *N Engl J Med*. 1990;322(6):352–358.

33. Efficacy of adjuvant fluorouracil and folinic acid in colon cancer. International Multicentre Pooled Analysis of Colon Cancer Trials (IMPACT) investigators. *Lancet*. 1995;345(8955):939–944.

34. Van Cutsem E, Labianca R, Bodoky G, et al. Randomized phase III trial comparing biweekly infusional fluorouracil/leucovorin alone or with irinotecan in the adjuvant treatment of stage III colon cancer: PETACC-3. *J Clin Oncol*. 2009;27(19):3117–3125.

35. André T, Boni C, Navarro M, et al. Improved overall survival with oxaliplatin, fluorouracil, and leucovorin as adjuvant treatment in stage II or III colon cancer in the MOSAIC trial. *J Clin Oncol*. 2009;27(19):3109–3116.

36. Chau I, Norman AR, Cunningham D, et al. A randomised comparison between 6 months of bolus fluorouracil/leucovorin and 12 weeks of protracted venous infusion fluorouracil as adjuvant treatment in colorectal cancer. *Ann Oncol*. 2005;16(4):549–557.

37. Twelves C, Wong A, Nowacki MP, et al. Capecitabine as adjuvant treatment for stage III colon cancer. *N Engl J Med.* 2005;352(26):2696–2704.

38. Haller DG, Tabernero J, Maroun J, et al. Capecitabine plus oxaliplatin compared with fluorouracil and folinic acid as adjuvant therapy for stage III colon cancer. *J Clin Oncol.* 2011;29(11):1465–1471.

39. Allegra CJ, Yothers G, O'Connell MJ, et al. Phase III trial assessing bevacizumab in stages II and III carcinoma of the colon: results of NSABP protocol C-08. *J Clin Oncol.* 2011;29(1):11–16.

40. Efficacy of adjuvant fluorouracil and folinic acid in B2 colon cancer. International Multicentre Pooled Analysis of B2 Colon Cancer Trials (IMPACT B2) investigators. *J Clin Oncol.* 1999;17(5):1356–1363.

41. Quasar Collaborative Group; Gray R, Barnwell J, McConkey C, et al. Adjuvant chemotherapy versus observation in patients with colorectal cancer: a randomised study. *Lancet.* 2007;370(9604):2020–2029.

42. Sargent DJ, Marsoni S, Monges G, et al. Defective mismatch repair as a predictive marker for lack of efficacy of fluorouracil-based adjuvant therapy in colon cancer. *J Clin Oncol.* 2010;28(20):3219–3226.

43. Gray RG, Quirke P, Handley K, et al. Validation study of a quantitative multigene reverse transcriptase-polymerase chain reaction assay for assessment of recurrence risk in patients with stage II colon cancer. *J Clin Oncol.* 2011;29(35):4611–4619.

44. Krishnan S, Janjan NA, Skibber JM, et al. Phase II study of capecitabine (Xeloda) and concomitant boost radiotherapy in patients with locally advanced rectal cancer. *Int J Radiat Oncol Biol Phys.* 2006;66(3):762–771.

45. Sauer R, Becker H, Hohenberger W, et al.; German Rectal Cancer Study Group. Preoperative versus postoperative chemoradiotherapy for rectal cancer. *N Engl J Med.* 2004;351(17):1731–1740.

46. Gérard JP, Azria D, Gourgou-Bourgade S, et al. Comparison of two neoadjuvant chemoradiotherapy regimens for locally advanced rectal cancer: results of the phase III trial ACCORD 12/0405-Prodige 2. *J Clin Oncol.* 2010;28(10):1638–1644.

# 12

## *Anal Cancer*

RUILING XU YUAN, MUHAMMAD A. TARAKJI, AND ELIZABETH YU CHIAO

## EPIDEMIOLOGY, RISK FACTORS, NATURAL HISTORY, AND PATHOLOGY

Anal canal cancer (ACC) is an uncommon gastrointestinal malignancy and accounts for only a small percentage (4%) of all cancers of the lower alimentary tract. According to the American Cancer Society Cancer Facts and Figures, there was an estimated incidence of 7060 new cases in the United States, and approximately 880 deaths, in 2013. Most anal cancers are squamous cell cancers or cloacogenic cancers, with a few adenocarcinomas (estimated to represent 2.9–10% of all ACC). In addition, melanoma and lymphomas also account for a small percentage of cancers found in the anal canal; however, because squamous cell cancer of the anus (SCCA) is by far the most common type of anal cancer, this chapter will focus on SCCA.

Over the last 30 years, the incidence of SCCA has been increasing among men (particularly, among black men) (1). The annual incidence among men and women was similar between 1994 and 2000 (2.04 and 2.06 per 100,000, respectively), which is in contrast to the period between 1973 and 1979 (1.06 and 1.39 per 100,000, respectively) (1). When broken down by race, a remarkable increase was observed among black men increasing from 1.09 per 100,000 to 2.71 per 100,000 in the same time period (1973–2000). The incidence has also significantly increased in other specific populations such as HIV-infected homosexual men. This finding is particularly noteworthy because several studies have shown that the incidence of SCCA among HIV-infected men continues to increase despite the widespread utilization of highly active antiretroviral treatment (HAART), indicating that the incidence of SCCA among HIV-infected individuals is unlikely to decrease in the future (2).

Several risk factors have been implicated in the development of SCCA (Table 12.1). The strongest risk factor is human papillomavirus (HPV) infection, which is the most common sexually transmitted disease worldwide (3). HPV infection is particularly prevalent among persons engaging in certain sexual practices such as receptive anal intercourse and among those with a high lifetime number of sexual partners (3). Certain HPV types (primarily types 16 and 18) have been identified in the majority of anal cancer specimens (4), and infection with these oncogenic types is strongly associated with cancer carcinogenesis along a pathway in which high-grade anal intraepithelial neoplasia (AIN) precedes SCCA (5).

Chronic immunosuppression, including iatrogenic causes such as solid organ transplant recipients and HIV infection, has been shown to increase the risk of SCCA. A large meta-analysis found that the standardized incidence ratio (SIR) for SCCA was 4.85 (95% confidence interval [CI] [1.36–17.3]) among renal transplant recipients (6) and 28.75 (95% CI [21.6–38.3]) among HIV-infected individuals (6). Sites of chronic inflammation have also been implicated as a risk factor and a recent systematic review of the literature found that there is a higher incidence of anal SCC in patients with Crohn's disease compared to the general population (7). Finally, cigarette smoking is significantly associated with an increased risk of anal cancer (RR = 1.9 for 20 pack-years, RR = 5.2 for 50 pack-years) (8).

The incidence of SCCA will likely continue to rise because of increased efforts in earlier detection of precancerous AIN through the use of anal cytology screening for anal cancer precursor lesions in high-risk individuals (9). In 2013, the Lower Anogenital Squamous Terminology (LAST) project work groups recommended a 2-tiered classification system, including low-grade squamous intraepithelial lesion (LSIL), which includes previously categorized AIN 1 lesions, and high-grade squamous intraepithelial lesion (HSIL), which includes previously categorized AIN 2 and 3, in order to standardize lower anogenital squamous pathology (10).

**Table 12.1** SCCA Risk Factors Associated With Sexual Behavior

| SCCA Risk Factors Associated With Sexual Behavior | Relative Risk |
|---|---|
| Never-married men | 8.6 |
| Homosexual men | 50 |
| Genital Warts | 27 |
| Gonorrhea | 17 |

SCCA, squamous cell cancer of the anus.
*Source*: Adapted from Ref. (3). Daling JR, Weiss NS, Hislop TG, et al. Sexual practices, sexually transmitted diseases, and the incidence of anal cancer. *N Engl J Med*. 1987;317(16):973–977.

**Table 12.2** Five-Year Overall Survival for SCCA

| Stage | Percentage (%) |
|---|---|
| I | 70 |
| II | 59 |
| III | 41 |
| IV | 19 |

SCCA, squamous cell cancer of the anus.
*Source*: Adapted from Ref. (14). Bilimoria KY, Bentrem DJ, Rock CE, et al. Outcomes and prognostic factors for squamous-cell carcinoma of the anal canal: analysis of patients from the National Cancer Data Base. *Dis Colon Rectum*. 2009;52(4):624–631.

Recent published reports have shown that use of the HPV vaccine reduced the rates of AIN and may help to reduce the risk of anal cancer in males (11). In 1 study, among males aged 16–26 years, the rates of grade 2 or 3 AIN related to infection with HPV-16 and -18 were reduced by 54% (95% CI [18.0–75.3]) in the intention-to-treat population and by 74.9% (95% CI [8.8–95.4]) in the per-protocol efficacy population (11). In October 2011, these finding prompted the Advisory Committee on Immunization Practices to recommend the routine use of quadrivalent HPV vaccine in males aged 11–12 years (12). For those not vaccinated at the target age, catch-up vaccination is recommended up to age 26 years (13).

## STAGING

SCCA tumors tend to spread by local extension, but have the potential to metastasize. The 3 major prognostic factors are site (anal canal vs. perianal skin), size, and nodal status. The staging of SCCA, unlike most gastrointestinal malignancies, is not dependent on the degree of tumor tissue penetration but rather on the size of the primary tumor.

| American Joint Committee on Cancer (AJCC) Staging System for Anal Carcinoma | |
|---|---|
| Stage | Definition |
| I | Tumor confined to anal canal, ≤2 cm (T1) |
| II | Tumor confined to anal canal, >2 cm, <5 cm (T2), or >5 cm (T3) |
| IIIA | Tumor of any size with metastasis to perirectal lymph nodes (N1), or tumor of any size with invasion of adjacent organs (e.g., vagina, urethra, bladder) (T4) without lymph node metastases |
| IIIB | Tumor invading adjacent organs (T4) and perirectal lymph node metastases (N1) or tumor of any size with metastases to internal iliac and/or inguinal lymph nodes (N2, N3) |
| IV | Tumor of any size with or without lymph node metastases with distant metastases (e.g., liver, lung, etc.) |

The prognosis of SCCA was stratified in a recent cohort of 19,195 patients, which showed that patients with SCCA had a higher risk of death if they were males ≥65 years old, black, living in lower median incomes areas, and had more advanced T stage tumors, nodal or distant metastases, or poorly differentiated cancers ($P < .0001$) (14). The 5-year overall survival is shown in Table 12.2.

## CASE SUMMARIES

### Limited Stage Anal Carcinoma

P.G. is a 61-year-old white HIV-negative female with a past medical history of hypertension and hyperlipidemia. She presented to her local gynecologist complaining of bright red blood per rectum. Digital rectal examination showed nodularity in the anal canal, and subsequent colonoscopy revealed a smooth anterolateral anal canal nodule, which was 1–1.5 cm in greatest dimension, and involved the anal sphincter. Biopsies were consistent with invasive squamous cell carcinoma. Staging CT scans of the chest, abdomen, and pelvis were unremarkable for other lesions or lymphadenopathy and the staging at presentation was T1, N0, M0 (stage I).

### Evidence-Based Case Discussion

P.G. has stage I squamous anal carcinoma, which was staged clinically by digital rectal examination. Palpation of inguinal lymph nodes is an indication for fine needle aspiration (FNA) or excisional biopsy to determine whether there is inguinal lymph node involvement. A CT scan or MRI of the abdomen and pelvis is generally necessary to evaluate the pelvic nodes for metastases. In addition, chest imaging with chest x-ray or CT scan is also recommended as a part of the initial staging workup. The use of PET scanning is not generally accepted as a routine method for initial staging. See Figure 12.1 for a diagnostic and therapeutic algorithm.

HIV testing is recommended because of the increased risk for SCCA among HIV-infected individuals, and measurement of CD4 count and HIV viral load is recommended

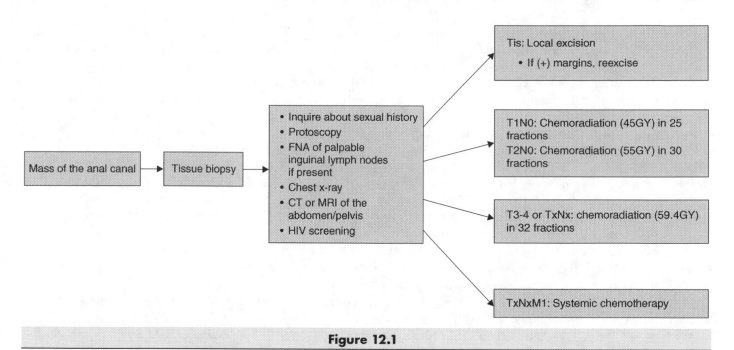

**Figure 12.1**

Diagnostic evaluation for anal canal mass. FNA, fine needle aspiration. *Source*: Adapted from Ref. (15). Ang C. Chapter 17: Anal cancer. In: Anderson MD, ed., *Manual of Medical Oncology*. The McGraw-Hill Companies Inc; 2006.

for all HIV-infected patients. In addition, gynecological examination and screening for HPV and cervical cancer are suggested for female patients.

The 5-year overall survival for this patient is up to 70% and currently the recommended treatment for patients with stage I–III ACC is concurrent chemotherapy and external beam radiation therapy (XRT) according to the Nigro protocol (16). This regimen consists of 5-fluorouracil (5-FU; 1000 mg/m²/d by continuous infusion days 1 through 4 and 29 through 32); mitomycin (10–15 mg/m² on day 1 only); and intermediate-dose XRT (45 Gy) given in 25 fractions over 5 weeks. Patients with stage II or III ACC are treated with the same chemotherapy regimen but with higher XRT doses (55–59 Gy). Surgery with abdominoperineal resection (APR) is only needed in patients who have residual tumor at the time of postradiation biopsy.

A number of studies have addressed the efficacy and safety of chemotherapy and XRT regimens. A phase III intergroup study done by the Radiation Therapy Oncology Group (RTOG 87–04) showed that patients who received concurrent XRT plus 5-FU and mitomycin had a lower APR rate (9% vs. 22%, $P$ = .002), and a higher 4-year disease-free survival (DFS; 73% vs. 51%, $P$ = .0003) compared with patients receiving XRT with 5-FU alone (17).

A more recent study done by the intergroup RTOG 98–11 compared the use of cisplatin in place of mitomycin, each along with 5-FU and concurrent XRT, and although there were no differences in primary end points of DFS (54% vs. 60%, $P$ = .17) and 5-year overall survival (70% vs. 75%: $P$ = .10) between the 2 regimens, the APR rate in

the group that received cisplatin was significantly higher (19% vs. 10%: $P$ = .02) (18). HIV-positive patients with anal cancer can be treated with standard chemoradiotherapy with the same tolerability and toxicity as HIV-negative patients. Long-term local control and survival rates are not significantly different between these groups (19).

The potential utility of maintenance chemotherapy after concurrent chemoradiation therapy (CRT) was explored in a recently published randomized phase III ACT II study that demonstrated no progression-free survival (PFS) benefit associated with the addition of maintenance therapy: the 3-year PFS was 74% (95% CI [69–77]) vs. 73% (95% CI [68–77]), maintenance versus no maintenance, respectively (20).

Thus, the current standard of care for early-stage SCCA (stages I–III) is concurrent 5-FU plus mitomycin chemotherapy with XRT.

## Metastatic Anal Carcinoma

F.A. is a 49-year-old Hispanic male with a history of HIV/AIDS (CD4 = 63 cells/µL), hepatitis B, and pulmonary cryptococcosis. He presented with an 8-month history of an enlarging perianal mass that had become increasingly painful over the 2 months prior to presentation. He also reported nonpurulent drainage with subjective fever and was evaluated by general surgery for possible incision and drainage. Anal examination under anesthesia showed an anal abscess, and a hard, palpable, 6-cm nodule associated with severe anal stenosis. Excision of the abscess along with multiple core biopsies was performed and showed pathology consistent with moderately differentiated, invasive squamous cell carcinoma. A CT scan of the chest, abdomen, and pelvis was performed and showed an increased number of enlarged perirectal and unilateral internal iliac lymph nodes in addition to the anal mass. The patient was staged as T3 N2 M0 (IIIB). He was started on fluconazole treatment for his pulmonary cryptococcosis, and on discharge he was referred to an outpatient HIV clinic, where a highly active antiretroviral therapy (HARRT) was initiated. Six weeks later, the patient had an undetectable HIV viral load and was started on the Nigro protocol with concurrent chemotherapy and XRT (59 Gy). The patient tolerated the treatment well without the need for any delays or dose reductions. Anoscopy performed 2 months later showed a complete resolution of the anal mass and CT scanning of the abdomen and pelvis demonstrated no lymphadenopathy, consistent with a complete response to therapy.

A posttreatment surveillance CT scan at 6 months showed a new 6.0-cm hypodense mass in the right hepatic lobe along with the reappearance of retroperitoneal lymphadenopathy. A liver biopsy was performed and the pathology was consistent with invasive squamous carcinoma. He did not return for any chemotherapy appointments, and was subsequently lost to follow-up.

### Evidence-Based Case Discussion

F.A. initially had stage IIIB SCCA and, after an initial complete response to therapy, subsequently developed stage IV SCCA. Of note, he completed standard dose concurrent chemotherapy and XRT while on HAART despite having a low CD4 count and an opportunistic infection 6 weeks before. This case demonstrates that HIV-infected patients with low CD4 counts can often tolerate standard dose therapy, as long as the patients demonstrate a response to HAART therapy, resulting in an undetectable HIV viral load.

Although concurrent chemotherapy and XRT in the treatment of early stages of SCCA is generally effective, there is up to a 40% rate of locoregional failure (21) and salvage surgery with an APR would then be the next appropriate step unless the recurrence is associated with distant metastasis. The most common sites of metastases outside the pelvis are the liver, lung, and extrapelvic lymph nodes. For metastatic disease, systemic treatment with cisplatin combined with 5-FU is generally the most active and effective palliative treatment regimen with an overall response rate of approximately 66% (22) and a 5-year survival of 19% (Table 12.2).

HIV-infected patients with SCCA should be treated similar to those who are HIV uninfected. However, patients with active opportunistic infections and/or with poorly controlled HIV as reflected by low CD4 counts or detectable HIV viral loads (due to poor compliance or drug resistance) may not be able to tolerate full doses of mitomycin. In a retrospective study that compared 20 HIV-infected patients

versus 24 HIV-uninfected patients, both the objective initial response rate and median overall survival were superior in HIV-uninfected patients (50% vs. 88% and 18 vs. 28 months, respectively; P < .01). However, patients who were HIV infected had a higher incidence of lymph node metastases (60% vs. 17%, respectively) and were less likely to have received combined-modality therapy (25% vs. 54%, respectively), which likely accounted for the inferior results (23).

A more recent series compared 17 immunodeficient (ID) HIV-infected patients with 19 immune competent (IC) HIV-uninfected patients and concluded that there was no significant relationship between the CD4 count and treatment-related acute toxicities even when CD4 counts were <200 cells/µL. In addition, there was also no difference in terms of overall survival, with 3-year overall survival reported as 83.6% (95% CI [68.2–100]) and 91.7% (95% CI [77.3–100]) in the IC and ID groups, respectively. The disease-specific survival was 88.2% (95% CI [74.2–100]) in the IC group and 91.7% (95% CI [77.3–100]) in the ID group. Finally, APR-free survival was 78.3% (95% CI [61.5–99.5]) and 80.9% (95% CI [63.4–100]) in the IC and ID groups, respectively (24).

### FUTURE DIRECTIONS

Epidermal growth factor receptor (EGFR) expression in anal carcinoma is observed in approximately 80–90% of cases. Moreover, some studies have demonstrated that *KRAS* mutations, the principal mechanism of resistance to anti-EGFR therapy, are virtually absent in this tumor (25). Clinical trials incorporating target agent cetuximab with current chemoradiotherapy for stages I–III anal cancer are ongoing.

### *Other Special Considerations for HIV-Infected Patients*

Given the fact that the risk for SCCA is significantly higher among HIV-infected individuals, and the fact that HIV-infected patients who are not on effective HIV therapy may not tolerate chemotherapy and XRT, screening of all new SCCA cases for HIV should be considered as a part of any standard SCCA diagnostic work up (Figure 12.1). In addition, for individuals already known to be HIV-infected, SCCA screening among high-risk patient populations, using anal cytology, has been advocated. In particular, it has been shown that yearly Pap testing of HIV-infected men who have sex with men is cost-effective and has a cost per quality adjusted life year (QALY) similar to other accepted cancer screening programs such as colon cancer screening with colonoscopy (26). Finally, a recent study found that while several different chemotherapy treatment regimens did not significantly influence CD4 cell count recovery, XRT did cause significant and prolonged decline of CD4+ T cells, for which the use of infection prophylaxis was recommended in patients with preexisting low CD4 counts (27).

## REVIEW QUESTIONS

1. A 20-year-old male college student presents to the college health clinic complaining about the recent development of anogenital warts and anal irritation. During his visit, he indicates that he is sexually active with other men. His physical examination, which includes a digital rectal examination, is unremarkable except for the presence of several perianal warts. In response to his health concerns, what reasonable advice can you give him to reduce his risk of developing human papillomavirus (HPV)-related malignancy?

   (A) Initiate a "catch-up" quadrivalent HPV vaccination
   (B) Undergo anal cytology screening for precancerous anal intraepithelial neoplasia
   (C) Use condoms when engaging in sexual activity
   (D) Avoid smoking
   (E) All of the above

2. A 41-year-old man with AIDS (CD4 count = 155) on highly active antiretroviral treatment (HAART) with a prior history of anal condyloma reported rectal bleeding and discharge for the past year for which he had sought no medical attention until now. In the emergency department, he was found to have a 9-cm fungating anal mass with inguinal lymphadenopathy (as also seen on CT of the pelvis) and a biopsy demonstrated an anal squamous cell carcinoma. His physical examination was otherwise unremarkable and his CT showed no evidence of distant disease. His renal and liver function was normal, and his performance status was 0. What is your recommendation regarding his management?

   (A) Surgical resection
   (B) Chemotherapy alone
   (C) Concurrent chemoradiation therapy
   (D) Palliative care and hospice referral
   (E) Observation and continue HAART therapy for his AIDS

3. The patient in Question 2 completed concurrent chemoradiation therapy and, after 10 weeks' follow-up, he returned for a restaging evaluation, which included a digital rectal examination (DRE), an anoscopy, and a CT scan of the abdomen and pelvis. This restaging demonstrated a complete clinical response to his treatment. What would you recommend as the next step in his management?

   (A) Initiate maintenance chemotherapy
   (B) Begin surveillance with periodic DRE, anoscopy, and annual CT scans
   (C) Administer a radiation therapy boost to the primary site
   (D) Discharge from your clinic advising the patient that he is cured

4. The patient in Question 3 does well for 2 years, but then presents to emergency department with rectal bleeding. His physical examination is unremarkable except tachycardia, and his laboratory evaluation demonstrates anemia with a Hgb of 7.0, for which he received 2 units of packed red blood cells. A restaging sigmoidoscopy shows a 2-cm perianal mass fixed to pelvic wall, with no lymphadenopathy found on physical examination or CT scans. Re-biopsy shows recurrent anal squamous cell carcinoma. What is your next step of management?

   (A) Radiation to the tumor bed
   (B) Systemic chemotherapy with cisplatin-based regimen
   (C) Repeat concurrent chemoradiation therapy
   (D) Surgical (abdominoperitoneal) resection

5. A 55-year-old woman had previously been diagnosed with stage II (T3N0M0) squamous cell carcinoma of the anal canal 2 years ago. She completed concurrent chemoradiation therapy with 45 Gy in 1.8 Gy fractions and 5-fluorouracil (5-FU)/mitomycin with no evidence of disease recurrence. She now presents with right upper quadrant abdominal pain of 3 months' duration accompanied by an unintentional weight loss of 10 kg. A restaging abdominal-pelvic CT showed a new 6-cm hypodense mass in the right hepatic lobe along with perihepatic and paraortic lymphadenopathy. An iridium-guided liver biopsy showed invasive squamous carcinoma. Her physical examination was not remarkable except a mild tenderness to palpation in RUQ. Her lab studies showed a Hgb of 10.3, and mildly elevated liver function tests. Her Eastern Cooperative Oncology Group performance status is 1, and she wishes to explore every treatment options at this time. What is your recommendation?

   (A) *KRAS* testing, if positive, start cetuximab
   (B) Referral for port placement and start FOLFOX
   (C) Consult surgery to evaluate for possible resection of the liver lesion
   (D) Cisplatin plus 5-FU
   (E) Observation with continuation of highly active antiretroviral treatment

## REFERENCES

1. Johnson LG, Madeleine MM, Newcomer LM, et al. Anal cancer incidence and survival: the surveillance, epidemiology, and end results experience, 1973–2000. *Cancer*, 2004;101(2): 281–288.
2. Kan M, Wong PH, Press N, Wiseman SM. Colorectal and anal cancer in HIV/AIDS patients: a comprehensive review. *Expert Rev Anticancer Ther*. 2014;14(4):395–405.
3. Daling JR, Weiss NS, Hislop TG, et al. Sexual practices, sexually transmitted diseases, and the incidence of anal cancer. *N Engl J Med*. 1987;317(16):973–977.

4.  Ouhoummane N, Steben M, Coutlée F, et al. Squamous anal cancer: patient characteristics and HPV type distribution. *Cancer Epidemiol.* 2013;37(6):807–812.

5.  Smyczek P, Singh AE, Romanowski B. Anal intraepithelial neoplasia: review and recommendations for screening and management. *Int J STD AIDS.* 2013;24(11):843–851.

6.  Grulich AE, van Leeuwen MT, Falster MO, Vajdic CM. Incidence of cancers in people with HIV/AIDS compared with immunosuppressed transplant recipients: a meta-analysis. *Lancet.* 2007;370(9581):59–67.

7.  Slesser AA, Bhangu A, Bower M, et al. A systematic review of anal squamous cell carcinoma in inflammatory bowel disease. *Surg Oncol.* 2013;22(4):230–237.

8.  Holly EA, Whittemore AS, Aston DA, et al. Anal cancer incidence: genital warts, anal fissure or fistula, hemorrhoids, and smoking. *J Natl Cancer Inst.* 1989;81(22):1726–1731.

9.  Northfelt DW, Swift PS, Palefsky JM. Anal neoplasia. Pathogenesis, diagnosis, and management. *Hematol Oncol Clin North Am.* 1996;10(5):1177–1187.

10. Darragh TM, Colgan TJ, Thomas Cox J, et al.; Members of the LAST Project Work Groups. The Lower Anogenital Squamous Terminology Standardization project for HPV-associated lesions: background and consensus recommendations from the College of American Pathologists and the American Society for Colposcopy and Cervical Pathology. *Int J Gynecol Pathol.* 2013;32(1):76–115.

11. Palefsky JM, Giuliano AR, Goldstone S, et al. HPV vaccine against anal HPV infection and anal intraepithelial neoplasia. *N Engl J Med.* 2011;365(17):1576–1585.

12. Centers for Disease Control and Prevention (CDC). Recommendations on the use of quadrivalent human papillomavirus vaccine in males—Advisory Committee on Immunization Practices (ACIP), 2011. *MMWR Morb Mortal Wkly Rep.* 2011;60(50):1705–1708.

13. Committee on Adolescent Health Care of the American College of Obstetricians and Gynecologists; Immunization Expert Work Group of the American College of Obstetricians and Gynecologists. Committee opinion no. 588: human papillomavirus vaccination. *Obstet Gynecol.* 2014;123(3):712–718.

14. Bilimoria KY, Bentrem DJ, Rock CE, et al. Outcomes and prognostic factors for squamous-cell carcinoma of the anal canal: analysis of patients from the National Cancer Data Base. *Dis Colon Rectum.* 2009;52(4):624–631.

15. Eng C. *Chapter 17. Anal Cancer. MD Anderson Manual of Medical Oncology.* 1st ed. New York, NY: McGraw-Hill Companies; 2006:429–448.

16. Leichman L, Nigro N, Vaitkevicius VK, et al. Cancer of the anal canal. Model for preoperative adjuvant combined modality therapy. *Am J Med.* 1985;78(2):211–215.

17. Flam M, John M, Pajak TF, et al. Role of mitomycin in combination with fluorouracil and radiotherapy, and of salvage chemoradiation in the definitive nonsurgical treatment of epidermoid carcinoma of the anal canal: results of a phase III randomized intergroup study. *J Clin Oncol.* 1996;14(9):2527–2539.

18. Ajani JA, Winter KA, Gunderson LL, et al. Fluorouracil, mitomycin, and radiotherapy vs fluorouracil, cisplatin, and radiotherapy for carcinoma of the anal canal: a randomized controlled trial. *JAMA.* 2008;299(16):1914–1921.

19. Fraunholz I, Rabeneck D, Gerstein J, et al. Concurrent chemoradiotherapy with 5-fluorouracil and mitomycin C for anal carcinoma: are there differences between HIV-positive and HIV-negative patients in the era of highly active antiretroviral therapy? *Radiother Oncol.* 2011;98(1):99–104.

20. James RD, Glynne-Jones R, Meadows HM, et al. Mitomycin or cisplatin chemoradiation with or without maintenance chemotherapy for treatment of squamous-cell carcinoma of the anus (ACT II): a randomised, phase 3, open-label, 2 × 2 factorial trial. *Lancet Oncol.* 2013;14(6):516–524.

21. Mullen JT, Rodriguez-Bigas MA, Chang GJ, et al. Results of surgical salvage after failed chemoradiation therapy for epidermoid carcinoma of the anal canal. *Ann Surg Oncol.* 2007;14(2):478–483.

22. Faivre C, Rougier P, Ducreux M, et al. [5-fluorouracile and cisplatinum combination chemotherapy for metastatic squamous-cell anal cancer]. *Bull Cancer.* 1999;86(10):861–865.

23. Vatra B, Sobhani I, Aparicio T, et al. [Anal canal squamous-cell carcinomas in HIV positive patients: clinical features, treatments and prognosis]. *Gastroenterol Clin Biol.* 2002;26(2):150–156.

24. Seo Y, Kinsella MT, Reynolds HL, et al. Outcomes of chemoradiotherapy with 5-Fluorouracil and mitomycin C for anal cancer in immunocompetent versus immunodeficient patients. *Int J Radiat Oncol Biol Phys.* 2009;75(1):143–149.

25. Paliga A, Onerheim R, Gologan A, et al. EGFR and K-ras gene mutation status in squamous cell anal carcinoma: a role for concurrent radiation and EGFR inhibitors? *Br J Cancer.* 2012;107(11):1864–1868.

26. Goldie SJ, Kuntz KM, Weinstein MC, et al. The clinical effectiveness and cost-effectiveness of screening for anal squamous intraepithelial lesions in homosexual and bisexual HIV-positive men. *JAMA.* 1999;281(19):1822–1829.

27. Sankatsing SU, Hillebregt MM, Gras L, et al. Prolonged decrease of CD4+ T lymphocytes in HIV-1-infected patients after radiotherapy for a solid tumor. *J Acquir Immune Defic Syndr.* 2013;62(5):546–549.

# 13

# *Prostate Cancer*

LEONEL F. HERNANDEZ-AYA, JINGSONG ZHANG, KATHLEEN A. COONEY,
AND MAHA H. HUSSAIN

## EPIDEMIOLOGY, RISK FACTORS, AND NATURAL HISTORY

Prostate cancer is the most common noncutaneous cancer diagnosed among U.S. men with approximately 233,000 new cases annually. It remains the second leading cause of cancer deaths in men, with 29,480 estimated deaths in 2014 (1). On the basis of the data collected between 1975 and 2004 from the Surveillance Epidemiology and End Results (SEER), the lifetime risk of developing prostate cancer in American men is 16%, but the risk of dying of prostate cancer is only 2.9%. Therefore, although the disease is lethal for some men, the majority of men with prostate cancer die from of other causes.

Age, race, and positive family history are the most important recognized risk factors for prostate cancer. The probability of developing prostate cancer increases with age, from 0.3% in men younger than 49 years, increasing to 11% in men 70 years and older. African American men have the highest prostate cancer incidence and death rates among all races/ethnicities, about 3 times those of Asian Americans, who have the lowest rates (1).

Familial clustering of prostate cancer has been widely reported since the early 1990s. A number of different studies have been conducted to measure the impact of family history on the risk of prostate cancer. Important factors associated with increased risk of prostate cancer include young age at diagnosis, the number of affected relatives, and the degree of relatedness of affected relatives (2). In addition, having an affected brother is associated with a higher risk compared with only having an affected father. Elegant research using linkage analysis and next-generation sequencing technologies led to the discovery of a recurrent mutation in *HOXB13* that is associated with early age at diagnosis and family history of prostate cancer (3).

Prostate-specific antigen (PSA) is a serum protease that became widely used in the late 1980s to diagnose prostate cancer and to monitor disease activity. As a result of the widespread use of PSA for diagnosis, there has been stage migration toward more localized stage prostate cancer. The use of PSA in combination with digital rectal examination (DRE) as a screening method for prostate cancer is controversial due to conflicting data from prostate cancer screening trials (4). The main concern is that a widespread use of PSA screening may lead to overdiagnosis and overtreatment of prostate cancers that would never have become clinically apparent. The American Cancer Society (ACS) recommends PSA for screening in men who have at least a 10-year life expectancy after an informed decision-making process to balance the benefits, harms, and uncertainties related to the use of PSA in this setting (5). In 2012, the U.S. Preventive Services Task Force (USPSTF) recommended against PSA-based screening for all men (6). Prostate cancer is a heterogeneous disease with differences in biology and clinical course. Presently, treatment decisions are based on the individual's risk of developing metastases and dying from prostate cancer. Some patients with low-risk disease do not require immediate treatment as the likelihood of developing prostate cancer–related symptoms is low and the risk of dying from other causes exceeds that of the cancer; on the other hand, other patients are diagnosed with aggressive forms of prostate cancer and require multidisciplinary management.

## PATHOLOGY AND STAGING

More than 95% of all prostate cancers are adenocarcinomas. The remaining types of prostate cancer include

**Table 13.1** Prostate Cancer Prognostic State Groups

| Group | TNM | PSA | Gleason |
|---|---|---|---|
| I | T1a-c N0 M0 | <10 | ≤6 |
| | T2 N0 M0 | <10 | ≤6 |
| | T1–2a N0 M0 | Not available | Not available |
| IIA | T1a-c N0 M0 | <20 | 7 |
| | T1a-c N0 M0 | ≥10, <20 | ≤6 |
| | T2a N0 M0 | ≥10, <20 | ≤6 |
| | T2a N0 M0 | <20 | 7 |
| | T2b N0 M0 | <20 | ≤7 |
| | T2b N0 M0 | Not available | Not available |
| IIB | T2c N0 M0 | Any PSA | Any Gleason |
| | T1–2 N0 M0 | ≥20 | Any Gleason |
| | T1–2 N0 M0 | Any PSA | ≥8 |
| III | T3a-b N0 M0 | Any PSA | Any Gleason |
| IV | T4 N0 M0 | Any PSA | Any Gleason |
| | Any T N1 M0 | Any PSA | Any Gleason |
| | Any T Any N M1 | Any PSA | Any Gleason |

PSA, prostate-specific antigen; TNM, tumor node metastases.
*Source*: Modified from *AJCC Cancer Staging Handbook, 7th edition* (2010), published by Springer Science and Business Media LLC.

entities such as mucinous adenocarcinoma, large cell neuroendocrine tumors, small cell carcinoma, and sarcomatoid carcinoma. The Gleason histological grading system provides microscopic evaluation of prostate adenocarcinoma using a 5-point grading scale. Pattern 1 tumors are the most differentiated, whereas pattern 5 lesions are the most undifferentiated. The Gleason score is based on the sum of the score for the most common or primary pattern followed by the second most common or secondary pattern (e.g., 4 + 3 = 7). A higher Gleason score is associated with more aggressive disease. Since its introduction several decades ago, the Gleason score has been recognized as one of the most powerful prognostic factors for prostate adenocarcinoma, and it is now incorporated in the current edition of American Joint Committee on Cancer (AJCC's) prostate cancer staging and prognostic grouping. The current (7th edition) AJCC staging system for prostate cancer that incorporates both the Gleason score and the PSA is shown in Table 13.1.

## CASE SUMMARIES

### Clinically Localized Prostate Cancer

A.M. is a 60-year-old African American man who presented to his primary care physician with a several-month history of urinary hesitancy and dribbling. DRE was notable for bilateral nodularity of the prostate gland. His serum PSA was 12 ng/mL and the patient reported no prior PSA tests. The patient's past medical history was significant for coronary artery disease, insulin-dependent diabetes mellitus, hypertension, and obesity with a body

mass index (BMI) of 34. His family history was positive for prostate cancer diagnosis in one of his 2 brothers. An ultrasound-guided transrectal biopsy of the prostate revealed adenocarcinoma of the prostate, Gleason score 5 + 4 = 9, involving multiple bilateral prostate cores. A staging evaluation including CT scan of the abdomen and pelvis as well as a bone scan failed to reveal evidence of distant metastases. A.M. was considered to have a clinical stage IIB, T2c N0 M0 Gleason 9 adenocarcinoma of the prostate. After a multidisciplinary evaluation and discussion of therapeutic options, A.M. elected to have definitive external beam radiation therapy (EBRT) concurrent with androgen deprivation therapy (ADT) with leuprolide. The patient was recommended to continue on ADT for at least 3 years. A.M.'s PSA was <0.1 ng/mL when he finished radiation therapy (RT) and his PSA remained low during ADT. The main complications of treatment experienced by the patient were urinary leakage, fatigue, sexual difficulty, and hot flashes. He maintained his BMI around 34 during the 3 years of ADT.

## Evidence-Based Case Discussion

A.M. was at an increased risk of developing prostate cancer because he has a first-degree relative (brother) with prostate cancer and because he is an African American. For high-risk individuals such as A.M. (African American, positive family history), some medical groups such as the ACS recommend considering prostate cancer screening beginning at age 45 years. Whether prostate cancer screening beginning at age 45 years would have affected Mr. A.M.'s management and survival is uncertain.

The patient presented with clinically localized prostate cancer. Localized prostate cancers are confined to the prostate gland without evidence of nodal or distant metastasis. The options of management for localized prostate cancer include radical surgery, RT, or watchful waiting in low-risk patients. Men with low-risk prostate cancer (T1–T2a, Gleason score ≤6, and PSA <10 ng/mL) may be considered for active surveillance because the risk of dying from noncancer causes exceeds that of prostate cancer. Men with intermediate (T2b and/or Gleason 7 and/or PSA 10–20 ng/mL) and high risk (≥T2c or Gleason 8–10 or PSA >20 ng/mL) of recurrence are recommended to be treated definitively with radical prostatectomy or EBRT (7). Both options of definitive therapy are widely accepted, leaving the decision to consideration of side effects and patient preference for each modality. The role of postoperative ADT has not been well studied in localized prostate cancer. The Southwest Oncology Group (SWOG) S9921 study randomly assigned 983 men with high-risk features at prostatectomy to receive adjuvant therapy with ADT alone or in combination with mitoxantrone chemotherapy (8). ADT consisted of goserelin and bicalutamide for 2 years. The control arm of S9921 represents the largest prospective cohort of patients treated with adjuvant ADT and shows that the combination of radical prostatectomy and combined androgen blockade is associated with favorable disease-free survival (DFS) and overall survival (OS) (8). However, grade 1 evidence is lacking for adjuvant ADT after radical prostatectomy in localized prostate cancer; therefore, perioperative ADT in localized prostate cancer is not recommended unless as part of a clinical trial. On the other hand, in men with node-positive prostate cancer who have undergone radical prostatectomy and pelvic lymphadenectomy, immediate adjuvant ADT showed significant improvements in progression-free survival (PFS) and OS after 11.9 years of follow-up in a study by Messing et al. (9). Consequently, evidence supports the use of adjuvant ADT in patients with node-positive disease after radical prostatectomy although the timing of initiation of treatment is controversial.

## Evidence Supports Adding ADT to RT for High-Risk Prostate Cancer

The role of neoadjuvant and concurrent ADT for patients treated with definitive radiation is well established. For patients with intermediate-risk prostate cancer receiving EBRT, neoadjuvant and concurrent androgen deprivation is recommended for 3–4 months' duration (10). In patients with high-risk disease, several phase III clinical trials reported that adding ADT to RT improved survival of men with localized, high-risk prostate cancer. In the European Organization for Research and Treatment of Cancer (EORTC) study by Bolla et al. (11), 415 patients with T1–T4 disease were randomly assigned to EBRT alone or EBRT plus 3 years of goserelin starting at the first day of radiation. Cyproterone acetate (150 mg orally) was given for 1 month starting 1 week before the first goserelin injection. Among these patients, 82% had T3 disease, 9% had T4 disease, and rest of the participants had World Health Organization (WHO) grade 3 T1–T2 disease. At a median follow-up of 5.5 years, adding ADT to EBRT significantly improved the 5-year clinical DFS (primary endpoint; 74% vs. 40%; *P* = .0001) and the 5-year OS (secondary endpoint; 78% vs. 62%; *P* = .0002). Extended follow-up with a median of 9.1 years confirmed the improved DFS and OS without an increase in cardiovascular toxicity (12). For patients with node-positive disease after radical prostatectomy, the Radiation Therapy Oncology Group (RTOG) 85–31 study randomized 977 patients with either clinical T3 prostate cancer or regional lymph node involvement to either EBRT alone versus EBRT with indefinite goserelin starting at the last week of EBRT. Androgen suppression as an adjuvant to definitive radiotherapy was associated with improved OS in tumors with a Gleason score 8–10 and a significant improvement in local control and freedom from disease progression (13). Although there is no consensus on the

optimal duration of adjuvant ADT, this decision should be tailored to the patients' comorbidities, life expectancy, as well as expected tolerance to treatments. Available data support the use of long-term (generally 2–3 years) adjuvant ADT in high-risk prostate cancer patients who elect RT (12). Improving cure rate and survival with minimum toxicity would be the ultimate goal of adjuvant trials. The efficacy and safety of adding adjuvant chemotherapy with docetaxel and prednisone to adjuvant ADT for men with prostate cancer exhibiting unfavorable prognostic factors will be determined by the RTOG 0521 study.

## Recognizing and Managing Side Effects of Long-Term ADT

Although generally less toxic than cytotoxic chemotherapy, prolonged ADT is not without side effects, which include hot flashes, fatigue, loss of libido, decline in sexual function, weight gain, and loss of bone density. A number of studies in the past 2 decades have highlighted the increased risk of osteoporosis in men receiving ADT for prostate cancer. ADT has been shown to decrease bone mineral density (BMD) after as early as 6 months of treatment for either localized or metastatic prostate adenocarcinoma (14). Two large retrospective studies directly assessed the risks of fracture in men treated with gonadotropin-releasing hormone (GnRH) agonist. Smith et al. used claims-based cohort of Medicare beneficiaries and demonstrated a significantly increased fracture risk in men with nonmetastatic prostate cancer (mPC) treated with GnRH agonist (*n* = 3887) versus those who were not (*n* = 7774) during a 7-year follow-up (15). Shahinian et al. studied the SEER-Medicare records of 50,613 men with prostate cancer (AJCC stages I–IV) and demonstrated a statistically significant relationship between the number of doses of GnRH agonist received during the 12 months after diagnosis and the subsequent risk of fracture (14).

There are a number of strategies used in the clinic to minimize potential bone loss related to ADT. Men on ADT should be assessed for bone loss before initiating ADT and at regular intervals while continuing on treatment. Unless contraindicated, routine use of calcium (>1200 mg/d) and vitamin D supplements (800 IU/d) should be considered along with lifestyle modifications (participation in aerobic and/or resistance training exercise programs, smoking reduction, etc.). Bisphosphonates have been shown to inhibit osteoclast activities, and several studies have reported the role of bisphosphonates in preventing bone loss. Oral bisphosphonate therapy should be considered for men starting ADT who already have evidence of osteoporosis. In a small study of men with severe osteopenia or osteoporosis (T-score >2.0) and receiving ADT for prostate cancer, once-weekly 70-mg alendronate significantly improved the BMD and decreased the risk of femoral neck fracture compared to a control group of men who did not receive alendronate (16).

Denosumab is a fully humanized monoclonal antibody that specifically binds to the receptor activator of nuclear factor-κB ligand (RANKL), which is a key mediator of osteoclast formation, function, and survival. In a randomized, double-blind phase III study in men receiving ADT for non-mPC, denosumab at a dose of 60 mg subcutaneously every 6 months significantly increased BMD and reduced the incidence of new vertebral fractures at 36 months compared to placebo (1.5% vs. 3.9% with placebo, $P = .006$) (17). The significant differences in BMD between the 2 groups were seen as early as 1 month and sustained through 36 months. The adverse events reported at 24 months did not appear to be significantly different in the denosumab arm compared to the placebo arm.

Note that there are data supporting the use of both zoledronic acid and denosumab for men with castrate-resistant prostate cancer (CRPC) metastatic to bone with the goal of reducing skeletal-related events (SREs), which include radiation to bone, clinical fracture, spinal cord compression, or surgery to bone. However, a recent study by Smith et al. showed no benefit in time to first SRE or OS in men who received zoledronic acid versus placebo for androgen-sensitive mPC (18) suggesting that the benefit of these agents in preventing SREs is in the castrate-resistant setting.

Other complications of ADT relate to the observed decrease in lean body mass and increase in fat mass. These changes appear to be early adverse effects with minimal additional changes in body composition beyond 18 months of treatment. ADT also reduces insulin sensitivity while increasing low-density lipoprotein cholesterol, high-density lipoprotein cholesterol, and triglycerides. These metabolic changes are consistent with an increased incidence of cardiovascular diseases and diabetes mellitus reported by multiple large observational studies. Although no randomized trials have prospectively addressed the risks of cardiovascular diseases and diabetes associated with ADT, none of the prospective randomized trials demonstrated any increase in cardiovascular mortalities in the ADT arms, and cardiovascular mortalities were found to be nonsignificant in retrospective analyses of randomized trials (19).

### Adjuvant Radiotherapy for Pathologically Advanced Prostate Cancer

Adjuvant radiotherapy is often considered in men with any of the following adverse pathological features: positive surgical margins, extracapsular extension, and involvement of the seminal vesicles or a combination of these features. Both SWOG 8794 and EORTC 22911 compared radical prostatectomy alone to radical prostatectomy and immediate adjuvant RT for men with pT3 cancers or with positive surgical margins. Neither study excluded patients with detectable postoperative PSA levels. When the EORTC

22911 trial was reported after a median follow-up of 5 years, 60-Gy adjuvant radiotherapy significantly improved biochemical PFS and local control compared to observation, but not OS (20). SWOG 8794 had a longer follow-up and, with a median follow-up of 12.6 years, showed that adjuvant external beam radiotherapy with 60–64 Gy to the prostatic fossa significantly improved both metastasis-free and OS compared to observation (21). Notably, only one third of the patients originally assigned to observation received salvage RT at the time of a biochemical recurrence, and these results cannot be used to compare a strategy of adjuvant RT with observation followed by salvage RT at the first sign of PSA recurrence. Adverse effects of radiotherapy include rectal complications (3.3% vs. 0% in observation); urethral strictures (17.8% vs. 9.5%); and total urinary incontinence (6.5% vs. 2.8%) (20).

## PSA-Only (Biochemical) Recurrence

W.R. is a 58-year-old-white man initially diagnosed with localized prostate cancer during an evaluation for an elevated screening PSA of 8. His DRE was normal and a biopsy confirmed adenocarcinoma with Gleason 7 (3 + 4) histology. He underwent radical prostatectomy and the pathology report confirmed Gleason 7 adenocarcinoma with evidence of extracapsular extension and positive margins (stage III). Two of the dissected lymph nodes were negative for cancer. His PSA was undetectable 6 weeks after the operation. It was recommended to W.R. that he consider adjuvant RT but he declined.

W.R. was followed over the next several years and his PSA increased from below 0.1–0.6 ng/mL. Five years after radical prostatectomy, his PSA reached 2.3 ng/mL. Imaging studies including bone scan, abdominal CT, and pelvic CT were negative for metastatic disease. At this time, he underwent salvage RT (66.6 Gy total) to the prostatic bed. His PSA declined to 1.2 ng/mL, 4 months after completion of radiation; however, 3 months later it increased to 10.7. Radiological imaging for metastatic cancer was again negative. On further evaluation, W.R. remained completely asymptomatic from his prostate cancer. His repeat PSA in 8 weeks stabilized at around 11.0 ng/mL. W.R. expressed concerns about the potential side effects of ADT, and he subsequently enrolled into an immunotherapy trial combining prostate-specific membrane antigen (PSMA) and T-cell receptor γ alternate reading frame protein (TARP) peptide with poly IC-LC adjuvant in human leukocyte antigens (HLA)-A2 (+) patients with biochemical recurrence (NCT00694551).

## Evidence-Based Case Discussion

### Biochemical Recurrence: Definition and Risk Stratification

Serum PSA is very sensitive for detecting recurrence after definitive local treatment for prostate cancer, which leads to the identification of men with a PSA-only or biochemical recurrence. According to the American Urological Association (AUA) guidelines, a biochemical recurrence after radical prostatectomy is defined as a serum PSA of >0.2 ng/mL, with a second confirmatory level of PSA of >0.2 ng/mL in patients who have no detectable metastases. Because some prostatic glandular tissues remain after RT, serum PSA levels are unlikely to fall to undetectable levels and typically will not reach a nadir until 1 year after completion of RT. To account for the variable PSA kinetics after different forms of RT, a consensus committee proposed the "Phoenix Definition" of PSA failure, which is defined as a PSA rise by 2 ng/mL or more above the post-radiotherapy nadir. In most cases, a rising PSA level indicates micrometastatic disease. However, the time to detection of visible metastatic disease is highly variable. The median time to the detection of metastatic disease reported in 1 series was 8 years, with 63% of the patients remaining free of disease at 5 years (22).

Several studies have demonstrated that PSA doubling time (PSADT) at the time of PSA recurrence is an important marker to predict prostate cancer–specific mortality. Using multiinstitutional databases, D'Amico et al. analyzed the outcome of 8669 patients treated with radical prostatectomy or RT for clinical stage T1c-4 NX or N0 M0 prostate adenocarcinoma between 1988 and January 2002. For men with PSADT of <3 months, the hazard ratios (HRs) for the time to prostate cancer–specific and all-cause mortality were 19.6 and 6.9, respectively (23). Freedland et al. conducted a retrospective study of 379 men who underwent radical prostatectomy at Johns Hopkins Hospital between 1982 and 2000 and confirmed the value of PSADT for time to prostate cancer–specific mortality (HR of 27.48 for PSADT <3 months and 8.76 for PSADT between 3 and 8.9 months). Recurrence within 3 years of radical prostatectomy and Gleason score of 8 or above were also important predictors of time to prostate cancer-specific mortality (HR of 3.53 and 2.26, respectively) (24). The role of Gleason score of 8 or above in prostate cancer-specific mortality was also shown by Zhou et al. in a study of 1159 men who developed PSA failure after initial definitive treatment with surgery or radiation (25). No prospective randomized study has demonstrated the value of initiating ADT to patients with biochemical-only progression after definitive therapy.

## Salvage Radiotherapy

For some men with low-level PSA recurrences after radical prostatectomy and life expectancy >10 years, salvage RT can be considered. Salvage RT is typically limited to the prostatic fossa. Based on the available PSA data, W.R. had a PSA recurrence within 3 years of initial radical prostatectomy. Unfortunately, he was not evaluated for salvage radiotherapy until his PSA increased from 0.6 to 2.3.

Multiple retrospective studies have shown that PSA level prior to salvage radiotherapy is the most consistent variable associated with the PSA-relapse-free outcome after salvage radiotherapy; that is, the lower the PSA level at the time of salvage RT, the better the treatment outcome. On the basis of the available evidence prior to 1999, the American Society for Therapeutic Radiology and Oncology (ASTRO) consensus panel concluded that the appropriate PSA cut point for salvage radiotherapy "seemed to be 1.5 ng/mL." Stephenson et al. (26) developed a nomogram to predict outcome of salvage radiotherapy based on a pooled cohort of >1500 patients. Significant variables in the model were PSA level before salvage treatment, prostatectomy Gleason grade, PSADT, surgical margins, ADT before or during salvage RT, and lymph node status. This nomogram has a reported concordance index of 0.69 and is currently available at www.mskcc.org/applications/nomograms/prostate/PostRadicalProstatectomy.aspx

## Metastatic Prostate Cancer

J.T. is a 62-year-old Hispanic man who was referred to a multidisciplinary urological cancer clinic for treatment of mPC. The patient initially presented with a PSA of 39 ng/mL and he was diagnosed with clinical stage IIB, T2c, Gleason 8 (4 + 4) prostate adenocarcinoma. Imaging studies were negative for metastatic diseases. He underwent EBRT treatment (78 Gy) with the initial plan of a total of 2 years' ADT. His PSA was 3.2 ng/mL 3 months after completing RT. It then started to increase shortly afterward, and J.T. was maintained on continuous ADT. His PSA continued to increase despite the addition of bicalutamide and subsequent bicalutamide withdrawal. His PSA increased to 220 ng/mL and he was eventually found to have metastatic cancer to the bone and multiple enlarged lymph nodes (the largest diameter was 5 cm). Clinically, he experienced bone pain in sites of metastases and weight loss. Mr. J.T. was offered the option to be enrolled in a clinical trial; however, he decided to receive standard management. He was started on abiraterone/prednisone with improvement of his bone symptoms and decrease in PSA levels. However, after 8 months of treatment, he had disease progression evidenced by enlargement of lymphadenopathy. J.T. was started on enzalutamide, which he continues up to now. He has experienced mild fatigue and mild diarrhea but overall, the treatment has been well-tolerated.

## Evidence-Based Case Discussion

### Metastatic Noncastrate Prostate Cancer

mPC has 2 different clinical states: the hormone-sensitive state and the castration-resistant state. The latter is the lethal phenotype of prostate cancer and has been the focus of prolific research and discovery of new treatment strategies. Prostate cancer is an androgen-dependent tumor and the majority of patients with newly diagnosed with mPC are initially responsive to ADT. Hormone-sensitive metastatic disease is defined by evidence of metastases on an imaging study. Although surgical and medical castration is equally effective, patient preference has made medical castration with GnRH-agonists/antagonists the most common treatment approach. Synthetic peptide analogs of GnRH such as leuprolide and goserelin, and GnRH-antagonists such as degarelix, are now part of the armamentarium for medical castration. The initial rise in testosterone after treatment with a GnRH-agonist can cause a clinical flare of the disease; therefore, GnRH-agonist is relatively contraindicated as monotherapy in patients with urinary symptoms, severe pain, or spinal cord compression. A GnRH-antagonist, lead in oral antiandrogens (bicalutamide or flutamide), or bilateral orchiectomy should be used as initial therapy in these patients. The use of GnRH-agonists in combination with an antiandrogen is believed to be a more potent strategy because antiandrogens can block the effects of nongonadal androgens synthesized in the adrenal glands.

The majority of patients initially respond to ADT. Up to 70% of patients will have normalization of PSA value of <4 ng/mL after castration and approximately 30–50% of tumor masses will regress by 50% or more. The PSA value measured at 7 months after initiating therapy was shown to be predictive of outcomes, with a median survival of 13 months for patients with a PSA nadir of >4 ng/mL, 44 months for patients with a PSA nadir of 0.2–4 ng/mL, and 75 months for patients with PSA nadir of <0.2 ng/mL (27). The research on hormone-sensitive disease has focused on investigating optimal and more effective ways to use the available therapies. Treatment strategies such as combining androgen receptor (AR) blockade with GnRH agonists, the use of intermittent versus continuous ADT, and the addition of chemotherapy to ADT have been tested. Based on the recently published results from SWOG 9346, continuous ADT remains standard, and patients willing to consider intermittent ADT should be carefully counseled (28). Although data for improved outcome with combination of AR blockade with GnRH agonist are not confirmed in every trial, combined ADT has become a widely used treatment strategy for hormone-sensitive mPC.

This approach will change for some patients with the results of the E3805 trial (CHAARTED: ChemoHormonal Therapy Versus Androgen Ablation Randomized Trial for Extensive Disease in Prostate Cancer). In this study, 790 men with mPC previously untreated received either ADT alone or ADT with the chemotherapy drug docetaxel at 75 mg/m² every 3 weeks for 6 cycles. The addition of docetaxel to ADT significantly improved OS especially in patients with high volume of disease (visceral metastasis and/or 4 or more bone metastases including at least 1 bone metastasis beyond the pelvis or axial skeleton). The median OS was 57.6 months in the ADT plus docetaxel arm and 44.0 months in the ADT arm (HR = 0.61, 95% CI [0.47–0.80]; P = .0003). In men with high-volume disease, the median OS was 49.2 months with docetaxel plus ADT compared with 32.2 months with ADT, a difference of 17 months (HR = 0.60, 95% CI [0.45–0.81]; P = .0006). In men with low-volume disease, median OS had not been reached at the time of the analysis (29).

## Castration-Resistant Prostate Cancer

CRPC is defined as disease progression evidenced by increasing serum PSA values and/or progressive disease by radiological imaging studies despite a castrate level of testosterone (<50 ng/dL or 17 nmol/dL). In men with CRPC who are asymptomatic, antiandrogen withdrawal (AAW) is often attempted. Withdrawal responses have been reported in approximately 20% of men treated with a variety of antiandrogens including both flutamide and bicalutamide. The phase III CALGB 9583 study showed that AAW and immediate addition of ketoconazole compared to AAW alone can result in approximately 30% PSA response rates; however, it has no impact on survival (30).

The last decade has witnessed an exponential increase in treatment options for metastatic CRPC (mCRPC) patients. Multiple agents targeting key pathways in carcinogenesis are now approved for the management of advanced disease. Chemotherapy agents (docetaxel, cabazitaxel); agents targeting the androgen signaling pathway (abiraterone, enzalutamide); bone-targeting radiopharmaceutical agents (radium-223); and immunotherapy (Sipuleucel-T) have demonstrated OS benefits in mCRPC (Table 13.2).

In 2004, Tannock et al. reported that docetaxel-based chemotherapy improves OS and health-related quality of life (HRQL) in men with mCRPC (31). Cabazitaxel is a novel taxane that also binds and stabilizes tubulin, inducing cell cycle arrest and inhibiting cell proliferation. In a phase III trial in patients with CRPC progressing on docetaxel, cabazitaxel improved median OS compared with mitoxantrone (15.1 vs. 12.7 months; 95% CI [0.61–0.84]) leading to its Food and Drug Administration (FDA) approval for mCRPC after docetaxel therapy (32).

New insights in the pathophysiology and mechanisms of resistance to ADT led to the development of novel drugs with survival benefit in the post- and pre-docetaxel mCRPC setting. A potent suppression of the androgen signaling pathway is effective in CRPC. Abiraterone is an oral irreversible inhibitor of the CYP-17A enzyme critical in the testosterone biosynthesis pathway. The COU-AA-301 (Cougar 301) phase III trial in CRPC patients post-docetaxel demonstrated a statistically significant improvement in survival of patients treated with abiraterone/prednisone

**Table 13.2** Medications With OS Benefit in Metastatic Castration-Resistant Prostate Cancer

| Drug | Clinical Trial | Clinical Setting | Main Study Results | FDA Approval |
|---|---|---|---|---|
| **Targeting the Microtubule** | | | | |
| Docetaxel | TAX327 Docetaxel vs. mitoxantrone | mCRCP | Docetaxel improved OS 18.9 vs. 16.5 mo | 2004 |
| | SWOG 9916 Docetaxel/estramustine vs. mitoxantrone | mCRPC | Docetaxel improved OS 17.5 vs. 15.6 mo | |
| Cabazitaxel | TROPIC ($n = 755$) Cabazitaxel vs. mitoxantrone | mCRPC Post-docetaxel | Cabazitaxel improved OS 15.1 vs. 12.7 mo (HR = 0.70) | 2010 |
| **Targeting the Immune System** | | | | |
| Sipuleucel-T | IMPACT ($n = 512$) Sipuleucel vs. placebo | mCRPC Asymptomatic or minimally symptomatic | Sipuleucel-T improved OS 25.8 vs. 21.7 mo HR = 0.77 | 2010 |
| **Targeting the Androgen Pathway** | | | | |
| Abiraterone | COU-AA-301 ($n = 1195$) Abiraterone/prednisone vs. placebo/prednisone | mCRPC Post-docetaxel | Improved OS 15.8 vs. 11.2 mo HR = 0.74 | 2011 |
| | COU-AA-302 ($n = 1088$) Abiraterone/prednisone vs. placebo/prednisone | mCRPC Chemotherapy-naive | Improved PFS 16.5 vs. 8.3 mo HR = 0.53 | 2012 |
| Enzalutamide | AFFIRM ($n = 1199$) Enzalutamide vs. placebo | mCRPC Post-docetaxel | Improved OS 18.4 vs. 13.6 mo HR = 0.63 | 2012 |
| | PREVAIL ($n = 1717$) Enzalutamide vs. placebo | mCRPC Chemotherapy-naive | Improved OS 32.4 vs. 30.2 mo HR = 0.71 | Pending for chemo-naive |
| **Targeting Bone Metastasis** | | | | |
| Radium-223 (Xofigo) | ALSYMPCA ($n = 921$) Placebo-controlled | mCRPC Post-docetaxel or unfit for docetaxel. Symptomatic Bone metastases | Improved OS 14.9 vs. 11.2 mo HR = 0.69 | 2013 |

AFFIRM, A Study Evaluating the Efficacy and Safety of the Investigational Drug MDV3100; ALSYMPCA, Alpharadin in Symptomatic Prostate Cancer Patients; FDA, Food and Drug Administration; HR, hazard ratio; mCRPC, metastatic castration-resistant prostate cancer; OS, overall survival; PREVAIL, a Safety and Efficacy Study of Oral MDV3100 in Chemotherapy-Naive Patients With Progressive Metastatic Prostate Cancer; PFS, progression-free survival; SWOG, Southwest Oncology Group; TROPIC, Cabazitaxel Plus Prednisone Compared to Mitoxantrone Plus Prednisone in Hormone Refractory Metastatic Prostate Cancer.

compared to that of patients treated with prednisone alone (15.8 vs. 11.2 months, respectively; HR = 0.74; 95% CI [0.64–0.86]) (33). In chemotherapy-naive patients, treatment with abiraterone/prednisone showed better radiographic PFS and a trend for OS benefits (34). Abiraterone in combination with prednisone is now approved in both post-docetaxel and pre-docetaxel setting. This regimen is very well tolerated with a few side effects, which include liver function test (LFT) abnormalities, high blood pressure, and lower extremity edema.

Enzalutamide (previously known as MDV3100) is an oral high-affinity selective AR inhibitor that potently binds to the AR, decreases nuclear translocation, impairs AR binding to DNA and coactivators, and blocks cell proliferation. Unlike bicalutamide, enzalutamide has no agonistic properties. Enzalutamide was approved by the FDA in the post-chemotherapy setting based on the results from the Atrial Fibrillation (AF) Follow-up Investigation of Rhythm Management (AFFIRM) trial. In men with mCRPC previously treated with docetaxel and enzalutamide showed a median OS of 18.4 versus 13.6 months of placebo (P < .001) representing a 37% reduction in risk of death (35). More recently, in the pre-docetaxel setting, the PREVAIL (enzalutamide in Chemotherapy-Naive Patients With

Progressive Metastatic Prostate Cancer) phase III trial in chemotherapy-naive patients also demonstrated OS benefit for enzalutamide compared to placebo. Enzalutamide significantly reduced the risk of death by 29% (HR = 0.706, 95% CI [0.60–0.84]; $P < .0001$). The median OS was estimated at 32.4 months in the enzalutamide group and 30.2 months in the placebo group. In addition, the rate of radiographic PFS at 12 months of follow-up was 65% among patients treated with enzalutamide, as compared with 14% among patients receiving placebo (36). The most common side effects of enzalutamide are fatigue, diarrhea, hot flashes, and rarely seizures.

Drugs targeting androgen-independent pathways have also shown clinical benefits in patients with CRPC. Sipuleucel-t, a dendritic cell-based vaccine, demonstrated a modest improvement in OS in the IMPACT (Sipuleucel-T immunotherapy for castration-resistant prostate cancer) trial. The median OS in the sipuleucel-T arm was 25.8 versus 21.7 months in the placebo group. However, there was no significant effect on PSA responses, radiological responses, or time to progression (37). Sipuleucel-T received FDA approval in April 2010 for asymptomatic or minimally symptomatic mCRPC.

Metastasis to bone is a major source of disease-related morbidity and mortality, and therapies targeting the bone have been a clinical and research focus for several decades with multiple trials testing agents targeting different key pathways. However, prior to 2013, the bone-targeted agents studied, including strontium, samarium, zoledronic acid, and denusomab, did not result in survival or PFS benefits. These agents have received FDA approval based on pain control or reduction of SREs. Radium-223 is a first-in-class radiopharmaceutical, an alpha emitter and calcium mimetic, which selectively binds to areas of bone metastasis. In a recently published phase III study, radium-223 improved OS by almost 4 months (11.3 vs. 14.9 months, $P = .00007$) and delayed time to first SRE in patients with symptomatic bony metastases pretreated with docetaxel or unfit for docetaxel (38). Based on these results, radium-223 was FDA approved in 2013.

Despite the multiple therapeutic options available, mCRPC remains a universally lethal disease, and there are important issues to clarify in order to maximize the benefits of current treatments. For example, in most practices, docetaxel is reserved for patients who have progressed on abiraterone and/or enzalutamide. However, upfront use of docetaxel should be considered in newly diagnosed CRPC patients who are symptomatic and presenting with extensive bone and/or visceral disease. On the other hand, the data on sipuleucel-T suggest that this therapy can be considered early in the course of mCRCP in asymptomatic or minimally symptomatic patients with low PSADT, and before corticosteroid use with other therapies. In regard to the androgen signaling targeting agents, most of the studies of these drugs were conducted in the pre- or post-docetaxel setting, and not in relation to prior use of these agents. Therefore, it is unclear if the activity of abiraterone and enzalutamide is preserved when used sequentially. Because there is no solid evidence to guide clinicians in how to sequence or combine these medications, it is essential to discover and validate predictive biomarkers to identify potential "responders" to specific drugs.

## REVIEW QUESTIONS

1. The patient is a 45-year-old male with 3 first-degree family members with prostate cancer, who had a screening prostate-specific antigen of 10 ng/mL. He underwent an ultrasound-guided biopsy and was found with a Gleason 3 + 4 = 7 prostate adenocarcinoma in multiple cores bilaterally. What genetic alteration is associated with hereditary prostate cancer and early age at diagnosis? (Select only one.)

   (A) *KRAS* amplification
   (B) EGFR mutation
   (C) *HOXB13* mutation
   (D) BRCA1
   (E) *PTEN* deletion

2. Mr. J.S. is a 68-year-old white male with a past medical history of obesity, hypertension, and coronary artery disease, had a screening prostate-specific antigen of 8 ng/mL ordered by his primary care physician. The patient is asymptomatic and digital rectal examination is unremarkable. He underwent an ultrasound-guided biopsy that showed a Gleason 3 + 3 = 6 prostate adenocarcinoma in 1 of 12 scores. CT scan of the abdomen and pelvis and bone scan were negative for metastatic disease. Which of the following would be the best treatment approach?

   (A) Androgen deprivation therapy (ADT) with gonadotropin-releasing hormone (GnRH) analogs
   (B) GnRH analogs followed by radical prostatectomy
   (C) External beam radiation followed by ADT
   (D) Radical prostatectomy
   (E) Watchful waiting

3. A.M. is a 60-year-old African American male diagnosed with localized prostate cancer during an evaluation for an elevated screening prostate-specific antigen (PSA) of 9 ng/mL. Biopsy confirmed adenocarcinoma with Gleason 3 + 4 = 7 histology. Imaging studies including bone scan, abdominal CT, and pelvic CT were negative for metastatic disease. He underwent radical prostatectomy and pathology confirmed Gleason 7 adenocarcinoma with evidence of extracapsular extension and positive margins (stage III).

Lymph nodes were negative for cancer. His PSA was undetectable 6 weeks after the operation. What is the next best treatment approach?

(A) Adjuvant androgen deprivation therapy with GnRH agonist
(B) Adjuvant radiation therapy (RT)
(C) Adjuvant abiraterone and prednisone
(D) Observation
(E) Start bicalutamide

4. C.A. is a 60-year-old white male who initially presented with a prostate-specific antigen (PSA) of 39 ng/mL, was diagnosed with clinical stage IIB, T2c, Gleason 8 (4 + 4) prostate adenocarcinoma. Imaging studies were negative for metastatic disease. He underwent external beam radiation therapy treatment and was started on androgen deprivation therapy (ADT) planning for a total of 2 years. His PSA was 3.2 ng/mL 3 months after completing radiation therapy. C.A. continued on ADT. His PSA continued to increase despite the addition of bicalutamide. His PSA increased to 20 ng/mL. Imaging studies were negative for metastatic disease. Which one of the following laboratory studies should be ordered next?

(A) Testosterone level
(B) Dehydroepiandrosterone level
(C) Liver function tests
(D) Renal function tests
(E) Cortisol level

5. E.M. is a 59-year-old male with metastatic prostate cancer receiving treatment with combined antiandrogen therapy with leuprolide and bicalutamide for the last year. E.M. is presenting with worsening pain over his lower back and his prostate-specific antigen is rising on current therapy. Bone scan and CT scan of abdomen and pelvis confirmed progression of appendicular metastatic bone lesions. After confirming castrate levels of testosterone, the patient elects to receive standard therapy. The patient is otherwise healthy and has good performance status. Which of the following medications has shown survival benefits prior to docetaxel therapy in patients with castrate-resistant prostate cancer fit for chemotherapy?

(A) Cabazitaxel
(B) Enzalutamide
(C) Denosumab
(D) Radium-223
(E) Orteronel (TAK-700)

6. Mr. D.P. is a 66-year-old male recently diagnosed with metastatic prostate cancer (mPC) when he presented with a prostate-specific antigen (PSA) of 120 ng/mL. He was found with bone metastasis and enlarged pelvic lymph nodes. A bone marrow biopsy confirmed mPC. Mr. D.P. was started on bicalutamide and 2 weeks later received a leuprolide injection. His PSA levels are decreasing and he is asymptomatic. Which of the following best describes the plan of care for this patient?

(A) The patient should have continuous androgen deprivation therapy (ADT) until disease progression
(B) The patient can consider intermittent ADT because it is equally effective to continuous ADT
(C) The patient can start abiraterone and prednisone for hormone-sensitive prostate cancer
(D) Immunotherapy with sipuleucel-T improves survival in hormone-sensitive prostate cancer
(E) Adding denosumab to his current therapy will improve overall survival

7. Which of the following medications are FDA approved for metastatic castration resistant prostate cancer based on overall survival benefits?

(A) Sipuleucel-t
(B) Abiraterone/prednisone
(C) Enzalutamide
(D) Docetaxel
(E) Cabazitaxel
(F) All of the above

## REFERENCES

1. Siegel R, Naishadham D, Jemal A. Cancer statistics, 2013. *CA Cancer J Clin.* 2013;63(1):11–30.
2. Zeegers MP, Jellema A, Ostrer H. Empiric risk of prostate carcinoma for relatives of patients with prostate carcinoma: a meta-analysis. *Cancer.* 2003;97(8):1894–1903.
3. Ewing CM, Ray AM, Lange EM, et al. Germline mutations in HOXB13 and prostate-cancer risk. *N Engl J Med.* 2012;366(2):141–149.
4. Ilic D, Neuberger MM, Djulbegovic M, Dahm P. Screening for prostate cancer. *Cochrane Database Syst Rev.* 2013;1:CD004720.
5. Smith RA, Manassaram-Baptiste D, Brooks D, et al. Cancer screening in the United States, 2014: a review of current American Cancer Society guidelines and current issues in cancer screening. *CA Cancer J Clin.* 2014;64(1):30–51.
6. Moyer VA; U.S. Preventive Services Task Force. Screening for prostate cancer: U.S. Preventive Services Task Force recommendation statement. *Ann Intern Med.* 2012;157(2):120–134.
7. NCCN Clinical Practice Guidelines in Oncology—Prostate Cancer. *NCCN Guidelines & Clinical Resources Version 1*; 2013. Retrieved from http://www.nccn.org/professionals/physician_gls/pdf/prostate.pdf
8. Dorff TB, Flaig TW, Tangen CM, et al. Adjuvant androgen deprivation for high-risk prostate cancer after radical prostatectomy: SWOG S9921 study. *J Clin Oncol.* 2011;29(15):2040–2045.
9. Messing EM, Manola J, Yao J, et al.; Eastern Cooperative Oncology Group study EST 3886. Immediate versus deferred androgen deprivation treatment in patients with node-positive prostate cancer after radical prostatectomy and pelvic lymphadenectomy. *Lancet Oncol.* 2006;7(6):472–479.

10. Jones CU, Hunt D, McGowan DG, et al. Radiotherapy and short-term androgen deprivation for localized prostate cancer. *N Engl J Med*. 2011;365(2):107–118.

11. Bolla M, Van Tienhoven G, Warde P, et al. External irradiation with or without long-term androgen suppression for prostate cancer with high metastatic risk: 10-year results of an EORTC randomised study. *Lancet Oncol*. 2010;11(11):1066–1073.

12. Bolla M, de Reijke TM, Van Tienhoven G, et al.; EORTC Radiation Oncology Group and Genito-Urinary Tract Cancer Group. Duration of androgen suppression in the treatment of prostate cancer. *N Engl J Med*. 2009;360(24):2516–2527.

13. Pilepich MV, Winter K, Lawton CA, et al. Androgen suppression adjuvant to definitive radiotherapy in prostate carcinoma—long-term results of phase III RTOG 85-31. *Int J Radiat Oncol Biol Phys*. 2005;61(5):1285–1290.

14. Shahinian VB, Kuo YF, Freeman JL, Goodwin JS. Risk of fracture after androgen deprivation for prostate cancer. *N Engl J Med*. 2005;352(2):154–164.

15. Smith MR, Lee WC, Brandman J, et al. Gonadotropin-releasing hormone agonists and fracture risk: a claims-based cohort study of men with nonmetastatic prostate cancer. *J Clin Oncol*. 2005;23(31):7897–7903.

16. Planas J, Trilla E, Raventós C, et al. Alendronate decreases the fracture risk in patients with prostate cancer on androgen-deprivation therapy and with severe osteopenia or osteoporosis. *BJU Int*. 2009;104(11):1637–1640.

17. Smith MR, Egerdie B, Hernández Toriz N, et al.; Denosumab HALT Prostate Cancer Study Group. Denosumab in men receiving androgen-deprivation therapy for prostate cancer. *N Engl J Med*. 2009;361(8):745–755.

18. Smith MR, Halabi S, Ryan CJ, et al. Randomized controlled trial of early zoledronic acid in men with castration-sensitive prostate cancer and bone metastases: results of CALGB 90202 (alliance). *J Clin Oncol*. 2014;32(11):1143–1150.

19. Levine GN, D'Amico AV, Berger P, et al.; American Heart Association Council on Clinical Cardiology and Council on Epidemiology and Prevention, the American Cancer Society, and the American Urological Association. Androgen-deprivation therapy in prostate cancer and cardiovascular risk: a science advisory from the American Heart Association, American Cancer Society, and American Urological Association: endorsed by the American Society for Radiation Oncology. *CA Cancer J Clin*. 2010;60(3):194–201.

20. Bolla M, van Poppel H, Collette L, et al.; European Organization for Research and Treatment of Cancer. Postoperative radiotherapy after radical prostatectomy: a randomised controlled trial (EORTC trial 22911). *Lancet*. 2005;366(9485):572–578.

21. Thompson IM, Tangen CM, Paradelo J, et al. Adjuvant radiotherapy for pathological T3N0M0 prostate cancer significantly reduces risk of metastases and improves survival: long-term followup of a randomized clinical trial. *J Urol*. 2009;181(3):956–962.

22. Pound CR, Partin AW, Eisenberger MA, et al. Natural history of progression after PSA elevation following radical prostatectomy. *JAMA*. 1999;281(17):1591–1597.

23. D'Amico AV, Moul JW, Carroll PR, et al. Surrogate end point for prostate cancer-specific mortality after radical prostatectomy or radiation therapy. *J Natl Cancer Inst*. 2003;95(18):1376–1383.

24. Freedland SJ, Humphreys EB, Mangold LA, et al. Risk of prostate cancer-specific mortality following biochemical recurrence after radical prostatectomy. *JAMA*. 2005;294(4):433–439.

25. Zhou P, Chen MH, McLeod D, et al. Predictors of prostate cancer-specific mortality after radical prostatectomy or radiation therapy. *J Clin Oncol*. 2005;23(28):6992–6998.

26. Stephenson AJ, Scardino PT, Kattan MW, et al. Predicting the outcome of salvage radiation therapy for recurrent prostate cancer after radical prostatectomy. *J Clin Oncol*. 2007;25(15):2035–2041.

27. Hussain M, Goldman B, Tangen C, et al. Prostate-specific antigen progression predicts overall survival in patients with metastatic prostate cancer: data from Southwest Oncology Group Trials 9346 (Intergroup Study 0162) and 9916. *J Clin Oncol*. 2009;27(15):2450–2456.

28. Hussain M, Tangen CM, Berry DL, et al. Intermittent versus continuous androgen deprivation in prostate cancer. *N Engl J Med*. 2013;368(14):1314–1325.

29. *E3805: CHAARTED: ChemoHormonal Therapy Versus Androgen Ablation Randomized Trial for Extensive Disease in Prostate Cancer*. ASCO, 2014 late breaking abstract #2.

30. Small EJ, Halabi S, Dawson NA, et al. Antiandrogen withdrawal alone or in combination with ketoconazole in androgen-independent prostate cancer patients: a phase III trial (CALGB 9583). *J Clin Oncol*. 2004;22(6):1025–1033.

31. Tannock IF, de Wit R, Berry WR, et al.; TAX 327 Investigators. Docetaxel plus prednisone or mitoxantrone plus prednisone for advanced prostate cancer. *N Engl J Med*. 2004;351(15):1502–1512.

32. de Bono JS, Oudard S, Ozguroglu M, et al.; TROPIC Investigators. Prednisone plus cabazitaxel or mitoxantrone for metastatic castration-resistant prostate cancer progressing after docetaxel treatment: a randomised open-label trial. *Lancet*. 2010;376(9747):1147–1154.

33. de Bono JS, Logothetis CJ, Molina A, et al.; COU-AA-301 Investigators. Abiraterone and increased survival in metastatic prostate cancer. *N Engl J Med*. 2011;364(21):1995–2005.

34. Ryan CJ, Smith MR, de Bono JS, et al.; COU-AA-302 Investigators. Abiraterone in metastatic prostate cancer without previous chemotherapy. *N Engl J Med*. 2013;368(2):138–148.

35. Scher HI, Fizazi K, Saad F, et al.; AFFIRM Investigators. Increased survival with enzalutamide in prostate cancer after chemotherapy. *N Engl J Med*. 2012;367(13):1187–1197.

36. Beer TM, Armstrong AJ, Rathkopf DE, et al.; PREVAIL Investigators. Enzalutamide in metastatic prostate cancer before chemotherapy. *N Engl J Med*. 2014;371(5):424–433.

37. Kantoff PW, Higano CS, Shore ND, et al.; IMPACT Study Investigators. Sipuleucel-T immunotherapy for castration-resistant prostate cancer. *N Engl J Med*. 2010;363(5):411–422.

38. Parker C, Nilsson S, Heinrich D, et al.; ALSYMPCA Investigators. Alpha emitter radium-223 and survival in metastatic prostate cancer. *N Engl J Med*. 2013;369(3):213–223.

# 14

# *Testicular Cancer*

DIEGO J. BEDOYA, MARTHA PRITCHETT MIMS, SHAMAIL BUTT,
AND COURTNEY N. MILLER-CHISM

## EPIDEMIOLOGY, RISK FACTORS, NATURAL HISTORY, AND PATHOLOGY

In many ways, testicular cancer represents a break from the common paradigm of solid malignancies. First, as the most common solid malignancy in males between the ages of 15 and 35 years, it usually affects a much younger population. Second, long-term survival is expected even in the presence of advanced disease with <400 deaths annually in the United States. Finally, staging of testicular cancer incorporates an additional element to the common Tumor, Node, and Metastasis (TNM) staging system: serum tumor markers (STMs).

An estimated 7920 new testicular cancer cases were observed in the United States in 2013 representing < 1% of all solid tumors in men (1). Testicular cancer is most common in white males, with a lower incidence in Hispanics, and the disease is relatively rare in African Americans. Data suggest an increasing incidence of testicular cancer over the last several decades, mostly restricted to seminoma in white males. The reasons for this increase are poorly understood.

Abdominal cryptorchidism is responsible for approximately 10% of testicular tumors (2). Interestingly, malignancy arises in the normally descended testicle in 25% of these cases. Prophylactic orchiectomy is generally recommended for cases of cryptorchidism presenting after puberty, especially when the undescended testis is intra-abdominal. The cumulative risk of a contralateral testicular cancer in men with a previous diagnosis of testicular cancer is 1.9% at 15 years, whereas the incidence of bilateral tumors at presentation is 1–5% (3). Risk is also increased in patients presenting with an extragonadal germ cell tumor (EGCT) especially those with retroperitoneal presentation. The relative risk of testicular cancer

increases 6- to 10-fold in first-degree relatives of a patient diagnosed with testicular cancer. Intratubular germ cell neoplasia (carcinoma in situ) is commonly found in patients at risk of testicular cancer; the risk of progression is 50% at 5 years when left untreated. An increased incidence of testicular cancer has also been described in patients with hypospadias, HIV infection (seminomas), testicular microlithiasis, Klinefelter and Down syndromes, and following exposure to exogenous estrogens in utero. Sertoli cell tumors have association with Peutz–Jegher syndrome and Carney complex.

Most patients present with an incidental finding of a painless mass; however, about one third complain of a heavy sensation in the lower abdomen or perianal area. Acute pain and symptoms secondary to metastatic disease are each reported by about 10% of patients at presentation.

Germ cell tumors (GCTs) account for 95% of testicular cancer. Most of the remainder are sex cord stromal tumors. Other tumor types including lymphoma, leukemia, or plasmacytoma are exceedingly rare and will not be discussed in this chapter. For management purposes, GCTs are divided into seminomas and nonseminomatous germ cell tumors (NSGCTs), each accounting for roughly half of the cases. By definition, seminomas exist only in their pure form, whereas NSGCTs are usually composed of a mixture of different subtypes (including seminomatous components). Table 14.1 summarizes the primary differences among the subtypes. These data highlight the high prevalence of the most specific cytogenetic abnormality in testicular cancer, the gain of 12p-sequences, most commonly through isochromosome formation (i12p) (4). This cytogenetic abnormality has also been shown in some cases of testicular carcinoma in situ, suggesting a role in the early development of this malignancy. Although GCTs

**Table 14.1**  Major Subtypes of Germ Cell Tumors

| | Average Age at Diagnosis (Years) | Contribution to Mixed NSGCTs (%) | Serum Tumor Markers | i12p (%)[a] |
|---|---|---|---|---|
| Seminoma | 40 | 20 | AFP: normal[b]; βhCG: normal or mildly elevated | 50 |
| Spermatocytic seminoma[c] | >60 | 0 | | 0 |
| NSGCTs | 30 | | | 80 |
| Embryonal carcinoma | | 85 | AFP: normal or mildly elevated; βhCG: normal or mildly elevated | |
| Choriocarcinoma[d] | | 10 | AFP: normal; βhCG >1000 IU/L | |
| Yolk sac tumor | | 40 | AFP: >100 ng/mL[e]; βhCG: normal | |
| Teratoma | | 30 | | |

[a]Isochromosome of the short arm of chromosome 12.
[b]If AFP is elevated, the diagnosis of pure seminoma should be doubted.
[c]Accounts for 1–4% of pure seminomas. Shows a different behavior. Good prognosis.
[d]Most aggressive subtype. Hematogenous spread occurs early.
[e]Levels correlate with disease extent.
AFP, alpha-fetoprotein; βhCG, beta human chorionic gonadotropin; NSGSTs, nonseminomatous germ cell tumors.

**Table 14.2**  Immunohistochemical Patterns of Germ Cell Tumors

| | Cytokeratin | CD 30 | PLAP[a] | OCT3/4[b] | NANOG | SOX2[c] | CD 117[d] | AFP | βhCG |
|---|---|---|---|---|---|---|---|---|---|
| Seminoma | +/– | – | ++ | + | + | – | ++ | – | +/– |
| Spermatocytic seminoma | – | – | +/– | | | | +/– | – | |
| Embryonal carcinoma | ++ | + | + | + | + | + | +/– | +/– | |
| Choriocarcinoma | +/– | | – | – | – | – | – | | ++ |
| Yolk sac tumor | ++ | +/– | +/– | – | – | – | +/– | + | |

[a]Placental-like alkaline phosphatase.
[b]Octamer-binding transcription factor.
[c]Sex-determining region Y-box 2.
[d]c-KIT receptor.

are usually differentiated and classified according to their morphology, occasionally immunohistochemical stains are required (Table 14.2) (5).

Unlike other solid malignancies, STMs have important implications in the diagnosis, management, prognosis, and monitoring of GCTs. Three STMs are clinically important: beta human chorionic gonadotropin (βhCG), alpha-fetoprotein (AFP), and lactate dehydrogenase (LDH) (6). The likelihood of having abnormally increased levels of one or more of these markers increases with tumor volume and the severity of the disease. As a consequence, they have been included as part of the TNM staging system and the International Germ Cell Cancer Collaboration Group (IGCCCG) prognostic model (see the Staging section). As most patients with suspected GCTs undergo orchiectomy for diagnostic and therapeutic purposes, tumor markers are not routinely used for diagnosis. However, increased levels of βhCG and/or AFP associated with a testicular mass may be

highly suggestive of a GCT, especially considering that the causes of false positive elevation of these markers are few and relatively rare (namely hypogonadism for the former and hepatocellular carcinoma in the latter). Nevertheless, in the unusual case in which obtaining tissue for diagnosis is not possible without significant risk for the patient (e.g., primary mediastinal tumor) or the pathology report is nondiagnostic, STMs may be used to support the diagnosis and initiate treatment. Pure seminomas do not secrete AFP; thus, elevated AFP in a patient with a diagnosis of pure seminoma should raise questions about the accuracy of the diagnosis. Patients in this situation are considered to have NSGCTs and are treated as such.

More frequently, STMs are used for monitoring both the response to a given treatment and the possibility of relapse after a complete response. It is important to note that βhCG and AFP have different half-lives; that of βhCG is 18–36 hours, whereas AFP has a significantly longer half-life of 4–5 days. Thus, depending on the initial STM values, a 10-fold decrease or normalization of these levels should be evident after 2 weeks and/or 25 to 30 days, respectively, of successful treatment. A slower response is considered unsatisfactory and a likely marker of treatment failure, which may prompt the clinician to consider early salvage therapy. If on the other hand the response is adequate and a complete response is achieved, periodic measurement of the STMs is of the utmost importance. Indeed, in more than half the cases, an elevation of βhCG and/or AFP is the first and sometimes the sole evidence of disease relapse.

## STAGING

As previously stated, the American Joint Committee on Cancer (AJCC) TNM staging system for GCTs incorporates STMs as part of the classification.

It is important to note that the STM values to be considered for staging and prognosis purposes are those obtained after orchiectomy and before other treatment begins (surgery, radiation therapy [RT], or chemotherapy), and not those obtained at the time of diagnosis. Briefly, stage I includes those patients with no regional node or metastasis, regardless of the size of the tumor. Stage II includes those with regional node involvement and only a mild elevation in the STMs, whereas stage III comprises those patients with metastatic disease or those with regional lymph node involvement and a more significant elevation of the STMs. In addition to the TNM system, GCTs are classified into good, intermediate, or poor prognosis (Table 14.3) on the basis of the validated prognostic model from the IGCCCG (7).

## CASE SUMMARIES

### Early-Stage Seminoma

D.L. is a 32-year-old business man who presents with lower abdominal discomfort, noticed initially after a long international flight. Physical examination revealed a painless swelling of his right testicle and scrotal ultrasound showed a 6-mm well-defined hypoechoic lesion. No abnormalities were found in the contralateral testicle. LDH, βhCG, and AFP levels were all within normal limits, and chest x-ray (CXR) was unremarkable. A radical inguinal orchiectomy was performed, with pathology confirming the diagnosis of pure seminoma, with no lymphovascular invasion (LVI) but involving the tunica vaginalis. A CT scan of the abdomen was then performed, with no evidence of enlarged lymph nodes. Therefore, the patient was diagnosed with a stage IB pure seminoma.

### Evidence-Based Case Discussion

The aforementioned case describes the initial diagnostic evaluation of any suspected GCT. After a thorough history and physical examination, a scrotal ultrasound should be pursued. Ultrasound can identify intrinsic testicular lesions as small as 1 mm. Seminomas tend to have a more homogeneous appearance on ultrasound with well-defined margins compared to NSGCTs, although this is not always the case. Once a mass is confirmed, STMs should be obtained and patient referred for an inguinal radical orchiectomy. A transscrotal surgery or biopsy (scrotal violation) is contraindicated because of the increased risk of the tumor spreading locally. In general, a

## American Joint Committee on Cancer TNM Staging for Testicular Cancer

| Stage | Definition |
|---|---|
| I | No regional lymph node involvement or metastasis |
| IA | Tumor invades up to the tunica albuginea without vascular/lymphatic invasion and normal serum tumor markers |
| IB | Invasion beyond tunica albuginea (vascular/lymphatic invasion or involvement of tunica vaginalis) |
| IS | Any tumor size and elevated serum tumor markers |
| II | Any tumor size with regional lymph node (retroperitoneal) involvement but no distant metastasis. Serum tumor markers are normal or only mildly elevated[a] |
| IIA | Clinical; N1 = lymph node mass 2 cm or less <br> Pathological; pN1 = lymph node mass 2 cm or less and up to 5 lymph nodes positive |
| IIB | Clinical; N2 = lymph node mass >2 cm in diameter, but <5 cm <br> Pathological; pN2 = lymph node mass >2 cm in diameter, but <5 cm, or >5 lymph nodes positive or extranodal extension of tumor |
| IIC | Clinical /pathological (N3/pN3); lymph node mass >5 cm in diameter |
| III | Distant metastasis or significantly elevated serum tumor markers |
| IIIA | Nonregional nodal (including pelvic nodes) or pulmonary metastasis, with normal or only mildly elevated serum tumor markers[a] |
| IIIB | Moderate elevation in serum tumor markers[b] with regional lymph node involvement without distant metastasis, or those with nonregional nodal or pulmonary metastasis regardless of regional lymph node status |
| IIIC | Similar to stage IIIB but with markedly elevated serum tumor markers[c] or those with nonpulmonary metastasis |

[a]LDH <1.5 × upper limits of normal; βhCG <5000 IU/L; AFP <1000 ng/mL.
[b]LDH =1.5–10 × upper limits of normal; βhCG = 5000–50,000 IU/L; AFP = 1000–10,000 ng/mL.
[c]LDH >10 × upper limits of normal; βhCG >50,000 IU/L; AFP >10,000 ng/mL.

**Table 14.3**  Prognostic Features of Germ Cell Tumors

| Prognosis | Percent of Total | Seminoma | | NSGCT | | 5-Year Survival (%) |
| | | Features | TNM | Features | TNM | |
| --- | --- | --- | --- | --- | --- | --- |
| Good prognosis | 60 | No nonpulmonary visceral metastasis | I, II, IIIA, IIIB | Testicular or retroperitoneal primary<br>No nonpulmonary visceral metastasis<br>Normal or mildly elevated serum tumor markers | I, II, IIIA | 91 |
| Intermediate prognosis | 26 | Nonpulmonary visceral metastasis | IIIC | Same as good prognosis but with moderately elevated serum tumor markers | IIIB | 79 |
| Poor prognosis | 14 | N/A | | Mediastinal primary<br>Nonpulmonary visceral metastasis<br>Markedly elevated serum tumor markers | IIIC | 48 |

NSGSTs, nonseminomatous germ cell tumors; TNM, tumor, node, and metastasis staging system.

biopsy of the contralateral testicle is not indicated unless there is an increased suspicion of synchronous GCT based on ultrasound findings (e.g., a hypoechoic mass or marked atrophy) or in the setting of cryptorchidism. If any of these were present, an open inguinal approach should be elected for the biopsy. Imaging studies should also be obtained as part of the initial workup. These include a CT scan of abdomen and pelvis and a CXR. Although routinely ordered as part of the initial workup by many physicians, the current guidelines recommend that a CT scan of the chest should only be requested if the CXR shows abnormalities or if retroperitoneal lymphadenopathy is apparent on the abdominal CT scan. Similarly, other imaging studies like bone scan or brain MRI are not routinely ordered, unless the symptoms reported by the patient are concerning for metastasis to these sites (8). Finally, STMs should be repeated postoperatively if they were elevated before the orchiectomy. As mentioned previously, the postoperative values should be used for both staging and IGCCCG prognosis classification.

The overall prognosis of stage I seminoma after orchiectomy is excellent, with almost 100% of patients being cured regardless of the treatment strategy adopted. There are 3 treatment alternatives currently accepted: surveillance, RT, and chemotherapy (Figure 14.1). One of the main advantages of surveillance is that it avoids unnecessary treatment for a significant percentage of patients. Despite a higher relapse rate with surveillance alone (15–20% compared with <5% for both RT and chemotherapy), overall survival (OS) is not affected with this approach since most relapses, if detected early, can be salvaged with RT or chemotherapy. Therefore, surveillance is preferred if the patient will adhere to the close follow-up schedule. In a pooled analysis of 638 patients from Europe, 2 factors were found to be predictive of a higher relapse rate in patients managed by surveillance; tumor size >4 cm (HR = 2.0) and invasion of the rete testis (HR = 1.7) (9). However, even in the presence of 1 or both of these risk

factors, surveillance is not contraindicated as long as the patient is motivated and compliant with the surveillance schedule. Unfortunately, there is no absolute consensus regarding the frequency of follow-up. Most relapses will occur within the first 2 years, which justifies a more frequent monitoring during this period. Similarly, given its longer natural history and higher incidence of late relapses compared with NSGCTs, most experts agree that follow-up should be extended for at least 10 years. For example, the National Comprehensive Cancer Network (NCCN) guidelines recommend obtaining STMs and abdominal/pelvic CT scan every 3–4 months for the first 3 years, every 6 months from years 4 to 7 and yearly thereafter. Other authors propose a less strict imaging schedule with CT scan every 4–6 months for the first 3 years, considering the relatively indolent course of seminomas. The usefulness of frequent STM measurement is even more controversial as they are not reliable in detecting disease recurrence in pure seminomas.

RT has been historically the adjuvant therapy of choice in stage I seminoma (and it is still the preferred management for stage Is seminoma). However, late toxicity (primarily the development of second malignancies), suggested by the long-term follow-up data, has made surveillance a more attractive option in recent years. In fact, a long-term, worldwide, retrospective analysis of >28,000 testicular cancer patients (15,000 with seminoma) treated from 1935 to 1993 showed an increased incidence of solid tumors diagnosed 5 or more years after the diagnosis of testicular cancer (cumulative risk at 25 years of 18.2%). Prior RT was significantly associated with those patients developing bladder, stomach, pancreas, and rectal cancer, as well as kidney cancer (in 20-year survivors) (10). This observation prompted changes in the radiation dose and field with attempts to reduce toxicity while maintaining efficacy (risk of relapse <4%). RT evolved from the "hockey-stick" or "dog-leg" field, which involves radiation to the renal hilum, pelvic lymph nodes, and para-aortic lymph

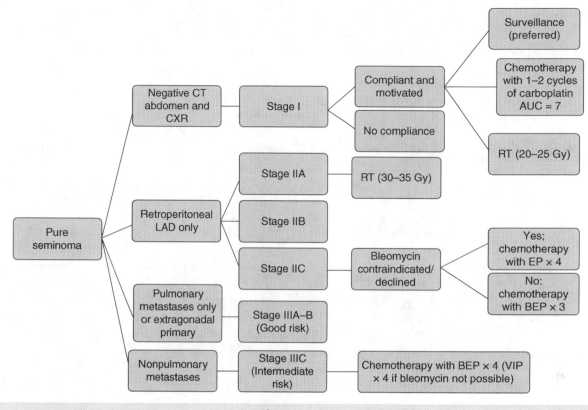

**Figure 14.1**

Management algorithm for pure seminoma. AUC, area under the curve; BEP, bleomycin, etoposide, and cisplatin; CXR, chest radiograph; EP, etoposide and cisplatin; LAD, lymphadenopathy; RT, radiation therapy.

nodes, to the so-called PA-strip radiation, which is limited to the para-aortic lymph nodes. This was based on data showing that the other sites included on the hockey-stick field are rarely involved at the time of diagnosis of a stage I seminoma. A direct comparison of these 2 approaches (40) showed that while pelvic relapses were more common with PA-strip compared with the hockey-stick field (1.7% vs. 0%), the total number of relapses was the same (4% on each arm) and the acute toxicity was less pronounced in the PA-strip group. Moreover, there was no difference in the OS at 3 years (96%). Although the median follow-up on this study (4.5 years) does not allow for an adequate assessment of long-term toxicity, most radiation oncologists currently use the PA strip as the standard field of choice in stage I seminoma.

Traditionally, a radiation dose of 30 Gy divided in 15 fractions has been used for the treatment of GCTs. More recent data supports the use of lower radiation doses, which are associated with similar relapse rates and decreased morbidity, compared to higher doses (11). In addition to second malignancies, there are concerns regarding the risk of cardiac toxicity and impaired fertility in those patients receiving RT. Although the data for these risks are either insufficient or conflicting, the use of smaller radiation fields (with no prophylactic radiation to mediastinum) and the use of scrotal shielding to the contralateral testicle

(even in those patients receiving PA-strip fields) are likely reducing these risks.

The use of chemotherapy as an alternative to RT in men with stage I seminoma has been evaluated more recently, given the success of cisplatin in treating advanced GCTs. Due to the higher risk of toxicity with cisplatin, carboplatin has been used as a single dose (AUC of 7) with excellent results. When compared against RT, carboplatin showed similar relapse rates at 5 years (12).

Although the relapse rates remained similar, there was a significant difference in the incidence of new contralateral GCTs, favoring carboplatin over RT (0.2% vs. 1.2%), resulting in an approximately 80% risk reduction in the rate of contralateral GCTs.

Given the excellent and quite similar outcomes, choice is usually based on the individual patient preferences or personal circumstances (Figure 14.1). For example, the patient described in this first case is a business man who travels frequently making him unable to comply with a tight surveillance protocol. He would likely benefit from either RT or chemotherapy.

### Early-Stage NSGCTs

R.M. is a 28-year-old man who presented with a painless testicular mass, confirmed with ultrasound. AFP levels were mildly elevated (500 ng/mL), whereas βhCG and LDH were within normal limits. After radical orchiectomy, pathology reported an NSGCT (60% embryonal, 40% yolk sac) invading tunica albuginea with LVI present. A CT scan of the abdomen/pelvis and CXR were unremarkable. AFP levels were markedly decreased 2 weeks after surgery and normalized after 4 weeks.

## Evidence-Based Case Discussion

This patient was also diagnosed with stage I testicular cancer, in this case an NSGCT. The treatment of stage I NSGCT is a contentious topic (Figure 14.2). Like stage I seminoma, surveillance alone is an attractive option in stage I NSGCTs as it can potentially prevent unnecessary treatment in a subset of patients. Unlike seminoma, however, the overall chance of relapse in a patient with stage I NSGCTs undergoing surveillance is approximately 30%, likely due to undetected micrometastasis at the time of diagnosis. In fact, 30% of patients undergoing retroperitoneal lymph node dissection (RPLND) for clinical stage I disease are eventually upstaged to stage II after this procedure. Also, unlike seminoma, late relapses are not common, with most occurring within the first 2 years. In a large European series, 373 patients with stage I NSGCTs

were followed by surveillance only (13). A relapse rate of 27% was observed with 80% occurring in the first year (61% in the retroperitoneal nodes and 25% in lungs).

Efforts are underway to define which patients have a higher probability of relapse and are thus more likely to benefit from adjuvant treatment with either RPLND or chemotherapy. Two features from this patient's primary tumor have been demonstrated to be useful in the stratification of patients into low risk and high risk of relapse: the presence of LVI and an embryonal carcinoma component. A retrospective Dutch study showed that the relapse rate in the absence of LVI was 11% compared to 51% when LVI was present (14). In addition, 50% of patients undergoing RPLND in this study were upstaged to stage II disease when LVI was present in the primary tumor (only 26% of those without LVI were upstaged). These results, as well as those in previous studies suggest that LVI is the single most important predictor of relapse in stage I NSGCTs. Similarly, the presence of embryonal carcinoma has been demonstrated to be an independent risk factor for relapse. Recent studies suggest that the predictive power is higher with increasing proportions of embryonal carcinoma, and not its mere presence. A cutoff of 45% has been used in some studies. If both LVI and embryonal carcinoma predominance are present, the risk of relapse increases

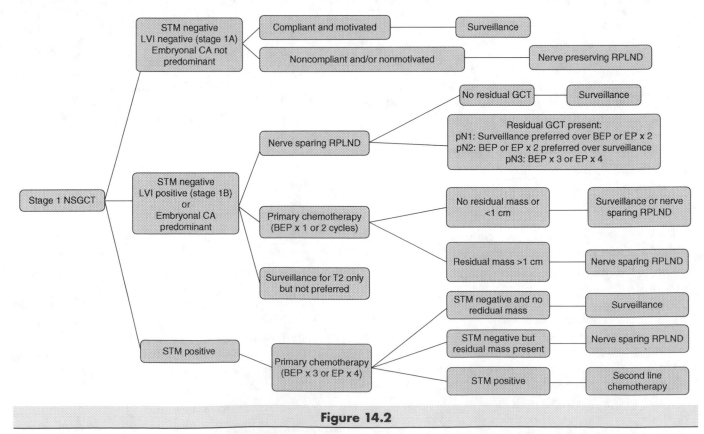

**Figure 14.2**

Management algorithm for stage I NSGCTs. BEP, bleomycin, etoposide, and cisplatin; CA, carcinoma; EP, etoposide, cisplatin; GCT, germ cell tumor; LVI, lymphovascular invasion; NSGCTs, nonseminomatous germ cell tumors; RPLND, retroperitoneal lymph node dissection; STM, serum tumor marker.

significantly. When 105 patients with stage I NSGCTs were followed at a single institution in the United States, the overall relapse rate after 11 years was 25.7%, with 3 patients dying after relapse (2.8%). The relapse rate was 12% for those patients without LVI or embryonal carcinoma ($n = 66$), compared with 71% when both factors were present ($n = 7$) (15).

Other factors linked to a higher risk of relapse are the absence of yolk sac component, tumor size, and the immunohistochemical analyses of proliferative rates of MIB1 antibody. Their overall importance does not seem to be as significant as the presence of LVI or embryonal carcinoma, but may be taken into consideration at the time of counseling a patient.

Although surveillance can prevent unnecessary treatment in 70–75% of patients with stage I NSGCTs (and close to 90% in low-risk patients), when relapse occurs, these patients are exposed to at least 3 cycles of chemotherapy. Furthermore, this approach requires close follow-up (especially during the first 2 years) and reliable imaging (CT scan) to decrease the risk of false-negative staging. The results of PET scan in this setting had been disappointing, and its use for stage I NSGCTs is not advocated.

Nevertheless, surveillance is a reasonable approach—and preferred in many centers—for patients with low-risk stage I NSGCTs (stage 1A). However, patients with high-risk features (stage IB) could benefit from adjuvant treatment. The choice of optimal treatment in this setting, between RPLND and chemotherapy, is still a matter of controversy.

Proponents of RPLND (the preferred method in the United States) claim that it has therapeutic benefit and allows for accurate staging. In fact, as previously mentioned, almost half of patients with clinical stage I NSGCTs with embryonal carcinoma predominance and/ or LVI will be upstaged to pathological stage II disease. Many of these men will be cured with RPLND alone. In a retrospective analysis of 292 patients with clinical stage I NSGCTs treated with RPLND, 66 (22.6%) had retroperitoneal nodal involvement (16). Thirty-one of these 66 patients were followed with surveillance alone, with relapse occurring in 7 (23%) patients, compared with no relapses in the group receiving chemotherapy. While the benefits from post-RPLND chemotherapy seem evident, the authors conclude that 77% of patients remained relapse free with RPLND alone, and thus RPLND alone remains an option for patients able to comply with surveillance who want to avoid chemotherapy toxicity. On the basis of these studies, the NCCN consensus guidelines propose that further treatment after RPLND be considered depending on the individual patient's compliance and the extent of the retroperitoneal nodal involvement. Two cycles of BEP (bleomycin, etoposide, and cisplatin) chemotherapy are recommended for noncompliant patients with pN1 or pN2 disease (positive nodal involvement up to 5 cm) and 3 or 4 cycles of chemotherapy for pN3 disease (>5 cm).

Although it can potentially prevent exposure to chemotherapy toxicity, RPLND is not exempt from complications, especially outside centers with extensive experience with this procedure. Laparoscopic RPLND has been advocated by some, given its reported low complication rate and decrease in hospital stay. However, few surgeons have enough experience with this procedure and its efficacy has come into question, particularly due to concerns about inadequate sampling. For this reason, an open nerve-sparing RPLND is still favored by most centers. The major morbidity associated with this procedure is the infertility due to retrograde ejaculation. However, new techniques in experienced hands result in preservation of antegrade function in >90% of cases.

Some centers, especially in Europe, advocate the use of chemotherapy as the initial adjuvant treatment after orchiectomy, based on the very low relapse rate (<3%) seen in most studies. Currently, 2 cycles of BEP are recommended for stage I NSGCTs in this setting. This recommendation is based on results of relatively small studies, although more recent studies suggest that only 1 cycle may have similar efficacy. A risk-stratified approach was used in a study from Scandinavia in 745 men with stage I NSGCTs. Based on the presence of LVI, patients were recommended to receive 1 cycle of BEP if LVI was present (but patients could opt to receive 2 cycles or just surveillance) or to undergo surveillance if no LVI was observed (patients could choose to receive chemotherapy) (17). The overall relapse rates in those receiving 2 cycles ($n = 70$), 1 cycle ($n = 312$), and surveillance ($n = 350$) were 0%, 2%, and 13%, respectively. In the presence of LVI, the relapse-free survival was significantly better for those patients receiving 2 cycles and 1 cycle of adjuvant chemotherapy compared with surveillance (100%, 96.5%, and 58.3%, respectively). A significant difference was observed in patients without LVI receiving chemotherapy (98.6%) versus those on surveillance (86.5%).

In summary, stage I NSGCT carries an excellent prognosis regardless of the post-orchiectomy strategy, with an OS of 98% because the vast majority of patients with relapse can be cured with salvage treatment. Therefore, the decision of adjuvant treatment should be based on the individual's circumstances including the risk of relapse. In low-risk patients, surveillance is the preferred method, with RPLND or chemotherapy left for noncompliant patients. Surveillance is still an option in high-risk patients (like the patient in our vignette) as long as the patient is willing to accept a 50% risk of relapse. If adjuvant treatment is pursued, RPLND is preferred in those centers with extensive experience that lowers the risk of complications. Otherwise, adjuvant chemotherapy is a good alternative with 1 cycle of BEP being probably as effective as the 2 cycles previously recommended (Figure 14.2).

The patient described in our vignette also reflects the most common pattern in stage I disease: the normalization of STMs after the orchiectomy. Rarely, however, the STMs will remain persistently high or will increase. Even in the absence of supporting imaging, it should be assumed that metastatic disease is present in these cases and treatment should be given accordingly with 3 cycles of BEP or 4 cycles of EP (etoposide and cisplatin).

## Locally Advanced Seminoma

B.C. is a 37-year-old man who presents with a painless mass incidentally found in his left testicle. Scrotal ultrasound showed a 23-mm lesion with no abnormalities seen on the contralateral testicle. LDH, βhCG, and AFP levels were all within normal values and CXR was unremarkable. A radical inguinal orchiectomy was performed, with pathology confirming the diagnosis of pure seminoma. A CT scan of abdomen showed enlarged para-aortic lymph nodes, with the largest diameter of 6 cm. Patient was diagnosed with a stage IIC pure seminoma. B.C. received 3 cycles of chemotherapy with BEP. Six weeks after the last cycle, a repeat CT scan of the abdomen showed that the para-aortic lymphadenopathy had decreased in size, and now was 3 cm in diameter.

## Evidence-Based Case Discussion

Stage II disease is defined as one limited to regional (retroperitoneal) lymph nodes. Unlike stage I disease, surveillance is not considered an appropriate option for these patients as the majority can expect to be cured with modern RT or chemotherapy. RPLND is not used as primary treatment, given the sensitivity of seminoma to both chemotherapy and RT. Stage II seminomas are subclassified according to the diameter of the involved lymph node mass. Radiation and chemotherapy are both acceptable adjuvant options patients with stage IIA and IIB disease (lymph node mass <5 cm in diameter). However, the preference for stage IIA seminomas (lymph node mass <2 cm) is RT, and chemotherapy is evolving as the treatment of choice for stage IIB disease (lymph node mass of 2–5 cm in diameter). Stage IIC disease should receive adjuvant chemo.

As stated previously, RT is considered the treatment of choice for men with stage IIA seminoma. A total of 30–36 Gy is administered to the infradiaphragmatic areas, including para-aortic lymph nodes and ipsilateral pelvic nodes, with a boost given to affected nodal areas. Scrotal and inguinal node shielding is indicated unless scrotal violation occurred during orchiectomy. Likewise, prophylactic mediastinal radiation is no longer performed. Recent data from a study of stage II testicular seminomas over 40 years reported a 10-year disease-free specific survival of 98% for stage IIA seminoma versus

79% of stage IIB seminomas (18). Moreover, another group reported a 30% relapse rate in stage IIB patients who were predominantly treated with adjuvant radiation (19). These data have increased the support for adjuvant chemotherapy in stage IIB, although the counterargument still remains that this subset population can still be salvaged with chemotherapy at time of relapse, nevertheless with increased risk of toxicity with the use of radiation and chemotherapy.

For stage IIB patients, those who do not wish to undergo RT, those with previous radiation to the retroperitoneum, or those with a relative contraindication to RT (e.g., horseshoe kidney or inflammatory bowel disease), chemotherapy with 4 cycles of EP or 3 cycles of BEP can be given as an alternative. Single-agent carboplatin has also been evaluated, given its success in stage I seminoma; however, this approach is associated with high relapse rate and thus not recommended.

In men who present with para-aortic lymph nodes >5 cm in diameter, RT alone resulted in relapse rates of 35%, with 5-year OS of 77% after salvage chemotherapy. Although newer RT techniques and improvements in salvage chemotherapy improved these outcomes, these patients fare better with upfront chemotherapy, with cure rates near 90%. Furthermore, several reports suggest that response to chemotherapy is significantly better for patients without prior exposure to radiation. The extent of radiation also seems to affect the outcomes, with patients with more limited exposure having better responses. At this time, either EP × 4 or BEP × 3 are considered the treatment of choice for stage IIC. Both are considered equivalent for the treatment of stage II as well as for stage IIIA and IIIB seminoma (good-risk disease on the IGCCCG classification; Table 14.3), although most centers will favor BEP given a trend toward improved outcomes when full doses of bleomycin are used. The evolution of this regimen started in the 1970s with the introduction of cisplatin, currently the most active drug for the treatment in GCTs. Cisplatin (20 mg/m² from day 1 to 5), was initially combined with bleomycin (30 units weekly) and vinblastine (0.4 mg/kg) for a total of 4 cycles followed by maintenance vinblastine. While this regimen (PVB) had remarkable results when compared with historical controls, the development of vinblastine-induced neuromuscular toxicity was a limiting factor. Eliminating maintenance vinblastine helped reduce this risk without affecting efficacy, but still remained a concern. Around this time, the activity of etoposide against GCTs and its synergism with cisplatin was demonstrated. This led to its use in combination with cisplatin and bleomycin instead of vinblastine. When both regimens were compared head to head, BEP showed a significantly better response rate, particularly in those with bulky disease. Furthermore, neurotoxicity was significantly more common in those receiving PVB, whereas no difference in myelosuppression was noted. Later, 4 cycles of BEP were compared to only 3 cycles in patients with good-risk disease. No differences in OS or disease-free survival (DFS) were reported; so currently a fourth cycle of BEP is considered unnecessary for patients with good-risk GCTs. However, patients with intermediate-risk disease, which include nonpulmonary visceral metastases, should receive 4 cycles of BEP, similar to intermediate- and poor-risk NSGCTs.

The choice between 3 cycles of BEP or 4 cycles of EP depends mostly on the pulmonary function of the individual. Although most patients with testicular cancer (usually young patients without comorbidities) are able to tolerate 3 doses of bleomycin, older patients and those with prior pulmonary damage or who cannot afford the risk of pulmonary toxicity (e.g., certain athletes) may be better served with 4 cycles of EP. Nevertheless, as stated previously, most trials comparing BEP with EP showed a nonsignificant difference in DFS and mortality favoring BEP. Similarly, dose reductions in bleomycin or etoposide produced inferior results. Therefore, BEP should be the treatment of choice in this setting unless a clear indication to avoid bleomycin is present.

Many patients with stage II seminoma, especially those with bulky disease, will have a residual mass seen on CT scan after chemotherapy. Unlike NSGCTs, where any residual mass should be surgically resected, a subset of patients with residual seminoma can be followed by surveillance. Before the advent of PET scan, the distinction between which patients should undergo further treatment and who can be followed up with surveillance alone was based on size parameters, with 3 cm used as the cutoff. Several reports showed that many of the masses of <3 cm will disappear during surveillance and therefore no further treatment was recommended. Conversely, the risk of disease progression was higher for those patients with a residual mass >3 cm as they frequently would have residual seminoma (20). Moreover, the radiographic appearance of the residual mass has been used by some to predict the presence of residual disease. Two distinct radiographic patterns had been described. In the first one, the residual tumor obliterates radiographic planes, merging with great vessels, psoas muscles, and retroperitoneal structures. These are considered unresectable and usually represent fibrotic tissue. The second clinical presentation shows well-delineated masses that, especially when >3 cm, have a high incidence of residual seminoma. In those cases, surgical resection is justified although a complete RPLND is frequently not possible.

This led to recommendations of surgical resection of the residual mass for patients with residual masses >3 cm, particularly when well defined on CT scan. Alternative, second-line chemotherapy or RT can be considered. However, in the appropriate setting and selected patients, surveillance alone is a viable option when only the size

criterion is used. PET scan is a helpful modality to assist with decision making in this setting. When performed at least 6 weeks after chemotherapy (to avoid false positives), PET scan has shown to be a better predictor of residual seminoma than size criteria. In the largest multicenter study that included 51 patients, PET scan correctly predicted all 19 cases with residual masses >3 cm, and 35 of the 37 with residual lesions of ≤3 cm (21). The specificity (100% vs. 74%), sensitivity (80% vs. 70%), positive predictive value (100% vs. 37%), and negative predictive value (96% vs. 92%) all favored PET scan over size criteria.

Therefore, PET scan is currently recommended for those patients with residual mass and negative STMs after chemotherapy for locally advanced seminoma, such as the patient described in the clinical vignette. If PET scan is negative, surveillance is suggested, while further treatment (surgery, second-line chemotherapy, or RT) should be considered for those patients with positive PET scan regardless of the size of the mass. If PET scan is not readily available, patients with a residual mass >3 cm should be considered for surgery or RT, with surveillance being a reasonable option for selected patients. For a residual mass <3 cm, surveillance alone is recommended. Patients with growing lymphadenopathy or positive tumor markers should be treated for progressive disease with second-line chemotherapy.

## Locally Advanced NSGCTs

X.N. is a 29-year-old man who presents with scrotal pain. On physical examination, a testicular mass is noted and confirmed with ultrasound. βhCG levels were mildly elevated (4000 IU/L), whereas AFP and LDH were within normal limits. After radical orchiectomy, pathology reports an NSGCT (60% yolk sac, 30% choriocarcinoma, 10% mature teratoma). CT scan of the abdomen and pelvis showed a 1.5-cm pelvic lymph node and the CXR was unremarkable. STMs returned to normal baseline after surgery. X.N. is diagnosed with a stage IIA NSGCT. On discussion of further management, he expresses that he does not want to have more children and, moreover, he is concerned about long-term effects of chemotherapy. Based on this, RPLND is performed with plans for surveillance after this. The pathology report confirms the presence of NSGCTs in 7 lymph nodes, with a maximum diameter of 1.8 cm. After being informed of these results, X.N. asks if surveillance is still a reasonable option.

## Evidence-Based Case Discussion

This clinical vignette reflects the frequent disconnect between clinical and pathological staging. This patient was classified as stage IIA based on imaging (N1, no lymph node >2 cm), and received primary RPLND. Given the relapse-free survival of approximately 90% for stage IIA NSGCTs after RPLND, this procedure is favored by many, especially if done at a specialized center. Alternatively, 3 cycles of BEP or 4 cycles of EP can be used (Figure 14.3). However, the numbers of positive lymph nodes upstages him to a pathologic stage IIB (pN2).

Although surveillance is still a reasonable option after RPLND in stage IIB disease, many argue in favor of adjuvant chemotherapy in this setting based on the higher relapse rate (35% compared with 10–15% in those with stage IIA). Indeed, the choice between surveillance and chemotherapy in patients with pathologic stage II disease depends on the volume of nodal disease burden. In a previous section, the NCCN recommendations for adjuvant chemotherapy for patients upstaged to stage II after RPLND for suspected stage I NSGCTs were reviewed. The same principles apply to patients who undergo RPLND for clinical stage II, such as the patient in the vignette. Briefly, surveillance is recommended for those with pN0, whereas 2 cycles of BEP are recommended for pN2 disease and 3 cycles (or 4 cycles of EP) for those with pN3. For patients with pN1, either surveillance or 2 cycles of BEP are considered appropriate,

and the decision based on patient's preference or compliance (Figure 14.3). These recommendations are aimed at decreasing the risk of relapse without impacting OS as most patients who relapse during surveillance can be successfully cured with 3 cycles of chemotherapy. The patient in this vignette could potentially benefit from 2 cycles of chemotherapy, since this will significantly decrease his risk of relapse. However, if he is motivated, surveillance is not contraindicated as his survival will not be affected.

Primary chemotherapy (BEP × 3 or EP × 4) is favored for patients with stage IIB, especially if there is multifocal involvement in the retroperitoneum. This also applies to patients with stage IIC and patients with positive STMs after orchiectomy. Similarly, patients with stage IIIA (good-risk disease, Table 14.3) should undergo primary chemotherapy. Relapse-free survival and OS are excellent after chemotherapy. If complete response is seen after chemotherapy, including negative markers, surveillance is considered appropriate.

However, some authors recommend RPLND after chemotherapy regardless of response (i.e., normal post-chemotherapy scans). Although this recommendation is somewhat controversial, it may improve outcomes if a

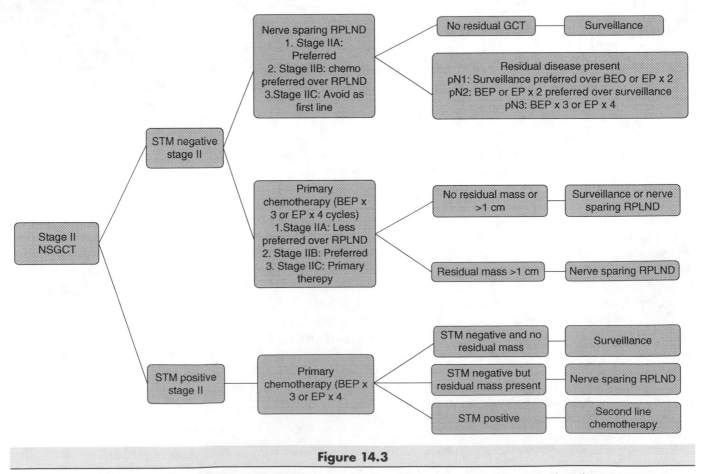

**Figure 14.3**

Management algorithm for stage II NSGCTs. BEP, bleomycin, etoposide, and cisplatin; EP, etoposide and cisplatin; NSGCTs, nonseminomatous germ cell tumors; RPLND, retroperitoneal lymph node dissection; STMs, serum tumor markers.

teratoma component is present as this is relatively resistant to chemotherapy. In fact, this aggressive surgical approach may decrease the rate of growing teratoma syndrome (GTS), a phenomenon considered to be rare although its true incidence is largely unknown. It was first described almost 30 years ago and since then it has been described mostly as case reports or case series (22). It should be suspected in the presence of a metastatic lesion (most commonly retroperitoneal, but has been described in other locations) that increases in size during chemotherapy, while STMs decline or normalize. Suspicion should also arise when a mixed response to treatment is seen on imaging during chemotherapy or if an isolated mass grows after chemotherapy despite normal STMs, especially if a teratoma component was present in the primary tumor. Surgery should be considered as soon as this process is suspected and is curative if a complete resection is possible.

If markers return to normal but a residual mass is seen at follow-up CT scan, RPLND should be performed. It should be kept in mind that small lymph nodes are usually detected after chemotherapy with current high-resolution imaging techniques. PET scan does not have a role in this setting as it does in seminoma as it cannot reliably differentiate fibrosis from teratoma. What constitutes a normal size residual lymph node varies from institution to institution, but most centers will perform post-chemotherapy RPLND for any residual mass >1 cm. For those with masses <1 cm, surveillance may be considered as results seem to be excellent. A retrospective analysis of the long-term outcomes of 141 patients with advanced GCT treated at Indiana University between 1984 and 2005 who achieved complete remission (CR) (normal STMs and residual mass <1 cm) after chemotherapy alone (23). Median follow-up was 15.5 years. A total of 12 patients relapsed, 6 of the relapses occurred in the retroperitoneum. The DFS was 90% and the OS reached 97% as 8 of the 12 patients showed no evidence of disease (NED) after salvage treatment. Five patients relapsed >3 years posttreatment, which reinforces the need for prolonged follow-up in these patients. The authors concluded that patients achieving a CR after chemotherapy alone can be safely monitored without RPLND.

In those patients in whom post-chemotherapy resection is performed, further treatment after surgery is based on pathology findings. In most patients (approximately 85%), teratoma or fibrosis will be reported after residual mass resection. In these patients, surveillance can be safely started. Conversely, if residual viable tumor is found, 2 more cycles of combination chemotherapy are currently recommended. EP, etoposide/ifosfamide/cisplatin (VIP), vinblastine/ifosfamide/cisplatin (VeIP), or paclitaxel/ifosfamide/cisplatin (TIP) are all acceptable options in this setting. Similarly, if markers remain positive, patient should be treated with second-line chemotherapy, like the ones mentioned previously, for refractory disease.

## Intermediate Risk, Advanced NSGCTs

T.R. is a 39-year-old man who presented to his primary care physician with 3 weeks history of dry cough, worsening over the previous week. He denied any fever associated with these symptoms. On review of systems, he reported an occasional abdominal discomfort and bloating for the last several months, worse after meals, but otherwise no other symptoms were reported. His past medical history was positive for smoking and obesity. He denied any significant family history. Auscultation of the lungs was unremarkable and abdominal examination did not reveal any tenderness, organomegaly, or masses. His symptoms were attributed to gastroesophageal reflux and a trial of proton pump inhibitors was given. T.R. returned 2 weeks later with a report that his cough was somewhat worse. His physical examination was unchanged. His physician ordered a CXR that showed multiple nodules in both lungs, concerning for malignancy. Laboratory data showed an increased LDH (2 times the upper limits of normal), with normal blood counts and basic metabolic panel. A CT scan of the chest, abdomen, and pelvis confirmed multiple lung nodules, with the largest measuring 4.5 cm. In addition, bulky lymphadenopathy was noted in the retroperitoneum. Given this presentation, STMs and a scrotal ultrasound were ordered. The ultrasound showed a 1-cm hypoechoic mass on the right testicle that was missed on physical examination. βhCG and AFP were elevated at 10,000 IU/L and 8000 ng/mL, respectively. Immediate orchiectomy was performed and pathology confirmed the presence of a GCT with 70% yolk sac tumor, 25% choriocarcinoma, and 5% teratoma. After surgery, βhCG and AFP levels fell to 5000 IU/L and 2000 ng/mL, respectively. T.R. was diagnosed with stage IIIB NSGCT and received 4 cycles of BEP. Repeat scans obtained 6 weeks after completion of chemotherapy showed that all pulmonary nodules had resolved except for the largest one, now 1.5 cm, as well as a residual 2.5-cm para-aortic mass. STMs were within normal limits.

## Evidence-Based Case Discussion

This patient was diagnosed with stage IIIB NSGCT which, along with stage IIIC seminoma, constitutes an intermediate-risk advanced disease (Table 14.3). This case encompasses 2 important concepts: the use of 4 cycles of BEP for intermediate-risk disease and the possibility of residual masses in >1 anatomical location, which creates a challenge for both the oncologist and the surgeon.

Currently, 4 cycles of BEP are considered the treatment of choice for intermediate-risk metastatic disease. With this approach, a DFS between 70% and 80% can be expected. Although this survival could be considered to be quite good, up to 30% of patients will relapse after being exposed to 4 cycles of chemotherapy including bleomycin. About a third of these patients can be salvaged with an ifosfamide-based regimen. This success led to the study of ifosfamide as a possible first-line agent for the treatment of intermediate-risk and poor-risk disease. Several studies addressing this question were conducted in the late 1980s and early 1990s. The largest study performed within several cooperative groups compared 4 cycles of BEP to 4 cycles of VIP essentially substituting ifosfamide for bleomycin. While equivalent in efficacy, the incidence of clinically important hematologic and genitourinary toxicity was significantly higher in the ifosfamide group. On the basis of these results, the authors concluded that 4 cycles of BEP were still the standard of care for advanced disseminated GCTs (24).

Another alternative that has been studied is the addition of paclitaxel to BEP. An initial phase I/II study showed a complete response in all 13 patients receiving escalating doses of paclitaxel combined with BEP. A randomized phase III (EORTC 30983) intent to treat study compared paclitaxel-BEP (with granulocyte-colony stimulating factor [G-CSF] support) to standard BEP in intermediate prognosis germ cell cancer failed to accrue enough patients and also included nearly 10% ineligible patients. The primary statistical analysis failed to show benefit in taxane arm, although the subset

analysis excluding ineligible patients showed a progression free survival (PFS) benefit, but no OS benefit (25).

On the basis of these results, 4 cycles of BEP are still the standard of care for intermediate-risk advanced GCT. Treatment with VIP can be considered as a good alternative in those patients with lung disease or those who can be expected to need an extensive pulmonary resection (Figure 14.4). It is important to mention that the presence of lung metastasis by itself, such as in the patient described, is not a contraindication for bleomycin.

A persistent mass after chemotherapy is a relatively frequent occurrence in patients with advanced disease, being more common with higher disease burden at the time of presentation. Whenever possible, resection of all residual masses is recommended after chemotherapy, as long as STMs return to normal. In patients with metastatic disease, the retroperitoneum is also the most common site for a residual mass. Most commonly, this will represent either necrosis or teratoma.

In patients with intrathoracic residual masses after chemotherapy, efforts should be aimed toward a complete surgical resection. When this is achieved, good outcomes can be expected as reported in some early studies. The

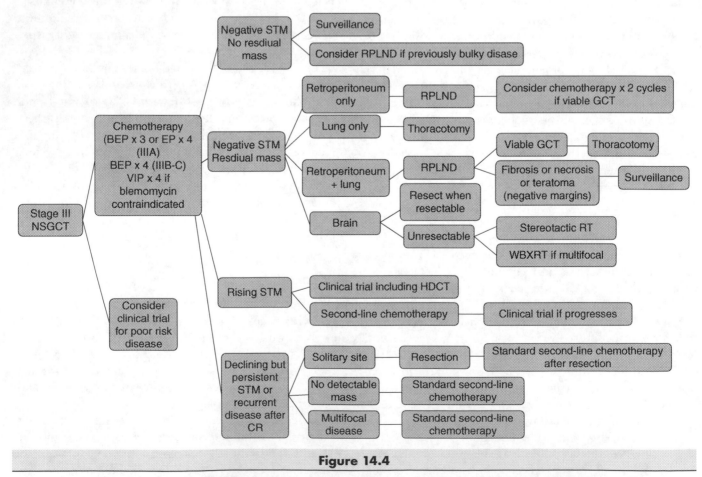

**Figure 14.4**

Management algorithm for stage III NSGCTs and disease relapse. BEP, bleomycin, etoposide, and cisplatin; CR, complete remission; EP, etoposide, cisplatin; GCT, germ cell tumor; HDCT, high-dose chemotherapy; NSGCTs, nonseminomatous germ cell tumors; RPLND, retroperitoneal lymph node dissection; RT, radiation therapy; STMs, serum tumor markers; VIP, etoposide, ifosfamide, and cisplatin; WBXRT, whole brain radiation therapy.

outcomes of 141 patients who underwent thoracic metastasectomy for GCT at a single institution in England from 1980 to 1997 had been described (26). Of these, 104 had lung metastasis at the time of presentation, whereas 37 developed them after initial chemotherapy. Eighty-seven percent (123 patients) received chemotherapy prior to surgery. At the time of surgery, 51% had lung-only metastasis, 24% had both lung and mediastinum metastasis, and 24% had residual disease only in the mediastinum. Complete resection was possible in 123 patients (87%). There were 2 perioperative deaths. Pathological analysis of the resected metastasis revealed necrosis or fibrosis (23%), mature teratoma (45%), and viable malignancy (32%). Sixty-seven patients recurred after surgery, with recurrence being more common in patients with viable GCT (33 of 46; 72%) than in those with fibrosis (10 of 32; 31%) or teratoma (24 of 63; 38%). Many of these patients received a second thoracotomy successfully and the OS was 78% at 5 years after the initial metastasectomy surgery. In a multivariate analysis, a significantly increased risk of death from disease was found for those with viable malignancy in the surgical sample (response rate [RR] = 5.7), residual disease at resection (RR = 4.0), and multiple metastases (RR = 4.1). It is important to mention that less than half the patients included in this study received the current standard regimen of BEP. With modern therapy, even better outcomes should be expected.

As stated previously, close to 50% of patients undergoing thoracotomy for a residual pulmonary mass are found to have fibrosis or necrosis. Because relapse is unusual in these patients, surveillance would have been appropriate for them, avoiding the risks associated with surgery. Unfortunately, imaging alone cannot predict which patients will have residual disease (GCT or teratoma) on resection. As previously stated, PET scan cannot differentiate between teratoma and fibrosis. Attempts to create predictive models led to the observation that histology at RPLND was the most useful predictor of the histology of a residual pulmonary mass. A retrospective, international, multicenter study evaluated the outcomes of 215 patients undergoing thoracotomy after chemotherapy (27). More than half of these patients (54%) had necrosis found after pathology evaluation, while mature teratoma and viable GCTs were found in 33% and 13%, respectively. In addition, when RPLND was performed prior to pulmonary resection, the finding of necrosis in the retroperitoneum predicted necrosis in the pulmonary tissue in 89% of the cases, thus constituting the strongest predictor of pulmonary histology. Conversely, if mature teratoma or persistent cancer was found after RPLND, the probability of finding necrotic tissue only after thoracotomy was 38% and 30%, respectively. Other predictors of necrosis in the residual pulmonary mass were a teratoma negative primary tumor, normal AFP before chemotherapy and the presence of a single, unilateral residual lung nodule. As expected, an increase in size of a lung nodule during chemotherapy predicted a low likelihood of necrosis. The authors concluded that thoracotomy can be reconsidered if RPLND shows necrosis only, especially if other predictive factors of necrosis are present, unless the patient or the treating physician feels that the risk of missing teratoma or active cancer at thoracotomy is too high. A sequential rather than concurrent surgical approach is recommended by most experts when both retroperitoneal and pulmonary residual disease is present after initial chemotherapy. Thoracotomy should be pursued when teratoma or viable carcinoma is found after RPLND. This procedure can be delayed and patient placed in surveillance if only necrosis is found. However, current NCCN guidelines still advocate for the concurrent surgical approach with resection of all residual masses.

## Poor-Risk, Advanced GCT With Extrapulmonary Metastases

C.P. is a 31-year-old marathon runner with a past medical history of migraine headaches who noted some heaviness on his lower abdomen during his last race. He had also felt that he was tiring more easily while training over the past 2 months, and was experiencing postprandial epigastric pain. His family history was unremarkable. His physical examination revealed mild tenderness on palpation of right upper quadrant of the abdomen, as well as an enlarged right testicle. Scrotal ultrasound confirmed presence of a mass and CT scan showed diffuse retroperitoneal lymphadenopathy, multiple pulmonary nodules as well as 3 nodules in the liver ranging in size from 1 to 3 cm. STMs revealed an LDH 5 times the upper limits of normal, a βhCG of 68,000 IU/L, and an AFP of 8000 ng/mL. Orchiectomy confirmed the diagnosis of NSGCTs (50% embryonal, 30% yolk sac, 20% choriocarcinoma). Tumor markers decreased postoperatively, but did not reach normal values (LDH 2 times upper limits of normal, βhCG = 53,000 IU/L, AFP = 3500 ng/mL). Chemotherapy options were discussed with C.P., and he refused to receive bleomycin due to concerns of its effect on his lung capacity. Therefore, 4 cycles of VIP were given without immediate complications. STMs returned to normal after the third cycle and remained within normal limits 4 weeks after chemotherapy was completed. CT scan revealed residual masses, with a 1-cm pulmonary nodule, a 1.2-cm pelvic lymph node, as well as a 1.1-cm liver nodule. C.P. underwent an RPLND and resection of the liver nodule. Both masses were reported to contain fibrotic tissue only and the patient chose to begin surveillance of the pulmonary nodule. Repeat CT scans at 3 and 6 months showed no changes and STMs remained within normal limits. C.P. presented for an 8-month follow-up visit and tumor markers revealed a βhCG level of 20,000 IU/L. He denied any new symptoms, but did report that his migraine headaches had become more frequent and less responsive to usual measures. CT scans were ordered, including a head CT scan. CT of chest, abdomen, and pelvis reported no significant changes compared with previous scans, but the CT head showed a 2-cm lesion in the right parieto-occipital region.

## Evidence-Based Case Discussion

This vignette focuses our attention on few key issues in the management of GCTs, namely the initial management of patients with poor prognosis, the management of a residual liver mass after chemotherapy, the treatment for relapsing or refractory disease, and the approach to brain metastasis, either at initial presentation or, as in this case, as a manifestation of recurrence. If available, inclusion in a clinical trial should be considered for patients with poor-risk prognosis. The patient described in the vignette was initially offered chemotherapy with BEP (4 cycles), which, as described in the previous section, is the standard regimen of choice for intermediate or poor-prognosis patients with advanced GCTs. Owing to concerns of his lung function, VIP was used. As previously described, this is an adequate alternative regimen in this setting, although hematologic toxicity is higher.

In the poor-risk population, the 5-year OS is approximately 50% with conventional chemotherapy. Therefore, more intense regimens have been studied trying to improve survival, including regimens with dose intensification of cisplatin as well as induction-sequential chemotherapy schedule with bleomycin, vincristine, and cisplatin followed by etoposide, ifosfamide, cisplatin, and bleomycin (BOP/VIP-B). Both regimens offered no DFS or OS benefit and resulted in increased toxicity.

More promising was the experience of 54 patients with poor-risk prognosis treated with an intensive 6-week induction regimen of CBOP (carboplatin in weeks 2 and 4, cisplatin 40 mg/m$^2$ in weeks 2 and 4, and 100 mg/m$^2$ in weeks 1 and 3; vincristine was given weekly until week 6 and bleomycin was also given weekly). This was followed by 3 cycles of BEP (28). OS was 91% at 3 years and 87.6% at 5 years. Whereas these numbers compare favorably with historical data, the sample was relatively small and there was a lack of a control arm. Similarly, the favorable experience (OS = 75% at 3 years) in patients with poor-risk prognosis treated with POMB/ACE (cisplatin, vincristine, methotrexate, bleomycin, actinomycin D, cyclophosphamide, and etoposide) over 20 years at 2 institutions in England has been described (29). Although the results of these 2 trials may be enticing, a prospective phase III randomized study is needed to confirm the results as none of them has proven to be superior to BEP.

Finally, the use of high-dose chemotherapy (HDCT) with stem cell rescue has been evaluated as a possible first-line treatment for low-risk patients. Two small noncontrolled studies showed some promising results when compared with historical data. In these studies HDCT was offered to those patients with a suboptimal response to the first 2 cycles of conventional chemotherapy. However, a phase III trial using BEP disclosed somewhat disappointing results

(30). In this study, 219 patients were randomly assigned to receive 4 cycles of BEP versus 2 cycles of BEP followed by 2 cycles of HDCT with carboplatin and etoposide and stem cell rescue. The primary end point was durable CR at 1 year, which was observed in 52% (HDCT arm) compared with 48% (conventional dose arm), a nonsignificant difference. After a median follow-up of 51 months, no difference in the OS was observed either. A planned subset analysis evaluated the response in those patients with elevated STMs at baseline. In those who showed an inadequate decline in STMs prior to the third cycle (early chemotherapy resistance), HDCT provided a significant benefit in durable CR at 1 year (61% vs. 34% in those who received conventional chemotherapy) as well as in OS at 2 years (78% vs. 55%, respectively). This difference was not observed in those who had an adequate decline in their STMs after the first 2 cycles of chemotherapy. However, because random assignment did not occur within this subset and the benefit of HDCT in the patients with early chemotherapy resistance was based on a small sample size of 70 patients, data were not considered robust enough to be translated into conventional treatment. The authors concluded that 4 cycles of BEP remain the standard chemotherapy for this population, but early referral for clinical studies should be considered for patients with a suboptimal decline in STMs after 2 cycles of conventional cisplatin-based chemotherapy.

In summary, patients diagnosed with a poor-risk prognosis NSGCTs (seminomas are never classified as poor-risk prognosis) should be treated within the scope of clinical trial if available for them. Otherwise, 4 cycles of BEP (or VIP) are considered the standard first-line regimen. More intensive treatments, including HDCT, should be considered in those patients with early resistance to chemotherapy as part of clinical studies only (Figure 14.4). However, regardless of the treatment, a significant proportion of patients are expected to relapse.

## Therapeutic Options at Relapse

The management of relapsed stage I and stage II disease and the excellent results with standard chemotherapy as salvage modality have been described in a previous section. Conversely, approximately half of patients with intermediate and poor-risk disease are expected to relapse, and only 25% of these will have a prolonged response to standard salvage chemotherapy.

Our patient also reflects the most common type of presentation at relapse. Indeed, the majority of relapses are detected by an increase in the STMs during routine follow-up (even in patients with normal STMs at original presentation), and most relapses will occur within 2 years of the original chemotherapy. Patients who experience relapse within 4 weeks of receiving cisplatin-based chemotherapy are considered to have cisplatin-refractory disease that carries a particularly poor prognosis. Likewise, those who relapse after 2 years have a tendency for chemotherapy resistance and a worse prognosis unless aggressive surgical resection of residual masses is possible.

Both paclitaxel and ifosfamide had shown activity as salvage treatment after platinum-based chemotherapy. For this reason, for those patients who relapse within 2 years, standard dose chemotherapy options include VeIP (vinblastine, 0.11 mg/kg/d for 2 days; ifosfamide, 1200 mg/m²/d for 5 days; and cisplatin, 20 mg/m²/d for 5 days) and TIP (paclitaxel, 250 mg/m² on day 1 followed by ifosfamide 1500 mg/m²/d and cisplatin 25 mg/m²/d on days 2–5). If etoposide was not given during initial chemotherapy (rare occurrence nowadays), VIP chemotherapy becomes an alternative. For patients who relapse after VIP therapy (like the one described here), second-line therapy is less defined. Although TIP is still a reasonable option, regimens including gemcitabine and/or oxaliplatin (both of which have showed activity in cisplatin-refractory disease) have also been utilized.

Loehrer et al. evaluated 135 patients who received VeIP for relapsed disease after etoposide- and cisplatin-based chemotherapy. A CR was achieved in 49.6% of patients. At 6 years of follow-up, 23.7% were continuously free of disease (31). Results with paclitaxel had been even more promising. A small phase I/II study included a selected population of 30 patients with relapsing GCTs with favorable prognostic factor as per Memorial Sloan Kettering Cancer Center (MSKCC) criteria (testicular primary, <6 previous cycles of cisplatin, and a CR to initial chemotherapy) (32). Paclitaxel was started at a dose of 175 mg/m² and increased up to 250 mg/m² in a subsequent cohort (24 out of 30 patients received the latter dose). They reported a CR in 77% of the patients, with a durable response in 73% (at 33 months). Results were less encouraging in the 43 evaluable patients included in a multicenter study in England (33). This study, however, also included patients with less favorable prognostic factors, used a lower dose of paclitaxel and ifosfamide, and allowed dose reductions based on cytopenias. In the whole cohort, a favorable response (CR or partial response with negative STMs) was recorded in 60%, but only a 38% failure-free survival (FFS) after 1 year. When only the 26 patients meeting similar good-prognosis criteria as those from the MSKCC study were analyzed, favorable response rate and FFS were somewhat better (73% and 43%, respectively) but still less impressive than those at MSKCC.

On the basis of these results, chemotherapy with TIP (with paclitaxel dose of 250 mg/m²) or VeIP is the preferred treatment strategy for patients who relapse after initial cisplatin-based chemotherapy and good-risk features (testicular primary, low STMs and disease volume, and complete response to first-line chemotherapy). In centers with adequate expertise, HDCT with stem cell rescue can be considered. Conversely, for those patients with poor-prognosis features, inclusion in a clinical trial should be considered, given the suboptimal results with conventional chemotherapy. If no clinical trial is available, conventional chemotherapy or HDCT should be pursued. Poor-prognosis

features include an extratesticular primary, high-volume disease or markedly increased STMs, as well as patients considered cisplatin refractory and those with late relapse.

Patients who progress within 4 weeks of receiving a cisplatin-based chemotherapy or during chemotherapy cycles are defined as refractory and absolutely refractory, respectively, and have a distinctly poor prognosis. These patients are candidates for palliative gemcitabine/oxaliplatin (GEMOX)-based chemotherapy or HDCT. The former is based mostly in phase II studies that began after gemcitabine and later oxaliplatin had shown single-agent activity against GCTs. The use of oxaliplatin in combination with gemcitabine in 35 patients (63% cisplatin refractory and 89% relapsed after HDCT) yielded an overall response of 46% (16 patients), including 3 patients with a CR (all of whom remained disease free at the end of follow-up). Seven of the 16 responders were cisplatin refractory, including 1 patient who achieved CR (34). More recently, paclitaxel was used in combination with both gemcitabine and oxaliplatin by the German Testicular Cancer Study Group, resulting in an approximately 50% RR and a CR rate approaching 20% following resection of residual disease (35). Although each of these regimens is considered palliative for patients with very poor prognosis, a small number of patients may achieve a significant survival.

## The Use of High-Dose Therapy With Autologous Stem Cell Support

Another treatment option for advanced GCT involves the use of HDCT regimens followed by stem cell rescue. This strategy has been tested in different settings, and currently HDCT is considered part of the armamentarium of second-line treatment for patients who relapse after initial chemotherapy and a reasonable third-line treatment in those who relapse after conventional dose salvage chemotherapy. Some patients will respond to conventional chemotherapy, and are thus spared from the potential toxicity of HDCT. Identifying patients unresponsive to conventional therapy who are more or less likely to respond to HDCT remains an important challenge. The first attempt to define these prognostic factors came from a multicenter retrospective analysis of 310 patients treated with HDCT for relapsing or refractory disease (36). In a multivariate analysis, progressive disease before HDCT, mediastinal NSGCT primary, refractory disease, and HCG levels before HDCT >1000 IU/L correlated with worse prognosis. The Beyer prognostic model used these factors to classify patients with good, intermediate, and poor prognoses, with FFS rates at 2 years of 51%, 27%, and 5%, respectively. Subsequent studies have validated as well as challenged the Beyer model.

The appropriate timing for HDCT as well as the choice of agents or the use of single versus tandem HDCT should had been the focus of several studies over the past 2 decades. These questions, unfortunately, remain mostly unanswered despite these efforts because of the relatively small numbers, lack of randomization, different regimens used, and differences in the population selected for these studies.

A phase I/II study employing a dose-intensive regimen with 2 cycles of ifosfamide/paclitaxel (given 2 weeks apart) followed by 3 cycles of high-dose etoposide and carboplatin (with increasing dose of carboplatin between cohorts) included 37,108 patients considered unlikely to respond to conventional chemotherapy as second-line treatment (37). Seventy-four percent of patients were platinum refractory and 20% had mediastinal primary tumors. Most of these patients had incomplete response to first-line treatment, and 8 patients had mediastinal primary tumors. After a median of 61 months of follow-up, 50% patients achieved CR. Fifty-one patients remained disease free at 5 years with DFS if 47%, including 5 of 21 patients with primary mediastinal NSGCTs. These findings, therefore, discourage the exclusion of patients for HDCT and autologous rescue, based purely on a prognostic score or model (i.e., primary mediastinal NSGCTs). A different approach was used at Indiana University, where 2 cycles of HDCT are given upfront and patients with primary mediastinal tumors were excluded. One hundred eighty-four patients underwent 2 cycles of high-dose carboplatin and etoposide followed by stem cell rescue as initial salvage therapy (38). At a median follow-up of 48 months, 116 patients from the whole cohort were still in CR (63%). In a subset analysis, 70% of those who received HDCT in first relapse were disease free (94 out of 135) compared with 45% of those receiving it after 2 or more previous regimens (22 out of 49). Moreover, 18 out of 40 patients with cisplatin-refractory disease were still in CR. The multivariate analysis revealed that the timing of HDCT (best when used as second-line rather than third-line treatment), cisplatin refractoriness, and IGCCCG poor-risk stage were independent predictors of response. When a scoring algorithm was applied using these factors, different OS curves (low, intermediate, and high risk) were statistically significant.

## Management of Brain Metastases

Finally, the patient (C.P.) described in this vignette presented with a single site of recurrence, in this case a solitary brain mass. CNS metastases are a relatively rare occurrence, being diagnosed in about 1% of patients with metastatic GCTs at the time of original presentation, whereas up to an additional 4% will develop them during the course of the disease. Given its rarity, most of our knowledge arises from small retrospective series. These studies identified 3 subsets with distinct prognosis. First, in patients with brain metastasis as part of their initial presentation, disease-specific survival ranges from 43% to 86% in the different series. A second group comprises those with brain metastasis as a manifestation of relapse after a CR with conventional chemotherapy, and the final group includes those who develop brain metastasis after an incomplete response

to chemotherapy and those with additional metastatic sites. Although the former can show survival rates between 39% and 44%, the latter group usually has poor outcomes with survival rates between 2% and 26%. Patients with a single metastatic site that is amenable for local therapy tend to have significantly better prognosis that explains the wide range of survival rates reported in the different series.

Owing to the lack of prospective data, the optimal management of brain metastasis in metastatic GCTs is unclear. Currently, most centers and guidelines advocate the use of chemotherapy as an initial step. The rationale of this approach is based on the adequate penetration through the brain–blood barrier, in the presence of macroscopic intracerebral metastasis, of the most common chemotherapy agents used for treatment of GCTs, including cisplatin. Moreover, the majority of these patients present with additional metastatic foci, either as part of the initial presentation or as relapse, therefore requiring adequate systemic treatment. Patients who are chemotherapy naive tend to have better responses to chemotherapy, hence the better survival rates seen in this group. The development of chemotherapy resistance within clinically silent brain metastases during initial conventional chemotherapy may explain the inferior outcomes of chemotherapy when used in patients with brain lesions as a manifestation of relapse. Whether HDCT could overcome the development of these resistant clones is debatable.

The appropriate approach after chemotherapy is controversial. Whole-brain radiation therapy (WBXRT) has been used as part of the management of brain metastases in a variety of malignancies. However, given the usual young age of onset and the possibility of long-term survival in patients with GCTs, concerns of late toxicity, such as progressive multifocal leukoencephalopathy and cognitive impairment, are a priority. Furthermore, questions had arisen regarding its usefulness in the absence of multifocal residual disease as surgical resection seems to provide similar results without delayed toxicity. A small study reported the outcomes of 22 patients treated at a single institution comparing WBXRT after resection of easily accessible solitary brain lesions against a more aggressive surgical approach without WBXRT (39). They concluded that cure can be achieved with induction chemotherapy and aggressive surgery without WBXRT. Similarly, a retrospective pooled analysis of 139 patients treated for brain metastasis between 1979 and 1995 in Europe showed that the use of WBXRT did not translate into good prognosis in those patients with brain metastasis found at the initial presentation, but did seem to benefit those receiving it as part of relapse treatment (40). Delayed toxicity was not addressed in this study.

Given these questions, many centers have abandoned the routine use of post-chemotherapy WBXRT, with further treatment now being given according to the response to chemotherapy. If no residual disease is seen, a careful surveillance approach is adopted. Conversely, if limited residual disease is noted on post-chemotherapy imaging, local therapy is used, which includes surgical resection and focal RT. The use of WBXRT is reserved for those patients with more extensive residual disease or those who failed to respond to chemotherapy. Although there is no absolute consensus on this matter, the most recent NCCN guidelines recommends brain RT as optional, depending on the individual clinical setting.

In summary, C.P. would benefit from inclusion in a clinical trial for management of relapsed disease, including the possibility of HDCT. If no trial is available, conventional salvage chemotherapy with VeIP or TIP should be given. Despite the seemingly limited disease at the time of relapse, systemic chemotherapy should be given initially, especially considering his increased STMs. After completing chemotherapy, repeat imaging studies should be obtained. If a residual mass is present, surgical resection (or focal radiation if surgery is contraindicated or not feasible) should be pursued. This can be followed by WBXRT (especially in the relapse setting, more likely to be chemotherapy resistant) or surveillance (Figure 14.4).

## Extragonadal NSGCTs

E.N. is a previously healthy 22-year-old college student who presents to the free clinic during the fall with 3 weeks of dyspnea and cough. Initially he thought he had contracted a common cold from his niece on a recent trip home, but symptoms worsened and he now reports fever and night sweats. He is unsure about weight loss. He is up-to-date with his vaccinations and he is a lifelong nonsmoker. Physical examination is unremarkable and he is given a short course of antibiotics with no improvement in symptoms. A CXR showed a wide mediastinum. A CT of the chest showed a 7-cm mass in the anterior mediastinum. No other masses were found on imaging. Laboratory data were within normal limits except for increased STMs: AFP (2943 ng/mL), βhCG (11 IU/L), and LDH (523 IU/L). Scrotal ultrasound was unremarkable. These results strongly suggested a GCT and tissue obtained from the mediastinal mass confirmed the diagnosis of extragonadal NSGCT, with predominance of yolk sac tumor. E.N. received 4 cycles of VIP with STMs returning to normal. CT scan images showed a partial response, with the mediastinal NSGCT now measuring 4 cm. Surgical resection was then performed, with the pathology report showing necrosis and elements of teratoma with negative margins. STMs and CT scans remained within normal parameters on the subsequent follow-up visit. Seven months after the initial diagnosis, he returned to the clinic complaining of weight loss, progressive weakness, and easy bruising. A CT scan did not show any evidence of recurrence and STMs were again normal but routine laboratory data showed pancytopenia (hemoglobin = 8.1 g/dL, platelets = 16,000, and WBC = $4.1 \times 10^9$). Bone marrow biopsy was consistent with acute megakaryoblastic leukemia and fluorescence in situ hybridization (FISH) analyses demonstrated the presence of an isochromosome 12p (i12p).

He received induction chemotherapy, but limited response was seen. He died 3 weeks later due to complications of neutropenic fever.

## Evidence-Based Case Discussion

This patient was diagnosed with an EGCT. These tumors represent up to 5% of all GCTs, and are usually found in the midline on the body, mostly in the mediastinum or retroperitoneum, with other locations such as the pineal gland being much less common. The histogenesis of these tumors is unclear. It has been hypothesized that they may derive from germ cells that fail to complete their migration along the urogenital ridge during the embryonal development or that they may represent transformed testicular germ cells that undergo reverse migration (41). In some cases, testicular calcifications can be seen in scrotal ultrasound, leading to the theory that EGCTs are really metastatic GCTs with a "burnt-out" testicular primary. However, the fact that testicular GCT rarely metastasize to the anterior mediastinum and the reported association between mediastinal NSGCT with Klinefelter syndrome as well as the increased incidence of hematological malignancies (not seen with testicular primary tumors) support an independent origin. There is, nevertheless, an increased risk of developing a metachronous testicular GCT, especially in cases with a retroperitoneal primary.

There are no significant differences in the histology of these tumors compared with their gonadal counterparts, but there is a difference in their relative frequencies. Teratomas are the most common mediastinal GCT (60–70%), with mature teratomas being more common than immature. Pure seminomas represent less than one third of the remainder of EGCTs, and there is a higher incidence of yolk sac tumor among the nonseminomatous EGCTs. Features of GCT or teratoma are usually clearly defined in biopsy samples, but occasionally only a poorly differentiated tumor is reported. STMs are elevated in 85% of patients, with more pronounced AFP levels. Elevations of βhCG are usually less marked. In rare instances, some centers will treat a poorly differentiated mediastinal tumor as GCT based on the concurrent elevation of STMs in a young male. As with testicular primary tumors, cytogenetic analyses frequently reveal an isochromosome i(12p).

Unlike primary testicular mature teratomas, which have some degree of metastatic potential and malignant transformation, mediastinal mature teratomas have a rather benign behavior and are frequently found incidentally unless symptoms related to compression of surrounding structures occur first. Resection is almost always curative. On the other hand, immature teratomas have a poor prognosis overall and are frequently incurable unless a complete resection is possible.

Most patients with either seminoma or nonseminomatous EGCTs are symptomatic at the time of diagnosis.

Dyspnea, cough, chest pain, or discomfort are usual complaints among patients with mediastinal tumors, with weight loss, superior vena cava syndrome, fever, and nausea being less frequent, but reported presentations. Patients with retroperitoneal primaries will frequently present with abdominal and/or back pain.

Pure extragonadal seminomas are rare, with most data coming from relatively small series. Both mediastinal and retroperitoneal seminomas occur with rather similar frequencies, although mediastinal primaries had been considered more common by some series. They tend to grow slowly, and are usually bulky or metastatic by the time they cause symptoms and are diagnosed. Nevertheless, prognosis is still excellent for both mediastinal and retroperitoneal primaries, with no significant differences in PFS or OS between these 2 presentations (approximately 92% and 88% at 5 years, respectively). Primary chemotherapy is the treatment of choice in extragonadal seminoma. On the basis of the presence or absence of nonpulmonary metastasis, these tumors will have a good- or intermediate-risk prognosis (Table 14.3). The choice of agents and number of cycles to be used in good- and intermediate-risk disease had been previously described. In the case of mediastinal primaries, however, the use of bleomycin is sometimes avoided as there is a chance that thoracic surgery to remove residual masses may be required following chemotherapy. When residual masses are resected after treatment of extragonadal seminoma, necrosis is usually found. For this reason, as with stage II seminoma, many will observe masses of <3 cm, especially if resection is technically difficult. However, size criterion alone is even less reliable in this setting compared to those with gonadal primaries; so this recommendation is controversial. The use of PET scan is not yet recommended because false positives seem to be an issue. Occasionally, after resection, teratoma is found that may indicate the presence of nonseminomatous elements in the original tumor. Frequently used in the past as initial treatment for extragonadal seminoma, RT has fallen out of favor against primary chemotherapy. Since most of the times bulky disease is present at the time of the initial diagnosis, the use of RT results in high relapse rates (approximately 30%). Furthermore, patients initially treated with radiation may have a decreased response to subsequent chemotherapy.

Unlike seminomas, patients with extragonadal NSGCTs carry a worse prognosis (42). This is particularly true for those with a mediastinal primary who are classified in the poor-risk prognosis group regardless of the STM levels or the absence of distant metastases. Before the cisplatin era, survival rates for these patients were usually <5%. With the current chemotherapy regimens plus aggressive surgical management of residual masses, survival rates around 50% are common.

Patients with relapsing extragonadal mediastinal primary tumors have dismal responses to salvage therapy, including HDCT. In fact, many centers will exclude these patients from HDCT trials. In general, survival rates of approximately 10% are expected for this population. Although long-term survival had been reported, this usually occurred in cases where complete resection of the mass was achieved. This highlights the important role surgery has in the salvage treatment of these patients even in the presence of increased tumor markers.

Although the prognosis of patients with retroperitoneal primaries is not as poor as those with mediastinal primaries, they usually have worse survival rates than their gonadal counterparts when matched by the IGCCCG prognostic classification, especially for those with good or intermediate prognosis. In the largest retrospective series to date, which included 283 patients with retroperitoneal primary tumors, the survival rate for those with good or intermediate prognosis was 61%, a result clearly inferior compared to those expected in those groups. The authors suggested that these patients may benefit from 4 cycles of chemotherapy instead of the standard recommendation of 3 cycles. This study also showed that patients with a retroperitoneal primary who relapsed after chemotherapy had similar long-term salvage rates to those reported for patients with relapsed metastatic gonadal GCT.

The patient described in the vignette was successfully treated with 4 cycles of chemotherapy for a mediastinal primary GCT. However, he died shortly afterward due to acute leukemia. The short period between chemotherapy and the development of leukemia argues against treatment toxicity, since chemotherapy-induced second malignancies usually take years to develop. Hematologic disorders associated with EGCTs, especially in the megakaryocytic line, had been described in the literature with relative frequency. These had been reported almost exclusively in association with mediastinal NSGCTs, with an incidence in this subset of patients as high as 6%. These disorders are usually diagnosed within months of the diagnosis of mediastinal GCT (median time to onset of 6 months), and sometimes are diagnosed concurrently. They follow a rather aggressive course with a poor response to treatment, with a median survival time of 5 months. Cytogenetic analysis of leukemic cells frequently reveals an isochromosome i(12p), which suggests a common carcinogenesis pathway with the original GCT.

## DEVELOPING CONCEPTS IN GCT RESPONSIVENESS TO CONVENTIONAL THERAPY

Chemo-refractory GCTs are associated with poor outcomes; thus management of this population remains challenging. Recent studies have begun to shed more insight on testicular cancer at the molecular level, which may have future therapeutic implications. The association of mismatch repair (MMR) deficiency and microsatellite instability (MSI) is being evaluated in cisplatin resistance in human GCTs. A control–cohort study analyzed MSI, BRAF, and KRAS mutations in 100 control GCTs (50 seminomas and 50 nonseminomas) and 35 cisplatin-based chemotherapy-resistant

GCTs. Resistant tumors showed a higher incidence of MSI than controls: 26% versus 0% in 2 or more loci ($P < .0001$). All resistant tumors were wild-type KRAS, and 2 controls (2%) contained a KRAS mutation. There was a significantly higher incidence of BRAF V600E mutation in resistant tumors compared with controls: 26% versus 1% ($P < .0001$). BRAF mutations were highly correlated with MSI ($P = .006$), and MSI and mutated BRAF were correlated with weak or absent staining for human mutL homolog 1 (hMLH1) ($P = .017$ and $P = .008$). Low or absent staining of hMLH1 was correlated with promoter hypermethylation ($P < .001$). Tumors lacking expression of hMLH1 or MSH6 were significantly more frequent in resistant GCTs than in controls ($P = .001$ and $.0036$, respectively). Further studies are needed to validate findings (43).

A single institution study evaluating data on 304 GCT patients treated with bleomycin containing chemotherapy from 1997 to 2003 has shown potential role of a gene polymorphism involving bleomycin hydrolase (BLMH), an enzyme that inactivates bleomycin. BLMH gene single nucleotide polymorphism (SNP) A1450G showed a significant effect on GCT-related survival. The homozygous variant (G/G) genotype was associated with decreased GCT-related survival compared with the heterozygous and wild-type variants. Furthermore, the G/G genotype showed a higher relapse rate compared to the other genotypes (44).

## REVIEW QUESTIONS

Normal laboratory values

| | |
|---|---|
| AFP, serum | <10 ng/mL |
| βhCG | <3 mIU/mL |
| LDH, serum | 80–225 U/L |

1. A 32-year-old male presents to his primary care physician with dragging sensation in his left testicle. Testicular examination is normal but scrotal ultrasound reveals a 1.0-cm hypoechoic lesion. His contralateral testicle is normal. Routine lab work is normal. Serum alpha-fetoprotein (AFP) is 780 ng/mL, beta human chorionic gonadotropin 50 IU/L, and lactate dehydrogenase 260 IU/L. CT scan does not show any other masses or lymphadenopathy. Left inguinal orchiectomy is performed. Pathology shows 99% seminoma and 1% yolk sac component and involves tunica albuginea but not tunica vaginalis. Serum tumor markers are normal when checked after 4 weeks. Which of following statements is correct?

   (A) Patient has a pure seminoma
   (B) Patient has stage 1B germ cell tumor (GCT) because AFP is mildly elevated (<1000 ng/mL) before orchiectomy
   (C) Post-orchiectomy, the best approach is to give 3 cycles of bleomycin, etoposide, and cisplatin to this patient

   (D) Surveillance or retroperitoneal lymph node dissection (RPLND) is a reasonable option at this point
   (E) Presence of yolk sac component makes this a high-risk stage 1 GCT

2. A 19-year-old male presents to his primary care provider with slight enlargement of his right testicle. He is monogamous and denies any urethral discharge. Physical examination shows slight enlargement of his right testicle. His left scrotum is empty. Scrotal ultrasound shows a 1.5-cm mass in his right testicle, whereas the left testicle could not be visualized. The patient says he has always had 1 testicle. Alpha-fetoprotein (AFP) is 976 ng/mL, beta human chorionic gonadotropin 4336 IU/L, and lactate dehydrogenase (LDH) 376 IU/L. CT scan of abdomen confirms undescended testicle and no other masses or lymph nodes identified. Chest radiograph is clear. The patient is counseled about sperm banking prior to orchiectomy because his left testicle is undescended and likely nonfunctional. Sperm banking is expedited and patient undergoes right inguinal orchiectomy within 1 week. Pathology shows nonseminomatous germ cell tumor with no lymphovascular invasion. Four weeks after orchiectomy, serum tumor markers (STMs) are improving (AFP = 428 ng/mL, βhCG = 677 IU/L, and LDH = 122 IU/L). What should be next step in management of this patient?

   (A) Surveillance with repeat STMs and CT scan of abdomen in 6 weeks because there is no other evidence of disease and tumor markers are improving after orchiectomy.
   (B) retroperitoneal lymph node dissection
   (C) Bleomycin, etoposide, and cisplatin (BEP) × 1–2 cycles
   (D) BEP × 3 cycles or etoposide, cisplatin (EP) × 4 cycles and removal of undescended testicle
   (E) Liver MRI to evaluate for occult hepatocellular carcinoma given persistent elevation of AFP

3. A 29-year-old law student presented to the emergency department with left testicular pain. Physical examination shows slight enlargement of his left testicle. Scrotal ultrasound does not show torsion but a 2-cm testicular mass is identified. Contralateral testicle is normal. CT scan of abdomen shows a 1.7-cm retroperitoneal lymph node with no other masses. Chest radiograph is clear. Serum tumor markers (STMs) show alpha-fetoprotein = 826 ng/mL, beta human chorionic gonadotropin = 7435 IU/L, and lactate dehydrogenase = 301 IU/L. Left inguinal radical orchiectomy is performed, which shows nonseminomatous germ cell tumors (70% yolk sac, 20% seminoma, and 10% teratoma). STMs checked 4 weeks after orchiectomy are normal. Patient undergoes retroperitoneal lymph node dissection and 6 lymph nodes are involved with metastases. Pulmonary function tests reveal diffusing

capacity of the lung for carbon monoxide 60% of the predicted value as patient reports a prior diagnosis of bronchiolitis obliterans organizing pneumonia in past. What should be the next step in management?

(A) Bleomycin, etoposide, and cisplatin (BEP) × 3 cycles or etoposide and cisplatin (EP) x 4 cycles
(B) Gemcitabine/oxaliplatin x 3 cycles
(C) BEP × 4 cycles
(D) EP × 2 cycles
(E) Surveillance because all retroperitoneal lymph nodes involved are apparently removed and STMs have normalized

4. A 39-year-old male presents to the emergency room with a 4-week history of progressively worsening dry cough, chest pressure, and lower back pain. Chest x-ray reveals multiple lung nodules. He is a lifelong nonsmoker and lives a healthy lifestyle. CT chest, abdomen, and pelvis show retroperitoneal lymphadenopathy. Serum lactate dehydrogenase (LDH) is 799 IU/L. Scrotal ultrasound reveals 1.4-cm hypoechoic lesion in the right testicle. The alpha-fetoprotein (AFP) level is 9420 ng/mL and beta human chorionic gonadotropin (βhCG) is 41550 IU/L. An urgent R inguinal orchiectomy is performed, which shows nonseminomatous germ cell tumors (60% choriocarcinoma, 30% yolk sac tumor, and 10% teratoma). Post-orchiectomy tumor markers are AFP: 1760 ng/mL, LDH: 327 IU/L, and βhCG: 6650 IU/L. Patient receives 4 cycles of bleomycin, etoposide, and cisplatin (BEP). Post-chemotherapy CT scans show partial response, but there are residual 2-cm solitary R lung mass and 2.2-cm solitary retroperitoneal lymph node. Serum tumor markers have normalized. What should be the most appropriate next step in management?

(A) Thoracotomy and resection of lung lesion
(B) Retroperitoneal lymph node dissection (RPLND) and resection of lung lesion
(C) PET CT scan
(D) Second-line chemotherapy

5. A 27-year-old male presents to his primary care physician with a 4-week history of dry cough, chest pressure, and night sweats. A chest radiograph performed in the office does not show evidence of pneumonia but the mediastinum is widened. CT scans confirm a 6-cm mediastinal mass without any other masses. Routine lab work is within normal limits. Testicular ultrasound is normal. Alpha-fetoprotein is 3746 ng/mL, beta human chorionic gonadotropin 13 IU/L, and lactate dehydrogenase 476 IU/L. Biopsy reports nonseminomatous germ cell tumor. Which statement is correct about this tumor?

(A) Flourescence in situ hybridization (FISH) analysis frequently reveals an isochromosome i(12p)

(B) This tumor carries a better prognosis than pure seminoma
(C) This patient is at risk of developing chronic myeloid leukemia
(D) This tumor is expected to respond well to mediastinal irradiation
(E) Surgery will not play a significant role in salvage treatment of this patient

6. A 21-year-old male presents with a 4-month history of progressive swelling of his right testicle. Physical examination and ultrasound reveal a 5-cm testicular mass. Tumor markers are drawn, revealing lactate dehydrogenase: 250 IU/L, alpha-fetoprotein: 100 ng/mL, and beta human chorionic gonadotropin: 15 IU/L. A right inguinal radical orchiectomy is performed and final pathology confirms pure seminoma. Staging CT scan of abdomen and pelvis as well as chest radiograph are normal. Which is the next best step of management?

(A) Surveillance
(B) Adjuvant carboplatin × 1 cycle
(C) Obtain a second pathology consultation
(D) Adjuvant radiation

7. A 25-year-old male presents with a 2-month history of left testicular swelling. His workup revealed a 4.5-cm mass in his left testicle. Staging scans were negative for retroperitoneal and abdominal adenopathy. Chest radiograph was normal. Postoperative tumor markers were normal and final pathology revealed pure seminoma. The patient is an international student who wishes to resume his studies abroad once he completes his therapy and does not feel that he will be able to comply with a rigorous surveillance scheduled. Which adjuvant therapy is best for this patient?

(A) Surveillance
(B) Adjuvant bleomycin, etoposide, and cisplatin × 3 cycles
(C) Adjuvant carboplatin (AUC 7) × 3 cycles
(D) Adjuvant radiation

8. A 26–year-old male has been recently diagnosed with testicular cancer. He has undergone a right inguinal orchiectomy, which revealed a 5-cm pure seminoma. His staging scans revealed a 7-cm retroperitoneal lymph node as well as pulmonary and liver metastases. The most appropriate therapy in this patient is:

(A) Bleomycin, etoposide, and cisplatin (BEP) × 4 cycles
(B) BEP × 3 cycles
(C) Adjuvant carboplatin (AUC 7) × 2 cycles
(D) Etoposide, cisplatin × 3 cycles

9. A 25-year-old male presents to your office for a new patient evaluation after he was discharged from the

local hospital with a diagnosis of testicular carcinoma. He underwent a left radical orchiectomy. Upon presentation, his complete blood counts and complete metabolic profile were within normal limits. Prior to orchiectomy, his lactate dehydrogenase was 700 IU/L, beta human chorionic gonadotropin 7,000 IU/mL, and alpha-fetoprotein 1250 ng/mL. His pathology was consistent with nonseminomatous germ cell tumor (50% embryonal carcinoma, 35% choriocarcinoma, and 30% teratoma). His staging scans revealed a 3-cm retroperitoneal mass. There were no other sites of metastasis. Which is the next best step of management?

(A) Proceed with adjuvant bleomycin, etoposide, and cisplatin x 3 cycles
(B) Retroperitoneal lymph node dissection
(C) Repeat tumor markers
(D) Radiation therapy

10. A 29-year-old male presented with progressive shortness of breath and dyspnea on exertion, as well as abdominal and back pain. Chest imaging revealed innumerable bilateral pulmonary nodules and bulky mediastinal adenopathy. On further review, the patient also mentioned that his right testicle was swollen for the past 6 months, which developed after a groin injury after playing soccer. Physical examination and testicular examination revealed a 4-cm testicular mass; CT abdomen and pelvis also revealed bulky retroperitoneal adenopathy. He was instantly taken to OR for radical orchiectomy, which revealed a mixed germ cell tumor (50% choriocarcinoma, 40% embryonal carcinoma, and 10% seminoma). Post-orchiectomy, lactate dehydrogenase was 462 IU/L, beta human chorionic gonadotropin was 120,000 IU/mL, and alpha-fetoprotein was 7,350 ng/mL. The best normal management for this patient is:

(A) Etoposide, cisplatin × 4 cycles
(B) Bleomycin, etoposide, and cisplatin × 3 cycles
(C) Etoposide, ifosfamide, cisplatin × 4 cycles
(D) High-dose chemotherapy, followed by autologous stem cell transplant

11. The aforementioned patient completes bleomycin, etoposide, and cisplatin × 4 cycles. The patient has an excellent response with normalization of tumor markers and resolution of disease on CT scans. The patient undergoes bilateral retroperitoneal lymph node dissection with no evidence of residual disease and proceeds to surveillance. Six months later, his tumor markers begin to slowly rise. Restaging scans reveal 3 pulmonary masses, the largest 3 cm. Which of the following is appropriate for next step of management?

(A) Stereotactic body radiation therapy to pulmonary nodules

(B) Paclitaxel, ifosfamide, cisplatin
(C) Surgical resection of pulmonary nodules
(D) Gemicitabine/oxaliplatin

12. A 21-year-old male is diagnosed with stage IIC seminoma. Post-orchiectomy, he was treated with bleomycin, etoposide, and cisplatin × 3 cycles. After completion of adjuvant chemotherapy, the tumor markers are now normal but restaging CT scans reveal a 2-cm mass in the retroperitoneum. Which is the best next step of management?

(A) Surgical resection
(B) Radiation therapy
(C) PET CT
(D) Surveillance

13. Which of the following statements regarding brain metastases in testicular cancer is *true*?

(A) Radiation therapy should always be included in the initial management of brain metastases
(B) Because some of the chemotherapy agents in first-line regimens for testicular cancer have blood–brain barrier penetrance, it may be reasonable to manage brain metastases with systemic chemotherapy, particularly in chemotherapy-naïve-patients with limited central nervous system (CNS) compromise
(C) Patients who present with nonsolitary brain metastases at relapse usually have a better prognosis than patients who present with brain metastases at diagnosis
(D) Whole-brain radiation therapy is the best management for a solitary brain metastasis that persists after initial chemotherapy

## REFERENCES

1. Siegel R, Naishadham D, Jemel A, et al. Cancer statistics, 2013. *CA Cancer J Clin.* 2013;63:11–30.
2. Oh J, Landman J, Evers A, et al. Management of the postpubertal patient with cryptorchidism: an updated analysis. *J Urol.* 2002;167:1329.
3. Fossa SD, Chen J, Schonfeld SJ, et al. Risk of contralateral testicular cancer: a population-based study of 29,515 U.S. men. *J Natl Cancer Inst.* 2005;97:1056.
4. Bosl GJ, Ilson DH, Rodriguez E, et al. Clinical relevance of the i(12p) marker chromosome in germ cell tumors. *J Natl Cancer Inst.* 1994;86:349.
5. Ulbright, TM. Germ cell tumors of the gonads: a selective review emphasizing problems in differential diagnosis, newly appreciated, and controversial issues. *Mod Pathol.* 2005;18(suppl 2):S61.
6. Bosl GJ, Motzer RJ. Medical progress: testicular germ-cell cancer. *N Engl J Med.* 1997;337:242.
7. International Germ Cell Cancer Collaborative Group. International germ cell consensus classification: a prognostic factor-based staging system for metastatic germ cell cancers. *J Clin Oncol.* 1997;15:594–603.
8. National Comprehensive Cancer Network. NCCN clinical practice guidelines in oncology: testicular cancer V.1.2014. http://

www.nccn.org/professionals/physician_gls/ f_guidelines.asp. Accessed April 20, 2014

9. Warde P, Specht L, Horwich A, et al. Prognostic factors for relapse in stage I seminoma managed by surveillance: a pooled analysis. *J Clin Oncol.* 2002;20:4448.

10. Travis LB, Curtis RE, Storm H, et al. Risk of second malignant neoplasms among long-term survivors of testicular cancer. *J Natl Cancer Inst.* 1997;89:1429.

11. Jones WG, Fossa SD, Mead GM, et al. Randomized trial of 30 versus 20 Gy in the adjuvant treatment of stage I testicular seminoma: a report on Medical Research Council Trial TE18, European Organization for the Research and Treatment of Cancer Trial 30942 (ISRCTN18525328). *J Clin Oncol.* 2005;23:1200.

12. Oliver RT, Mead GM, Rustin GJ, et al. Randomized trial of carboplatin versus radiotherapy for stage I seminoma: mature results on relapse and contralateral testis cancer rates in MRC TE19/EORTC 30982 study (ISRCTN 27163214). *J Clin Oncol.* 2011;29:957.

13. Read G, Stenning SP, Cullen MH, et al. Medical Research Council prospective study of surveillance for stage I testicular teratoma. Medical Research Council Testicular Tumors Working Party. *J Clin Oncol.* 1992;10:1762–1768.

14. Spermon JR, Roeleveld TA, van del Poel HG, et al. Comparison of surveillance and retroperitoneal lymph node dissection in stage I nonseminomatous germ cell tumors. *Urology.* 2002;59: 923–929.

15. Sogani PC, Perrotti M, Herr HW, et al. Clinical stage I testis cancer: long-term outcome of patients on surveillance. *J Urol.* 1998;159(3):855–858.

16. Hermans BP, Sweeney CJ, Foster RS, et al. Risk of systemic metastases in clinical stage I nonseminoma germ cell testis tumor managed by retroperitoneal lymph node dissection. *J Urol.* 2000;163(6):1721–1724.

17. Tandstad T, Dahl O, Cohn-Cedermark G, et al. *Risk-Adapted Treatment in Clinical Stage I Nonseminomatous Germ Cell Testicular Cancer: The SWENOTECA Management Program.* J *Clin Oncol.* 2009;27:2122–2128.

18. Detti B, Livi L, Scoccianti S, et al. Management of stage II testicular seminoma over a period of 40 years. *Urol Oncol: Semin Ori Investig.* 2009;27:534–538.

19. Domont J, Massard C, Patrikidou A, et al. A risk-adapted strategy of radiotherapy or cisplatin-based chemotherapy in stage II seminoma. *Urol Oncol: Semin Ori Investig.* 2013;31:697–705.

20. Herr HW, Sheinfeld J, Puc HS, et al. Surgery for a postchemotherapy residual mass in seminom? *J Urol.* 1997;157:860–862.

21. De Santis M, Becherer A, Bokemeyer C, et al. 2–18 Fluoro-deoxy-d-glucose positron emission tomography is a reliable predictor for viable tumor in postchemotherapy seminoma: an update of the prospective multicentric SEMPET trial. *J Clin Oncol.* 2004;22:1034–1039.

22. Spiess PE, Kassouf W, Brown GA, et al. Surgical management of growing teratoma syndrome: the M. D. Anderson Cancer Center experience. *J Urol.* 2007;177(4):1330–1334.

23. Ehrlich Y, Brames MJ, Beck SDW, et al. Long-term follow-up of cisplatin combination chemotherapy in patients with disseminated nonseminomatous germ cell tumors: is a postchemotherapy retroperitoneal lymph node dissection needed after complete remission? *J Clin Oncol.* 2010;28(4):531–536.

24. Nichols CR, Catalano P, Crawford ED, et al. Randomized comparison of cisplatin and etoposide and either bleomycin or ifosfamide in treatment of advanced disseminated germ cell tumors; an Eastern Cooperative Oncology Group, Southwest Oncology Group, and Cancer and Leukemia Group B study. *J Clin Oncol.* 1998;16:1287–1293.

25. De Wit R, Skoneczna I, Daugaard G, et al. Randomized phase III study comparing paclitaxel–bleomycin, etoposide, and cisplatin (BEP) to standard BEP in intermediate-prognosis germ-cell cancer: intergroup study EORTC 30983. *J Clin Oncol.* 2012;30:792–799.

26. Cagini L, Nicholson AG, Horwich A, et al. Thoracic metastasectomy for germ cell tumors: long term survival and prognostic factors. *Ann Oncol.* 1998;9:1185–1991.

27. Steyerberg EW, Keizer HJ, Messemer JE, et al. Residual pulmonary masses after chemotherapy for metastatic nonseminomatous germ cell tumor. Prediction of histology. ReHiT Study Group. *Cancer.* 1997;79:345–355.

28. Christian JA, Huddart RA, Norman A, et al. Intensive induction chemotherapy with CBOP/BEP in patients with poor prognosis germ cell tumors. *J Clin Oncol.* 2003;21:871–877.

29. Bower M, Newlands E, Holden L, et al. Treatment of men with metastatic non-seminomatous germ cell tumours with cyclical POMB/ACE chemotherapy. *Ann Oncol.* 1997;8:477–483.

30. Motzer RJ, Nichols CJ, Margolin KA, et al. Phase III randomized trial of conventional-dose chemotherapy with or without high-dose chemotherapy and autologous hematopoietic stem-cell rescue as first-line treatment for patients with poor-prognosis metastatic germ cell tumors. *J Clin Oncol.* 2007;25(3):247–256.

31. Loehrer PJ Sr, Gonin R, Nichols CR, et al. Vinblastine plus ifosfamide plus cisplatin as initial salvage therapy in recurrent germ cell tumor. *J Clin Oncol.* 1998;16:2500–2504.

32. Motzer RJ, Sheinfeld J, Mazumdar M, et al. Paclitaxel, ifosfamide, and cisplatin second-line therapy for patients with relapsed testicular germ cell cancer. *J Clin Oncol.* 2000;18:2413–2418.

33. Mead GM, Cullen MH, Huddart R, et al. A phase II trial of TIP (paclitaxel, ifosfamide and cisplatin) given as second-line (post-BEP) salvage chemotherapy for patients with metastatic germ cell cancer: a medical research council trial. *Br J Cancer* 2005;93:178–184.

34. Kollmannsberger C, Beyer J, Liersch R, et al. Combination chemotherapy with gemcitabine plus oxaliplatin in patients with intensively pretreated or refractory germ cell cancer: a study of the German testicular cancer study group. *J Clin Oncol.* 2004;22:108–114.

35. Bokemeyer C, Oechsle K, Honecker F. Combination chemotherapy with gemcitabine, oxaliplatin, and paclitaxel in patients with cisplatin-refractory or multiply relapsed germ-cell tumors: a study of the German Testicular Cancer Study Group. *Ann Oncol.* 2008;19(3):448–453.

36. Beyer J, Kramar A, Mandanas R, et al. High-dose chemotherapy as salvage treatment in germ cell tumors: a multivariate analysis of prognostic variables. *J Clin Oncol.* 1996;14:2638–2645.

37. Feldman DR, Sheinfeld J, Bajorin DF, et al. TI-CE high-dose chemotherapy for patients with previously treated germ cell tumors: results and prognostic factor analysis. *J Clin Oncol.* 2010;28;1706–1713.

38. Einhorn LH, Williams SD, Chamness A, et al. High-dose chemotherapy and stem-cell rescue for metastatic germ-cell tumors. *N Engl J Med.* 2007;357(4):340–348.

39. Gremmer R, Schröder ML, Bokkel ten Huinink WW, et al. Successful management of brain metastases from malignant germ cell tumors with standard induction chemotherapy. *J Neurooncol.* 2008;90:335–339.

40. Fossa SD, Bokemeyer C, Gerl A, et al. Treatment outcome of patients with brain metastases from malignant germ cell tumors. *Cancer.* 1999;85:988–997.

41. Bokemeyer C, Nichols CR, Droz JP, et al. Extragonadal germ cell tumors of the mediastinum and retroperitoneum: results from an international analysis. *J Clin Oncol.* 2002;20:1864–1873.

42. Vuky J, Bains M, Bacik J, et al. Role of postchemotherapy adjunctive surgery in the management of patients with nonseminoma arising from the mediastinum. *J Clin Oncol.* 2001;19:682–688.

43. Honecker F, Wermann H, Mayer F, et al. Microsatellite instability, mismatch repair deficiency, and BRAF mutation in treatment-resistant germ cell tumors. *Clin Oncol.* 2009;27:2129–2136.

44. de Haas EC, Zwart N, Meijer C, et al. Variation in bleomycin hydrolase gene is associated with reduced survival after chemotherapy for testicular germ cell cancer. *J Clin Oncol.* 2008;26:1817–1823.

# 15

## Kidney Cancer

BENJAMIN Y. SCHEIER, JENNY J. KIM, AND BRUCE G. REDMAN

## EPIDEMIOLOGY, RISK FACTORS, NATURAL HISTORY, AND PATHOLOGY

Renal cell carcinoma (RCC) comprises approximately 3–5% of all malignancies with an expected 63,920 new cases and 13,860 deaths in the United States in 2014. It is the sixth most common malignancy in U.S. men and the eighth most common malignancy in U.S. women (1). The median age at diagnosis of RCC is 60 years. Although the gap is narrowing, there is a male predominance in incidence with a male:female ratio of 2:1. Over the last 50 years, the number of new cases of RCC has also steadily increased, largely due to noninvasive imaging studies that permit detection of small, organ-confined disease amenable to definitive therapy. The incidence of advanced disease has also increased over the same period, although the reason for this increase remains unclear.

Several risk factors have been implicated in the development of RCC. Smoking has been shown to double the risk of developing RCC. Obesity (specifically increased body mass index) is also associated with an increased risk of RCC, although specific dietary associations are not well defined. Exposure to chemical carcinogens such as cadmium, asbestos, and petroleum by-products is linked to an increased risk of RCC as well. Furthermore, individuals with end-stage renal disease and acquired renal cystic disease have a higher risk of developing RCC as compared to the general population. Despite these associations, most patients with RCC are without clearly identifiable environmental and/or lifestyle risk factors.

Kidney cancer can also be a feature of several recognizable genetic syndromes and approximately 5% of all RCC cases may be considered to have a strong heritable component. For example, hereditary papillary renal carcinoma is an autosomal dominant hereditary syndrome marked by the occurrence of multifocal, bilateral kidney tumors with a papillary histology. This syndrome has been shown to be due to mutations in the MET proto-oncogene (2). Another well-recognized genetic syndrome is von-Hippel Lindau (VHL) disease, which is an autosomal dominant disorder with a wide spectrum of vascular tumors, including hemangioblastomas of the central nervous system, retinal angiomas, serous cystadenomas, and neuroendocrine tumors of the pancreas, as well as clear cell RCCs. Renal cell tumors associated with VHL syndrome tend to be early onset and multifocal. VHL is caused by mutations in the VHL tumor suppressor gene on chromosome 3p25 (3). The incidence of VHL syndrome is approximately 1 in 36,000 births.

The prognosis of RCC depends largely on the extent of disease (see the American Joint Committee of Cancer [AJCC] staging system subsequently), nuclear differentiation (Fuhrman grade), and clinical factors (performance status). Several prognostic models have been developed over the years, including the University of California at Los Angeles (UCLA)-Integrated Staging System (UISS), the mostly widely and extensively studied model, which takes into account several factors mentioned earlier in predicting patients' long-term outcome (4) (Table 15.1).

RCC consists of several histological subtypes, with the clear cell subtype comprising approximately 80% of all RCC. Other histological subtypes include papillary, chromophobe, oncocytic, collecting duct, unclassified, and medullary, each with its distinct genetic, histological, and clinical characteristics (5,6) (see Figure 15.1).

**Table 15.1** UCLA Integrated Staging System (UISS)

| UISS Stage | 1997 TNM Stage | Fuhrman Grade | ECOG PS | 2-Year Survival (%) | 5-Year Survival (%) |
|---|---|---|---|---|---|
| I | I | 1,2 | 0 | 96 | 94 |
| II | I | 1,2 | >1 | 89 | 67 |
|  | I | 3,4 | Any |  |  |
|  | II | Any | Any |  |  |
|  | III | Any | 0 |  |  |
|  | III | 1 | >1 |  |  |
| III | III | 2–4 | >1 | 66 | 39 |
|  | IV | 1,2 | 0 |  |  |
| IV | IV | 3,4 | 0 | 42 | 23 |
|  |  | 1–3 | >1 |  |  |
| V | IV | 4 | >1 | 9 | 0 |

ECOG, Eastern Cooperative Oncology Group; PS, performance status; TNM, Tumor, Node, Metastasis; UISS, UCLA Integrated Staging System.

| | Clear cell | Papillary | Chromophobe |
|---|---|---|---|
| Histology | 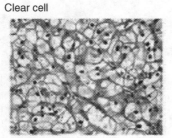 | 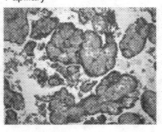 | 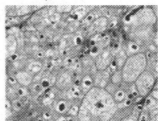 |
| Frequency | 70–80% | 10–15% | 3–5% |
| Genetic abnormalities | • Deletions of chromosome 3p segments<br>• Inactvation of VHL gene by mutation and promoter hypermethylation<br>• Gain of chromosome 5q<br>• Loss of chromosomes 8p, 9p, and 14q | • Trisomy of chromosomes 7 and 17<br>• Loss of chromosome Y in men<br>• Gain of chromosomes 12, 16, and 20<br>• Rare mutations of MET proto-oncogene | • Loss of chromosomes Y, 1, 2, 6, 10, 13, 17, and 21 |
| Characteristics | • Compact nests of tumor cells with clear cytoplasm separated by delicate vasculature<br>• Several architectural patterns, including solid, alveolar, and acinar | • Microscopically variable proportions of papillae, tubulopapillae, and tubules<br>• Type I: papillae lined with one layer of tumor cells with scant pale cytoplasm and low-grade nuclei<br>• Type II: abundant eosinophilic cytoplasm and large pseudostratified nuclei with prominent nucleoli | • Cells are large, polygonal with finely reticulated cytoplasm, distinct cell borders, and atypical nuclei with perinuclear halo<br>• Cells can have intensely eosinophilic cytoplasm |

**Figure 15.1**

Major histological subtypes of RCC. VHL, von-Hippel Lindau.

## STAGING

## CASE SUMMARIES

### Limited-Stage RCC

P.A. is a 42-year-old white man with no significant past medical history who presented to his local emergency department with left flank pain and gross hematuria. He had a history of kidney stones; thus, a CT scan of the abdomen and pelvis was performed to rule out a recurrence. The CT scan showed a 7.7 × 6.7 cm enhancing interpolar left renal mass. A CT of the chest revealed no evidence of metastatic disease. P.A. underwent left radical nephrectomy that showed a 7.5 × 6.6 × 4.3 cm RCC, clear cell type, Fuhrman nuclear grade 3 out of 4. The perirenal and renal sinus fat as well as soft tissue resection margins were free of tumor. No angiolymphatic invasion was identified. The pathologic staging was pT2a N0 M0. No additional treatment was recommended and the patient was followed every 6 months by his surgeon without clinical or radiological evidence of disease recurrence.

### Evidence-Based Case Discussion

The classic triad of symptoms of RCC includes flank pain, hematuria, and a palpable mass in the abdomen. However, <10% of patients with kidney cancer have all 3 features, which are typically associated with more advanced disease. Notably, P.A. had hematuria that suggests invasion of the tumor into the collecting system. Staging is mainly accomplished by CT imaging where contrast enhancement correlates with malignant disease in about 80% of cases. Chest imaging is also recommended as part of the initial staging evaluation. Further staging including brain MRI and bone scan are indicated only if there is clinical suspicion of metastases to these sites. This patient has stage II disease, and according to the UISS model, has a 60–70% probability of 5-year survival (Table 15.1). Currently, the recommended treatment for stage I–III RCC is surgical resection (7). Traditional surgical management of RCC is radical nephrectomy that includes resection of the kidney, perirenal fat, regional lymph nodes (LNs), and ipsilateral adrenal gland. However, more recent approaches aim to achieve adequate tumor control while minimizing removal of structures unlikely to be involved with cancer. For example, the National Comprehensive Cancer Network (NCCN) Kidney Cancer panel recommends adrenal gland resection only when involvement is suspected by preoperative CT or in the presence of a large upper pole tumor (7). Other contemporary trends in resection of kidney cancer include an increased use of partial nephrectomy (also known as "nephron sparing surgery") using open as well as laparoscopic and robotic approaches, thereby maximally preserving the patient's renal function.

| Staging System for Renal Cell Carcinoma | |
| --- | --- |
| Stage | Description |
| I | Tumor ≤7 cm in greatest dimension, limited to the kidney |
| II | Tumor >7 cm in greatest dimension, limited to the kidney |
| III | Tumor limited to kidney with 1 regional LN involvement<br>*or*<br>Tumor extends into major veins or perinephric tissues but *not* into the ipsilateral adrenal gland and *not* beyond Gerota's fascia with or without regional LN involvement |
| IV | Tumor involves ipsilateral adrenal gland and/or extends beyond Gerota's fascia<br>*or*<br>Involvement of >1 regional LNs<br>*or*<br>Presence of distant metastasis |

LN, lymph node.
*Source: AJCC Cancer Staging Handbook, 7th Edition.*

Radiation therapy to the nephrectomy site as well as systemic immunotherapy with interferon (IFN) or interleuken-2 (IL-2) have been evaluated in the adjuvant setting, but have demonstrated no significant impact on relapse or survival. The recent success of anti-vascular endothelial growth factor (VEGF) therapy in advanced disease has also led to evaluation of these agents in the adjuvant setting. At present, however, there are no data to support routine use of local or systemic adjuvant therapy. Thus, outside of a clinical trial, postsurgical observation remains the standard of care.

Recommended clinical monitoring following primary therapy for RCC should be individualized according to patient factors as well as specific features of the tumor, including grade and stage as they relate to the risk of recurrence (Table 15.1). The majority of recurrences are detected within 3 years of surgery. According to NCCN guidelines, patients should be evaluated at least every 6 months for 2 or 3 years and then annually.

### Locally Advanced RCC

T.D. is a 56-year-old white man who presented to his physician with vague left flank pain of 1-week duration. His physical examination was unremarkable. Urine analysis showed microscopic hematuria without evidence of urinary tract infection. A CT scan of the abdomen showed a 10-cm heterogeneous left renal mass with retroperitoneal lymphadenopathy, the largest of which was 2.5 cm in diameter. A CT scan of the chest was negative for evidence of metastatic disease. T.D. underwent a radical nephrectomy with LN dissection, and pathology review showed a 9.5-cm clear cell RCC, Fuhrman grade 3 or 4 with tumor involvement of the renal vein, and 1 of 10 LNs.

## Evidence-Based Case Discussion

Renal vein invasion of the primary tumor and 1 LN posi-tivity denote pT3 N1, and therefore a stage III disease. In localized disease, routine lymphadenectomy is not generally recommended as evidenced by the European Organization for Research and Treatment of Cancer (EORTC) 30881 trial that randomized 772 patients to nephrectomy with or without regional lymphadenectomy. After 12 years of follow-up, there was no difference in disease-specific mortality with lymphadenectomy (8). However, only 4% of the patients in the lymphadenec-tomy group had positive LNs on pathology review, sug-gesting that majority of patients enrolled in the study may have been low-risk patients who likely did not need lymphadenectomy. Currently, however, patients with sus-pected LN involvement on preoperative imaging studies are candidates for extended LN dissection, which may provide a survival advantage in this subset of patients. As in the previous case of localized RCC, standard of care after nephrectomy is surveillance. The potential benefit of adjuvant therapy using targeted agents is currently under investigation in ongoing clinical trials.

## Advanced RCC

T.M. is a 67-year-old white woman who presented with left lower quadrant pain. Diverticulitis was suspected. However, a CT scan of the abdomen and pelvis revealed an 8-cm left renal mass suspicious for RCC. CT of the chest showed no evidence of metastatic disease. T.M. under-went a left radical nephrectomy that revealed a 7.7-cm, Fuhrman grade 2 or 3 clear cell RCC. She embarked on surveillance postoperatively and remained free of recur-rence. Two years postnephrectomy, however, the patient complained of right buttock discomfort and a surveillance CT scan revealed a 7.7 × 5.6 cm lesion in the right ilium. A CT-guided biopsy of the right iliac bone confirmed metastatic RCC. A bone scan showed increased uptake in the right iliac bone and in the left proximal femur sugges-tive of metastases. A CT scan of the chest showed mul-tiple bilateral lung nodules. Aside from elevated alkaline phosphatase at 296 IU/L, all laboratory studies including hemoglobin, platelet count, and absolute neutrophil count, along with serum calcium, albumin, and lactate dehydro-genase (LDH), were normal. Her Karnofsky performance status (KPS) was 90%.

## Evidence-Based Case Discussion

T.M. has metastatic clear cell RCC with lesions in the ilium, left femur, and lungs after definitive nephrectomy 2 years earlier. With regard to prognosis, a large retrospec-tive multivariate analysis from Memorial Sloan Kettering Cancer Center (during a time period when cytokines were often used in the treatment of metastatic RCC) defined the

following negative prognostic variables in advanced RCC patients (9):

- A KPS <80%
- Serum LDH level >1.5 times the upper limit of normal
- Corrected serum calcium >10 mg/dL (2.5 mmol/L)
- Hemoglobin concentration below the lower limit of normal
- Absence of nephrectomy (i.e., no disease-free interval)

These prognostic factors subdivide patients into 3 risk groups: a favorable-risk group (no risk factors), an intermediate-risk group (1 or 2 risk factors), and a poor-risk group (3 or more risk factors). Survival rates at 1 year for favorable-, intermediate-, and poor- patients are 71%, 42%, and 12%, respectively, and at 3 years are 31%, 7%, and 0%, respectively.

Prognostic factors for survival of advanced RCC in the targeted therapy era have also been reported. A multivari-ate analysis of baseline characteristics seen in 645 patients who were treated with sunitinib, sorafenib, or bevacizumab also confirmed the relevance of KPS < 80, time from origi-nal diagnosis to treatment of <1 year, hemoglobin less than the lower limit of normal, and elevated serum calcium. Two other laboratory parameters including neutrophil count and platelet count greater than the upper limit of normal were also significantly related to prognosis. These prognostic factors may be helpful in patient care and coun-seling as well as proper patient stratification and selection in clinical trial design in the targeted therapy era (10).

In the past, treatment options for patients with advanced RCC were limited to cytokine therapy or participation in a clinical trial. Importantly, high-dose IL-2 still remains the only modality of therapy that can result in long-term disease remission in a small, but selective group of patients with advanced clear cell RCC. Favorable patient character-istics for high-dose IL-2 include a clear cell histology, good performance status ( Eastern Cooperative Oncology Group [ECOG] 0–1), minimal disease burden, and lung-only dis-ease. Recently updated data reported in a single-arm phase II study (SELECT) confirmed the association between an improved response outcome and these patient selection cri-teria—results that were reported at the American Society of Clinical Oncology 2010 Annual Meeting (11).

Furthermore, an improved understanding of the biol-ogy of renal cell cancer (including distinctive characteris-tics such as VHL silencing and resulting hypoxia-induced factor accumulation and a heavy dependence on angiogen-esis for viability and progression) has provided the mecha-nistic rationale for the development and Food and Drug Administration (FDA) approval of 7 new agents for the treat-ment of RCC (Table 15.2). These agents target the VEGF pathway (sunitinib, sorafenib, bevacizumab, pazopanib, and axitinib) and the mammalian target of rapamycin (mTOR) pathway (temsirolimus and everolimus), both of which have

**Table 15.2** Targeted Therapy in Advanced RCC

| Agent (Ref.) | PFS (Months) | OS (Months) | Setting |
|---|---|---|---|
| Sunitinib (12) | 11 vs. 5 | 26.4 vs. 21.8 | First line vs. IFN-α |
| Sorafenib (13) | 5.5 vs. 2.8 | 17.8 vs. 15.2 | Second line vs. placebo |
| Pazopanib (14) | 9.2 vs. 4.2 | 22.9 vs. 20.5 | First line vs. placebo |
| Bevacizumab + IFN-α (15,16) | 10.2 vs. 5.4 | 23.3 vs. 21.3 | First line with IFN-α vs. IFN-α alone |
|  | 8.5 vs. 5.2 | 18.3 vs. 17.4 |  |
| Temsirolimus (18) | 5.5 vs. 3.1 | 10.9 vs. 7.3 | First line, poor-risk patients vs. IFN-α |
| Everolimus (19) | 5.5 vs. 1.9 | 14.8 vs. 14.4 | Second line vs. placebo |
| Axitinib (20) | 6.7 vs. 4.7 | 20.1 vs. 19.2 | Second line vs. sorafenib |

IFN-α, interferon-alpha; OS, overall survival; RCC, renal cell carcinoma; PFS, progression-free survival.

been described to be critical pathways in tumor survival, proliferation, and angiogenesis in not only renal cell cancer but also several other solid tumors. Most of these agents have been tested in good- and intermediate-prognosis clear cell renal cell cancer patients and have shown proven superiority in progression-free survival (PFS) relative to IFN, a standard frontline therapy in the past. Currently, sunitinib, pazopanib, or the combination of bevacizumab plus IFN represent optimal choices as frontline agents in the treatment of patients with good- and intermediate-prognosis clear cell metastatic RCC, assuming they are not candidates for high-dose IL-2 (12,14–16). Comparison across clinical trials has indicated that the targeted therapies have similar efficacies. Understandably, due to the crossover design employed in the large phase III frontline trials and variability in eligibility criteria, survival advantage and superiority of any of these regimens have been difficult to elucidate. Recently, a head-to-head phase III trial involving >1000 patients compared sunitinib and pazopanib in the frontline setting for advanced RCC. The response rates, PFS, and overall survival were comparable. However, compared with patients receiving pazopanib, patients in the sunitinib arm had higher incidences of fatigue, myelosuppression, and severe palmar-plantar erythrodysesthesia (17).

Class toxicities from the VEGF tyrosine kinase inhibitors include fatigue, hypertension, rash, hand–foot syndrome, diarrhea, myelosuppression, congestive heart failure, and hypothyroidism. Pazopanib can also cause significant hepatotoxicity.

Temsirolimus, an mTOR inhibitor, is the only agent to have been tested in poor prognosis patients, and remains the only agent to have shown a significant survival benefit in poor-prognosis patients to date (18).

Everolimus (Afinitor), another mTOR inhibitor, is an agent of choice in patients with disease refractory to VEGF pathway targeting agents based on a large phase III randomized trial conducted against placebo (19). This study was the first phase III study to demonstrate efficacy of a second-line therapy in patients with progressive disease on a VEGF inhibitor. After studies indicated that patients whose disease progresses on VEGF inhibitors may still benefit from another targeted therapy, research efforts have shifted to optimizing the best treatment sequence of the targeted agents. The AXIS trial, a recent prospective randomized study, compared axitinib, a VEGF selective tyrosine kinase inhibitor, to sorafenib in patients whose disease had progressed on frontline therapy. The median PFS was 6.7 months for patients treated with axitinib compared to 4.7 months for patients receiving sorafenib. In subgroup analysis, the PFS for axitinib was 12 months (vs. 6.5 for sorafenib) in patients who received frontline cytokine therapy and 4.8 months (vs. 3.4 months for sorafenib) after prior sunitinib therapy, suggesting a greater benefit to second-line axitinib in patients previously treated with cytokine therapy. The most common adverse reactions seen with axitinib were diarrhea, hypertension, fatigue, nausea, dysphonia, and hand–foot syndrome (20). Based on the results of this trial, the U.S. FDA approved axitinib for the treatment of advanced RCC after failure of 1 prior systemic therapy.

Unfortunately, most of the non-clear cell histological subtypes tend to have a poorer prognosis as compared to the clear cell subtype, and furthermore, therapeutic recommendations for this subset of patients are not as well characterized. Temsirolimus is the first-line agent based on the result of the subanalysis of the randomized phase III trial that showed its activity across all histologies, although response as well as PFS benefit are modest at best (18). Alternatively, sunitinib and sorafenib also have been shown to exhibit modest activity as shown in retrospective analyses from expanded access trials (21,22). Further research and therapeutic options are much to be desired in this subset of patients at this time. Figure 15.2 represents a current treatment algorithm for the management of metastatic RCC.

Although recent advances in the development of targeted agents have greatly expanded the therapeutic options for the treatment of metastatic RCC, nevertheless durable responses still remain elusive. For example, the upfront combination of targeted therapies has not yielded positive results toward that end. Participation in clinical trials

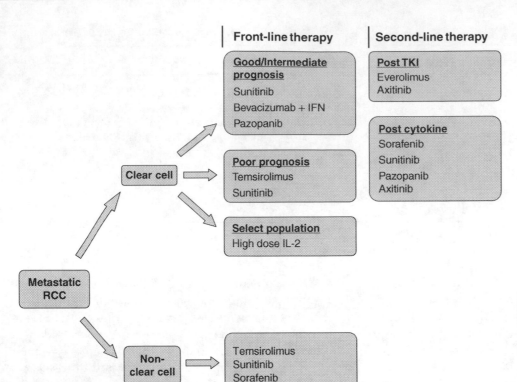

**Figure 15.2**

Treatment algorithm for the management of metastatic RCC. IFN, interferon; IL, interleukin; RCC, renal cell carcinoma; TKI, tyrosine kinase inhibitor.

evaluating new investigational therapies continues to remain an important option for patients with advanced RCC.

It is important to mention the role of cytoreductive nephrectomy in metastatic disease. Data from the IFN era support the use of debulking nephrectomy to improve survival in selected patients with metastatic disease (23). However, similar confirmatory data are lacking in the targeted therapy era. Prospective clinical trials are ongoing to address the issue of cytoreductive nephrectomy in the setting of targeted therapy in metastatic disease. Palliative nephrectomy in advanced disease can be considered for patients with pain, hypercalcemia, or other symptoms due to the primary kidney tumor.

## REVIEW QUESTIONS

1. A 69-year-old man with a past medical history of hypertension presents to his primary care physician with 3 months of fatigue and painless gross hematuria. A CT scan with intravenous contrast reveals a 12-cm mass in the superior pole of the right kidney. There is no radiographic evidence of metastatic disease at the time. He undergoes a right partial nephrectomy with pathology revealing high-grade clear cell carcinoma. He recovers from surgery, and 6 months later, is found to have scattered 1- to 2-cm lung nodules bilaterally on CT imaging. A lung nodule is biopsied and this confirms metastatic clear cell carcinoma. He is then initiated on sunitinib 50 mg by mouth daily for 4 weeks of 6-week cycles.

CT scan 3 months after treatment initiation shows disease response. At his return visit, he endorses grade 2 fatigue. He also endorses a 15-lb weight gain, generalized muscle weakness, and cold sensitivity. Routine lab evaluation reveals a normal complete blood count, kidney, and liver function. Which is the following is the most appropriate next step?

(A) Stop sunitinib and start sorafenib
(B) Stop sunitinib and start pazopanib
(C) Stop sunitinib and start everolimus
(D) Continue sunitinib and evaluate thyroid function
(E) Perform a stress echocardiogram

2. A 64-year-old woman underwent nephrectomy for a large right kidney mass 2 years ago identified by CT scan after the patient reported gross hematuria to her primary care physician. She underwent radical nephrectomy, with pathology revealing a 10-cm tumor, clear cell type, Furham grade III, with 2 of 10 lymph nodes involved. Recent CT of the chest revealed scattered 1- to 2-cm lung nodules and CT of the abdomen revealed two 2-cm lesions in the right hepatic lobe. She presents for recommendations for therapy. She has a history of hypertension, coronary artery disease with a non-ST elevation myocardial infarction requiring percutaneous coronary intervention 5 years ago, insulin-dependent diabetes, and chronic kidney disease, with a baseline creatinine of 1.8 mg/dL (normal: 0.5–1.0 mg/dL). Medications include aspirin, hydrochlorothiazide,

metoprolol, and lisinopril. Physical examination is unremarkable. What would you recommend next?

(A) Initiate high-dose interleukin-2 therapy

(B) Initiate axitinib 5-mg per mouth twice a day

(C) Recommend surgical referral for resection of low-volume hepatic metastases

(D) Initiate carboplatin (adjuvant carboplatin = 5) and paclitaxel (175 mg/m²) q3weeks

(E) Initiate pazopanib, 800 mg by mouth every day

3. You are seeing a 61-year-old man with a history of hyperlipidemia and cholelithiasis 1 week after he was seen in the local emergency department for new onset of right upper quadrant pain. He was diagnosed with recurrent cholelithiasis after CT scan of the abdomen revealed nonobstructing gallstones. CT scan of the abdomen also revealed a 9-cm complex mass of the right kidney. His symptoms were controlled with analgesics and he was discharged home. One week later, his primary care physician refers to you for evaluation. Which is the most appropriate next step in the management of this patient?

(A) Referral to IR for CT-guided fine needle aspiration of R kidney mass

(B) Repeated CT scan of the abdomen with IV contrast in 3 months

(C) Referral to urology for surgical resection of kidney mass

(D) Observation and further imaging based on symptoms

4. A 65-year-old man is seeing you in consultation after undergoing a radical nephrectomy 8 weeks ago for a 10-cm right kidney clear cell carcinoma. Staging CT scans of the chest, abdomen, and pelvis revealed no metastatic disease. Resection was complete and surgical margins were negative. Two of the 11 lymph nodes contained clear cell carcinoma. He has a past medical history of hypertension and diabetes mellitus. Examination is unremarkable. Complete blood count, liver function, and kidney function are within normal limit. What would you recommend next?

(A) Interferon-alpha for 6 months

(B) Sunitinib therapy for 1 year

(C) Adjuvant radiation to nephrectomy surgical bed

(D) Observation

5. Which of the following statements about risk factors associated with kidney cancer is true?

(A) Smoking, but not obesity, has been associated with an increased risk of kidney cancer

(B) Obesity, but not smoking, has been associated with an increased risk of kidney cancer

(C) Smoking and obesity have been associated with an increased risk of kidney cancer

(D) Neither smoking nor obesity has been associated with an increased risk of kidney cancer

6. A 71-year-old man with a history of atrial fibrillation, coronary artery disease, and peripheral artery disease presented to his primary care physician with fatigue, weight loss, and painless hematuria for 2 months. Two weeks ago, he developed acute rib pain and a plain radiograph revealed multiple rib and lung lesions suspicious for malignancy. CT imaging confirmed multiple lung, bone, and liver lesions with a 10-cm mass of the left kidney. Biopsy of 1 of the rib lesions was consistent with metastatic renal cell carcinoma, clear cell type. For the past 3 weeks, he has been quite limited in his ability to care for himself and maintain his home, and now is living with his son. His Karnofsky performance status is 70. Physical examination reveals a thin, chronically ill appearing man with tenderness to palpation on bilateral ribs and left femur. Vital signs are normal. Lab assessment reveals hemoglobin concentration of 10.0 g/dL (normal: 13.5–17.5 g/dL), normal creatinine, corrected serum calcium of 10.8 g/dL (normal: 8.9–9.8 g/dL), and lactate dehydrogenase of 540 U/L (normal: 105–230 U/L). He is interested in starting therapy. What would you recommend next?

(A) Interferon-alpha plus bevacizumab

(B) Everolimus

(C) Temsirolimus

(D) High dose interleuken-2

(E) Pazopanib

## REFERENCES

1. Siegel R, Ma J, Zou Z, et al. Cancer statistics, 2014. *CA Cancer J Clin.* 2014;64:9–29.

2. Schmidt L, Duh FM, Chen F, et al. Germline and somatic mutations in the tyrosine kinase domain of the MET proto-oncogene in papillary renal cancers. *Nat Genet.* 1997;16(1):68–73.

3. Latif F, Tory K, Gnarra J, et al. Identification of the von Hippel-Lindau disease tumor suppressor gene. *Science.* 1993;260(5112):1317–1320.

4. Zisman A, Pantuck AJ, Dorey F, et al. Improved prognostication of renal cell carcinoma using an integrated staging system. *J Clin Oncol.* 2001;19(6):1649–1657.

5. Rini BI, Campbell SC, Escudier B. Renal cell carcinoma. *Lancet.* 2009;373:1119–1132.

6. Linehan WM, Wlather MM, Zbar B. The genetic basis of cancer of the kidney. *J Urol.* 2003;170: 2163–2172.

7. National Comprehensive Cancer Network Guidelines™. Kidney cancer. Version 2.2011. http://www.nccn.org/professionals/physician_gls/pdf/kidney.pdf. Accessed August 12, 2014.

8. Blom JH, van Poppel H, Maréchal JM, et al. EORTC Genitourinary Tract Cancer Group. Radical nephrectomy with and without lymph-node dissection: final results of European Organization for Research and Treatment of Cancer (EORTC) randomized phase 3 trial 30881. *Eur Urol.* 2009;55(1):28–34.

9. Motzer RJ, Mazumdar M, Bacik J, et al. Survival and prognostic stratification of 670 patients with advanced renal cell carcinoma. *J Clin Oncol.* 1999;17(8):2530–2540.

10. Heng DY, Xie W, Regan MM, et al. Prognostic factors for overall survival in patients with metastatic renal cell carcinoma treated with vascular endothelial growth factor-targeted agents: results from a large, multicenter study. *J Clin Oncol.* 2009;27(34):5794–5799.

11. McDermott DF, Ghebremichael MS, Signoretti S, et al. The high-dose aldesleukin (HD IL-2) "SELECT" trial in patients with metastatic renal cell carcinoma (mRCC): ASCO annual meeting proceedings. *J Clin Oncol.* 2010;28(suppl; abstr 4514):15s.

12. Motzer RJ, Hutson TE, Tomczak T, et al. Sunitinib versus interferon alfa in metastatic renal-cell carcinoma. *N Engl J Med.* 2007;356: 115–124.

13. Escudier B, Eisen T, Stadler WM, et al. Sorafenib for treatment of renal cell carcinoma: final efficacy and safety results of the phase III treatment approaches in renal cancer global evaluation trial. *J Clin Oncol.* 2009;27:3312–3318.

14. Sternberg CN, Davis IN, Mardiak J, et al. Pazopanib in locally advanced or metastatic renal cell carcinoma: results of a randomized phase III trial. *J Clin Oncol.* 2010;28:1061–1068.

15. Escudier B, Bellmunt J, Negrier S, et al. Phase III trial of bevacizumab plus interferon alfa-2a in patients with metastatic renal cell carcinoma (AVOREN): final analysis of overall survival. *J Clin Oncol.* 2010;28:2144–2150.

16. Rini BI, Halabi S, Rosenberg JE, et al. Phase III trial of bevacizumab plus interferon alfa versus interferon alfamonotherapy in patients with metastatic renal cell carcinoma: final results of CALGB 90206. *J Clin Oncol.* 2010;28:2137–2143.

17. Motzer RJ, Hutson TE, Cella D, et al. Pazopanib versus sunitinib in metastatic renal-cell carcinoma. *N Engl J Med.* 2013; 369:722–731.

18. Hudes G, Carducci M, Tomczak, P, et al. Temsirolimus, interferon alfa, or both for advanced renal-cell carcinoma. *N Engl J Med.* 2007;356:2271–2281.

19. Motzer RJ, Escudier B, Oudard S, et al. Phase 3 trial of everolimus for metastatic renal cell carcinoma: final results and analysis of prognostic factors. *Cancer.* 2010;116(18):4256–4265.

20. Rini BI, Escudier B, Tomczak P, et al. Comparative effectiveness of axitinib versus sorafenib in advanced renal cell carcinoma (AXIS): a randomized phase III trial. *Lancet.* 2011;378:1931–1939.

21. Gore ME, Szczylik C, Porta C, et al. Safety and efficacy of sunitinib for metastatic renal cell carcinoma: an expanded-access trial. *Lancet Oncol.* 2009;10:757–763.

22. Stadler WM, Figlin RA, McDermott DF, et al. Safety and efficacy results of the advanced renal cell carcinoma sorafenib expanded access program in North America. *Cancer.* 2010;116:1272–1280.

23. Flanigan RC, Salmon SE, Blumenstein BA, et al. Nephrectomy followed by interferon α-2b compared with interferon α-2b alone for metastatic renal-cell cancer. *N Engl J Med.* 2001;345: 1655–1659.

# 16

# *Bladder Cancer*

ERIN F. COBAIN, COLIN J. MOONEY, AND DAVID C. SMITH

## EPIDEMIOLOGY, RISK FACTORS, NATURAL HISTORY, AND PATHOLOGY

Carcinoma of the bladder continues to pose a significant challenge to physicians and patients who attempt to balance the toxicity of overtreating highly curable lower-risk disease while avoiding undertreating lethal high-grade lesions. More than 70,000 patients are expected to be diagnosed with bladder cancer in 2014, whereas >15,000 will ultimately die from their disease (1). The median age of presentation is approximately 70 years, with rare occurrences in individuals younger than 40 years. Three out of four patients will be male; bladder cancer is the 4th and 11th most common cause of cancer in men and women, respectively, in the United States. The incidence of bladder cancer in white men is twice that of African American men; however, African Americans are more likely to die of the disease.

Environmental exposures are implicated in the majority of bladder cancers. In the Western world, tobacco exposure strongly correlates with bladder cancer risk, contributing to 66% of diagnoses in men and 30% in women. Smoking cessation results in an immediate decrease in cancer risk; however, even after 25 years, the risk does not reach that of never smokers. Occupational exposures account for approximately 20% of bladder cancer diagnoses and affect many groups including painters, truck drivers, aluminum workers, leather and textile workers, and others exposed to industrial chemicals. Several medications, such as chronic oral cyclophosphamide, have been implicated in increased risk of bladder cancer. Prolonged exposure to bladder irritants results in an increased incidence of squamous cell carcinoma (SCC) of the bladder rather than transitional cell carcinoma (TCC). Infectious and noninfectious chronic cystitis, often due to a chronic indwelling catheter, renal calculus, or neurogenic bladder,

results in a 25-fold increased risk of SCC bladder cancer. Outside the United States and Western Europe, schistosomiasis has been correlated with SCC and is considered a major public health issue.

The classic presentation of bladder cancer as painless microscopic or, more often, gross hematuria still occurs in the majority of patients. Hematuria is typically intermittent and occurs throughout micturation. All patients with gross hematuria require a urological evaluation. Approximately, one quarter of patients present with irritable bladder symptoms such as frequency, urgency, and dysuria; this is particularly common in those with carcinoma in situ (CIS) of the bladder. Unfortunately, these symptoms may inaccurately be ascribed to benign disorders (urinary tract infections, prostatitis, and passage of renal calculi) resulting in a delay of diagnosis. Advanced disease may present with bladder outlet obstruction from the tumor mass or clot, pelvic or flank pain from ureteral obstruction, lower extremity lymphedema, or deep venous thrombosis due to pelvic lymphatic involvement. Occasionally, advanced disease presents with constitutional symptoms such as weight loss or a symptomatic metastatic focus.

Screening tests to detect early bladder cancer have not been particularly useful, even in high-risk patient populations such as cigarette smokers. Screening tests available include urinalysis to detect microhematuria and urine cytology, which is generally regarded as the gold standard for noninvasive screening for bladder cancer. Detection of abnormal urine cytology has a sensitivity of 40–60% and a specificity >90% (2). While studies using urinalysis as a bladder cancer screening modality in men over the age of 50 years have reported a potential survival benefit for bladder cancer detected by screening as opposed to bladder cancer detected due to symptoms of disease, these studies have been criticized due to lack of randomization and

207

significant differences between the study patient population and the control arm (3). Thus, there remains no clear benefit to screening patients for bladder cancer, even those who are at higher risk of developing the disease.

According to the World Health Organization/ International Society of Urologic Pathology (WHO/ISUP), urothelial cancer is divided into low or high grade based on degree of nuclear anaplasia and architectural abnormalities; invasive urothelial cancer is almost always high grade. Bladder cancer comprises a heterogeneous group of histological entities with a vast majority being of epithelial origin. In Western countries, 90–95% of these are urothelial, also known as TCC. TCC originates from the urinary bladder in 90% of cases, but may also arise from the renal pelvis, ureters, and proximal two thirds of the urethra. SCC accounts for 3–5% of bladder cancer in the United States, but it may represent 75% of diagnoses in areas endemic with *Schistosoma haematobium* infection. Of the remaining subtypes, adenocarcinoma and small cell (neuroendocrine) carcinoma account for 2% and 1%, respectively. TCC with mixed histologies often occur; these should be treated as urothelial carcinomas, with the exception of small cell neuroendocrine cancer, which should be treated with a small cell regimen. Chemotherapy regimens most often used for TCC may be ineffective for pure nontransitional cell entities.

## STAGING

Clinically, bladder cancer is divided into 3 categories: non-muscle-invasive (superficial), muscularis propria-invasive, and metastatic disease, each with differing clinical behavior, approach to management, and prognosis. In the case of noninvasive disease, imaging of the upper tract collecting system should be performed prior to transurethral resection of the bladder tumor (TURBT). If a noninvasive lesion is sessile or of high grade, a pelvic CT should also be considered. In the setting of muscle-invasive disease, workup at the time of diagnosis should include a complete blood count and chemistry profile including alkaline phosphatase. Chest imaging as well as a CT scan of the abdomen/pelvis should be performed to rule out the possibility of metastatic disease. If alkaline phosphatase is elevated or if patients have symptoms suggestive of bone metastases, bone scan should also be performed (4).

### AJCC TNM Staging System for Bladder Cancer

| Stage | Definition |
|-------|------------|
| 0a | Noninvasive papillary carcinoma (Ta), usually low grade |
| 0is | Carcinoma in situ (Tis) |
| I | Subepithelial connective tissue invasion without muscle involvement (T1) |
| II | Invasion of the muscularis propria superficially (T2a) or deep (T2b) |
| III | Microscopic direct perivesicular adipose invasion (T3a) *or* Macroscopic direct perivesicular adipose invasion (T3b) *or* |
| IV | Direct pelvic organ invasion: prostatic stroma, uterus, or vagina (T4a) Direct extension to pelvic/abdominal walls or organ outside pelvis (T4b) *or* Metastasis to regional nodes; ≤2 cm (N1), >2 cm but ≤5 cm (N2), >5 cm (N3) *or* Distant metastasis (M1) |

AJCC, American Joint Committee on Cancer; TNM, tumor, node, metastasis.
*Source: AJCC Cancer Staging Handbook, 7th Edition,* 2010.

## CASE SUMMARIES

### Non-Muscle-Invasive Tumors (Ta, Tis, T1)

M.R. is a 71-year-old male non-smoker who developed painless gross hematuria. M.R. did not initially seek medical attention, attributing his symptoms to the warfarin he was taking for atrial fibrillation. The bleeding resolved spontaneously, but returned with progression to clot formation and irritable bladder symptoms. M.R.'s primary care physician initiated ciprofloxacin empirically for treatment of a presumed bacterial cystitis, but also ordered a urine cytology. This revealed atypical epithelial cells. His symptoms persisted and he was referred to a urologist.

M.R.'s medical history was notable for cardioversion of atrial fibrillation, hypertension, non-insulin dependent diabetes mellitus, dyslipidemia, obstructive sleep apnea, and morbid obesity. Other than a remote 20-pack-year smoking history, his social and family histories were unremarkable. Physical examination was limited due to significant obesity but was otherwise unrevealing. Laboratory evaluation was unremarkable with normal renal, liver, and hematopoietic function. Office cystoscopy revealed visible bladder tumors. CT urogram showed eccentric wall thickening in the right aspect of the urinary bladder, encompassing the right ureterovesicular junction without hydronephrosis or hydroureter. Staging workup showed no lymphadenopathy or evidence of hepatic or pulmonary metastases. Warfarin was held and cystoscopy and bimanual examination under anesthesia were performed with TURBT. A large solitary, sessile tumor was visualized on the right lateral wall. A complete resection was attempted. Pathology revealed invasive high-grade pure papillary urothelial carcinoma without angiolymphatic invasion. Muscularis propria was present in the sample but without invasion. Adjacent CIS was noted.

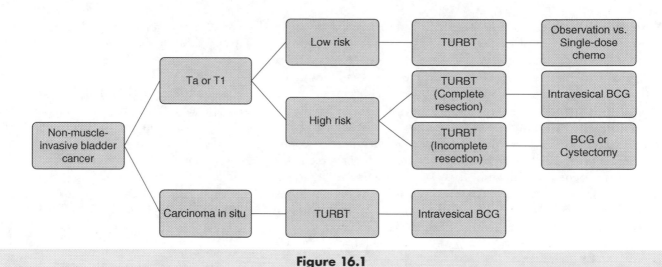

**Figure 16.1**

Treatment of non-muscle-invasive bladder cancer. BCG, bacillus Calmette-Guerin; TURBT, transurethral resection of the bladder tumor.

M.R. underwent a restaging cystoscopy and TURBT 10 weeks after his initial diagnosis, which revealed recurrent high-grade T1 TCC. The tumor was fully resected. The optimal therapy for his cancer was determined to be cystectomy with neobladder formation to prevent the development of muscle-invasive disease. Unfortunately, the risks of complications from the surgery for this patient with multiple comorbidities were felt to outweigh the benefits. After long deliberation with the patient, the decision was made to treat with 6 weeks of bacillus Calmette-Guerin (BCG) intravesical immunotherapy. Repeat TURBT revealed recurrent T1 disease. Consideration of cystectomy was again entertained but the risk of surgical complications remained too great. He underwent intravesicular BCG and follow-up cystoscopy with random biopsies demonstrated no malignant disease. A course of maintenance BCG therapy was completed and he was followed with close observation without evidence of recurrence to date.

## Evidence-Based Case Discussion

The patient described is representative of the average bladder cancer patient: an older man with multiple medical problems initially presenting with hematuria that, after thorough evaluation, revealed a T1 urothelial cancer. Though the term "superficial" is used for Ta, Tis, and T1 tumors, this is a misnomer as T1 lesions invade the submucosa or lamina propria; "non-muscle-invasive" is a more precise description. This group of tumors (Ta, Tis, T1) represent 70% of all new TCC diagnoses.

Cystoscopy with full evaluation of the bladder mucosa and urethra is the initial diagnostic test for bladder cancer detection. If the appearance of the mass on cystoscopy suggests a tumor that is high grade, solid, or muscle invasive, a CT scan of the abdomen and pelvis with and without contrast is recommended prior to TURBT. This allows

evaluation of the local tumor extent and abdominal lymph node involvement as well as synchronous or metachronous upper-tract tumors that occur in 1–4% of patients. Following visualization of a mass, TURBT is required to confirm the diagnosis and extent of disease. Determining gross invasion and differences between well and poorly differentiated cancers may be apparent to an experienced cystoscopist; however, pathological confirmation of a resected specimen is required.

An outline of the treatment of non-muscle-invasive bladder cancer is shown in Figure 16.1. The cornerstone of all non-muscle-invasive bladder cancer therapy is transurethral resection (TUR), utilized to diagnose, stage, and often cure. An inadequate TUR may lead to faulty decision making, undertreatment, and a poorer clinical outcome. Muscularis propria must be included in the resected tumor for the TUR to be considered adequate and complete. For low-grade Ta and low-risk T1 tumors, TUR alone may be sufficient. Large tumors (>3 cm), multifocal lesions, adjacent CIS, and recurrence within 2–3 months of initial resection are all associated with a poor prognosis. CIS is a high-grade intraurothelial neoplasia confined to the epithelium growing in a flat, disordered pattern that may be focal, multifocal, or diffuse. CIS increases the risk of subsequent muscle-invasive disease whether found alone or associated with a resected superficial tumor. In T1 disease, repeat TUR is recommended because up to 30% will be understaged even when initial resection appeared complete. Recurrence rates of T1 disease at 1, 3, and 5 years from TUR can be as high as 50%, 80%, and 90%, respectively. Though initially limited to the mucosa, Ta tumors may recur locally multiple times prior to eventually becoming invasive. Close observation with repeat cystoscopy initially every 3–6 months is recommended.

Intravesical therapy is used adjuvantly after TUR for noninvasive (high-grade Ta, Tis) or minimally invasive

(T1) disease to reduce the risk of recurrence. With direct infusion therapy into the bladder, high local concentrations of medication can be achieved without systemic side effects. This may eliminate residual and undetected disease, though reduced progression to more invasive cancer has not been demonstrated. Treatments historically have included cytotoxic and immune-mediated agents.

Studies investigating appropriate intravesical therapy tend to be flawed due to poor trial design, small patient numbers, heterogeneous populations, and poorly defined outcomes. A meta-analysis was performed reviewing published clinical trials that compared TUR alone to TUR plus 1 cycle of immediate instillation of chemotherapy (5). Seven trials, totaling 1476 patients with low-risk papillary disease (Ta or T1 without Tis) were reviewed; chemotherapies received included: epirubicin, mitomycin C, thiotepa, or pirarubicin. A decreased risk of recurrence from 48% to 37% was noted in the treatment group (odds ratio [OR] = 0.61). No difference was noted based on agent selected. Patients with multifocal disease also benefitted from intravesical chemotherapy, but the risk of recurrence was still high after treatment (62.5% for multifocal disease vs. 35.8% for a single focus tumor). Single-dose intravesical chemotherapy is insufficient for multifocal tumors. Theoretically, delivering therapy within 24 hours of resection interferes with the implantation process and is more commonly being applied clinically. In the United States, mitomycin C is most frequently used due to limited systemic absorption resulting in a preferred side-effect profile.

For high-risk, non-muscle-invasive tumors (CIS, multifocal, and recurrent disease), the treatment of choice is immunotherapy with BCG, a live attenuated strain of *Mycobacterium bovis*. Though the mechanism of BCG treatment is not clear, intravesical therapy triggers a variety of local immune responses that correlate with antitumor activity. The dose and schedule most commonly used is 120 mg intravesical weekly for 6 weeks. In a randomized trial of TUR versus TUR plus BCG involving patients with recurrent superficial disease, Herr et al. demonstrated a significant decrease in need for cystectomy and a 10-year survival advantage of 75% compared with 55.2% with the addition of BCG immunotherapy (6). Maintenance BCG for those with a complete response to induction, dosed weekly for 3 weeks every 6 months over 2–3 years, was superior to induction alone and trials showed that BCG was superior to mitomycin C (7). Although serious complications such as systemic infections and sepsis are rare, a self-limited localized BCG cystitis with increased urinary frequency, low-grade fever, and hematuria occur in most patients for approximately 24 hours after infusion. Symptoms persisting beyond 48 hours raise the concern for systemic infection. Rarely, deaths have occurred secondary to overwhelming BCG sepsis.

Surveillance in early-stage bladder cancer permits organ preservation. Low-grade, noninvasive papillary tumors may be managed with repeat TUR, even in recurrent disease. Early radical cystectomy remains an appropriate option for patients with high-grade histology, multiple tumors or frequent recurrences despite appropriate treatment with intravesical BCG. Patients considered high risk are likely to benefit from earlier cystectomy prior to the development of T2 or greater disease (8). Failures to control CIS with TUR and adjuvant BCG therapy or recurrence of T1 tumor 6–12 months after appropriate treatment are indications for cystectomy.

## Muscle-Invasive Disease (T2 or T3 or T4a)

J.K. is a 49-year-old healthy man who visited his primary care physician after an episode of painless, gross hematuria. An abdominal CT showed a calcified bladder mass. Urology was consulted for cystoscopy and TURBT, which yielded a high-grade papillary urothelial carcinoma invading the lamina propria with tumor adjacent to but not invading muscle. CIS was noted within the resected specimen but there was no angiolymphatic invasion. Re-resection was not completed at that time; instead the patient received 6 doses of BCG immunotherapy. Urine cytology was suspicious for urothelial carcinoma following treatment and repeat cystoscopy revealed persistent disease on the left bladder wall. CT urogram confirmed a 6- to 7-cm exophytic mass with associated hydronephrosis but no evidence of metastatic disease. Chest radiographs were normal. Repeat TURBT and bimanual examination under anesthesia demonstrated a large palpable muscle-invasive TCC; no attempt at complete resection was made. Clinically, J.K. was felt to have a stage III (cT3, Nx, M0) tumor due to hydronephrosis seen on CT.

J.K. was referred to medical oncology for consultation. Review of systems was positive only for urinary frequency, nocturia, and gross hematuria. The patient was well appearing with an excellent performance status, mild hypertension, and an otherwise unremarkable physical examination. Laboratory evaluations were normal including renal function, alkaline phosphatase, and blood counts.

J.K. underwent 3 cycles of neoadjuvant chemotherapy with methotrexate, vinblastine, doxorubicin, and cisplatin (MVAC) followed by radical cystoprostatectomy, bilateral pelvic lymph node dissection, and creation of an ileal neobladder. Pathology revealed a complete response within the bladder and incidental Gleason 3 + 3 = 6, pT2b, N0 prostate adenocarcinoma. His postoperative course was complicated by left lower extremity deep venous thrombosis. The urine cytology, CT abdomen, chest radiographs, and physical examination remain unrevealing for metastatic disease on follow-up.

### Evidence-Based Case Discussion

J.K. is a relatively young, otherwise healthy man without medical comorbidities who presents with muscle-invasive

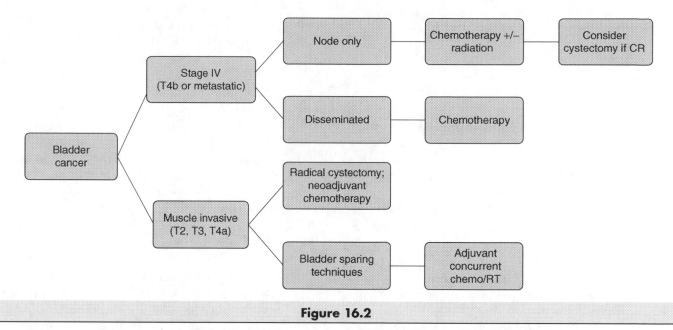

**Figure 16.2**

Treatment of muscle-invasive bladder cancer. CR, complete response; RT, radiation therapy.

bladder cancer without evidence of metastatic disease. He is therefore a candidate for aggressive treatment. Unfortunately for many patients, the advanced age and common comorbidities that share risk factors for bladder cancer, such as smoking, often complicate management and limit treatment options. The large mass palpable under anesthesia with hydronephrosis makes this a high-risk tumor; however, the pure urothelial histology and normal alkaline phosphatase predict a more favorable prognosis.

Figure 16.2 shows a treatment algorithm for treating muscle-invasive bladder cancer. For decades, the standard of care for muscle-invasive bladder cancer has been bilateral pelvic lymphadenectomy, radical cystectomy, and urinary diversion. In men, a radical cystectomy involves radical cystoprostatectomy and potentially a urethrectomy if the prostatic urethra is involved. Women undergo anterior exenteration that includes excision of the bladder, urethra, uterus, adnexa, and ventral vaginal wall. Options for urinary diversion include an ileal conduit, internal urinary reservoir with drainage to the abdominal wall or urethra, and orthotopic diversion or neobladder that more closely mimics a native bladder.

Although radical cystectomy is the most efficacious treatment to locally control bladder cancer, it is associated with high morbidity. Historically, postoperative mortality rates reached 40–50%, a number now reduced to 1–3%. Mortality in older patients (>80 years old) is 2–3 times higher than that for younger patients. Overall 5-year survival status postcystectomy is 50%, but this clearly varies with clinical stage. Organ-confined tumors ($\leq$T2b) have a significantly better prognosis than extravesical disease ($\geq$T3a). At a minimum, lymphadenectomy should include bilateral dissection of common, internal and external iliac,

and obturator nodes. A metastatic lymph node deposit predicts a much higher recurrence risk; however, cure remains possible especially after completion of an adequate lymph node dissection. Surgical factors negatively influencing survival following radical cystectomy include positive margins and <10 nodes removed (9).

Alternatives to radical cystectomy for those with significant comorbidities, advanced age, or strong desire for organ preservation may be considered, including partial cystectomy, radical TUR, and radiation techniques. Many consider these techniques inferior to radical cystectomy although limited direct comparisons exist. If the group considered for these procedures are carefully selected, outcomes may approach those of the more aggressive approach. Optimal patients include those only with urothelial histology, T2 and T3a tumors with a limited disease burden.

Partial cystectomy, removal of only a portion of the bladder wall to maintain bladder function, may be considered for patients with a T2 solitary lesion without Tis. Only 5% of patients considered for cystectomy will be candidates for this procedure. For this minority of patients, 5-year survival approaches 50%, similar to that of radical cystectomy. Importantly, even in this limited surgery, a bilateral pelvic lymphadenectomy is still required. The role of partial cystectomy is diminishing, given improved orthotopic neobladder formation.

Other alternatives to radical cystectomy include aggressive TUR alone or TUR followed by chemotherapy, radiation, or concurrent chemoradiation. These options are especially appealing for patients who are medically unfit for more aggressive surgeries. A major limitation of TUR is the inability to determine with certainty the completeness of tumor resection. Intensive, long-term cystoscopic follow-up is mandatory due to the high risk of recurrent tumors. TUR followed by single modality radiotherapy is only indicated for those unable to tolerate cystectomy or chemotherapy because of medical comorbidities. Similarly, chemotherapy alone is not adequate to control local disease.

Aggressive TUR followed by concurrent chemoradiation therapy with cisplatin is considered the standard for bladder preservation. Shipley et al. (10), the most heavily published author on this topic, advocates for neoadjuvant chemotherapy prior to concurrent chemoradiation, though this is debated. His regimen includes 2 cycles of neoadjuvant chemotherapy with cisplatin, methotrexate, and vinblastine (CMV) followed by concurrent chemoradiation. Patients are evaluated during treatment and those with a complete response as documented by transurethral cystoscopy and biopsies go on to complete concurrent therapy. One hundred ninety patients with T2–T4a urothelial bladder cancer were treated prospectively on sequential trials led by Shipley et al. with this basic protocol strategy after completion of optimal TURBT (7). The 5- and 10-year survival rates reached 54% and 36%, respectively. Of the surviving patients, 73% were able to maintain bladder preservation at 5 years. Assessment for complete response (CR) is critically important; if unable to achieve a CR due to chemo/radiation insensitive disease, the patient must go to immediate cystectomy barring contraindication. The most common approach to concurrent therapy following complete TURBT is cisplatin dosed weeks 1 and 4 plus 40 Gy external beam radiotherapy followed by cystoscopy with biopsy. If malignant disease is detected, the patient undergoes cystectomy; if biopsies are negative (T0), an additional 25 Gy of radiation and a third dose of cisplatin are delivered. Other chemosensitizing agents that may be considered include 5-fluorouracil (5-FU) or paclitaxel in combination with cisplatin or as single agents. Cystectomy may be difficult in patients who recur after receiving the full course of pelvic radiation.

Half of the patients with localized muscle-invasive disease will develop metastatic disease despite optimal surgical management including cystectomy. Given the high responses of TCC to chemotherapy (up to 75% to cisplatin-based regimens with 20% CR), adjuvant and neoadjuvant therapy have been explored to reduce this recurrence rate. The best evidence is for neoadjuvant chemotherapy. Theoretical advantages of this approach include the ability to assess the chemotherapy responsiveness of the tumor, immediate treatment of microscopic metastatic disease rather than waiting for postoperative healing, and better tolerance of therapy preoperatively allowing more chemotherapy to be delivered. In muscle-invasive urothelial cancer, neoadjuvant chemotherapy demonstrates a survival advantage. The largest neoadjuvant chemotherapy trial was a phase III collaborative group study including the Medical Research Council, the European Organization for Research and Treatment of Cancer (EORTC) (11). A total of 976 patients with cT2 to cT4a, N0 to Nx TCC were randomized to receive neoadjuvant CMV versus no chemotherapy, both followed by institutional choice of radical cystectomy or radiation therapy. The absolute survival benefit of neoadjuvant CMV at 3 years was 5.5% (55.5% vs. 50%; $P$ = .075). Although initially not significant, an update published with median follow-up of 7 years at the 2002 American Society of Clinical Oncology (ASCO) meeting demonstrated a significantly superior survival in those randomized to neoadjuvant chemotherapy compared with those with local treatment alone (12). A phase III SWOG trial (INT 0080) of 317 patients with cT2 to cT4a urothelial carcinoma randomized to either 3 cycles of MVAC followed by cystectomy versus cystectomy alone also demonstrated benefit for those that received chemotherapy. The patients receiving neoadjuvant chemotherapy had an improved median overall survival (OS = 77 vs. 46 months; $P$ = .06) and 5-year OS (57% vs. 43%; $P$ = .06). Not surprisingly, there was a significant increase in pT0 status at the time of cystectomy from 15% in the cystectomy alone group to 38% in the neoadjuvant group. Patients generally tolerated neoadjuvant therapy well without any treatment-related deaths (13). Several large meta-analyses have been performed that likewise determined a significant absolute 5-year OS advantage of >5% in patients treated with neoadjuvant cisplatin-based chemotherapy followed by radical cystectomy versus surgery alone.

Multiple studies have investigated the use of adjuvant chemotherapy in locally advanced bladder cancer but no statistically significant survival advantage has been demonstrated. The theoretical advantage of this approach is immediate local control followed by therapy for those with high-risk disease based on pathological criteria. Trials investigating this issue have been plagued by small sample size, difficult accrual, and methodologically flawed trial designs. The Advanced Bladder Cancer Meta-Analysis Collaboration reviewed 6 available randomized controlled trials of 491 individual patients comparing adjuvant cisplatin-based chemotherapy to local treatment alone in invasive urothelial cancer (14). The authors found a significant reduction in relative risk of death (25%, $P$ = .019) in the adjuvant chemotherapy group, but serious methodological flaws limit the interpretation of their results. In spite of the limitations of this trial and the others, the data suggest that it is reasonable to consider adjuvant therapy if no neoadjuvant therapy was delivered especially in higher-risk disease (T3–T4 tumors or positive nodes).

## Unresectable (T4b) or Metastatic Disease (N1–3 or M1)

F.T. is a 50-year-old woman who presented to her primary care physician complaining of dysuria and dyspareunia.

Her symptoms failed to resolve after a course of antibiotics for treatment of a presumed urinary tract infection. She then noted a vaginal mass. F.T. was referred to a urologist for cystoscopy and a TURBT revealed high-grade muscle-invasive TCC. A biopsy of the vaginal mass at the time of this procedure was positive for TCC confirming a T4a bladder cancer. A CT scan of the chest, abdomen, and pelvis revealed a tiny right middle lobe pulmonary nodule of uncertain significance, a large bladder mass, and a 2-cm ovoid soft tissue mass right and posterior to the bladder. A pelvic MRI confirmed the large bladder mass and questionable right perivesicular lymph node seen on CT. A bone scan had no evidence of metastatic disease. F.T. was referred to medical oncology for consideration of neoadjuvant chemotherapy.

At the clinic visit, F.T. complained of mild fatigue, slight fever, and decreased appetite with some weight loss. She also noted persistent dysuria, pelvic pain, and mild nausea. Past medical history was remarkable for idiopathic polyneuropathy and she was a 30-pack-year current smoker. Physical examination was remarkable only for mild right lower quadrant tenderness to deep palpation noted on examination. The possible pelvic lymph node discovered on imaging suggested possible stage IV disease and she was enrolled on a clinical trial of neoadjuvant paclitaxel, carboplatin, and gemcitabine. Cisplatin was considered but withheld due to her history of neuropathy. She completed 3 cycles of neoadjuvant therapy requiring minimal dose reductions and growth factor support due to cytopenias. A follow-up CT scan revealed a partial response without evidence of distant metastatic disease.

F.T. eventually underwent a radical cystectomy, hysterectomy, partial vaginectomy, bilateral pelvic lymph node dissection, and ileal neobladder reconstruction. She tolerated the procedure well. Pathology revealed a residual 20 × 15 mm high-grade urothelial tumor with extensive clear cell features. Margins were negative but angiolymphatic invasion was identified. Four of eight pelvic lymph nodes were involved bilaterally (pT3a, N2) confirming metastatic, locally advanced disease. There was no evidence of distant metastatic disease. Further therapy was considered for this patient with advanced, aggressive disease even though all visible disease had been resected. Her oncologist elected to administer 3 cycles of adjuvant carboplatin, paclitaxel, and gemcitabine.

F.T. remained without disease following her chemotherapy for almost a year when she developed low-grade fevers, night sweats, and new pelvic pain. She underwent biopsy of an isolated pelvic mass, which was consistent with a local recurrent TCC. Doublet therapy with cisplatin and gemcitabine was initiated resulting in tumor shrinkage. However, F.T. developed a progressive neuropathy and treatment was discontinued after 5 cycles. She had a 10-month progression-free interval off therapy and was eventually enrolled in a clinical trial at the time of further disease progression.

## Evidence-Based Case Discussion

F.T. is a relatively young woman with locally advanced bladder cancer and regional lymph node involvement who had only a partial response despite aggressive neoadjuvant chemotherapy. Findings of angiolymphatic invasion, multiple lymph node involvement, lack of complete response to neoadjuvant chemotherapy, and partial clear-cell histology are consistent with an aggressive, poor prognosis tumor. All macroscopic disease had been resected at the time of her surgery. Due to her very high-risk disease, adjuvant chemotherapy therapy was considered despite lack of evidence for increased survival.

Although response rates are high with urothelial carcinoma compared to other solid tumors, the median survival of patients with metastatic disease remains at only 14 months even with aggressive chemotherapy and only 15% of patients are alive at 5 years. Poor performance status and visceral organ metastases correspond to shortened survival. More interest in molecular markers have demonstrated increased resistance to MVAC, and other cisplatin-based chemotherapy in tumors with *p53* mutations and high excision repair cross-complementing 1 (ERCC1) levels (15).

First-line chemotherapy in the setting of metastatic disease is MVAC. Historically, cisplatin had been recognized as the most active agent in bladder cancer with objective remissions as high as 40%. Based on promising preliminary results, Loehrer et al. compared MVAC (methotrexate 30 mg/m$^2$, days 1, 15, and 22; vinblastine 3 mg/m$^2$, days 2, 15, and 22; doxorubicin 30 mg/m$^2$ and cisplatin 70 mg/m$^2$ on day 2) to single-agent cisplatin (70 mg/m$^2$) in 226 randomly assigned patients with advanced urothelial carcinoma (16). As expected, the multidrug combination had more toxicities than cisplatin alone including cytopenias, neutropenic fever, sepsis, mucositis, nausea, and treatment-related mortality. There were 5 (4%) deaths in the combination arm and none with cisplatin alone. Despite this, the MVAC group did significantly better than the single-agent group in response rates (39% vs. 12%; $P < .0001$), progression-free survival (PFS; 10.0 vs. 4.3 months) and OS (12.5 vs. 8.2 months). Multiple regimens have been compared to MVAC in an attempt to find a more effective or less toxic alternative. When compared directly to the combination of cisplatin, cyclophosphamide, and doxorubicin (CISCA) in a phase III clinical trial, MVAC had a superior response rate (65% vs. 46%) and OS time (median = 11 vs. 10 months) (17). In an attempt to increase response rates, MVAC was compared to 5-Fluorouracil, interferon alpha-2b, and cisplatin (FAP) in a phase III trial (18). MVAC had a superior response rate and complete response rate (24% vs. 10%), but identical OS times (12.5 months) and toxicity profile. Other trials evaluating high-dose MVAC with granulocyte colony stimulating factor support failed to demonstrate superiority of standard MVAC. Based on these studies and previous phase II trials, MVAC emerged as the standard of care for metastatic TCC.

Preliminary studies using the combination of gemcitabine and cisplatin (GC) demonstrated promising activity in metastatic urothelial cancer in chemotherapy-naive patients with less toxicity than seen with other regimens; this led to a phase III study directly comparing GC to MVAC in locally advanced or metastatic TCC (19). Four hundred five treatment-naive patients were randomized equally to either GC (gemcitabine 1000 mg/m$^2$, days 1, 8, and 15, and cisplatin 70 mg/m$^2$, day 2) or standard MVAC. The overall response rate (47% vs. 46%), time to progression (both 7.4 months), and median survival (13.8 vs. 14.8 months) were very similar in GC and MVAC arms, respectively. With the exception of grade 3 or 4 anemia and thrombocytopenia, the toxicity profile of GC was superior with more patients able to complete 6 cycles of chemotherapy without dose reductions and fewer treatment-related deaths (1% vs. 3%). This trial was not powered to demonstrate equivalency, but given the similar 5-year OS results (GC = 13%, MVAC = 15%) and a better safety profile and tolerability, many consider GC as the standard first-line regimen for patients with advanced TCC rather than MVAC.

Various other treatment combinations have been evaluated in an attempt to improve response rates and median survival. Taxanes have demonstrated promising single-agent activity in bladder cancer, although double-agent therapy of paclitaxel with cisplatin did not appear superior to standard therapy in subsequent studies. In a randomized phase III trial of 627 patients, the triplet paclitaxel/carboplatin/gemcitabine (PCG; paclitaxel 80 mg/m$^2$, days 1 and 8, cisplatin 70 mg/m$^2$, day 1, gemcitabine 1000 mg/m$^2$, days 1 and 8 of a 21-day cycle) was evaluated against standard GC (20). Overall (57.1% vs. 46.4%) and complete responses (15% vs. 10%) were significantly better in PCG compared with GC; however, the trend toward superiority of PCG to GC for median survival (15.7 vs. 12.8 months) was not statistically significant (P = .10). Both treatments were well tolerated with increased thrombocytopenia and febrile neutropenia in the triplet arm.

Standard salvage therapy in recurrent urothelial carcinoma is not defined. Multiple drugs demonstrate single-agent activity in bladder cancer with response rates of 20% or less in the second-line setting. These drugs include paclitaxel, docetaxel, gemcitabine, ifosfamide, and oxaliplatin. Biological therapies are currently under investigation. Epidermal growth factor receptor (EGFR) and angiogenesis pathways have demonstrated upregulation in urothelial cancers, and trials are ongoing to assess the incorporation of these targeted agents into standard regimens.

## REVIEW QUESTIONS

1. All of the following have been associated with an increased risk of bladder cancer *except*:

   (A) Tobacco use
   (B) Chronic use of oral cyclophosphamide
   (C) Chronic cystitis secondary to an indwelling Foley catheter
   (D) Schistosomiasis
   (E) Female gender

2. A 62-year-old man with a past medical history significant for hypertension and non-insulin dependent diabetes presents to his primary care physician after noticing blood in his urine for the past 5 days. He denies having any pain or difficulty urinating, but does state that he is urinating more often. According to his social history he has a 35-pack-year history of tobacco use and he is currently an active smoker. His physical examination is notable only for some mild end-expiratory wheezes on lung examination. The patient's hematuria fails to resolve despite treatment with a 7-day course of ciprofloxacin. He is ultimately referred to a urologist, who performed an office cystoscopy and noted a 4-cm solid-appearing mass originating from the right bladder wall. Which is the most appropriate next step in the management of this patient?

   (A) Obtain a CT urogram study
   (B) Schedule the patient to have repeat cystoscopy under anesthesia with transurethral resection of the bladder tumor and complete resection of the bladder mass
   (C) Perform cystectomy with neobladder formation
   (D) Administration of intravesical bacillus Calmette–Guerin

3. A 76-year-old man with no significant past medical history is referred for evaluation by urology due to a 3-week history of intermittent painless hematuria. A CT scan of the abdomen and pelvis obtained by his primary care physician revealed a calcified bladder mass, but no other abnormalities. He ultimately undergoes cystoscopy with transurethral resection of the bladder tumor. Pathology reveals a 2.9-cm high-grade papillary urothelial carcinoma. Muscularis propria was present in the sample but is without invasion. Which of the following is the most appropriate management of this patient following complete resection of the bladder mass via cystoscopy?

   (A) Radical cystectomy
   (B) Administration of adjuvant intravesical bacillus Calmette–Guerin in conjunction with surveillance cystoscopy every 3–6 months

(C) Administration of neoadjuvant methotrexate, vinblastine, doxorubicin, and cisplatin chemotherapy

(D) Observation with cystoscopy every 3–6 months

4. The same patient in Question 3 undergoes intravesical bacillus Calmette–Guerin (BCG) therapy and repeat cystoscopy 6 months following his original diagnosis of bladder cancer. The study reveals a recurrent lesion that is completely resected via cystoscopy. On pathology the lesion is again demonstrated to be consistent with high-grade papillary urothelial carcinoma and is 1.5 cm in size. At this point, what is the most appropriate management of this patient?

(A) Continue surveillance cystoscopy every 3–6 months along with intravesical BCG therapy

(B) Observation

(C) Adjuvant methotrexate, vinblastine, doxorubicin, and cisplatin chemotherapy

(D) Cystectomy

5. In muscle-invasive bladder cancer, randomized controlled clinical trials have demonstrated a survival advantage for both neoadjuvant and adjuvant chemotherapy administration. *True or false.*

6. A 66-year-old man with a 35-pack-year smoking history began to experience urinary frequency and urgency, which was subsequently followed by the development of gross hematuria. He underwent cystoscopy, which revealed the presence of a 6-cm bladder mass. He then underwent CT scan of the abdomen pelvis, which did not reveal any evidence of metastatic disease, but did show evidence of mild left-sided hydronephrosis. A transurethral resection of the bladder tumor was then performed, which confirmed the diagnosis of a high-grade transitional cell carcinoma invading the muscularis propria. No attempt at complete resection was made. Which of the following is the most appropriate management of this patient?

(A) Radical cystectomy followed by administration of adjuvant chemotherapy

(B) Administration of neoadjuvant chemotherapy followed by radical cystectomy or definitive radiotherapy

(C) Partial cystectomy followed by administration of adjuvant chemotherapy

(D) Administration of neoadjuvant chemotherapy followed by partial cystectomy

7. A 78-year-old woman with a long-standing smoking history and advanced chronic obstructive pulmonary disease (COPD) requiring 1–2 L of home oxygen is diagnosed with muscle-invasive transitional cell carcinoma of the bladder. CT scan of the abdomen/pelvis does not demonstrate any obvious evidence of metastatic disease. Although surgical options for treatment are considered,

it is ultimately determined that the patient's advanced COPD would place her at significant risk for surgical complications. Which of the following bladder-sparing treatment options would be most likely to achieve disease control?

(A) Aggressive transurethral resection (TUR) of the tumor followed by administration of concurrent chemotherapy and radiation therapy

(B) Aggressive TUR of the tumor alone

(C) Concurrent chemoradiotherapy

(D) Chemotherapy alone

## REFERENCES

1. American Cancer Society. *Cancer Facts & Figures 2014.* Atlanta: American Cancer Society; 2014.

2. Lokeshwar VB, Habuchi T, Grossman HB, et al. Bladder tumor markers beyond cytology: International Consensus Panel on bladder tumor markers. *Urology.* 2005;66(6 Suppl 1):35–63.

3. Messing EM, Madeb R, Young T, et al. Long-term outcome of hematuria home screening for bladder cancer in men. *Cancer.* 2006;107(9):2173–2179.

4. National Comprehensive Cancer Network. Bladder Cancer (Version 2.2014). http://www.nccn.org/professionals/physician_gls/pdf/bladder.pdf. Accessed August 17, 2014.

5. Sylvester RJ, Oosterlinck W, van der Meijden AP. A single immediate postoperative instillation of chemotherapy decreases the risk of recurrence in patients with stage Ta T1 bladder cancer: a meta-analysis of published results of randomized clinical trials. *J Urol.* 2004;171(6 Pt 1):2186–2190, quiz 2435.

6. Herr HW, Schwalb DM, Zhang ZF, et al. Intravesical bacillus Calmette-Guérin therapy prevents tumor progression and death from superficial bladder cancer: ten-year follow-up of a prospective randomized trial. *J Clin Oncol.* 1995;13(6):1404–1408.

7. Malmström PU, Sylvester RJ, Crawford DE, et al. An individual patient data meta-analysis of the long-term outcome of randomised studies comparing intravesical mitomycin C versus bacillus Calmette-Guérin for non-muscle-invasive bladder cancer. *Eur Urol.* 2009;56(2):247–256.

8. Lee CT, Dunn RL, Ingold C, et al. Early-stage bladder cancer surveillance does not improve survival if high-risk patients are permitted to progress to muscle invasion. *Urology.* 2007; 69(6):1068–1072.

9. Herr HW, Faulkner JR, Grossman HB, et al. Surgical factors influence bladder cancer outcomes: a cooperative group report. *J Clin Oncol.* 2004;22(14):2781–2789.

10. Shipley WU, Kaufman DS, Zehr E, et al. Selective bladder preservation by combined modality protocol treatment: long-term outcomes of 190 patients with invasive bladder cancer. *Urology.* 2002;60(1):62–7; discussion 67.

11. EORTC. Neoadjuvant cisplatin, methotrexate, and vinblastine chemotherapy for muscle-invasive bladder cancer: a randomized controlled trial. *Lancet.* 1999;254(9178):533–540.

12. Hall RR. Updated results of a randomized controlled trial of neoadjuvant cisplatin (C), methrotrexate (M) and vinblastine (V) chemotherapy for muscle-invasive bladder cancer. *Proc Annu Meet Am Soc Clin Oncol.* 2002;21:178a.

13. Grossman HB, Natale RB, Tangen CM, et al. Neoadjuvant chemotherapy plus cystectomy compared with cystectomy alone for locally advanced bladder cancer. *N Engl J Med.* 2003;349(9): 859–866.

14. Advanced Bladder Cancer (ABC) Meta-Analysis Collaboration. Adjuvant chemotherapy in invasive bladder cancer: a systemic review and meta-analysis of individual patient data Advanced

Bladder Cancer (ABC) Meta-analysis Collaborative. *Eur Urol.* 2005;48(2):199–201.

15. Bellmunt J, Paz-Ares L, Cuello M, et al.; Spanish Oncology Genitourinary Group. Gene expression of ERCC1 as a novel prognostic marker in advanced bladder cancer patients receiving cisplatin-based chemotherapy. *Ann Oncol.* 2007;18(3):522–528.

16. Loehrer PJ Sr, Einhorn LH, Elson PJ, et al. A randomized comparison of cisplatin alone or in combination with methotrexate, vinblastine, and doxorubicin in patients with metastatic urothelial carcinoma: a cooperative group study. *J Clin Oncol.* 1992;10(7): 1066–1073.

17. Logothetis CJ, Dexeus FH, Finn L, et al. A prospective randomized trial comparing MVAC and CISCA chemotherapy for patients with metastatic urothelial tumors. *J Clin Oncol.* 1990;8(6):1050–1055.

18. Siefker-Radtke AO, Millikan RE, Tu SM, et al. Phase III trial of fluorouracil, interferon alpha-2b, and cisplatin versus methotrexate, vinblastine, doxorubicin, and cisplatin in metastatic or unresectable urothelial cancer. *J Clin Oncol.* 2002;20(5):1361–1367.

19. von der Maase Hansen SW, Roberts JT, Dogliotti L, et al. Gemcitabine and cisplatin versus methotrexate, vinblastine, doxorubicin, and cisplatin in advanced or metastatic bladder cancer: results of a large, randomized, multinational, multicenter, phase III study. *J Clin Oncol.* 2000;18(17):3068–3077.

20. Bellmunt J, von der Maase H, Mead GM, et al. Randomized phase III study comparing paclitaxel/cisplatin/gemcitabine and gemcitabine/cisplatin in patients with locally advanced or metastatic urothelial cancer without prior systemic therapy; EORTC30987/ Intergroup Study. *Am Soc Clin Oncol Annu Meet.* 2007; (Abstract LBA 5030).

# 17

# *Cervical Cancer*

ANDREI MARCONESCU, CELESTINE S. TUNG, SHAN GUO,
CONCEPCION R. DIAZ-ARRASTIA, AND MARIAN YVETTE WILLIAMS-BROWN

## EPIDEMIOLOGY, RISK FACTORS, NATURAL HISTORY, AND PATHOLOGY

Cervical cancer is the second most common cause of cancer-related morbidity and mortality among women worldwide. Internationally, 500,000 new cases are diagnosed each year and 250,000 deaths occur each year, corresponding to a 50% mortality rate. In the United States, cervical cancer is relatively uncommon; the incidence of invasive cervical cancer has declined steadily over the past few decades due to a widely available screening program. It is estimated that in 2014, 12,360 cases of invasive cervical cancer will be diagnosed and that 4020 women will die of the disease in the United States (www.seer.cancer.gov/statfacts/html/cervix.html). Race and ethnicity are some of the many complex interacting biological and social risk factors for cervical carcinoma in the United States. African Americans, Hispanics, Native Americans, and Vietnamese Americans have a higher risk of death from cervical cancer than non-Hispanic white Americans. The mean age for cervical cancer is 51.4 years.

High-risk human papillomavirus (HPV) infection is the carcinogenic trigger for >99% of cervical cancers. The most common types of HPV implicated in cervical cancer are 16, 18, 31, 33, 45, 52, and 58, and types 16 and 18 are found in nearly 70% of all invasive cervical cancers. Approximately 75–80% of sexually active adults will have or have had an HPV genital tract infection by the age of 50 years. Roughly, 50% of women will contract the HPV virus within the first 3 years of coitarche. Despite a high prevalence of HPV infection, the majority of women will clear the HPV virus within 1–2 years from the time of infection. An HPV infection persisting for >2 years may develop into high-grade cervical intraepithelial neoplasia (CIN), the cancer precursor (discussed subsequently).

Annually, in the United States, the estimated cases of CIN in females are 2.7 per 1000. Therefore, although an infection with the carcinogenic HPV is necessary, it alone is not sufficient to cause cervical cancer. HPV infection is only the first step in a series of events that leads to invasive carcinoma. Integration of HPV DNA into the host cellular genome and overexpression of the viral *E6* and *E7* oncogenes lead to cervical carcinogenesis. The *E6* and *E7* proteins bind and inactivate tumor suppressors *p53* and retinoblastoma protein, thereby affecting multiple biological processes that lead to increased cellular proliferation. High-grade CIN usually occurs in the transformation zone of the cervix at the squamocolumnar junction. Currently, there are 2 vaccines available for protection against HPV: a bivalent vaccine (Cervarix) that protects against subtypes 16 and 18, and a quadravalent vaccine (Gardasil) that protects against subtypes 16 and 18 as well as 6 and 11.

Other risk factors for CIN and cervical carcinoma include a past medical history of abnormal Pap smears or CIN, lack of participation in Pap smear screening, early onset of sexual activity, multiple sexual partners, a high-risk sexual partner, history of sexually transmitted diseases, high parity, immunosuppression, low socioeconomic status, prolonged use of oral contraceptives, and previous history of anogenital dysplasia. Smoking is associated with an increased risk of squamous cell carcinoma but not with adenocarcinoma of the cervix (1).

In addition to the availability of HPV vaccines for primary prevention, prevention of invasive cervical cancer is possible by the application of highly effective screening procedures, which can lead to the detection and excision/ablation of premalignant CIN. At this time, there are 2 acceptable screening methods utilized today: (a) the Papanicolaou test that samples cervical cells from the transformation zone using a cytobrush and (b) HPV testing in

**Table 17.1** Cervical Cancer Screening Guidelines

| Patient Status | Recommended Screening Method |
|---|---|
| <21 yr old | No screening recommended |
| 21–29 yr old | Pap smear cytology alone every 3 yr |
| 30–65 yr old | HPV and Pap smear cytology co-testing every 5 yr (preferred) |
| | Pap smear cytology alone every 3 yr (acceptable) |
| >65 yr old | No screening if adequate prior negative results[a] (applies to women without a history of CIN 2,3, adenocarcinoma in situ or cancer in the past 20 yr) |
| Prior hysterectomy | No screening is necessary[a] (applies to women without a cervix and without a history of CIN 2,3, adenocarcinoma in situ or cancer in the past 20 yr) |
| Prior HPV vaccination | Follow age-specific recommendations (same as unvaccinated women) |

CIN, cervical intraepithelial neoplasia; HPV, human papillomavirus.
[a]Adequate negative prior screening: 3 consecutive negative Pap smear results or 2 consecutive negative co-test results within the past 10 years with the most recent within the past 5 years.
*Source*: Adapted from Ref. (2). Saslow D, Solomon D, Lawson HW, et al.; ACS-ASCCP-ASCP Cervical Cancer Guideline Committee. American Cancer Society, American Society for Colposcopy and Cervical Pathology, and American Society for Clinical Pathology screening guidelines for the prevention and early detection of cervical cancer. *CA Cancer J Clin.* 2012;62(3):147–172.

combination with the Pap test, also called co-testing. The recommended screening guidelines based on age are outlined in Table 17.1.

In countries where women are screened routinely such as the United States, the most common presentation of cervical cancer is an abnormal Pap smear. These asymptomatic patients usually have smaller tumors at an earlier stage of disease. Patients with advanced cervical cancer typically present with abnormal vaginal bleeding. Postcoital bleeding is the pathogonomonic symptom, although the bleeding can also be intermenstrual or postmenopausal. Patients can also present with a vaginal discharge due to an infected necrotic tumor or pelvic pain due to extension of the disease to the surrounding structures. In the presence of pelvic sidewall involvement, the patient can present with the triad of leg edema, pain, and hydronephrosis.

As indicated earlier, CIN is a precursor to the development of invasive cervical carcinoma. CIN is graded based on the extent of the atypical cellular changes in the stratified squamous epithelium. Mild dysplasia (CIN 1) refers to atypical cellular changes involving the basal third of the epithelium. Moderate dysplasia (CIN 2) is considered as a high-grade lesion characterized by atypical cellular changes extending to the basal two thirds of the epithelium. Severe dysplasia (CIN 3/carcinoma in situ or CIS) is also considered a high-grade lesion with atypical

cellular changes encompassing more than two thirds of the epithelial thickness (CIN 3) and includes full-thickness intraepithelial lesions (CIS). Most CIN 1 lesions regress spontaneously or persist, whereas 10% progress to CIN 2 and 3 over 2 years. If untreated, CIN 3/CIS ultimately progresses to cancer over a prolonged period of time, typically 8–13 years without any symptoms. Therefore, it is recommended that any CIN 2 and 3 be treated by ablation or excision.

Histologically, most cervical cancers are squamous cell carcinomas (70%), followed by adenocarcinomas (25%), and adenosquamous carcinomas (3–5%). Rarely neuroendocrine or small cell carcinomas can arise primarily from the cervix. Treatment strategies for adenocarcinoma and adenosquamous carcinoma are similar to that of squamous cell carcinoma. This chapter focuses on squamous cell carcinoma. Cervical cancer spreads primarily by direct extension to surrounding structures such as the vagina, parametria, uterosacral and cardinal ligaments, and the bladder or rectum. Cervical cancer is also characterized by early lymphatic metastasis. The obturator lymph nodes are the primary drainage of the cervix. From there, the lymphatic metastases follow the afferent lymphatics up the iliac nodal chain to the para-aortic lymph nodes, then ultimately to the scalene nodes via the thoracic duct. Hematogenous metastases to the lung, mediastinum, bone, and liver are found late in the disease process.

## STAGING

The International Federation of Gynecology and Obstetrics (FIGO) staging system is the widely used staging system for cervical cancer and was most recently updated in 2009. Because 80% of cervical cancers are diagnosed in developing countries where access to advanced imaging techniques is limited, the current staging system relies on clinical evaluation alone. However, the information obtained via CT, PET-CT, and MRI can be used to develop treatment plans and to counsel patients regarding prognosis.

## CASE SUMMARIES

### Early-Stage Cervical Cancer

C.T. is a 32-year-old Gravida 1 Para 1 (G1P1) woman who was referred to the gynecology service for a 6-month history of abnormal vaginal bleeding. The vaginal bleeding was initially postcoital, but then progressed to almost daily bleeding. She also reported generalized fatigue. She denied abdominal pain associated with bleeding. Her last Pap smear was 4 years previously. She had no history of sexually transmitted diseases. On pelvic examination she was found to have a 1 × 1.5 cm exophytic, friable mass at the posterior lip of the cervix without gross involvement

| Cervical Cancer | |
|---|---|
| **Stage** | **Description** |
| I | *Carcinoma is strictly confined to the cervix; extension to the uterine corpus would be disregarded.* |
| IA | Invasive carcinoma diagnosed only by microscopy. Stromal invasion with a maximum depth of 5.0 mm measured from the base of the epithelium and a horizontal spread of 7.0 mm or less. Vascular space involvement, venous or lymphatic, should not alter the staging. |
| IA1 | Measured invasion of the stroma is 3 mm or less in depth and 7 mm or less in horizontal spread. |
| IA2 | Measured invasion of stroma is >3 mm but <5 mm and 7 mm or less in horizontal spread. |
| IB | Clinically visible lesions confined to the cervix or preclinical lesions > stage IA. |
| IB1 | Clinically visible lesions 4 cm or less in size. |
| IB2 | Clinically visible lesions >4 cm in size. |
| II | *Carcinoma that extends beyond the uterus but has not extended to the pelvic sidewall or to the lower 3rd of the vagina.* |
| IIA | No obvious parametrial involvement |
| IIA1 | Clinically visible lesions 4 cm or less in size. |
| IIA2 | Clinically visible lesion >4 cm in size. |
| IIB | Obvious parametrial involvement but not to the pelvic sidewall |
| III | *Carcinoma that has extended to the pelvic sidewall and/or involves the lower third of the vagina. On rectal examination, there is no cancer-free space between the tumor and the pelvic sidewall. All cases with a hydronephrosis or nonfunctioning kidney should be included, unless they are known to be due to other causes.* |
| IIIA | No extension to the pelvic sidewall but involvement of the lower third of the vagina. |
| IIIB | Extension to the pelvic sidewall and/or hydronephrosis or nonfunctioning kidney. |
| IV | *Carcinoma that has extended beyond the true pelvis or has involved (biopsy proven) the mucosa of the bladder and/or rectum.* |
| IVA | Spread of the tumor to adjacent pelvic organs. |
| IVB | Spread to distant organs. |

of vaginal walls, parametria, or pelvic sidewall. Biopsy of the mass was consistent with invasive squamous cell carcinoma. MRI imaging of the pelvis showed a 1.5-cm posterior cervical mass with no evidence of involvement of surrounding structures or lymph nodes. A chest x-ray showed no evidence of distant metastasis. Her performance status was 0, and her baseline lab work showed mild anemia with a hemoglobin of 9.2 g/dL. She had normal renal and liver function tests.

## Evidence-Based Case Discussion

C.T. has stage IB1 squamous cell carcinoma of cervix. Various treatment options exist for early-staged cervical cancer. Treatment options for stage IA1 carcinoma without lymphovascular space invasion may include simple hysterectomy that can be performed via laparotomy, vaginally, or laparoscopically. For patients who strongly desire to preserve their fertility, an alternative treatment is conization alone (Figure 17.1).

Treatment options for stage IA2–IIA1 lesions include radical hysterectomy with pelvic lymphadenectomy with or without operative para-aortic lymph node assessment, or definitive concurrent chemotherapy and pelvic radiation therapy and brachytherapy. An alternative therapy for those interested in fertility preservation is the radical trachelectomy with pelvic lymphadenectomy where the cervix is removed radically while sparing the uterine body in order to allow for pregnancy (Figure 17.2).

The major difference between a simple hysterectomy or trachelectomy and a radical procedure is the removal of the parametrial tissue and the upper vagina. The parametria is the connective tissue immediately around the cervix that includes the cardinal and uterosacral ligaments. It contains the vascular supply and lymphatics of the cervix well as the distal ureter en route to the bladder. The major difference between a radical hysterectomy and a radical trachelectomy is that in the latter there is preservation of the upper cervix and uterine body allowing for future pregnancy. In both the radical trachelectomy and radical hysterectomy, after mobilization of the ureters, the parametria and upper vagina are removed as part of the radical resection of the cervical tumor in order to ensure adequate margins of resection.

Surgery and radiation therapy are equally effective for early-stage disease, resulting in cure rates of 75–80% (3). Landoni et al. conducted a randomized clinical trial involving 343 women with stage IB–IIA cervical cancer in which 172 underwent surgery and 171 received radiation therapy. After a median follow-up of 87 months, the 5-year overall survival (OS) and progression-free survival (PFS) were identical in the surgery and radiation therapy groups (83% and 74%, respectively, for both groups) (4).

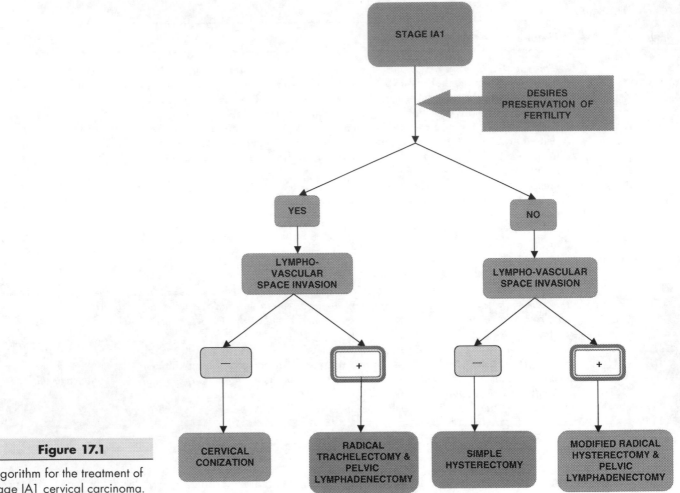

**Figure 17.1**

Algorithm for the treatment of stage IA1 cervical carcinoma.

Treatment decisions are usually based on patient factors and available local expertise. For most women with early cervical cancer, radical hysterectomy with pelvic lymphadenectomy with or without para-aortic lymph node assessment is preferred unless the patient has medical comorbidities precluding surgery or a poor functional status. The advantages of surgery include the preservation of vaginal function and the option to preserve ovarian function. If, at the time of surgery, the primary tumor is deemed unresectable or there is metastatic disease, the hysterectomy is usually aborted and chemoradiation is necessary. However, at that time, the ovaries can be transposed to the upper abdomen out of the pelvic radiation therapy field and/or bulky metastatic lymph nodes may be resected, which may be of therapeutic benefit. The downside of a surgical approach is the inherent surgical and anesthesia risks, especially in the patient with other comorbidities. The major disadvantages of primary chemoradiation are increased risk of bowel dysfunction and sexual dysfunction. However, if poor prognostic factors are identified in the surgical specimen, such as large tumor size, positive lymph nodes, positive margins, deep stromal invasion, and lymphovascular space invasion, then adjuvant radiation therapy with or without chemotherapy

is recommended. Women treated with both surgery and adjuvant radiation with or without chemotherapy have the highest complication rates and lowest quality of life (QOL) scores compared to women treated with 1 modality of therapy. Therefore, surgery should be reserved for well-selected candidates who may have a reasonable chance of cure from surgery alone.

The lymph nodes can be surgically evaluated via an open or laparoscopic approach and the laparoscopic approach can be either conventional or with robotic assistance. For tumors <2 cm in size, sentinel lymph node mapping may be a consideration. This technique involves injecting the cervix with a dye and/or a radiocolloid material such as technetium-99 (99Tc) to detect the sentinel lymph node(s) with direct visual inspection (if colored dye is used), a special florescent camera (if indocyanine green is used), or a gamma probe (if 99Tc is used). All mapped sentinel lymph nodes should be removed as well as any lymph nodes suspected to contain metastases. If a sentinel lymph node is not detected on 1 side of the pelvis, then a side-specific full lymph node dissection should be performed (5).

C.T. desired to have another child and inquired about treatment options that would preserve her fertility. This is

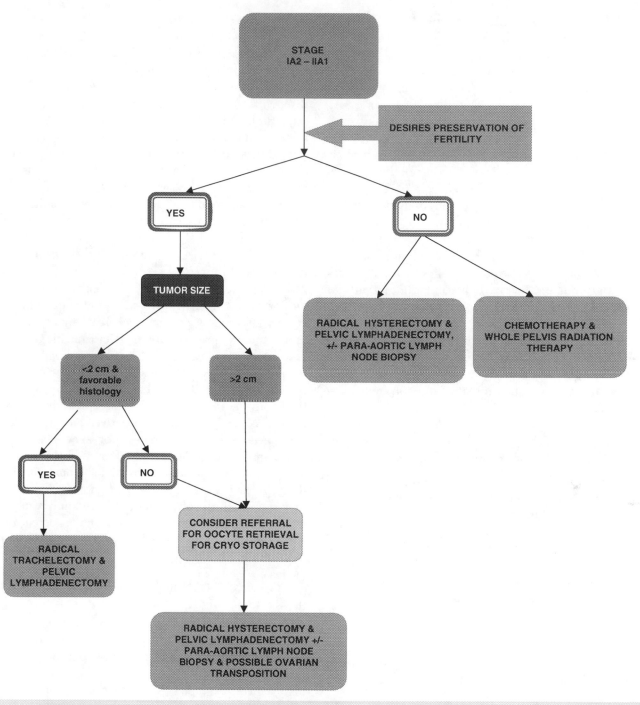

**Figure 17.2**

Algorithm for the treatment of stage IA2–IIA1 cervical carcinoma.

not an uncommon scenario because 42% of cases of cervical cancer are diagnosed in women prior to age 45 years.

As outlined in Figure 17.2, radical trachelectomy with pelvic lymphadenectomy and preservation of the uterine body is an option for a well-selected group of patients who desire to preserve fertility. The surgical approach can be vaginal, abdominal, or laparoscopic with robotic assistance. Selection criteria include patients with no clinical evidence of impaired fertility, stage IA2–IB1, lesion size <2 cm, limited endocervical involvement as evidenced

by direct visualization of the lesion by colposcopy or by MRI, squamous carcinoma or adenocarcinoma histology and no evidence of lymph node metastasis (6). Meeting all of these criteria, C.T. is a candidate for radical trachelectomy with pelvic lymphadenectomy.

MRI of the pelvis is useful before surgery to best define the endocervical tumor extension and determine the endocervical margin of resection. The initial surgical step is the lymph node evaluation. If the lymph nodes are negative, then the radical trachelectomy may proceed. A permanent cerclage is sutured in the remaining cervical stump and uterine body as a therapeutic measure for anticipated cervical incompetence in any future pregnancy. Other potential adverse effects of radical trachelectomy include premature labor, chronic vaginal discharge, irregular bleeding, dysmenorrhea, cerclage erosion, amenorrhea, and cervical stenosis (7). Approximately 10–12% of these patients are found to have more extensive disease or lymph node metastasis on intraoperative frozen section, contraindicating the fertility-preserving procedure (8).

In the young woman who remains interested in fertility but who is not a candidate for radical trachelectomy with preservation of the uterine body, oocyte retrieval for future fertilization and implantation into a surrogate uterus can be offered. In these circumstances, the best option is preoperative ovarian stimulation with retrieval of mature oocytes for immediate fertilization with donor sperm. These early embryos are cryopreserved for implantation into a surrogate uterus at a later time. If immediate in vitro fertilization is not acceptable to the patient, cryostorage of mature oocytes after ovarian stimulation for fertilization at a later time may be an alternative.

## Locally Advanced Cervical Cancer

L.S. is a 47-year-old healthy woman who presented with painful periods for 8 months. She took ibuprofen with some initial relief, but the pain progressed and she also developed vaginal bleeding between periods. Her last Pap smear was done approximately 10 years previously and was reported as normal. She denied a history of sexually transmitted diseases. Speculum examination showed blood clots in the vaginal vault and an ulcerative lesion replacing the cervix, extending to the upper third of the vagina. Bimanual examination confirmed an ulcerative lesion replacing the cervix and extending to the upper vagina circumferentially and to the parametrial tissues bilaterally. Biopsies of the cervical and upper vaginal lesion were consistent with invasive squamous cell carcinoma of the cervix.

A CT scan of the chest, abdomen, and pelvis showed irregular cervical margins and prominent parametrial strands suggesting parametrial involvement. Mild left hydronephrosis and diffuse bilateral pelvic lymphadenopathy were noted. No para-aortic lymphadenopathy or distant metastasis was identified on CT. As part of the staging procedure, cystoscopy and proctoscopy were performed and both were negative.

### Evidence-Based Case Discussion

L.S. has stage IIIB cervical cancer, which is categorized as locally advanced disease (stages IB2 and IIA2 to IVA).

Because squamous cell carcinoma of the cervix is both radiation and chemotherapy sensitive, the treatment of choice for locally advanced cervical cancer is concurrent chemotherapy and radiation therapy. Five landmark randomized clinical trials, involving nearly 1900 women, demonstrated a clear survival advantage for the use of cisplatin-based chemotherapy when administered concurrently with radiation therapy. Three of these trials demonstrated the benefit of cisplatin-based regimens when given concurrently with definitive radiation therapy for patients not amenable to surgery (9–11). These trials compared definitive radiation therapy regimens given either alone or in combination with hydroxyurea, cisplatin, or cisplatin–5-fluorouracil (5-FU) doublet. The cisplatin-containing regimens had better PFS and OS. In these trials, the relative risk of death at long-term follow-up was improved by 26–42%. The addition of 5-FU to cisplatin did not provide additional benefit. Two studies examined the role of concurrent therapy prior to hysterectomy or as adjuvant treatment after primary surgery. Keys and his Gynecologic Oncology Group (GOG) colleagues (12) randomized 369 women with stage IB2 disease to receive pelvic radiation therapy with or without concurrent cisplatin, and showed that both the PFS and OS were significantly better (relative risks of 0.51 and 0.54, respectively) for those receiving combined modality treatment prior to adjuvant hysterectomy. In the adjuvant setting after radical hysterectomy and pelvic lymphadenectomy, 243 women who were found to have positive margins, lymph node metastases, or parametrium involvement were randomized to receive either radiation therapy alone or with concurrent PF (13). At 4 years' follow-up, the concurrent radiation therapy/PF arm was associated with a superior PFS and OS: 80% versus 63% and 81% versus 71%, respectively.

The role of pelvic lymphadenectomy before chemoradiation is controversial. In addition to providing accurate treatment planning, lymphadenectomy also has the potential therapeutic survival benefit by resecting bulky nodes that do not respond well to chemoradiation (14,15). For patients with histologically confirmed para-aortic nodal involvement, extended field radiation therapy to include both pelvic and para-aortic nodes is recommended. For patients with locally advanced cervical carcinoma, disease stage is the most important prognostic factor, followed by lymph node status. Outcomes are worse for women with para-aortic lymph node metastasis.

## Distant Metastatic Cervical Cancer

N.S. is a 40-year-old woman, who emigrated from her home country in Central America 5 years ago never having had a Pap smear. She presented with episodes of heavy vaginal bleeding for 1 year and with a 4-month history of lower abdominal pain that extended to her back and radiated down her right leg. A pelvic examination revealed a 4.5 × 3.5 cm ulcerated cervical lesion extending down to the lower one third of the vagina, into both parametria and reaching the right pelvic sidewall. Biopsy of the cervical lesion was consistent with moderately differentiated invasive squamous cell carcinoma. A CT showed extensive pelvic and para-aortic lymph node enlargement, mild bilateral hydronephrosis, lytic lesions at right iliac wing, and pulmonary nodules. Biopsy of a pulmonary nodule was consistent with metastatic squamous cell carcinoma of the cervix. Laboratory studies showed severe anemia with a hemoglobin of 6.5 g/dL and mildly impaired renal function. Her performance status was 2.

## Evidence-Based Case Discussion

N.S. has disseminated stage IVB cervical cancer that is rare at initial diagnosis in the United States but common in developing countries. The most common sites of metastasis are lymph nodes followed by lung, liver, and bone. Treatment for stage IVB is focused on pallation of symptoms. For example, if vaginal bleeding is the main concern, an abbreviated course of pelvic radiation therapy at a higher dose per fraction can be administered to control acute bleeding. This pelvic palliative treatment can be followed by targeted radiation therapy to symptomatic lesions and/or chemotherapy to treat the systemic disease. Several chemotherapeutic drugs have shown activity in metastatic cervical cancer. Single-agent cisplatin has been used to treat recurrent and metastatic cervical cancer with a response rate of approximately 20%. A GOG phase III trial demonstrated a higher response rate (36% vs. 19%) and improved median PFS (4.8 vs. 2.8 months) in the treatment arm that received combination regimen with cisplatin and paclitaxel as compared to cisplatin alone; however, the OS was similar (16). Another phase III trial compared 4 cisplatin doublet regimens and found a trend in response rate, PFS, and OS that favored a cisplatin–paclitaxel combination. Specifically, response rates for cisplatin with either vinorelbine, gemcitabine, or topotecan were 25%, 22%, and 23%, respectively, which were not superior to cisplatin and paclitaxel with a response rate of 29% (17).

Another agent currently being studied is bevacizumab, a monoclonal anti-vascular endothelial growth factor receptor (VEGFR) agent. It has shown some promising results in a phase II trial (GOG 227C) where it was used as single agent after at least 1 prior chemotherapy line and had a better OS than historical controls (18). A recently published phase III randomized study (GOG 240) used a $2 \times 2$ factorial design to compare the best cisplatin doublet from GOG 204 (cisplatin/paclitaxel) with a non-platinum doublet (topotecan/paclitaxel). Each treatment combination was then randomized to either receive additional bevacizumab or not. None of the chemotherapy doublets had better outcome; however, the addition of bevacizumab to chemotherapy increased the overall response rate from 36% to 48%, with a doubling of CR from 6% to 12% ($P = .03$). With a follow-up of 20.8 months, bevacizumab groups had an increased OS from 13.3 to 17 months (death HR = 0.71, 0.54–0.94) and PFS from 5.9 to 8.2 months (HR = 0.67, 0.54–0.82). Importantly, bevacizumab seems to facilitate a response even in patients who have previously received platinum and radiotherapy, where retreatment with platinum doublets has little effect. As seen in other malignancies, addition of anti-VEGF was associated with increased hypertension, thromboembolic events (8%), and gastrointestinal (GI) fistulas and perforation (3%), but these have not led to a statistically significant decrease in QOL. The benefit was not seen in adenocarcinoma, where there was a trend toward worse outcome with additional bevacizumab (19). On the basis of this trial, the National Comprehensive Cancer Network (NCCN) now includes cisplatin/paclitaxel plus bevacizumab as first-line therapy (category 2A). A reasonable option is to replace cisplatin for carboplatin in the combination with paclitaxel, with similar outcome of PFS and OS and with an improvement in QOL and ease of administration (20). For patients whose performance status is poor, single-agent chemotherapy or best supportive care can be offered. In the case of N.S., a reasonable approach would be palliative pelvic radiation therapy to control symptomatic bleeding, followed by a platinum doublet and bevacizumab.

## REVIEW QUESTIONS

1. A 17-year-old high school student makes her first visit to the gynecologist and requests a contraception prescription because she is planning to become sexually active. Her body mass index is 31, she is not physically active, drinks rarely, and smokes several cigarettes a day. Her mother died of cervical cancer in her early 50s. She inquires how she can minimize cervical cancer risk. You counsel her that all of the following would decrease her risk of cervical cancer with the exception of:

   (A) Starting an exercise and weight-loss regimen
   (B) Obtaining a human papillomavirus vaccine against strains 6, 11, 16, and 18 immediately
   (C) Having routine Pap smear examination after age 21 years
   (D) Smoking cessation

2. A 29-year-old recently married woman has a preconception counseling visit, and a speculum examination shows a 1-cm posterior cervical lesion with a friable surface. A biopsy showed invasive squamous cell carcinoma with no lymphovascular invasion (LVI). A PET-CT scan does not reveal any distant metastases, and pelvic MRI shows that the mass is confined to the cervix only. She would like to have children. The best next step in her treatment plan is:

   (A) A cone biopsy and if negative margins, no further treatment

(B) Simple hysterectomy, pelvic lymph node dissection, and para-aortic lymph node sampling

(C) Simple trachelectomy

(D) Radical trachelectomy with pelvic lymph node dissection and possible para-aortic lymph node sampling

3. A 31-year-old woman, married with 1 child, presents to her gynecologist for postcoital bleeding. Her pelvic examination demonstrates a cervical lesion of 3 cm. A biopsy shows poorly differentiated squamous cell carcinoma. A PET-CT scan does not show any distant lesions. An MRI of the pelvis confirms that lesion is confined to the cervix. She undergoes radical hysterectomy with pelvic lymph node dissection and para-aortic lymph node sampling. The final pathology shows a 3.5-cm tumor invading the outer two thirds of the cervix with lymphovascular invasion. All the nodes are negative and margins are uninvolved with tumor. The most appropriate next step for the patient is the following:

(A) Surveillance with history and physical (H&P) examination every 3 months and CT scan as clinically indicated

(B) Surveillance with H&P examination every 3 months and CT scan for chest, abdomen, and pelvis every 6 months for the first 2 years, than annually for 3 years

(C) Adjuvant cisplatin-based chemotherapy

(D) Pelvic radiation therapy with or without concurrent cisplatin sensitization

4. A 50-year-old woman, obese, with diabetes mellitus type II, stage III chronic kidney disease, and well-controlled hypertension has a worsening cough of 3 months' duration. A chest x-ray shows bilateral pulmonary nodules and a subsequent CT of the chest, abdomen, and pelvis shows an ill-defined cervical mass extending into parametria bilaterally and reaching the left pelvic sidewall. There is also retroperitoneal lymphadenopathy, multiple bilateral subcentimeter lung nodules, and several lytic lesions in the vertebrae. She has never had a Pap smear. A biopsy of the cervical mass shows poorly differentiated squamous cell carcinoma. She has lost 10 kg over the last 6 months and is tired, but still able to work full time as a bus driver. You counsel her about her incurable condition and offer palliative chemotherapy. She is very determined to try any treatment offered. The most appropriate first-line chemotherapy regimen for her is:

(A) Cisplatin, paclitaxel, and bevazicumab

(B) Carboplatin, paclitaxel, and bevacizumab

(C) Topotecan and paclitaxel

(D) Carboplatin, gemcitabine, and bevacizumab

5. A 30-year-old woman has her first well-women examination in 10 years. A speculum examination shows a 2-cm cervical mass with extension into the upper third of the posterior vaginal wall. On bimanual examination, there was no evidence of parametrial involvement. A biopsy shows squamous cell carcinoma. Her Eastern Cooperative Oncology Group performance status is 0 and she has no other comorbidities. She is scheduled to have surgery in 2 weeks but meanwhile she is admitted with back pain. CT scan reveals left-sided hydronephrosis and lower ureteral obstruction due to lateral expansion of the tumor. No stone is noted. A percutaneous nephrostomy is placed and her symptoms improve. Her serum creatinine is 1.0. What is the next most appropriate step in her cervical cancer treatment?

(A) Proceed with radical trachelectomy, pelvic node dissection, and para-aortic lymph node sampling

(B) Proceed with radical hysterectomy, pelvic node dissection, and para-aortic lymph node sampling

(C) Cancel surgery and refer her to a radiation oncologist to proceed with concurrent pelvic radiation therapy with cisplatin sensitization

(D) Proceed with neoadjuvant chemotherapy with cisplatin-containing doublet prior to radical trachelectomy, pelvic node dissection, and para-aortic lymph node sampling

6. A 34-year-old woman has an abnormal Pap smear and normal appearing cervix. Her colposcopy reveals a very small aceto white lesion, and cervical biopsy is consistent with well-differentiated squamous cell carcinoma with stromal invasion to a depth of at least 1 mm. She is newly married and desires to have children. She undergoes a cold knife conization, which reveals a 5-mm tumor with stromal invasion of 2 mm. What do you offer her regarding further treatment options?

(A) Adjuvant chemotherapy with cisplatin, paclitaxel, and bevacizumab

(B) Radical trachelectomy with pelvic node dissection and possible para-aortic lymph node sampling

(C) Close surveillance with routine Pap smears

(D) Radical hysterectomy with pelvic node dissection and possible para-aortic lymph node sampling

## REFERENCES

1. International Collaboration of Epidemiological Studies of Cervical Cancer. Comparison of risk factors for invasive squamous cell carcinoma and adenocarcinoma of the cervix: collaborative reanalysis of individual data on 8,097 women with squamous cell carcinoma and 1,374 women with adenocarcinoma from 12 epidemiological studies. *Int J Cancer.* 2007;120:885–891.

2. Saslow D, Solomon D, Lawson HW, et al.; ACS-ASCCP-ASCP Cervical Cancer Guideline Committee. American Cancer Society,

American Society for Colposcopy and Cervical Pathology, and American Society for Clinical Pathology screening guidelines for the prevention and early detection of cervical cancer. *CA Cancer J Clin.* 2012;62(3):147–172.

3. Eifel PJ, Burke TW, Delclos L, et al. Early stage I adenocarcinoma of the uterine cervix: treatment results in patients with tumors less than or equal to 4 cm in diameter. *Gynecol Oncol.* 1991;41(3):199–205.

4. Landoni F, Maneo A, Colombo A, et al. Randomised study of radical surgery versus radiotherapy for stage Ib-IIa cervical cancer. *Lancet.* 1997;350(9077):535–540.

5. Cormier B, Diaz JP, Shih K, et al. Establishing a sentinel lymph node mapping algorithm for the treatment of early cervical cancer. *Gynecol Oncol.* 2011;122(2):275–280.

6. Alexander-Sefre F, Chee N, Spencer C, et al. Surgical morbidity associated with radical trachelectomy and radical hysterectomy. *Gynecol Oncol.* 2006;101(3):450–454.

7. Plante M, Renaud MC, François H, Roy M. Vaginal radical trachelectomy: an oncologically safe fertility-preserving surgery. An updated series of 72 cases and review of the literature. *Gynecol Oncol.* 2004;94(3):614–623.

8. Burghardt E, Baltzer J, Tulusan AH, Haas J. Results of surgical treatment of 1028 cervical cancers studied with volumetry. *Cancer.* 1992;70(3):648–655.

9. Whitney CW, Sause W, Bundy BN, et al. Randomized comparison of fluorouracil plus cisplatin versus hydroxyurea as an adjunct to radiation therapy in stage IIB-IVA carcinoma of the cervix with negative para-aortic lymph nodes: a Gynecologic Oncology Group and Southwest Oncology Group study. *J Clin Oncol.* 1999;17(5):1339–1348.

10. Rose PG, Bundy BN, Watkins EB, et al. Concurrent cisplatin-based radiotherapy and chemotherapy for locally advanced cervical cancer. *N Engl J Med.* 1999;340(15):1144–1153.

11. Morris M, Eifel PJ, Lu J, et al. Pelvic radiation with concurrent chemotherapy compared with pelvic and para-aortic radiation for high-risk cervical cancer. *N Engl J Med.* 1999;340(15):1137–1143.

12. Keys HM, Bundy BN, Stehman FB, et al. Cisplatin, radiation, and adjuvant hysterectomy compared with radiation and adjuvant hysterectomy for bulky stage IB cervical carcinoma. *N Engl J Med.* 1999;340(15):1154–1161.

13. Peters WA 3rd, Liu PY, Barrett RJ 2nd, et al. Concurrent chemotherapy and pelvic radiation therapy compared with pelvic radiation therapy alone as adjuvant therapy after radical surgery in high-risk early-stage cancer of the cervix. *J Clin Oncol.* 2000;18(8):1606–1613.

14. Hacker NF, Wain GV, Nicklin JL. Resection of bulky positive lymph nodes in patients with cervical carcinoma. *Int J Gynecol Cancer.* 1995;5(4):250–256.

15. Marnitz S, Köhler C, Roth C, et al. Is there a benefit of pretreatment laparoscopic transperitoneal surgical staging in patients with advanced cervical cancer? *Gynecol Oncol.* 2005;99(3):536–544.

16. Moore DH, Blessing JA, McQuellon RP, et al. Phase III study of cisplatin with or without paclitaxel in stage IVB, recurrent, or persistent squamous cell carcinoma of the cervix: a gynecologic oncology group study. *J Clin Oncol.* 2004;22(15):3113–3119.

17. Monk BJ, Sill MW, McMeekin DS, et al. Phase III trial of four cisplatin-containing doublet combinations in stage IVB, recurrent, or persistent cervical carcinoma: a Gynecologic Oncology Group study. *J Clin Oncol.* 2009;27(28):4649–4655.

18. Monk BJ, Sill MW, Burger RA, et al. Phase II trial of bevacizumab in the treatment of persistent or recurrent squamous cell carcinoma of the cervix: a gynecologic oncology group study. *J Clin Oncol.* 2009;27(7):1069–1074.

19. Tewari KS, Sill MW, Long HJ 3rd, et al. Improved survival with bevacizumab in advanced cervical cancer. *N Engl J Med.* 2014;370(8):734–743.

20. Kitagawa, R, Katsumata N, Shibata T, et al. A randomized, phase III trial of paclitaxel plus carboplatin (TC) versus paclitaxel plus cisplatin (TP) in stage IVb, persistent or recurrent cervical cancer: Japan Clinical Oncology Group study (JCOG0505). *J Clin Oncol.* 2012;30(Suppl, Abstract 5006).

# 18

# Uterine Cancer

KIRAN NAQVI, ATISHA P. MANHAS, AND MATTHEW L. ANDERSON

## EPIDEMIOLOGY, RISK FACTORS, NATURAL HISTORY, AND PATHOLOGY

Uterine cancer is the most common female genital tract malignancy in the United States (1) and includes both endometrial cancers (endometrial adenocarcinoma) and more rare cancers arising in the myometrium, such as uterine leiomyosarcomas (2). Endometrial cancers are most commonly diagnosed in women aged 50–65 years. Seventy-five percent of patients are postmenopausal. For many women, the pathogenesis of endometrial cancer appears to be related to prolonged exposure of unopposed estrogen (caused by obesity, diabetes mellitus, and/or high-fat diet), which promotes endometrial growth and ultimately causes poorly understood changes in endometrial glands. Other significant risk factors include early menarche and late menopause, nulliparity, Lynch syndrome, older age (≥55 years), and tamoxifen use (3).

Early estrogen-induced changes in the endometrium can lead to simple hyperplasia, which is typically reversible with hormonal treatment and is not considered to be a premalignant condition. However, more disorganized lesions, such as complex atypical hyperplasia (CAH), are now recognized to have significant malignant potential. The molecular basis of complex or atypical endometrial hyperplasia is poorly understood. About 25% of women with CAH will eventually develop an invasive endometrial cancer. In light of this issue, as well as the fact that as many as 30% of women diagnosed with CAH by endometrial biopsy are actually harboring an early-stage cancer, these lesions are often treated with hysterectomy. Surgical excision of premalignant lesions is almost always successful in preventing uterine cancer.

Hormonally driven cancers are generally categorized as type I endometrial cancers. Women taking tamoxifen have an approximately 3- to 7-fold higher risk of developing endometrial cancer (4). Hereditary nonpolyposis colorectal cancer (HNPCC) syndrome is also a risk factor, associated with a 20–60% lifetime risk of endometrial cancer. Genetic testing and counseling should be performed for all patients <50 years of age with endometrial cancer or with significant family history of endometrial and/or colon cancer (5). Factors that decrease the risk of type I endometrial cancer include combined oral contraceptive use, early menopause, multiparity, and smoking (likely through an antiestrogenic effect).

The vast majority (75%) of patients with type I endometrial cancer and traditional risk factors have disease confined to the uterus (stage I) at diagnosis (6). These are histologically similar to their tissue of origin and are categorized as endometrioid adenocarcinoma. A second category of endometrial cancers (type II) has been defined and includes less common but clinically more aggressive cancers such as serous adenocarcinoma, clear cell adenocarcinoma, and carcinosarcoma (malignant mixed Mullerian tumors). Although for many years, carcinosarcomas were considered to be a type of sarcoma, more recent evidence suggests that these pleomorphic cancers are actually metaplastic carcinomas and are treated similarly to other high-grade epithelial endometrial cancers (7). Despite comprising <10% of uterine cancers, serous adenocarcinomas account for >40% of uterine cancer deaths in the United States. These and other type II uterine cancers are found more frequently in African American women and are less likely to be associated with obesity or hormonal exposure. In large part, the mortality related to type II cancers is due to their propensity to metastasize early (8). There is increasing appreciation that type II uterine cancers arise via a distinct endometrial precursor known as endometrial intraepithelial neoplasia (EIN). The molecular events leading to EIN are poorly defined.

About 90% of patients with endometrial cancer present with postmenopausal bleeding. For these women, office endometrial biopsy often establishes the diagnosis (9), allowing patients to be triaged to appropriate surgical management. It is important to keep in mind that endometrial biopsies have a 10% false-negative rate. Hence, in symptomatic patients, a fractional dilation and curettage (D&C) should be performed to rule out cancer under circumstances where women continue to experience problems with postmenopausal bleeding. Currently, there is no validated screening test for endometrial cancer. Endometrial cancer is surgically staged. International Federation of Obstetricians and Gynecologists (FIGO) and American Joint Committee on Cancer (AJCC) updated the surgical–pathological staging criteria for uterine neoplasms in 2010 (Table 18.1) (10). Initial clinical management includes total abdominal hysterectomy with bilateral salpingo-oophorectomy (TAH/BSO) and a careful examination of the entire abdominopelvic cavity. Suspicious lesions identified at the time of surgery should be thoroughly sampled to establish the presence or absence of carcinoma. Historically, surgical staging procedures such as pelvic washings and pelvic and para-aortic lymph node dissections have been performed once size, grade, and depth of myometrial invasion are established by intraoperative frozen section. A number of investigators have advocated thorough surgical staging regardless of whether poorly differentiated tumor histology, deep myometrial invasion, or lymphovascular invasion are noted on frozen section. Peritoneal cytology is no longer a part of the updated FIGO staging. However, FIGO and AJCC continue to recommend that peritoneal cytology be assessed at hysterectomy, because a positive result may add to other risk factors and help to determine treatment plans. A second, ongoing issue is the extent of lymphadenectomy necessary to adequately stage endometrial cancers. Retrospective data suggest that thorough lymphadenectomies not only identify para-aortic lymph node metastases in approximately 20% of women with no radiographic evidence of metastases in pelvic lymph nodes, but may also have a therapeutic benefit. Despite this, there are currently no data from a randomized trial to support the use of routine lymphadenectomies as part of the initial surgical management of endometrial cancer (11). Pending further trials, many gynecologic oncologists recommend staging lymphadenectomies for patients found to have high-risk histological features on preoperative endometrial biopsy and/or frozen section (deeply invasive lesions, high-grade histology and tumors of serous or clear cell adenocarcinoma, or carcinosarcoma). The utility of sentinel lymph node mapping has been studied in women with patients with disease confined to the uterus, but at present this procedure is considered experimental (12).

**Table 18.1** 2010 FIGO Staging for Endometrial Carcinoma

| Stage | Definition |
|-------|-----------|
| I | Primary tumor is confined to the corpus uteri |
| IA | Tumor limited to endometrium or invades less than half of the myometrium |
| IB | Tumor invades one half or more of the myometrium |
| II | Primary tumor invades cervical stroma, but does not extend beyond uterus[a] |
| III | Local and/or regional spread of tumor is present |
| IIIA | Tumor invades serosa of the corpus uteri and/or adnexae[b] |
| IIIB | Vaginal and/or parametrial involvement is present[b] |
| IIIC | Metastasis to pelvic and/or para-aortic lymph nodes is present[b] |
| IIIC-1 | Positive pelvic nodes |
| IIIC-2 | Positive para-aortic nodes with or without positive pelvic lymph nodes |
| IV | Tumor invades bladder mucosa and/or bowel, or distant metastasis is present |
| IVA | Tumor invades bladder mucosa and/or bowel |
| IVB | Distant metastasis is present |

FIGO, International Federation of Obstetricians and Gynecologists.
[a]Endocervical glandular involvement is considered stage I and no longer is stage II.
[b]Positive peritoneal cytology should be reported separately and does not change the stage.

Five-year survival for endometrial cancer varies by stage: 83% for patients with stage I disease, 73% for those with stage II disease, 52% for those with stage III disease, and 27% for those with stage IV disease. Features associated with a worse prognosis include high-grade, type II histology, older age, and vascular invasion.

Several other malignant conditions may arise in the uterus as a result of the malignant transformation of gestational trophoblastic tissue. Collectively, the spectra of these diseases are defined as malignant gestational trophoblastic disease (GTD). These cancers commonly develop after molar pregnancy, but may develop after nonmolar pregnancy as well. Diagnosis is made when levels of serum beta human chorionic gonadotropin (βhCG) fail to decrease appropriately following uterine evacuation. Less commonly, the diagnosis is established by histological evaluation of evacuated uterine contents. An initial βhCG >100,000 mIU/mL, history of prior GTD, and age >40 years all increase the risk of malignant GTD following molar pregnancy. Subtypes of malignant GTD are quite heterogeneous in clinical behavior and include persistent–invasive gestational trophoblastic neoplasia (GTN), choriocarcinoma, and placental site trophoblastic tumor (PSTT). Persistent–invasive GTN follows approximately 20% of complete molar pregnancies and is rarely metastatic at presentation. Conversely, choriocarcinoma is a highly aggressive cancer. The majority of women

**Table 18.2** WHO Staging of Malignant Gestational Trophoblast Disease

| Prognostic Factor | Risk Score | | | |
| --- | --- | --- | --- | --- |
| | 0 | 1 | 2 | 4 |
| Age (yr) | <40 | ≥40 | | |
| Antecedent pregnancy | Hydatidiform mole | Abortion | Term pregnancy | |
| Interval months from pregnancy | <4 | 4–6 | 7–12 | >12 |
| Pretreatment serum βhCG (IU/mL) | <1000 | 1000 to <10,000 | 10,000 to <100,000 | |
| Largest tumor size, including uterus (cm) | <3 | 3–5 | >5 | |
| Site of metastases | Lung | Spleen, kidney | GI tract | Brain, liver |
| Number of metastases identified | | 1–4 | 5–8 | >8 |
| Previous failed chemotherapy | | | Single drug | 2 or more drugs |
| Total score | <6 = low risk, ≥7 = high risk | | | |

βhCG, beta human chorionic gonadotropin; GI, gastrointestinal; WHO, World Health Organization.

diagnosed with choriocarcinoma of trophoblastic origin present with metastases, most commonly to the lung. Fifty percent of choriocarcinomas develop after molar pregnancies, while the remaining 50% are diagnosed following nonmolar pregnancies (normal pregnancies, spontaneous abortions, and ectopic pregnancies). PSTT is a rare form of malignant GTD that develops from intermediate cytotrophoblast. PSTT may present months to years after a term gestation. These tumors secrete only small amounts of βhCG and are not nearly as sensitive to chemotherapy as other types of malignant GTD. Outcomes for this disease are typically guarded.

Staging of malignant GTD is clinical rather than surgical and has evolved to include elements that define the anatomic extent of disease as well as specific prognostic features. These elements have been incorporated by the World Health Organization (WHO) into a scoring system that is used to determine clinical care for women judged to be at intermediate risk (Table 18.2). Under this system, patients are given a number score and placed into "low-risk" or "high-risk" categories based on multiple factors including age, interval from antecedent pregnancy, and pretreatment βhCG. Significant clinical data support the validity of WHO prognostic scores for assessing risk and prospectively identifying patients most likely to require combination chemotherapy. Fortunately, with the exception of PSTT, even high-risk metastatic malignant GTD is highly sensitive to chemotherapy. With standard treatment, cure rates >90% are typically achieved (13).

## CASE SUMMARIES

### Early-Stage Endometrial Cancer

L.C., a 67-year-old retired accountant who was menopausal since age 59 years, presented to her gynecologist with a 2-week history of vaginal bleeding. She described her bleeding as mild and intermittent, occurring 1–2 times daily. She denied abdominal pain or weight loss. Her medical and surgical history were remarkable for hypertension, osteoporosis, and a right hip replacement 3 years earlier. She had 3 children from 3 pregnancies. She had not taken hormone replacement therapy, had no family history of cancer, and had smoked 1 pack of cigarettes daily for 40 years. General physical examination was significant for obesity. On pelvic examination, the uterus was normal in size and non-tender, and the cervix was smooth without lesions. Adnexae were normal.

An office endometrial biopsy was performed. Results of this biopsy revealed grade 2 moderately differentiated adenocarcinoma. Chest x-ray showed no evidence of metastatic disease. The patient underwent TAH, BSO, and pelvic and para-aortic lymph node sampling. Final pathology showed a moderately differentiated endometrioid adenocarcinoma with >50% invasion of the myometrium, including the outer third, and lymphovascular invasion (Figure 18.1). All lymph nodes were negative for malignancy. She was referred to an oncologist for recommendations regarding adjuvant therapy.

### Evidence-Based Case Discussion

Using updated FIGO criteria, this patient's tumor is classified as a stage IB endometrial cancer, because her disease is localized to corpus uteri, but invades through >50% of the myometrium. Under the previous version of FIGO staging, she would be considered to have stage IC disease. Her risk factors for endometrial cancer include obesity and late menopause. Smoking is not a risk factor for endometrial cancer, as it promotes the synthesis of steroid hormone–binding globulins protective for this disease.

Approaches to adjuvant therapy in early-stage endometrial cancer have been defined by randomized trials investigating the role of adjuvant pelvic irradiation. Interpretation of results from these trials is complicated by the fact that

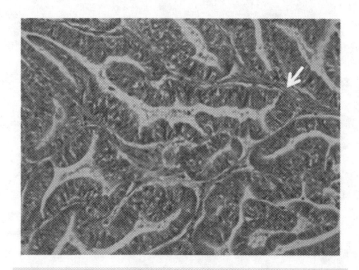

**Figure 18.1**

Endometrial adenocarcinoma. Uterine cancers are characterized by abnormal gland formation (arrow), diminished or absent stroma between glands, disordered chromatin distribution, nuclear enlargement, increased mitoses, and necrosis. Severity of histological features is used to grade tumors and is associated with prognosis.

FIGO recently updated its system for endometrial staging, incorporating former stage IA and IB tumors (invasion <half myometrial thickness) into a new stage IA. Former stage IC cancers are now defined as stage IB disease. Gynecologic Oncology Group (GOG) 99 compared adjuvant pelvic radiation to observation in 400 patients with stage I, IB, IC, and II disease. No difference in overall survival (OS) was found with use of pelvic radiation; however, local pelvic and/or vaginal recurrences occurred less frequently following pelvic radiation (3% vs. 12%). The Post-Operative Radiation Therapy in Endometrial Carcinoma-1 (PORTEC-1) trial, which randomized 714 patients with stage I disease to pelvic radiation or observation, also showed a decrease in local recurrences following pelvic radiation, again with no difference in OS. Similarly, the ASTEC/EN.5 study failed to show improvement in relapse-free survival (RFS) or OS with only a small improvement in local pelvic control. The latter study is controversial, as 51% of patients in the observation arm received vaginal brachytherapy, making it difficult to truly assess the outcomes of conservative management.

To determine which patients may benefit from adjuvant radiation, Creutzberg et al. used data from GOG 99 to define subgroups at "low-" and high–intermediate risk for local recurrence (14). Patients with stage IA or IB (current FIGO IA) and grade 1 or 2 tumors were defined as "low" risk, with a 6% chance of local recurrence. Patients in this subset are considered candidates for conservative management without adjuvant therapy. In patients with stage IC tumors (or grade 3 tumors in stage IA or IB), risk factors were used to determine high–intermediate risk patients who would benefit from radiotherapy. Factors considered to increase risk included advanced age, grade 2 or 3 tumors, outer third invasion of the myometrium, and lymphovascular space invasion. High–intermediate risk patients were categorized as patients 70 years or older with 1 other risk factor, patients between 50 and 70 years with 2 other risk factors, or any age with all 3 risk factors. Given that this patient has 3 risk factors, she would be classified as "high–intermediate" risk and should be considered for adjuvant radiation therapy (RT).

Vaginal brachytherapy appears to be equally effective as whole pelvic radiation for preventing recurrences with high–intermediate risk, stage I endometrial cancers. This conclusion is suggested by the PORTEC-2 trial, which showed no significant difference in local recurrence rates in patients assigned to either modality. In light of its favorable toxicity profile, vaginal brachytherapy has become the standard modality used for adjuvant RT for high–intermediate risk stage I uterine cancer patients. The role of adjuvant chemotherapy in early-stage endometrial cancer remains undefined and is being evaluated in several large clinical trials, including GOG 249 and PORTEC-3. A preliminary Japanese GOG trial has reported better OS for high–intermediate-risk patients (stage IC) patients receiving cyclophosphamide, doxorubicin, and cisplatin rather than radiation (90% vs. 74%) (15).

In summary, patients with stage IA and grade 1 or 2 cancers are considered low risk, and no adjuvant treatment is recommended. For all other patients with stage I disease, risk factors should be evaluated. Those patients deemed to be high–intermediate risk should be considered for adjuvant vaginal brachytherapy. Figure 18.2 outlines a suggested algorithm for the management of stage I disease.

The treatment of stage II endometrial cancer is more complex due to involvement of the cervical stroma. If surgeons are aware of cervical invasion prior to hysterectomy, 1 option potentially associated with an improved outcome is to perform a radical hysterectomy rather than the more standard simple extrafascial hysterectomy. Different treatment strategies, including primary radioactive implants have been used following hysterectomy for stage II disease. In patients who have undergone radical hysterectomy with negative margins and with no evidence of extrauterine disease, observation or vaginal brachytherapy are both valid options. Patients with stage II disease should be encouraged to enroll in clinical trials evaluating these various treatment approaches.

Although the primary treatment of endometrial carcinoma is surgery, continuous progestin-based therapy may be considered in certain patients with complex endometrial hyperplasia or stage-IA disease who wish to preserve their fertility (16). There are strict criteria for fertility-sparing therapy, and each 1 of them has to be fulfilled to qualify for this approach. These include well-differentiated (grade 1) endometrioid adenocarcinoma identified

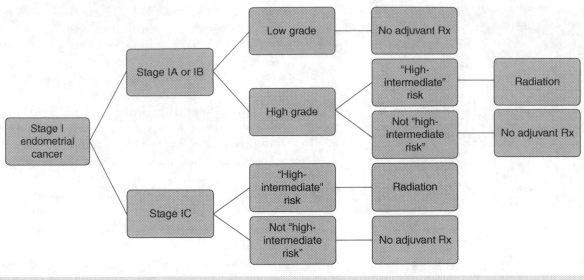

### Figure 18.2

Treatment algorithm for early-stage endometrial carcinoma. Adjuvant treatment is determined by the histological features of each cancer and other risk factors for recurrence. Factors that increase risk include age, increasing histological ($\geq$2) grade, presence of tumor in the outer third of the myometrium, and lymphovascular invasion. "High–intermediate"-risk patients are defined as patients older than 70 years with 1 other risk factor, older than 50 years with 2 other risk factors, or any age with all 3 risk factors.

on endometrial biopsy or uterine D&C, reviewed by an expert pathologist, disease limited to the endometrium on MRI, no evidence of extrauterine or metastatic disease on imaging, and no contraindication to medical therapy or pregnancy. It is particularly important to counsel patients considering this option that fertility-sparing medical management is not currently considered standard of care and that experience with this option, although growing, remains limited. Patients treated with continuous progestin-based therapy require endometrial sampling every 3–6 months. A durable complete response is seen in about 50% of patients (17). Surgical treatment with TAH/BSO and/or staging is recommended: (a) once childbearing is complete, (b) if the patient progresses on progestin therapy, or (c) if endometrial cancer persists after 6 months of treatment (18). Approximately 35% of females treated with progestin-based therapy with subsequent negative endometrial biopsy are able to become pregnant. However, it is also important to caution patients that recurrences of endometrial cancer after medical management are common, occurring in as many as 35% of women (19). It should also be noted that patients have been found to experience disease progression and metastasis while pursuing conservative management of their cancer in this manner.

## Locally Advanced Endometrial Cancer

Y.R. is a 48-year-old woman who presented to her gynecologist's office with a complaint of abnormal vaginal bleeding. She noted intermittent, mild bleeding between each menstrual cycle, as well as abnormally heavy menses for 3 months. Prior to this, she had increasing menstrual

irregularity for 1 year, but no abnormally heavy menses or spotting. In addition, she noted the development of a dull pain in her left abdomen 1 week prior to presentation. She had experienced a 10-pound weight loss over the last 3 months, but had no other constitutional symptoms. Her medical history was remarkable for type II diabetes and mild peripheral neuropathy. She had never been pregnant, did not smoke, and her only medication was metformin. Her family history was unremarkable for cancer or gynecological diseases. On general examination, she was overweight but had no other abnormalities. Pelvic examination revealed no external genital lesions, a smooth cervix without lesions, and a normal-sized uterus and normal adnexae. Transvaginal ultrasound showed an endometrial thickness of 6 mm. Endometrial biopsy was done, and results revealed endometrial adenocarcinoma.

Chest x-ray showed no abnormalities, but CT scan of the abdomen and pelvis revealed an isolated enlarged left pelvic lymph node (Figure 18.3). There was no para-aortic lymphadenopathy. The patient underwent surgical resection and staging, consisting of TAH, BSO, and lymph node dissection. Pathology revealed a grade 2 endometrioid adenocarcinoma, with 2 pelvic lymph nodes positive for malignancy. Peritoneal cytology was also positive for malignancy.

### Evidence-Based Case Discussion

This patient presents with a FIGO stage III endometrial cancer. Specifically, she has stage IIIC-1 disease, due to involvement of adjacent pelvic lymph nodes. Although the patient had positive peritoneal cytology, this finding does

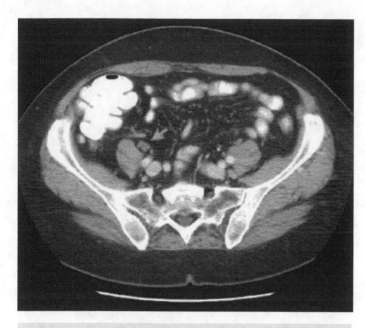

**Figure 18.3**

Imaging of lymphatic metastasis. An isolated pelvic lymph node metastasis (arrow) was visualized by CT in a patient with endometrial carcinoma.

not contribute to surgical stage according to updated 2010 FIGO guidelines. This patient's case highlights the fact that endometrial cancer frequently affects perimenopausal women in addition to women who have already undergone menopause. Younger women of reproductive age can also develop endometrial cancer. In fact, women younger than age 50 years constitute 10–15% of all endometrial cancer cases (1).

Many patients with stage III endometrial cancer (and selective patients with stage IV) are considered to have surgically resectable disease, with an estimated 50–80% chance of long-term survival. Randall and Reisinger evaluated data from recent studies with the goal of defining prognostic features in patients with surgical stage III and IV disease (20). Favorable characteristics included isolated adnexal or serosal involvement (stage IIIA) and isolated pelvic lymph node involvement with surgically confirmed negative para-aortic lymph nodes. Unfavorable features included the presence of gross residual tumor after surgery, para-aortic lymph node involvement, multiple sites of extrauterine spread, high histological grade, lymphovascular space invasion, peritoneal spread, and high-risk serous and clear cell histologies. These high-risk patients are at greater risk for both local failure and distant metastasis.

Optimal adjuvant treatment for surgically resected, advanced-stage endometrial cancer is a work in progress. RT and chemotherapy have both been studied in clinical trials. Although the use of whole abdominal irradiation (WAI) has been studied by a number of investigators, GOG 94, a large phase II trial evaluating WAI in 180 patients

with stage III or IV disease, found that 3-year RFS rates were relatively low (29% and 27% for typical and high-risk histologies, respectively). Half of the recurrences found in patients enrolled in GOG 94 consisted of distant relapses, underscoring the need to evaluate adjuvant systemic therapy. The role of chemotherapy in adjuvant treatment of stage III endometrial carcinoma is further underscored by the pivotal GOG 122 trial. This trial compared WAI to chemotherapy in patients with surgical stage III or IVA endometrial cancer with <2-cm gross residual disease. Chemotherapy consisted of doxorubicin 60 mg/m$^2$ and cisplatin 50 mg/m$^2$ every 3 weeks for 7 cycles, followed by 1 cycle of cisplatin. The chemotherapy arm demonstrated superior 5-year progression-free survival (PFS; 50% vs. 38%) and OS (55% vs. 42%). As a result of this trial, chemotherapy is now a mainstay of adjuvant treatment of advanced, surgically resectable endometrial cancer. However, the local recurrence rate in the trial was higher in the chemotherapy arm than in the radiation arm (32% vs. 29% of all recurrences), suggesting that radiation should still play a role in these patients. Acute toxicity such as peripheral neuropathy was also greater in the chemotherapy arm. Many clinicians will combine radiation with chemotherapy for patients who are thought to be at high risk for pelvic recurrence; however, this approach has not yet been validated. Two large trials are currently evaluating combination therapy, in which the modalities are given concomitantly (GOG 99–07) or sequentially (GOG 99–08).

The optimal chemotherapy regimen remains to be defined. Of note, GOG 122 was followed by GOG 184, a trial that compared the combination of cisplatin and doxorubicin to a regimen with cisplatin, doxorubicin, and paclitaxel. There was no difference in 3-year survival between the 2 arms, with greater toxicity in subjects receiving the 3-drug regimen. Although GOG 122 used doxorubicin and cisplatin, the TAP regimen (doxorubicin 45 mg/m$^2$ on day 1, paclitaxel 160 mg/m$^2$ on day 2, and cisplatin 50 mg/m$^2$ on day 1) is utilized by many clinicians due to a survival benefit seen in advanced or recurrent unresectable endometrial cancer. More recent evidence suggests that the use of carboplatin and paclitaxel (TC) combination may produce equivalent results. Due to its favorable toxicity profile, many oncologists now rely on this latter regimen for the adjuvant therapy of women at high risk of recurrence.

In summary, although optimal adjuvant treatment for stage III and IV endometrial cancer is evolving, the current standard of care is chemotherapy based on the GOG 122 trial data. Clinicians often incorporate radiation as part of the treatment plan for women thought to be at high risk for local failure, although this approach is still under investigation. In the case of the 48-year-old patient with stage IIIC endometrial cancer involving pelvic lymph nodes, the recommended adjuvant treatment would be chemotherapy. Her peripheral neuropathy would preclude the use of a taxane, so a reasonable regimen for her would be doxorubicin and cisplatin. Her isolated pelvic lymph node metastases place her in a favorable risk group, because her para-aortic nodes were unaffected. As she is not at particularly high risk of local failure, radiation may not offer additional benefit.

## Recurrent and Metastatic Endometrial Cancer

A 72-year-old postmenopausal woman presented to her primary care provider with intermittent vaginal bleeding of 6 months' duration. She described fatigue and dizziness on standing as well as a 9-pound unintentional weight loss over 3 months. She had no ongoing medical problems, took no medications, and did not smoke. She was a retired business woman but still volunteered fairly actively in her community. General physical examination was remarkable for slight abdominal fullness, but no discrete mass. On bimanual examination, the right adnexa were markedly tender. However, uterus and cervix were both normal. Transvaginal ultrasound showed increased endometrial thickness and an enlarged right ovary. Office endometrial biopsy revealed endometrial adenocarcinoma, grade 2. CT scan of the abdomen and pelvis showed a thickened uterus as well as discrete metastatic deposits on the right ovary and bladder, peritoneal implants, and 3 hypoattenuating lesions in the liver. Image-guided biopsy of 1 of the liver lesions was consistent with endometrial adenocarcinoma.

## Evidence-Based Case Discussion

This patient presents with a stage IVB uterine cancer (distant metastasis to the liver). For patients presenting with metastatic disease, several recent retrospective studies have examined the potential utility of debulking surgery. Results of these studies have been generally favorable, suggesting improved survival with optimal debulking of metastatic disease. Patients with metastatic or recurrent endometrial cancer have several different treatment options, depending on the extent of disease. For patients with isolated vaginal or pelvic relapse, radiation offers approximately 50–70% 5-year survival (21). In the PORTEC trial, 3-year survival rates in patients with local relapse were 51% for those who received radiation and 19% for those who did not (22). For those patients who have already undergone pelvic radiation, surgery can also provide an opportunity for long-term survival. Bristow et al. found that of the 35 patients who underwent surgery for locally recurrent endometrial cancer at 1 institution, 54% of women who underwent a complete resection were alive at 3 years, as opposed to none in the group of patients with residual disease following resection (23). Patients with isolated pelvic recurrence after RT may also be considered for pelvic exenteration.

Despite its associated morbidity, exenteration with complete tumor resection offers a 20–45% chance of long-term survival (24).

Widely metastatic disease may be treated with systemic therapy, including hormone therapy and chemotherapy. Progestational agents, including megestrol acetate, hydroxyprogesterone caproate, and medroxyprogesterone acetate, have each been found to produce clinical responses when used to treat uterine cancer. Objective response rates for women receiving high doses of these agents are typically between 10% and 30%. Although the average duration of response is 4 months, some patients remain progression free for over 2 years. The likelihood of a response is highly dependent on estrogen and/or progesterone–receptor expression. Progesterone–receptor negative tumors have very low response rates; thus, progestins are recommended as initial therapy only for women who have progesterone–receptor-positive tumors. Tamoxifen has also shown response in patients with hormone–receptor-positive cancers, with a 20% response rate in those who do not respond to standard progesterone therapy (24). In general, low-grade histology and a long disease-free interval between initial diagnosis and development of metastatic disease are associated with increased likelihood of a response (25).

Chemotherapy is the treatment of choice for patients with metastatic disease who have progesterone receptor (PR)-negative tumors or have failed hormonal therapy, and it is often considered for many patients, regardless of hormone receptor status. Doxorubicin, cisplatin, carboplatin, and paclitaxel are all active agents, with response rates of up to 30%. Each may be used as monotherapy. Combination chemotherapy has also been studied with some success. In GOG 107, the combination of cisplatin and doxorubicin was associated with higher PFS compared with doxorubicin alone (5.7 vs. 3.8 months) for 281 patients with advanced unresectable disease. However, there was no OS benefit. In a large phase III trial (GOG 177) comparing a paclitaxel-containing regimen (TAP, or paclitaxel, doxorubicin, and cisplatin) with doxorubicin and cisplatin, the paclitaxel-containing combination showed an improvement in median survival (15.3 vs. 12.3 months). However, this was at the cost of added toxicity. Another treatment option is paclitaxel and carboplatin, which, when compared with doxorubicin and cisplatin in a French study of 67 patients, was found to improve PFS (35% vs. 24%) and OS (41% vs. 27%) at 15 months without added toxicity (26). Most recent data from GOG 209 comparing the TAP regimen with TC have shown that TC is not inferior to TAP in terms of PFS (13.3 vs. 13.5 months; hazard ratio [HR] = 1.03) and OS (36.5 vs. 40.3 months; HR = 1.05). TC also has a better toxicity profile than TAP.

To summarize, patients with locally recurrent endometrial carcinoma can potentially be salvaged with radiation. For patients with an isolated vaginal recurrence who

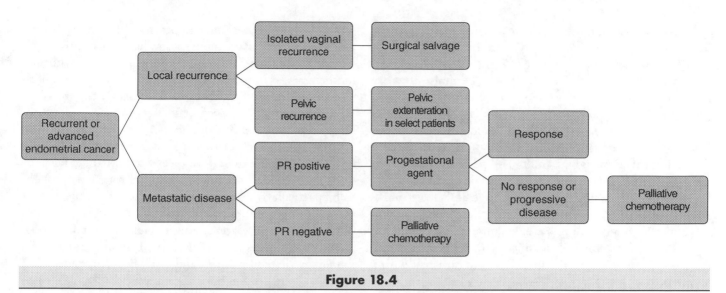

### Figure 18.4

Treatment algorithm for metastatic endometrial carcinoma. Salvage can sometimes be achieved for isolated recurrences of endometrial cancer with surgery and/or radiation. For more widespread disease, multimodality therapy can also be considered to palliate symptoms. Cure is less likely. PR, progesterone receptor.

previously had radiation, surgical salvage up to or including pelvic exenteration is an option when complete resection is deemed feasible. Progestational agents should be considered only if the tumor expresses PRs in patients with asymptomatic or low-grade metastatic disease. Otherwise, palliative chemotherapy should be employed. The most effective regimens appear to be paclitaxel–doxorubicin–cisplatin and paclitaxel–carboplatin. Figure 18.4 provides a treatment algorithm for recurrent or metastatic disease. In the case of the patient presented here, hormone receptor testing of the tumor is indicated. If the tumor expresses PR, a progestational agent could be considered as initial therapy. If the tumor is PR negative, palliative chemotherapy should be considered. Despite being elderly, the patient discussed appears to have excellent functional status, so a reasonable approach would be a standard chemotherapy with paclitaxel–carboplatin or TAP, with close monitoring for toxicity.

More recently, targeted therapies are being explored in the treatment of recurrent or metastatic disease. Aghajanian et al. conducted a phase II clinical trial where bevacizumab as a single agent showed a clinical response rate of 13.5%; PFS and OS were 4.2 and 10.5 months, respectively (27). Similarly, temsirolimus was evaluated in a phase II study as a single agent in recurrent and metastatic endometrial cancer in both chemotherapy-naive and chemotherapy-treated patients. Temsirolimus has shown a superior partial response in chemotherapy-naive compared to chemotherapy-treated patients (14% vs. 4%) (28).

For the more aggressive endometrial cancer histologies, serous and clear cell adenocarcinomas and carcinosarcoma, multimodality treatment is recommended. Given the aggressive nature of these cancers, most of the patients have extrauterine disease at presentation. Primary treatment includes TAH/BSO with surgical staging, peritoneal lavage with cytology, omental and peritoneal biopsies, and maximal tumor debulking for gross disease. For patients with disease localized to the endometrium, options include observation, chemotherapy or tumor-directed radiation, or a combination of the latter 2 modalities. For more advanced disease, chemotherapy with or without tumor-directed radiation is the preferred option. An adjuvant platinum/taxane-based regimen improves survival in serous and clear cell adenocarcinoma, whereas ifosfamide/paclitaxel is the preferred choice for carcinosarcoma. In a phase III trial, OS was 13.5 months with ifosfamide/paclitaxel versus 8.4 months with ifosfamide alone (29). A phase II trial has also shown TC as an effective regimen in carcinosarcoma, with a response rate of 54% (30). Currently GOG is conducting a trial comparing ifosfamide/paclitaxel versus carboplatin/paclitaxel (31).

## High-Risk Malignant GTD

T.R. is a 16-year-old woman, $G_1P_0$, who initially presented for evaluation of irregular menses. Four months earlier, she had experienced the onset of irregular vaginal bleeding. The patient described episodes of heavy bleeding that occurred 3–4 times per month, each lasting up to 4 days. Several weeks earlier, she had started oral contraceptives and iron supplements prescribed by a local primary care physician, with little improvement in her symptoms. For several days prior to her initial evaluation, she had been having problems with lightheadedness and shortness of breath, particularly upon standing. The patient reported a pregnancy had ended spontaneously in the first trimester slightly more than a year earlier. Uterine evacuation was not performed afterward and she had recovered uneventfully. She denied any sexual activity since her miscarriage.

Physical examination revealed the patient to be uncomfortable and dyspneic with a blood pressure of 104/70 mmHg, resting heart rate of 116, and oxygen saturation by pulse oximetry of 93%. Of note, her pulse rate rose to 160 on standing, with no significant change in her blood pressure. Breath sounds were normal bilaterally, there was no dullness to chest percussion, and abdominal examination was unremarkable. Pelvic examination revealed scant dark blood in the vaginal vault. The patient's cervix was visually closed. Her uterus was normal in size. A urine pregnancy test was positive. Quantitative $\beta$hCG was markedly elevated at 1,316,600 mIU/mL. Hemoglobin level was 6.8 g/dL. Pelvic ultrasound revealed minimal thickening of the endometrial stripe to 2 cm and a large ovoid mass arising from the left side of the uterus, most consistent with a leiomyoma. Adnexae were normal. A chest radiograph was performed, which revealed numerous solid lesions throughout the patient's lung fields bilaterally, some as large as 3 cm. Thyroid-stimulating hormone (TSH) was markedly suppressed at <0.01 mIU/mL. Testing for antithyroglobulin and anti-thyroperoxidase (TPO) was negative.

The patient was diagnosed with metastatic GTD and admitted to the hospital. She was transfused with 4 units of packed red blood cells, after which her hemoglobin rose to 10.2 g/dL. Because of her metastatic disease and WHO score of 12, she was started on a course of chemotherapy with etoposide, methotrexate, actinomycin D, cyclophosphamide, and vincristine (EMA-CO). On day 2 of her first infusion of this regimen, she experienced acute onset of worsening shortness of breath. Pulse oximetry was 80% on room air. Oxygen was administered, and a chest radiograph was obtained. This revealed acute pulmonary edema, which was successfully treated with a single dose of intravenous furosemide. Intravenous hydration was held. Her oxygen status improved quickly and returned to baseline. She experienced no further complications or issues associated with her chemotherapy infusion. During her initial hospital admission, she was also started on depot medroxyprogesterone for contraception.

The patient received a total of 5 cycles of EMA-CO. Immediately prior to her second cycle, her serum $\beta$hCG was 108 mIU/mL. This normalized prior to her third cycle. She received an additional 2 cycles of EMA-CO after normal serum $\beta$hCG levels were achieved. The pulmonary lesions resolved completely. The patient has now been followed for nearly a year and has remained healthy. Serum $\beta$hCG levels have remained <5 mIU/mL and her thyroid function tests have remained normal. Her menses have returned and are currently regular.

## Evidence-Based Case Discussion

For women diagnosed with malignant GTD, treatment with the goal of cure should be initiated in a timely fashion. The WHO scoring system is used to assess risk and triage patients to appropriate levels of treatment following the diagnosis of this disease. For most women, diagnosis is established by uterine evacuation, which also serves a therapeutic role, or by tissue biopsy. However, due to this young woman's precarious medical condition, treatment with chemotherapy was initiated without a tissue biopsy to establish the diagnosis. There were several reasons for this decision. First, the uterus was normal in size and no evidence of retained products of conception or GTD were identified by imaging within her uterus. The value of endometrial biopsy or D&C under these circumstances was thought to be questionable. Second, percutaneous tissue biopsies were thought to be particularly risky, given the propensity of metastases from this disease to bleed severely when disturbed. Serum $\beta$hCG is a sensitive and highly reliable marker for GTD, although not necessarily diagnostic. Due to the structural homology shared by $\beta$hCG and TSH, hyperthyroidism is a common complication of GTD. However, subclinical cases do not require treatment with thyroid suppression.

Single-agent regimens of either methotrexate or actinomycin D have been reported to be highly effective for curing nonmetastatic/low-risk GTD using the WHO scoring system. Although many clinicians prefer methotrexate, either agent can be used with similar efficacy, following serial serum $\beta$hCG levels until resolution of disease. Osborne et al. in 2011 published a phase III trial comparing actinomycin D with methotrexate in which response rates were better with actinomycin D (36). The dose of methotrexate used in the trial (30 mg/m$^2$) was lower than the recommended dose of 50 mg/m$^2$ utilized by many oncologists. Also, all patients who failed therapy with 1 drug received the other drug as salvage, complicating interpretation of study results. Currently, methotrexate is the drug of choice for nonmetastatic/low-grade GTD. In patients not desiring fertility, hysterectomy with chemotherapy is also a valid option, with cure rates approaching 100%. Diffuse pulmonary metastases as well as this patient's WHO score (=12) indicated that neither single-agent regimen would have been sufficient to adequately treat the extent of this young woman's disease. This score represents both the number of pulmonary lesions noted, the extremely high serum $\beta$hCG levels found at initial diagnosis, as well as the long interval between the patient's antecedent pregnancy and her diagnosis. Each of these characteristics is a poor prognostic feature. For this reason, she was started on EMA-CO. Initiation of this regimen resulted in a rapid and impressive resolution of the patient's pulmonary lesions, with improvement in her ability to breathe comfortably and rapid quantitative improvement in her serum $\beta$hCG levels. In general, EMA-CO is well tolerated. Modest depression of bone marrow function is often accepted with the goal of maintaining dose intensity with few complications such as neutropenic fever. A number of studies indicate that response rates for women diagnosed with high-risk GTD should be favorable, with a cure possible for the majority of patients (13,32). For patients who fail to respond to EMA-CO, various therapeutic regimens have been evaluated (33–35). Salvage rates for women with GTD who fail EMA-CO are much more guarded; however, durable remission rates of up to 80% have been reported with EMA-EP (33). Once normal βhCG levels have been achieved, treatment for an additional 2 cycles "past normal" has emerged as the standard of care. On completion of chemotherapy, women are followed monthly to bimonthly for 6–12 months, regularly checking serum βhCG levels.

An important aspect of care for women diagnosed with malignant GTD is contraception. Fertility typically returns following the successful treatment of this disease. However, subsequent pregnancy can significantly complicate posttreatment care by causing elevations in serum βhCG under circumstances where it can often be difficult to distinguish between a normal pregnancy and disease recurrence. For women with high-risk disease, recurrence rates are estimated to range from approximately 15 to 25%, but decline significantly after remaining disease free for at least 1 year (13,32). Options for contraception should be discussed with all patients, and a reliable method for birth control selected that can be realistically achieved. Many clinicians recommend that contraception be continued for at least 6 months following the conclusion of therapy.

## REVIEW QUESTIONS

1. Complete surgical staging of uterine cancer does not include which one of the following procedures:

   (A) Bilateral salpingo-oophorectomy
   (B) Pelvic washings
   (C) Pelvic lymphadenectomies
   (D) Omentectomy

2. Medical management of endometrial cancer can be considered when the following criteria are met:

   (A) Normal serum levels of cancer antigen (CA)-125
   (B) Disease confined to the endometrial cavity
   (C) No evidence of tumor invasion deeper than outer half of myometrium detected on pelvic MRI
   (D) Tumor histology that includes endometrioid and papillary serous carcinoma but not clear cell carcinoma

3. World Health Organization risk factors used to triage women diagnosed with gestational trophoblastic disease (GTD) for treatment include:

   (A) Number of pulmonary nodules
   (B) Serum-free T4 level
   (C) Time interval between antecedent pregnancy and diagnosis of GTD
   (D) Number of previous pregnancies

4. Risk factors for developing papillary scrous uterine cancer include

   (A) Obesity
   (B) Diabetes mellitus

   (C) African American race
   (D) Prior use of unopposed estrogens as naturopathic hormone replacement therapy

5. A 55-year-old woman presents to your office with a 2-month history of postmenopausal bleeding. After performing a pelvic examination, the next best step in evaluation of this patient is:

   (A) Endometrial biopsy
   (B) CT scan of abdomen and pelvis
   (C) PET scan
   (D) Dilation and curettage

6. A 65-year-old retired schoolteacher presented to her gynecologist with a 3-month history of vaginal bleeding. She is diabetic and hypertensive, has no children, and has been menopausal for 12 years. On examination, she has a diffusely enlarged uterus. An office endometrial biopsy shows grade II endometrioid endometrial carcinoma. What is the next best step in the management of her cancer?

   (A) Dilation and curettage
   (B) Total abdominal hysterectomy (TAH) and bilateral salpingo-oophorectomy (BSO)
   (C) Chemotherapy
   (D) Pelvic radiation

7. The same woman undergoes total abdominal hysterectomy and surgical staging and is found to have a grade II endometrioid endometrial carcinoma with tumor invading >50% of the myometrium. The pelvic and para-aortic lymph node sampling shows no tumor involvement. Peritoneal cytology is negative for malignancy. What is the next best step in the treatment of this patient?

   (A) Concurrent chemotherapy and radiation
   (B) Pelvic radiation
   (C) Observation
   (D) Vaginal brachytherapy

8. A 55-year-old otherwise healthy female who has never been pregnant presented with a 2-month history of intermittent vaginal bleeding and 15-pound weight loss. She has a 25-pack-year history of smoking. On examination, patient was noted to have an enlarged uterus. Endometrial biopsy showed high-grade endometrioid carcinoma. She underwent total abdominal hysterectomy and bilateral salpingo-oophorectomy with pelvic lymph node dissection positive for malignancy. Para-aortic lymph node sampling and peritoneal cytology were negative for disease. What should be the next step?

   (A) Whole abdominal irradiation
   (B) Chemotherapy
   (C) Concurrent chemoradiation
   (D) Hospice

# REFERENCES

1. Lu K, Slomovitz BM. Neoplastic diseases of the uterus: endometrial hyperplasia, endometrial carcinoma, sarcoma: diagnosis and management. In: Katz VL, Lentz GM, Lobo RA, Gershenson DM, eds. *Comprehensive Gynecology*. 5th ed. Philadelphia, PA: Mosley Elsevier; 2007:813–838.

2. D'Angelo E, Prat J. Uterine sarcomas: a review. *Gynecol Oncol.* 2010;116(1):131–139.

3. Obermair A, Youlden DR, Young JP, et al. Risk of endometrial cancer for women diagnosed with HNPCC-related colorectal carcinoma. *Int J Cancer.* 2010;127(11):2678–2684.

4. Fisher B, Costantino JP, Redmond CK, et al. Endometrial cancer in tamoxifen-treated breast cancer patients: findings from the National Surgical Adjuvant Breast and Bowel Project (NSABP) B-14. *J Natl Cancer Inst.* 1994;86(7):527–537.

5. Meyer LA, Broaddus RR, Lu KH. Endometrial cancer and Lynch syndrome: clinical and pathologic considerations. *Cancer Control.* 2009;16(1):14–22.

6. Creasman WT, Odicino F, Maisonneuve P, et al. Carcinoma of the corpus uteri. FIGO 26th Annual Report on the Results of Treatment in Gynecological Cancer. *Int J Gynecol Obstet.* 2006;95(suppl 1):S105–S143.

7. McCluggage WG. Uterine carcinosarcomas (malignant mixed Mullerian tumors) are metaplastic carcinomas. *Int J Gynecol Cancer.* 2002;12(6):687–690.

8. Cirisano FD Jr, Robboy SJ, Dodge RK, et al. The outcome of stage I-II clinically and surgically staged papillary serous and clear cell endometrial cancers when compared with endometrioid carcinoma. *Gynecol Oncol.* 2000;77(1):55–65.

9. McCluggage WG. My approach to the interpretation of endometrial biopsies and curettings. *J Clin Pathol.* 2006;59(8):801–812.

10. Creasman W. Revised FIGO staging for carcinoma of the endometrium. *Int J Gynaecol Obstet.* 2009;105(2):109.

11. Kumar S, Mariani A, Bakkum-Gamez JN, et al. Risk factors that mitigate the role of paraaortic lymphadenectomy in uterine endometrioid cancer. *Gynecol Oncol.* 2013;130(3):441–445.

12. Barlin JN, Khoury-Collado F, Kim CH, et al. The importance of applying a sentinel lymph node mapping algorithm in endometrial cancer staging: beyond removal of blue nodes. *Gynecol Oncol.* 2012;125(3):531–535.

13. Lurain JR, Singh DK, Schink JC. Primary treatment of metastatic high-risk gestational trophoblastic neoplasia with EMA-CO chemotherapy. *J Reprod Med.* 2006;51(10):767–772.

14. Creutzberg CL. GOG-99: ending the controversy regarding pelvic radiotherapy for endometrial carcinoma? *Gynecol Oncol.* 2004;92(3): 740–743.

15. Susumu N, Sagae S, Udagawa Y, et al. Randomized phase III trial of pelvic radiotherapy versus cisplatin-based combined chemotherapy in patients with intermediate- and high-risk endometrial cancer: a Japanese Gynecologic Oncology Group study. *Gynecol Oncol.* 2008;108(1):226–233.

16. Ushijima K, Yahata H, Yoshikawa H, et al. Multicenter phase II study of fertility-sparing treatment with medroxyprogesterone acetate for endometrial carcinoma and atypical hyperplasia in young women. *J Clin Oncol.* 2007;25(19):2798–2803.

17. Gunderson CC, Fader AN, Carson KA, et al. Oncologic and reproductive outcomes with progestin therapy in women with endometrial hyperplasia and grade 1 adenocarcinoma: a systematic review. *Gynecol Oncol.* 2012;125(2):477–482.

18. Mehasseb MK, Latimer JA. Controversies in the management of endometrial carcinoma: an update. *Obstet Gynecol Int.* 2012;2012: 676032.

19. Park JY, Seong SJ, Kim TJ, et al. Pregnancy outcomes after fertility-sparing management in young women with early endometrial cancer. *Obstet Gynecol.* 2013;121(1):136–142.

20. Randall ME, Reisinger S. Radiation therapy and combined chemo-irradiation in advanced and recurrent endometrial carcinoma. *Semin Oncol.* 1994;21(1):91–99.

21. Jhingran A, Burke TW, Eifel PJ. Definitive radiotherapy for patients with isolated vaginal recurrence of endometrial carcinoma after hysterectomy. *Int J Radiat Oncol Biol Phys.* 2003;56(5): 1366–1372.

22. Creutzberg CL, van Putten WL, Koper PC, et al. Surgery and postoperative radiotherapy versus surgery alone for patients with stage-1 endometrial carcinoma: multicentre randomised trial. PORTEC Study Group. Post Operative Radiation Therapy in Endometrial Carcinoma. *Lancet.* 2000;355(9213):1404–1411.

23. Bristow RE, Santillan A, Zahurak ML, et al. Salvage cytoreductive surgery for recurrent endometrial cancer. *Gynecol Oncol.* 2006;103(1): 281–287.

24. Barakat RR, Goldman NA, Patel DA, et al. Pelvic exenteration for recurrent endometrial cancer. *Gynecol Oncol.* 1999;75(1): 99–102.

25. Lentz SS. Advanced and recurrent endometrial carcinoma: hormonal therapy. *Semin Oncol.* 1994;21(1):100–106.

26. Weber B, Mayer F, Bougnoux P, et al. What is the best chemotherapy regimen in recurrent or advanced endometrial carcinoma? Preliminary results. *Proc Am Soc Clin Oncol.* 2003;22:453. Abstract 1819.

27. Aghajanian C, Sill MW, Darcy KM, et al. Phase II trial of bevacizumab in recurrent or persistent endometrial cancer: a Gynecologic Oncology Group study. *J Clin Oncol.* 2011;29(16): 2259–2265.

28. Oza AM, Elit L, Tsao MS, et al. Phase II study of temsirolimus in women with recurrent or metastatic endometrial cancer: a trial of the NCIC Clinical Trials Group. *J Clin Oncol.* 2011;29(24):3278–3285.

29. Homesley HD, Filiaci V, Markman M, et al. Phase III trial of ifosfamide with or without paclitaxel in advanced uterine carcinosarcoma: a Gynecologic Oncology Group Study. *J Clin Oncol.* 2007;25(5):526–531.

30. Powell MA, Filiaci VL, Rose PG, et al. Phase II evaluation of paclitaxel and carboplatin in the treatment of carcinosarcoma of the uterus: a Gynecologic Oncology Group study. *J Clin Oncol.* 2010;28(16):2727–2731.

31. Cantrell LA, Havrilesky L, Moore DT, et al. A multi-institutional cohort study of adjuvant therapy in stage I-II uterine carcinosarcoma. *Gynecol Oncol.* 2012;127(1):22–26.

32. Bower M, Newlands ES, Holden L, et al. EMA/CO for high-risk gestational trophoblastic tumors: results from a cohort of 272 patients. *J Clin Oncol.* 1997;15(7):2636–2643.

33. Newlands ES, Mulholland PJ, Holden L, et al. Etoposide and cisplatin/etoposide, methotrexate, and actinomycin D (EMA) chemotherapy for patients with high-risk gestational trophoblastic tumors refractory to EMA/cyclophosphamide and vincristine chemotherapy and patients presenting with metastatic placental site trophoblastic tumors. *J Clin Oncol.* 2000;18(4):854–859.

34. Gordon AN, Kavanagh JJ, Gershenson DM, et al. Cisplatin, vinblastine, and bleomycin combination therapy in resistant gestational trophoblastic disease. *Cancer.* 1986;58(7):1407–1410.

35. Lurain JR, Nejad B. Secondary chemotherapy for high-risk gestational trophoblastic neoplasia. *Gynecol Oncol.* 2005;97(2):618–623.

36. Osborne RJ, Filiaci V, Schink JC, et al. Phase III trial of weekly methotrexate or pulsed dactinomycin for low-risk gestational trophoblastic neoplasia: a gynecologic oncology group study. *J Clin Oncol.* 2011;29(7):825–831.

# 19

# Ovarian Cancer

LAN COFFMAN, KAREN McLEAN, AND RONALD J. BUCKANOVICH

## EPIDEMIOLOGY, RISK FACTORS, NATURAL HISTORY, AND PATHOLOGY

Ovarian cancer is the fifth leading cause of cancer death in women, and the most lethal gynecologic malignancy. Roughly 22,000 women were newly diagnosed with ovarian cancer in 2014 with >14,000 ovarian cancer deaths. For sporadic epithelial ovarian cancers, the average age at diagnosis is 59 years.

Multiple risk factors for ovarian cancer have been identified, including reproductive factors, genetic factors, and environmental factors. The theory of "incessant ovulation" postulates that a woman's risk of ovarian cancer increases with the number of lifetime ovulatory cycles. This is supported by epidemiologic data demonstrating that oral contraceptives, increased parity, and breastfeeding all decrease a woman's risk of ovarian cancer, while nulliparity and infertility are associated with increased ovarian cancer risk. The cellular damage occurring during the wound-repair cycle of the ovarian epithelium at the time of follicle rupture and ovulation may explain the correlation between ovulatory cycles and risk of ovarian cancer.

Genetic factors also clearly play a role in the risk of developing ovarian cancer. Although the risk is 1 in 70 in the general population, this rises to approximately 1 in 25 when 1 first-degree relative is affected and 1 in 15 when 2 first-degree relatives are affected. Overall, 10–15% of ovarian cancers arise in the setting of a hereditary cancer syndrome. These include the hereditary breast–ovarian cancer (HBOC) syndrome and the hereditary nonpolyposis colorectal cancer (HNPCC) syndrome, also known as Lynch II syndrome. The majority of cases of the HBOC syndrome are due to mutations in either the *BRCA1* or the *BRCA2* gene, 2 tumor suppressor genes that play a role

in the repair of DNA double-strand breaks. Studies have demonstrated a genotype–phenotype correlation, with the specific mutation within either *BRCA1* or *BRCA2* altering the risk of ovarian cancer in mutation carriers. The risk for *BRCA1* mutation carriers ranges from 10% to 60% and the risk for *BRCA2* mutation carriers ranges from 20% to 40%. Reports suggest that patients with ovarian carcinoma arising in the setting of a *BRCA* mutation have improved survival as compared to those patients with nonhereditary ovarian cancer. HNPCC is a genetic syndrome resulting from a mutation in 1 of a number of genes, all of which have a protein product that functions in DNA mismatch repair, including *MSH2*, *MLH1*, *MSH6*, *PMS1*, and *PMS2*. Patients with HNPCC have approximately 10% lifetime risk of developing epithelial ovarian cancer, in addition to their increased risk of colon and other cancers. Several additional gene loci that are associated with increased ovarian cancer susceptibility have recently been reported and hopefully these loci will add to our understanding of the genetic etiology of ovarian cancer. In addition, a variant of the *KRAS* oncogene has been shown to be associated with >25% of ovarian cancer cases and a marker for increased risk of ovarian cancer in unaffected individuals. The *KRAS* variant was present in >60% of hereditary ovarian cancer pedigrees that did not harbor *BRCA* mutations. This led to Food and Drug Administration (FDA) approval of the PreOvar test to assess for the presence of this gene variant.

Although it is not possible to change one's genetics, it is possible to reduce an individual's ovarian cancer risk even in the setting of genetic mutation. Several recent studies have reported that prophylactic oophorectomy can reduce ovarian cancer risk by 90–95% in *BRCA* mutation carriers (1). Environmental factors are potentially more easily modifiable risk factors for cancer development. Unfortunately, none has clearly been linked as causative. The finding that tubal ligation decreases the risk of ovarian cancer has led to the hypothesis that there may be retrograde factors increasing the risk of ovarian cancer. However, it has also been suggested that tubal ligation may reduce ovarian cancer risk by decreasing blood flow to the ovary and/or the development of epithelial carcinomas that are actually arising in the fallopian tube. Vitamin D deficiency has been correlated with increased ovarian cancer risk in some, but not all studies. Obesity and high-fat diet are associated with higher rates of ovarian cancer in industrialized nations, but a causative association remains unproven.

The vast majority of epithelial ovarian cancers are diagnosed at advanced stage, because early-stage disease is often asymptomatic. When patients do ultimately develop symptoms, they are usually vague symptoms related to disease spread, including abdominal, pelvic, or back discomfort or pain, bloating, and urinary symptoms. Increasing data suggest that persistent non-specific symptoms are correlated with an increased risk of malignancy (2), and the use of a symptom index to screen women has been proposed. In patients with multiple symptoms, it is recommended that ovarian cancer be considered as a possible etiology. Typically, the patient should undergo a pelvic ultrasound and Cancer Antigen 125 (CA125) testing. In 2009, the FDA approved the OVA1 test, a blood test that combines the results of 5 immunoassays to give a likelihood of ovarian cancer in someone with an ovarian mass. This test has application in helping triage patients who should be referred to a gynecologic oncologist for further management. Several studies indicate that ovarian cancer patients who have surgery performed by a gynecologic oncologist, as compared to a general gynecologist or a surgical oncologist, are more likely to be appropriately staged and optimally debulked, resulting in better patient outcomes.

In patients with ovarian cancer, standard therapy includes surgical debulking followed by chemotherapy for all but the earliest stage, and overall survival is dependent on both the stage at the time of debulking and the degree to which optimal surgical debulking is obtained. Overall, prognosis remains poor largely due to advanced stage at diagnosis and the development of chemoresistant disease; overall 5-year survival is currently approximately 45%.

There are many histological subtypes of ovarian cancer based on their cell of origin: coelomic epithelial cell, mesenchyme (stromal and sex-cord), and germ cell. More than 90% of ovarian tumors are epithelial, and these will be the focus of this chapter. For practical purposes, fallopian tube carcinoma and primary peritoneal carcinoma are considered "epithelial ovarian carcinoma"; tumors arising from these sites share coelomic epithelial embryonal origins and have similar staging, management, and prognosis. In fact, increasing data suggest that some "ovarian cancers" may actually originate in the fallopian tube.

Within the subtype of epithelial ovarian cancer, there are several histological variants. Serous histology represents the vast majority of cases (>70%), followed in descending order of frequency by endometrioid, mucinous, and clear cell histologies. Tumors with endometrioid histology typically portend a better prognosis, whereas clear cell histology predicts a poorer outcome. Although the vast majority of ovarian tumors are invasive, 15% of ovarian cancers are of low malignant potential (LMP). LMP tumors can spread within the peritoneum and even metastasize to lymph nodes; however, they do not invade tissue stroma. LMP tumors generally demonstrate low mitotic activity, rendering them largely chemoresistant. Therefore, even advanced-stage LMP tumors are typically treated with surgical debulking alone, and repeat surgery in the setting of recurrent disease. Given that LMP tumors pose fewer clinical dilemmas than invasive epithelial ovarian cancers and have a generally favorable prognosis, they are not further discussed in this chapter.

## STAGING

Ovarian cancer is surgically staged, with the staging system defined by the International Federation of Gynecology and Obstetrics (FIGO), which was updated in January 2014.

| FIGO Ovarian Cancer Staging, January 2014 | |
|---|---|
| Stage | Definition |
| IA | Tumor limited to 1 ovary, capsule intact, no tumor on surface, negative washings |
| IB | Like IA, but tumor involves both ovaries |
| IC | One or both ovaries with: |
| IC1 | Surgical spill |
| IC2 | Preop capsule rupture or surface involvement |
| IC3 | Malignant ascites or positive washings |
| IIA | Extension or implant on uterus or tubes |
| IIB | Extension to other pelvic intraperitoneal (IP) tissues |
| IIIA1 | Positive retroperitoneal nodes only |
| | IIIA1(i)  Metastasis ≤ 10 mm |
| | IIIA1(ii) Metastasis > 10 mm |
| IIIA2 | Microscopic intra-abdominal peritoneal involvement ± positive retroperitoneal nodes |
| IIIB | Intra-abdominal peritoneal involvement ≤ 2 cm involvement ± positive retroperitoneal nodes Includes extension to capsule of liver/spleen |
| IIIC | Macroscopic, extrapelvic, peritoneal metastasis >2 cm ± positive retroperitoneal lymph nodes. Includes extension to capsule of liver/spleen |
| IVA | Pleural effusion with positive cytology |
| IVB | Hepatic or splenic parenchymal metastasis, or extra-abdominal organs including inguinal nodes and nodes outside abdominal cavity |

Include histology and site of origin (ovary, tube, or peritoneum). bx positive adhesions upstage I–II.

bx, biopsy; FIGO, International Federation of Gynecology and Obstetrics.

## CASE SUMMARIES

### Early-Stage Disease

D.N. is a 43-year-old premenopausal woman who presents to her gynecologist for an annual examination, and on bimanual examination is noted to have an 8-cm, freely mobile left adnexal mass. She is sent for an ultrasound that demonstrates a left ovarian mass measuring 8 cm with 2 thick septations and a 1-cm nodular area. Imaging also demonstrates a 3-cm cystic structure on the right adnexus. She is counseled to undergo surgical resection. Preoperative CA125 is 26.3 U/mL (normal < 35 U/mL) and chest x-ray is unremarkable. Laparoscopic left salpingo-oophorectomy is performed and pelvic washings are obtained. Intraoperative pathology frozen section demonstrates serous invasive epithelial ovarian carcinoma (Figure 19.1). She therefore undergoes comprehensive surgical staging consisting of hysterectomy, bilateral salpingo-oophorectomy, bilateral pelvic lymphadenectomy, para-aortic lymphadenectomy, staging biopsies, diaphragm scrapings, and omentectomy. Final pathology demonstrates grade 3 serous ovarian cancer in both ovaries, without surface involvement, and no other disease spread. Pelvic washings are negative for cancer cells.

### Evidence-Based Case Discussion

D.N. has stage IB, grade 3 serous ovarian adenocarcinoma. From a surgical standpoint, her 8-cm mass had a <5% chance of resolving spontaneously, and by ultrasound, it demonstrated multiple concerning findings, including septations and nodularity. CA125 is elevated

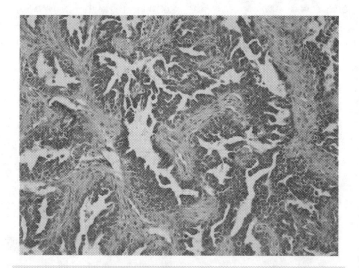

**Figure 19.1**

Serous epithelial ovarian cancer. Hematoxylin and eosin stain demonstrating the microscopic features characteristic of this tumor type. Papillae are noted as well as slit-like spaces. Stromal invasion and resultant desmoplastic response are common.

in approximately 55% of early-stage disease, and plays a limited role in triaging premenopausal patients with an adnexal mass. Likewise, CT imaging is not necessary in the preoperative setting in this case. It was appropriate to proceed with the surgical staging and debulking procedure. Although fertility sparing surgery can be safely performed in the setting of the earliest stage disease (stage IA, grade 1), a complete staging procedure is recommended whenever possible. Up to 30% of patients with apparent early-stage disease will be upstaged with appropriate surgery and > 20% are upstaged to stage III disease. Serous tumors are bilateral in up to one third of cases at the time of diagnosis.

For patients with early-stage disease (stage I or II), it is important to determine if they have high-risk or low-risk disease. Although the number of observational studies is limited, the primary risk factors for recurrent disease appear to be tumor grade (grade 2 or 3) and the presence of extra-ovarian disease (stage IC or II). Patients with stage IA or IB grade 1 tumors, who have had appropriate surgical treatment, have an estimated 5-year overall survival of 90–95%. Thus, the lack of a need for chemotherapy in these patients is generally well accepted (3). In fact, an Italian study concluded that for patients with low-risk disease, adjuvant therapy and salvage therapy were equally effective.

For patients with high-risk early-stage disease, treatment guidelines are based primarily on 2 large trials, the European Organization for Research and Treatment of Cancer (EORTC) ACTION trial and International Collaborative Ovarian Neoplasm Trial (ICON1), which investigated the benefit of adjuvant platinum-based chemotherapy in women with high-risk early-stage ovarian cancer. Both trials had limitations with regard to how the patient populations were defined and the quality of surgical staging. However, both trials suggested a non-statistically significant trend favoring overall survival in the women receiving adjuvant platinum-based chemotherapy. When the results of the 2 studies were combined, the outcomes suggested a statistically significant absolute increase in 5-year overall survival of 8% (4). Serial phase III clinical trials performed by the Gynecologic Oncology Group (GOG) have established the efficacy of platinum and taxane chemotherapy for epithelial ovarian cancer, with the standard intravenous (IV) regimen now consisting of carboplatin and paclitaxel. Given the increased risk of recurrence with increasing tumor grade, it is reasonable and preferred by these authors to administer adjuvant chemotherapy in the setting of all early-stage disease other than stage IA, grade 1 and stage IB, grade 1 disease.

The number of cycles of adjuvant therapy necessary for the treatment of early-stage ovarian cancer was addressed in the GOG Trial 157 that compared 3 versus 6 cycles of adjuvant carboplatin and paclitaxel for this patient population. This study concluded that 6 cycles increased toxicity without significantly altering recurrence risk (5).

However, there was a nonstatistically significant trend for a 5% improvement in 5-year overall survival in the group receiving 6 cycles of adjuvant therapy. Subsequent subset analysis of this patient data set, in the effort to identify specific factors suggesting higher risk of recurrence for which 6 cycles of chemotherapy would be indicated, suggested that patients with serous histology who received 6 cycles of carboplatin and paclitaxel had a statistically significant decrease in recurrence-free survival, but no difference in overall survival (6). Although recent data suggest a role for intraperitoneal (IP) chemotherapy in the adjuvant setting for optimally debulked, advanced-stage ovarian cancer (7, discussed in further detail later), currently no randomized, controlled studies exist for IP chemotherapy in stage I or II disease. Taken together, it would be our recommendation that the patient in this case, with stage IB, grade 3 disease, receive 3 cycles of IV carboplatin and paclitaxel chemotherapy.

## Advanced-Stage Disease

K.H. is a 56-year-old who presents to the emergency department with persistent nausea and vomiting. She reports a 2-month history of progressive bloating and abdominal distension. She is otherwise healthy with no significant past medical or surgical history. In the emergency department, she undergoes a CT scan (Figure 19.2), with findings including an adnexal mass, omental cake, and ascites. Her CA125 is 3221 U/mL. She is consented for surgery and undergoes exploratory laparotomy, total abdominal hysterectomy, bilateral salpingo-oophorectomy, omentectomy, staging biopsies, and argon beam tumor ablation, with optimal tumor debulking to microscopic residual disease. An IP port is placed at the time of her surgery.

## Evidence-Based Case Discussion

K.H.'s presentation is typical of many ovarian cancers. She presented with vague abdominal symptoms, and imaging demonstrates a large burden of disease consistent with advanced stage. The patient undergoes optimal surgical debulking, with findings demonstrating stage IIIC papillary serous ovarian cancer. The fundamental components of ovarian cancer treatment are surgical debulking and chemotherapy. Therefore, following her surgery, adjuvant chemotherapy is advisable.

The first management decision in this case is actually whether to attempt surgical debulking or to proceed with neoadjuvant chemotherapy followed by surgery. Currently, there are no good preoperative predictors of which patients will be optimally debulked at the time of surgery. A preoperative CA125 should be obtained, because the value has prognostic implications as well as utility in tracking disease response and recurrence. However, preoperative CA125 has not been shown to predict patients in whom optimal debulking can be achieved. In the absence of specific contraindications to initial surgical debulking, such as medical comorbidities, current data support an attempt at surgical debulking. In settings in which this is not possible, one can begin with neoadjuvant chemotherapy followed by a debulking surgery if the patient demonstrates a good disease response. The majority of data support improved patient outcomes with surgery first and then adjuvant chemotherapy rather than neoadjuvant chemotherapy (8).

For the past decade, the standard of care for epithelial ovarian cancer chemotherapy had been a 2-drug regimen consisting of a platinum and a taxane (Figure 19.3). The efficacy of carboplatin and paclitaxel has been demonstrated in randomized, controlled trials, with lower toxicity than earlier regimens. In these regimens, paclitaxel

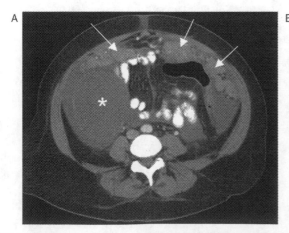
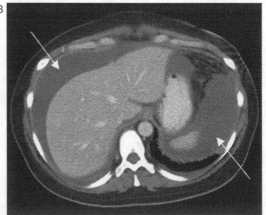

### Figure 19.2

CT imaging. (A) Right adnexal mass and omental cake. CT scan in the midpelvis reveals a cystic mass in the right adnexa measuring 9 × 10 × 11.7 cm (indicated by the asterisk), as well as omental caking (indicated by white arrows) and mesenteric nodularity.
(B) Ascites. CT imaging high in the abdomen demonstrates ascites (indicated by white arrows), particularly evident around the liver.

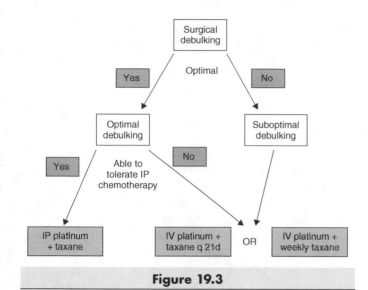

**Figure 19.3**

Decision analysis for adjuvant chemotherapy in advanced epithelial ovarian cancer. Adjuvant chemotherapy in advanced epithelial ovarian cancer consists of a regimen containing both a platinum drug and a taxane. The choice of specific regimen is dependent on whether optimal surgical cytoreduction was achieved as well as the performance status of the patient. IP, intraperitoneal.

and carboplatin are given intravenously on day 1 of a 21-day cycle, for 6 cycles. However, several studies have reported that IP chemotherapy can increase overall survival when compared to IV chemotherapy. Most recently, GOG Trial 172 randomized patients with optimally debulked stage III ovarian cancer to receive either IV cisplatin or paclitaxel (day 1 of a 21-day cycle for 6 total cycles) or to receive IV paclitaxel over a 24-hour period followed by IP cisplatin day 2 and IP paclitaxel on day 8 of a 21-day cycle. GOG 182 demonstrated that IP chemotherapy resulted in an 8% improvement in progression-free survival (PFS) at 5 years, and a >10% improvement in overall survival at 5 years (7). This is the most dramatic improvement in survival for ovarian cancer patients since the discovery of paclitaxel. IP treatment in this trial was associated with increased toxicity, with only 42% of patients able to complete the planned 6 cycles due to side effects, including port complications, pain, fatigue, and gastrointestinal, hematologic, and neurologic toxicities. However, several single-institution studies have reported modifications to the IP chemotherapy protocol to reduce side effects. These modifications include the addition of hematologic growth factor support, aggressive anti-emetic regimens, preventive IV hydration, and the use of IV docetaxel instead of paclitaxel to reduce neurotoxicity. With these modifications, >85% of patients can successfully complete all 6 cycles of IP chemotherapy (9). It is possible that with a reduction in side effects and more patients capable of completing IP chemotherapy, even greater improvements in patient survival may be seen. Thus, with judicious patient selection with regard to risk

of toxicities, IP chemotherapy represents an excellent adjuvant chemotherapy approach and one that we would favor in the patient in this case study.

The IP chemotherapy trials have included patients with optimal tumor debulking at the time of surgery, but this route of chemotherapy administration has not been validated in patients with suboptimal surgical debulking. Conceptually, the IP approach could be less effective due to decreased penetration of the chemotherapy into large tumor deposits. Therefore, alternative approaches must be considered in the patient with suboptimal tumor debulking. A study from the Japanese GOG investigated a regimen of dose-dense chemotherapy in which carboplatin is given on day 1 and paclitaxel is given weekly on a 21-day cycle. This study included suboptimally debulked patients and reports an 11-month increase in PFS as well as an increase in overall survival with this regimen (10). Of note, subgroup analysis demonstrated this benefit was not seen in patients with clear cell or mucinous histology; therefore, this regimen is not appropriate for patients with those histological subtypes. However, dose-dense carboplatin/paclitaxel is an alternative regimen that may play a role in patients who would not be treated with IP chemotherapy. A decision analysis schema for adjuvant chemotherapy in advanced-stage epithelial ovarian cancer is shown in Figure 19.3.

Recent clinical studies support a role for targeted biological therapies in the treatment of some epithelial ovarian cancers. The anti-vascular endothelial growth factor (VEGF) antibody bevacizumab has shown promise in clinical trials. GOG 218 investigated outcomes when bevacizumab is added to carboplatin and paclitaxel during the initial 6 cycles of adjuvant chemotherapy and then either continued or not for an additional 12 months of consolidation. Patients who received bevacizumab both with their adjuvant chemotherapy and for consolidation showed a 4-month improvement in PFS. However, there was no improvement in overall survival. Importantly, only the arm with maintenance bevacizumab demonstrated benefit. ICON7 also investigated the role of bevacizumab in adjuvant treatment of high-risk stage I–IV ovarian cancer with standard Q3 week carboplatin/paclitaxel for 6 cycles and continuing with maintenance bevacizumab for 12 additional cycles. PFS was approximately 2 months. However, in a planned subgroup analysis of stage IIIc suboptimally debulked or stage IV patients, PFS increased to 4.1 months with an overall survival advantage of 4.8 months. There was no survival advantage when assessing the entire study population. It is important to note that crossover was not allowed in this study as it was in GOG218, which may account for the difference in survival advantage. Bevacizumab in combination with chemotherapy has also been studied in recurrent, platinum-sensitive and platinum-resistant ovarian cancer (Ovarian Cancer Study Comparing Efficacy and Safety of

Chemotherapy and Anti-angiogenic Therapy in Platinum-Sensitive Recurrent Disease [OCEANS] trial and Avastin Use in Platinum-Resistant Epithelial Ovarian Cancer [AURELIA] trial, respectively) with demonstration of a 3- to 4-month improvement in PFS without overall survival benefit. Thus, bevacizumab has activity in ovarian cancer; however, the timing of use (either upfront with adjuvant therapy or at time of recurrence) is still under debate. Another group of targeted therapy currently under investigation is that of poly-adenosine diphosphate (ADP) ribose polymerase (PARP) inhibitors, such as olaparib. These inhibitors block the PARP enzyme that functions in DNA repair. Data suggest that this inhibition may be particularly effective in patients that have germ-line mutations in a *BRCA* gene that normally functions in DNA repair. PARP inhibitors are currently under active investigation in the clinical setting with encouraging phase II data and active phase III trials. Additionally, in low-grade serous ovarian cancer, which is generally chemoresistant, there are phase II data demonstrating the efficacy of targeting the MAPK pathway with use of the mitogen-activated protein kinase kinase 1/2 (MEK1/2) inhibitor, selumetinib (11).

## Recurrent Disease

K.H. from the aforementioned case completes 6 cycles of adjuvant chemotherapy using an outpatient IP regimen, with normalization of her CA125 before the fifth cycle. She undergoes a CT scan after completion of therapy that shows no evidence of disease, and her CA125 is 12.4 U/mL. She returns to the office every 3 months for surveillance visits with a physical examination and CA125. Nine months after completion of chemotherapy, her CA125 had risen to 30.6 U/mL. She is asymptomatic. She therefore has her CA125 checked again 1 month

later, with levels now increased to 124.3 U/mL, and she is starting to have vague abdominal pain. She undergoes a CT scan to assess for recurrent disease, with the finding of liver metastases (Figure 19.4). She elects to restart chemotherapy.

## Evidence-Based Case Discussion

Unfortunately, despite initial responses to chemotherapy, recurrent disease is common in epithelial ovarian cancer, and with few exceptions, is incurable. The next step in treatment is dependent on disease-free interval following the completion of initial adjuvant chemotherapy. If the interval is 6 months or longer, the patient has platinum-sensitive disease, and is typically retreated with a platinum-based regimen, most commonly carboplatin and paclitaxel, based on results of the ICON4 trial (12). For patients with late disease recurrences, >1 year since the completion of chemotherapy, an interval debulking procedure could be considered (see further discussion). If a patient develops recurrent disease in <6 months, the patient is categorized as having platinum-resistant disease and is therefore typically treated with nonplatinum-based regimens.

Multiple studies have investigated the role of CA125 during chemotherapy. A rapid fall in the CA125 level during chemotherapy has been correlated with a more favorable prognosis in the majority of studies (13). In patients in whom the CA125 is not falling during initial adjuvant chemotherapy, an earlier change in chemotherapy regimens may be indicated. The role of CA125 in monitoring patients in the surveillance setting is currently disputed. In the United States, standard practice is to check a CA125 level at every surveillance visit, whereas in Europe CA125 is not routinely checked. A recent European trial reports that women who restart chemotherapy based on an asymptomatic rise in CA125 do not live longer than women who wait until the development of symptoms before the reinitiation of chemotherapy (14). The clinical use of CA125 for monitoring recurrent disease and triggering reinitiation of chemotherapy remains an area of active investigation.

Before reviewing chemotherapy options for recurrent epithelial ovarian cancer, it is important to address the role of surgical exploration and secondary cytoreduction. Secondary cytoreduction has only been shown to have potential benefit in selective patients with platinum-sensitive recurrent disease. Factors predicting a survival benefit for secondary cytoreduction include disease-free interval >12 months, few recurrence sites, a lack of ascites, and surgical debulking to <0.5 cm on secondary cytoreduction (15). Given that our patient in this case study has cancer that recurred in <12 months with multifocal disease including liver lesions, she would not be a good candidate for attempted secondary cytoreduction.

The chemotherapy regimen of choice for patients with platinum-sensitive recurrent disease is carboplatin and paclitaxel (Figure 19.5). This is based on results of the

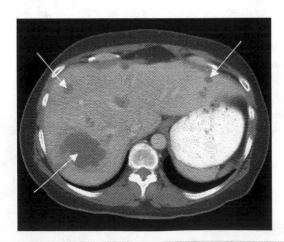

**Figure 19.4**

CT imaging demonstrating liver metastases. Areas of decreased signal intensity are noted within the liver, consistent with parenchymal metastatic disease (indicated by white arrows). Hepatomegaly is also appreciated on this image.

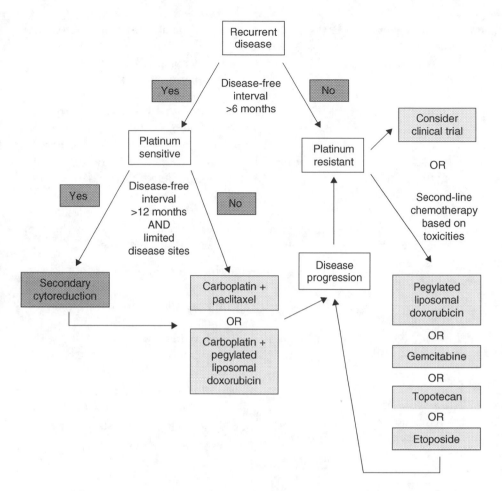

**Figure 19.5**

Decision analysis for recurrent epithelial ovarian cancer. Appropriate treatment of recurrent epithelial ovarian cancer is largely dependent on the disease-free interval. Once patients develop platinum-resistant disease, there are a number of second-line chemotherapies that have shown similar efficacy. An increasing number of clinical trials exist, and enrollment should be considered for any patient with recurrent disease.

ICON4 trial, which compared treatment of these patients with carboplatin alone versus carboplatin and paclitaxel (12). In this study, patients treated with carboplatin and paclitaxel had a 7% absolute increase in overall survival at 2 years. Response rates were approximately 65%. If paclitaxel side effects such as persistent neuropathy limit the use of this agent in the recurrent disease setting, an alternative regimen would be carboplatin and pegylated liposomal doxorubicin. In the CAeLYx in Platinum Sensitive Ovarian patients (CALYPSO) trial, this drug combination demonstrated improved PFS compared to carboplatin and paclitaxel in patients with platinum-sensitive recurrent disease. However, there was no difference in overall survival (16). Alternatively, carboplatin and gemcitabine also have been shown to have significant activity, although this has not been compared to carboplatin and paclitaxel as a standard of care.

Patients with recurrent platinum-sensitive disease are typically treated with systemic therapy. In addition to cytotoxic chemotherapies, as discussed previously, there is also a role for hormonal agents such as tamoxifen and aromatase inhibitors in the treatment of recurrent ovarian cancer. However, the objective response rates to hormonal agents are relatively low, 10–20%, and patients generally demonstrate stable disease rather than a partial or complete response. Given the low side-effect profile and the fact that some patients can have prolonged stable disease on the agents, hormonal therapy should be considered in any patient with recurrent disease. Most commonly, these agents are used in asymptomatic patients desiring therapy.

Once a patient recurs with platinum-resistant disease, there are still many chemotherapeutic options to consider (Figure 19.5). Studies have demonstrated multiple regimens with equivalent efficacy in this setting; response rates are typically low (15–30%) and the duration of response is often short. Because of the relative lack of efficacy of approved agents in platinum-resistant disease, clinical trials of novel agents should be considered for this patient population. When choosing among possible chemotherapeutic agents, given no clear survival advantage of a given regimen, chemotherapy choice should be driven by the side-effect profile of the specific agents as they apply to the individual patient. The use of multi-agent chemotherapeutic regimens is not recommended. Although doublet regimens can improve response rates and PFS, they have significant increased toxicity, and no phase III trial to date has demonstrated an improvement in overall survival rates with doublet therapy. Doublets can be considered when a rapid disease response is necessary. Due to the nature of epithelial ovarian cancer with multiple recurrences, most patients ultimately receive all of these potential "second-line" agents. Specific agents that have been shown to be effective include pegylated liposomal doxorubicin, gemcitabine, topotecan, and etoposide.

## REVIEW QUESTIONS

1. A 46-year-old female presents with a pelvic mass. She undergoes a surgical staging procedure with optimal debulking. Pathology demonstrates a 2.3-cm ovarian epithelial serous ovarian tumor of low malignant potential with capsular rupture and multiple peritoneal implants without evidence of invasion. The patient recovers well from surgery and presents to discuss adjuvant treatment options. Which of the following is the next best step?

   (A) Three to six cycles of adjuvant intravenous (IV) carboplatin/paclitaxel
   (B) Six cycles intraperitoneal (IP) cisplatin and IV/IP paclitaxel
   (C) Observation
   (D) Six cycles of IV carboplatin/paclitaxel/bevacizumab with 6 months of bevacizumab maintenance therapy

2. A 62-year-old female undergoes surgical staging for a newly diagnosed ovarian cancer. Pathology demonstrates a clear cell ovarian cancer limited to the right ovary with intact capsule, negative peritoneal washings, negative peritoneal and omental biopsies, and negative pelvic and periaortic lymph nodes. The patient is otherwise healthy, with good functional status. Which is the best option for adjuvant treatment?

   (A) Observation with Q3 month physical examination and CA125 measurement
   (B) Six cycles of dose-dense intravenous (IV) carboplatin/paclitaxel
   (C) Three to six cycles Q3 weekly IV carboplatin/paclitaxel

3. Patient M.S. has a new diagnosis of high-grade serous adenocarcinoma of the ovary involving both of the ovaries and pelvic lymph nodes with omental implants. Surgical debulking was performed with <1 cm of residual disease. The patient has recovered well from surgery. She is without significant comorbidities and has good performance status. Which of the following adjuvant treatment options have demonstrated the greatest overall survival advantage compared to 6 cycles of intravenous (IV) carboplatin and paclitaxel?

   (A) Six cycles of intraperitoneal (IP) cisplatin and IV/IP paclitaxel

   (B) Six cycles of IV carboplatin/pegylated liposomal doxorubicin
   (C) Nine cycles of IV carboplatin/paclitaxel
   (D) Six cycles of IV cisplatin/paclitaxel

4. K.C. presents with abdominal distention, early satiety, and constipation. She has a history of stage IIIC ovarian serous adenocarcinoma status postsurgical debulking followed by 6 cycles of intravenous (IV) carboplatin/paclitaxel completed 1 year ago. CA125 is 1500. Imaging demonstrates ascites, enlarged pelvic lymph nodes, and multiple peritoneal nodules consistent with recurrent ovarian cancer. Which is the next best step to improve overall survival?

   (A) Surgical debulking followed by 6 cycles of every 3 week IV carboplatin/paclitaxel
   (B) Every 4 week IV pegylated liposomal doxorubicin until disease progression
   (C) Aromatase inhibitor therapy
   (D) Six cycles of every 3 week IV carboplatin/paclitaxel

5. Ms. V. presents to discuss indications for genetic testing. She was diagnosed at age 60 years with high grade serous adenocarcinoma of the ovary. Her mother died in her 80s from a myocardial infarction. She has 2 sisters and 1 daughter who are alive and healthy. She denies a family history of breast or ovarian cancer. Which of the following is consistent with current national comprehensive cancer network guidelines?

   (A) Ms. V. does not meet criteria for genetic testing, as she has no family history of breast or ovarian cancer
   (B) Ms. V. does meet criteria for genetic testing, given her personal history of ovarian cancer
   (C) Ms. V. does meet criteria for genetic testing, as approximately 30% of the patients diagnosed with ovarian cancer have a mutation in either *BRCA1* or *BRCA2*
   (D) Ms. V. does not meet criteria for genetic testing, as *BRCA* mutational status is not prognostic in ovarian cancer

6. A 72-year-old female with recurrent serous ovarian cancer presents with abdominal pain and bloating with a rising CA125 2 months after completion of 6 cycles of intravenous (IV) carboplatin/paclitaxel. CT scan confirms recurrent disease. What is an appropriate next step in therapy?

   (A) Start every 4 week IV pegylated liposomal doxorubicin
   (B) Restart every 3 week IV carboplatin/paclitaxel

(C) Start every 3 week IV carboplatin/paclitaxel/bevacizumab

(D) Surgical debulking

7. A 51-year-old female presents with pelvic pain and is found to have bilateral adnexal masses and a CA125 of 646. She undergoes a surgical debulking and staging procedure that reveals endometrioid ovarian cancer involving both ovaries. The right ovarian mass extends from the ovary and into the uterus. Pelvic and periaortic lymph nodes are negative for disease. What adjuvant therapy has been demonstrated to most improve her overall survival?

(A) Six cycles of intravenous (IV) carboplatin every 3 weeks and gemcitabine days 1, 8

(B) Three to six cycles of every 3 week IV carboplatin/paclitaxel

(C) Six cycles of every 3 week IV carboplatin/paclitaxel/bevacizumab

(D) Six cycles of intraperitoneal (IP) cisplatin and IV/IP paclitaxel

## ACKNOWLEDGMENT

We thank Dr. Jonathan Dillman in Radiology at the University of Michigan for his assistance with the images for Figures 19.2 and 19.4.

## REFERENCES

1. Domchek SM, Friebel TM, Singer CF, et al. Association of risk-reducing surgery in BRCA1 or BRCA2 mutation carriers with cancer risk and mortality. *JAMA*. 2010;304(9):967–975.
2. Goff BA, Mandel LS, Melancon CH, et al. Frequency of symptoms of ovarian cancer in women presenting to primary care clinics. *JAMA*. 2004;291(22):2705–2712.
3. Young RC, Walton LA, Ellenberg SS, et al. Adjuvant therapy in stage I and stage II epithelial ovarian cancer. Results of two prospective randomized trials. *N Engl J Med*. 1990;322(15):1021–1027.
4. Trimbos JB, Parmar M, Vergote I, et al. International Collaborative Ovarian Neoplasm trial 1 and Adjuvant Chemotherapy in Ovarian Neoplasm trial: two parallel randomized phase III trials of adjuvant chemotherapy in patients with early-stage ovarian carcinoma. *J Natl Cancer Inst*. 2003;95(2):105–112.
5. Bell J, Brady MF, Young RC, et al. Randomized phase III trial of three versus six cycles of adjuvant carboplatin and paclitaxel in early stage epithelial ovarian carcinoma: a Gynecologic Oncology Group study. *Gynecol Oncol*. 2006;102(3):432–439.
6. Chan JK, Tian C, Fleming GF, et al. The potential benefit of 6 vs. 3 cycles of chemotherapy in subsets of women with early-stage high-risk epithelial ovarian cancer: an exploratory analysis of a Gynecologic Oncology Group study. *Gynecol Oncol*. 2010;116(3):301–306.
7. Armstrong DK, Bundy B, Wenzel L, et al. Intraperitoneal cisplatin and paclitaxel in ovarian cancer. *N Engl J Med*. 2006;354(1):34–43.
8. Bristow RE, Eisenhauer EL, Santillan A, et al. Delaying the primary surgical effort for advanced ovarian cancer: a systematic review of neoadjuvant chemotherapy and interval cytoreduction. *Gynecol Oncol*. 2007;104(2):480–490.
9. Berry E, Matthews KS, Singh DK, et al. An outpatient intraperitoneal chemotherapy regimen for advanced ovarian cancer. *Gynecol Oncol*. 2009;113(1):63–67.
10. Katsumata N, Yasuda M, Takahashi F, et al. Dose-dense paclitaxel once a week in combination with carboplatin every 3 weeks for advanced ovarian cancer: a phase 3, open-label, randomised controlled trial. *Lancet*. 2009;374(9698):1331–1338.
11. Farley J, Brady WE, Vathipadiekal V, et al. Selumetinib in women with recurrent low-grade serous carcinoma of the ovary or peritoneum: an open-label, single-arm, phase 2 study. *Lancet Oncol*. 2013;14:134–140.
12. Parmar MK, Ledermann JA, Colombo N, et al. Paclitaxel plus platinum-based chemotherapy versus conventional platinum-based chemotherapy in women with relapsed ovarian cancer: the ICON4/AGO-OVAR-2.2 trial. *Lancet*. 2003;361(9375):2099–2106.
13. Meyer T, Rustin GJ. Role of tumour markers in monitoring epithelial ovarian cancer. *Br J Cancer*. 2000;82(9):1535–1538.
14. Rustin GJ, van der Burg ME, Griffin CL, et al. Early versus delayed treatment of relapsed ovarian cancer (MRC OV05/EORTC 55955): a randomised trial. *Lancet*. 2010;376(9747):1155–1163.
15. Chi DS, McCaughty K, Diaz JP, et al. Guidelines and selection criteria for secondary cytoreductive surgery in patients with recurrent, platinum-sensitive epithelial ovarian carcinoma. *Cancer*. 2006;106(9):1933–1939.
16. Wagner, U, Marth, C, Largiller, R, et al. Final overall survival results of phase III GCIG CALYPSO trial of pegylated liposomal doxorubicin and carboplatin vs paclitaxel and carboplatin in platinum-sensitive ovarian cancer patients. *Br J Cancer*. 2012;107(4):588–591.

# 20

## Melanoma

ANN W. SILK, KEVIN McDONNELL, AND CHRISTOPHER D. LAO

## EPIDEMIOLOGY, RISK FACTORS, NATURAL HISTORY, AND PATHOLOGY

In 2014, there will be approximately 76,100 new cases of melanoma and 9710 deaths secondary to this disease (1). The median age at diagnosis of melanoma is 62 years, but it is the most common malignancy diagnosed in women between the ages of 25 and 29 years. The incidence of melanoma is highest among whites, with a rate of approximately 24 per 1000 persons, with a 1.5:1 male-to-female predominance (2).

Melanoma is a malignancy originating from the neural crest-derived melanocytes. Thus, it can develop in sites where these neural crest cells migrate, including the skin, mucosal membranes of the aerodigestive system, and uveal tissues of the eye. An association between sun exposure and melanoma exists; however, it appears more strongly associated with intermittent exposure resulting in sunburn. Recognized risk factors for the occurrence of melanoma include a previous personal or family history of melanoma, history of multiple (>50 nevi) benign and atypical nevi, a history of intermittent severe sunburns during adolescence, increased sensitivity to the sun, and an inherited susceptibility.

The most common histological subtype of melanoma is superficial spreading melanoma, representing up to three quarters of all diagnoses of the disease. This subtype often occurs in sun-exposed areas and appears as the classic irregular pigmented macule. Nodular melanomas represent the second most frequent histological subtype, accounting for between 20% and 30% of melanoma cases. Nodular melanomas usually appear as rapidly growing, homogeneous darkly pigmented nodules; microscopically, malignant cells may be either spindled or epithelioid. The third most frequent subtype is lentigo maligna, which most often originates in chronically solar-damaged skin, typically in older patients on skin of the head and neck. Acral lentiginous melanoma is a less-frequent histological subtype in whites, representing <10% of cases. However, among patients of Asian and African descent, acral lentiginous melanomas occur more frequently than other subtypes. Acral lentiginous melanomas typically occur subungually and on the palms and soles. This subtype is not clearly related to sun exposure.

Less-frequently occurring subtypes of melanoma include desmoplastic, mucosal, and uveal melanomas. Desmoplastic melanoma is a rare variant that is aggressive and deeply invasive. The desmoplastic melanoma is often amelanotic and therefore is often not initially appreciated as pathologic. It often occurs on areas of sun-exposed skin. Melanomas may also arise in nonsolar-exposed tissues such as the mucosal surfaces of the nose, esophagus, oral cavity, genitourinary tract, anus, and rectum. Melanomas uncommonly arise from the uvea of the eye. Uveal melanomas may manifest as pain or as a change in visual acuity, and are often diagnosed without a biopsy. Metastasis from uveal melanoma is usually hematogenous, with a characteristic predilection for liver involvement.

The recognition of unique genetic events in certain subtypes of melanoma will likely result in the future molecular or genetic characterization of melanoma instead of histological subtyping. Activating mutations of *BRAF* or *NRAS* have been found to be altered in 50% and 15% of melanomas, respectively (3). *BRAF* mutations are associated with melanomas arising from intermittently solar-damaged skin, as opposed to chronically solar-damaged skin. In subsets of melanomas that are associated with minimal ultraviolet exposure, such as mucosal and acral melanomas, the predominant foundational mutation may be an activating mutation in *KIT* rather than *BRAF* or

*NRAS* (4). An inherited genetic susceptibility is present in approximately 5–10% of patients with melanoma. Such melanoma families can harbor alterations in the tumor suppressor gene *CDKN2A* that encodes for p16INK4A and p19ARF. *GNAQ* or *GNA11* mutations have recently been recognized to occur in nearly 50% of uveal melanomas, and genotyping that can distinguish high-risk uveal melanoma is currently available for clinical risk stratification.

## STAGING

### Melanoma Pathologic Staging

| Stage | Definition |
|---|---|
| 0 | Primary tumor is confined to epidermis without lymph node or distant metastatic disease |
| IA | Primary tumor ≤1.00-mm thick, without ulceration and mitosis <1/mm² without lymph node or distant metastatic disease |
| IB | Primary tumor ≤1.00-mm thick, with ulceration or mitoses ≥1/mm² *or* 1.01- to 2.00-mm thick without ulceration without lymph node or distant metastatic disease |
| IIA | Primary tumor 1.01- to 2.00-mm thick with ulceration *or* 2.01- to 4.00-mm thick without ulceration without lymph node or distant metastatic disease |
| IIB | Primary tumor 2.01- to 4.00-mm thick with ulceration *or* 4.00-mm thick without ulceration without lymph node or distant metastatic disease |
| IIC | Primary tumor >4.00-mm thick with ulceration without lymph node or distant metastatic disease |
| IIIA | Primary tumor ≤1.00-mm thick and mitosis <1/mm² *or* >1.00-mm thick without ulceration, with 1–3 micrometastatic-positive lymph nodes and no distant metastatic disease |
| IIIB | Any tumor with 1–3 micro- or macrometastatic lymph nodes or in-transit metastases/satellites with no distant metastatic disease |
| IIIC | Any tumor with ulceration or mitoses ≥1/mm² with 1–3 macrometastatic-positive lymph nodes or in-transit metastases/satellites without distant metastatic disease *or* any tumor with >4 metastatic lymph nodes, matted nodes, or in-transit metastases/satellites with metastatic nodes without distant metastatic disease |
| IV | Primary tumor of any size without or without lymph node disease, with distant metastases |

*Source*: Adapted from *AJCC Cancer Staging Handbook, 7th Edition.*

## CASE SUMMARIES

### Early-Stage Melanoma (Stage II or III)

S.K. is a 36-year-old previously healthy man who noted an enlarging, pigmented lesion on his right upper back. He reported a long history of a nevus that began to increase in size and bleed over the preceding few months. He subsequently sought care from his primary care physician. The patient had no significant past medical history and no family history of melanoma or other cancers. He reported a past history of nonblistering sunburns, with occasional tanning bed use and a history of smoking approximately 1 pack of cigarettes per day for 15 years. Physical examination was remarkable only for an approximately 8-mm raised, pigmented lesion on the right upper back. There were <10 clinically atypical nevi, none meeting criteria for removal. He subsequently underwent an excisional biopsy of the index lesion, which demonstrated a superficial spreading-type melanoma, Breslow depth of 5.6 mm, with ulceration, a focus of angiolymphatic invasion, and satellitosis (Figure 20.1). The patient underwent a radical excision of the melanoma with 2-cm margins and sentinel node mapping. The wide excision margins were negative, but a 0.9-mm tumor nodule was also noted in the resection specimen. One sentinel lymph node was identified in the right axilla and was positive for melanoma. No extracapsular extension was seen. The patient then underwent complete right axillary lymph node dissection, which demonstrated 1/12 lymph nodes to be positive for melanoma. A CT scan of the chest, abdomen, and pelvis and an MRI of the brain were obtained for staging and were negative for distant metastatic disease.

### Evidence-Based Case Discussion

#### Prognostic Variables and Surgical Management

S.K. has a thick melanoma (≥4 mm), a focus of satellitosis, and a total of 2 lymph nodes positive for micrometastatic disease. He had no evidence of distant metastatic disease on staging workup. Overall, this patient is presenting with stage IIIC melanoma that has been completely resected.

Several prognostic variables associated with primary cutaneous melanoma have been identified, which include lymph node positivity, Breslow depth (tumor thickness), microscopic ulceration, and mitotic rate for thin primary melanomas (<1-mm thick). Clark level is no longer considered an independent prognostic variable, unless the lesion is thin and the mitotic rate is not available (5). Shave biopsies are often performed as a less invasive and more efficient means of biopsying suspicious lesions for diagnosis. If the deep margin is positive for melanoma, then the T stage cannot be accurately determined from the shave biopsy. Wide local excision specimens should always be examined for residual melanoma. When there is residual melanoma in the specimen, it is difficult to assess the T stage accurately.

If no lymph nodes are involved, then the primary treatment modality is surgery with adequate margins. The extent of the resection depends on the initial tumor thickness, and several clinical trials have been performed to determine the most appropriate surgical margins. For

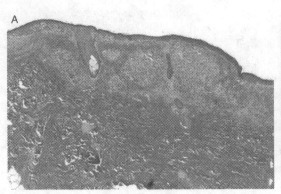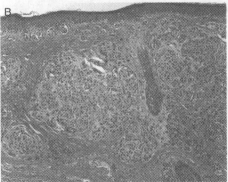

### Figure 20.1

(A) Invasive superficial spreading-type melanoma (low power view, hematoxylin and eosin stain). Nodular areas of dense accumulations of malignant cells noted in the dermis. (B) Magnified view (10×) of the same melanoma. Aggregates of uniformly, large, atypical melanocytes with abundant cytoplasm are evident. Scant melanin pigment dispersed throughout the lesion.

**Table 20.1**  Standard Workup, Evaluation, and Management of Cutaneous Melanoma

| Melanoma | Surgical Margins | Sentinel Lymph Node | Radiologic Imaging | Labs |
|---|---|---|---|---|
| In situ | 0.5 cm | No | No | No |
| <0.75 mm | 1 cm | No | No | No |
| 0.75–1 mm | 1 cm | Consider | No | No |
| 1–2 mm | 1–2 cm | Yes | If LN positive | No |
| >2 mm | 2 cm | Yes | If LN positive | No |
| In-transit disease | Negative margin | Consider | Consider | Consider LDH |
| Stage IV | N/A | N/A | Yes | LDH |

LDH, lactate dehydrogenase; LN, lymph node; N/A, not applicable.

melanoma in situ, standard recommendations are for surgical margins of 0.5 cm; for a tumor between 0.5- and 1-mm thick, the surgical margin should be 1.0 cm; for lesions >1 mm and up to 2 mm, surgical margins should be 1–2 cm; and for all tumors >2 mm a surgical margin of 2.0 cm should be obtained (Table 20.1).

Sentinel lymph node biopsy or mapping has proven to be an informative prognostic procedure for lesions ≥1 mm in Breslow depth. In the Multicenter Selective Lymphadenectomy Trial-1 (MSLT-1), in which patients with primary lesions ≥1-mm thick were randomized to sentinel lymph node mapping or observation, there was a 10-year disease-free survival advantage to sentinel lymph node mapping, but no overall survival advantage (6). Documentation of lymph node involvement identifies patients at higher risk for recurrence; therefore, adjuvant therapy, including enrollment in clinical trials, can be considered for such patients. For lesions between 0.75 and 1 mm, sentinel lymph mapping can also be considered if additional higher-risk features are identified, including young age, ulceration of the primary lesion, lymphovascular invasion, or a mitotic rate ≥1/mm$^2$ (Table 20.1). When positive nodes are identified on sentinel lymph

node mapping, a complete lymphadenectomy remains the standard of care. The importance of a subsequent completion node dissection following sentinel node biopsy is being evaluated in a randomized clinical trial (MSLT-II), in which patients are randomized to completion node dissection or surveillance. In the present clinical case, the Breslow depth of 5.6 mm was an indication for sentinel node lymph node biopsy.

Satellitosis can be defined as at least 1 separate focus of melanoma adjacent to the primary lesion. The presence of satellitosis increases the risk of recurrence. When disease is clinically detected in between the expected draining nodal basin and the primary lesion, but not immediately adjacent to the primary melanoma, it is considered in-transit metastasis. In-transit disease is typically managed with complete surgical excision if possible. Sentinel lymph biopsy for in-transit disease is controversial, as the lymphatics may be altered and unreliable.

### Adjuvant Therapy

Lymph node involvement defines stage III disease. The 5-year survival rates are approximately 80%, 60%, and 40% for stages IIIA, IIIB, and IIIC, respectively (5). Following surgical management of the primary lesion, adjuvant therapy can be considered and includes enrollment in a clinical trial if available, high-dose interferon alpha-2b, or observation. There is evidence from 1 randomized clinical trial performed by an intergroup (Australia and New Zealand Melanoma Trials Group [ANZMTG] and Trans-Tasman Radiation Oncology Group [TROG]) that adjuvant radiation when compared to observation can improve control of the lymph node field, but not disease-free survival or overall survival (7). Thus, in instances where regional control is required, radiotherapy may be considered.

The only Food and Drug Administration (FDA)-approved adjuvant therapy is high-dose interferon alpha-2b. Multiple randomized interferon trials have been performed comparing interferon to placebo or vaccine, but 3 U.S. cooperative group trials (Eastern Cooperative Oncology Group [ECOG] 1684, ECOG 1690, and ECOG 1694) have been performed with the high-dose regimen (20 million units/m$^2$ IV daily Monday through Friday for 4 weeks followed by 10 million units/m$^2$ subcutaneously 3 times a week for 48 weeks). ECOG 1684 was a randomized trial of high-dose interferon alpha-2b versus observation for patient with stages ≥ IIB (T4) and III disease. A statistically significant difference in overall and disease-free survival was observed at 5 years (8). This trial was the primary reason for the FDA approval of interferon for adjuvant therapy of melanoma in 1995. However, results from a meta-analysis of the interferon trials and in a pooled analysis of high-dose regimens in which patients were followed for a median of 12.6 years showed that an overall survival advantage was no longer statistically significant, although a relapse-free survival advantage remained significant (9,10). Interferon therapy is associated with a number of adverse effects that must be kept in mind when considering this therapy. In addition to generalized symptoms, such as anorexia, fatigue, malaise, headaches, nausea, vomiting, fever, chills, myalgias, and rash, interferon therapy may also induce liver dysfunction, myelosuppression, and depression. The latter is of concern particularly when contemplating this therapy for patients with a preexisting psychiatric condition. Given the toxicities of treatment and the controversy surrounding the benefit of adjuvant interferon, observation has more recently been considered an appropriate option, including acceptance of observation as the control arm of clinical trials.

In the current case, after undergoing a lymph node dissection, the patient opted to proceed with clinical observation. Standard follow-up after surgical excision in the absence of additional adjuvant therapy includes a history and physical examination every 3–4 months for the first 2 years, every 6 months for the next 3 years, and then annually as clinically appropriate thereafter. No standard recommendation exists for imaging studies. Chest x-ray,

CT, or PET scan as well as a brain MRI can be obtained at the discretion of the treating physician, but there is no evidence of a survival advantage with aggressive radiologic surveillance at this time. The lactate dehydrogenase (LDH) level is the only laboratory result with prognostic significance, and thus can be checked periodically during follow-up as well. After 5 years, interval laboratory testing and imaging are performed as clinically indicated.

## Locoregional and Metastatic (Stage IV) Melanoma

M.M. is a 70-year-old woman with a past history of coronary artery disease, hypertension, and a stage IB melanoma on her left lower leg (superficial spreading type, Breslow depth of 0.6 mm, no ulceration, and mitotic rate of 2/mm$^2$). The lesion was treated with wide excision and sentinel lymph node biopsy was not performed due to the thin nature of the melanoma. The patient proceeded with follow-up physical examinations every 6 months with dermatology. Three years after her original diagnosis, the patient discovered a mass in the left groin. Physical examination confirmed a palpable mass, without other nodules or masses concerning for melanoma at that time. She underwent fine needle aspiration (FNA) of this mass, which confirmed malignant melanoma. Staging workup including a PET-CT demonstrated an $^{18}$F-fludeoxyglucose (FDG)-avid mass in the groin, but failed to reveal any evidence of distant metastatic disease. Her regional recurrence was treated with left superficial inguinal lymph node dissection. This revealed 1 lymph node completely replaced with tumor. Following surgery, she chose to continue with observation alone. Approximately, 1 year after surgery, the patient noticed multiple nodules on her leg developing over several weeks (Figure 20.2). Excision of 1 of these nodules confirmed recurrent melanoma. Repeated PET-CT again failed to reveal distant metastases, but multiple subcutaneous nodules were identified. She was not considered a candidate for isolated limb perfusion (ILP) due to the proximal nature of her disease. She was being evaluated for participation in a clinical trial, but during the screening period, she had repeated imaging studies that revealed findings concerning for metastatic disease in her lungs, mediastinum, and liver. Brain MRI was negative. CT-guided biopsy of her liver confirmed metastatic disease. Measurement of the LDH was performed and was elevated to a level of 300 IU/L.

### Evidence-Based Discussion

She is a patient initially diagnosed with low-risk stage IB disease who presents with a palpable lymph node 3 years after her original diagnosis. She was being considered for management of her apparent unresectable regional disease, but developed biopsy-proven distant metastatic (stage IV) disease within a short follow-up interval.

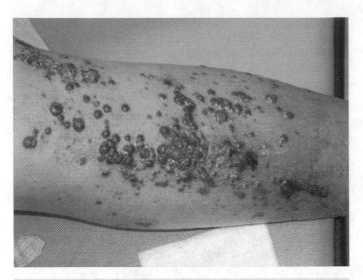

**Figure 20.2**

Representative photograph of multiple cutaneous and subcutaneous nodules of melanoma on an extremity of a patient.

## Locoregional Melanoma

Interval follow-ups are performed to detect recurrent disease, which if discovered within the locoregional area, defined as disease confined to the area of the primary lesion and the primary nodal basin, is still potentially curable with surgery. Recurrence can occur as either local recurrence at the primary tumor site, in-transit disease, nodal involvement, or distant metastatic disease. Imaging is at the discretion of the treating physician, but CT scans are standard and can pick up small volume disease. Melanoma tends to be FDG-avid, and thus PET-CT is also an acceptable test, particularly when the extremities are involved. Brain MRI is a preferred test for ruling out brain involvement, as the sensitivity is higher for detecting metastasis, and melanoma can have a distinct resonance on MRI.

If recurrence occurs in the regional lymph node basin, complete surgical resection of the node should be performed, which may be incorporated into a complete lymph node dissection if not previously performed. For lymph node disease in the groin, consideration should be given to iliac or obturator node dissection, particularly if CT imaging documents pelvic disease, Cloquet's node is involved, or 3 or more lymph nodes are involved.

If the recurrence is considered unresectable, then hyperthermic ILP or isolated limb infusion (ILI) with melphalan (if isolated to an extremity), clinical trial participation, local ablation therapy, radiotherapy, systemic therapy, or topical imiquinod can be considered. These options are dependent on the location of the disease, whether previous treatment to the area was given (e.g., radiotherapy); characteristics of the disease (e.g., epidermotropic metastases); and comorbidities of the patient. In a large, randomized, phase III clinical trial, ILP did not demonstrate

an improvement in overall survival in the adjuvant setting. The response rate to ILP, however, is between 50% and 90%, with a large proportion being complete responses. Therefore, this approach can be useful to control unresectable disease in appropriately selected patients. The use of surgery and/or radiation for regional recurrence in the setting of metastatic disease is based on whether a significant amount of morbidity would be expected from disease that could potentially grow uncontrolled. The current patient was not a candidate for ILP due to the proximal nature of the disease in her extremity. Also, given the pace of her metastatic disease, systemic therapy was indicated and locoregional treatment was deferred.

## Stage IV Melanoma

Systemic therapy options for unresectable stage III and IV melanoma are similar. Stage IV disease is further classified based on the location of the disease and whether the LDH is elevated, as they are independent predictors of survival (5). Stage IV, M1a disease is defined as distant skin, subcutaneous, or nodal metastatic disease with a normal LDH. M1b disease includes lung metastases with a normal LDH, and M1c includes visceral metastases or any distant metastases with an elevated LDH value. The 5-year survival rates for stage IV patients with normal and elevated LDH values are 30% and 10%, respectively. Survival rates at 5 years for patients with M1a, M1b, and M1c disease are approximately 30%, 20%, and 10%, respectively.

The initial management decision in patients presenting with stage IV melanoma is whether the metastatic disease can be completely resected (see Figure 20.3 for workup and management algorithm). If the patient is surgically rendered free of disease from stage IV melanoma, the standard of care following surgery is observation or enrollment in a clinical trial. Survival in this cohort of patients is significantly better than in patients whose disease could not be resected, as demonstrated in at least 2 clinical trials (11,12).

In the case of disseminated, unresectable disease, several therapeutic options exist. Prior to 2011, there were only 2 FDA-approved agents for stage IV melanoma: dacarbazine and high-dose interleukin-2 (IL-2). Both agents were approved for the treatment of stage IV melanoma based on clinical activity (with some durability of responses for IL-2) and absence of other effective therapies at the time, despite a lack of randomized phase III clinical trial evidence of a survival advantage. High-dose IL-2 is a specialized treatment for appropriately selected patients. The toxicities are significant with this therapy and include signs and symptoms mimicking sepsis. Treatment requires hospitalization for administration. For patients who are candidates for IL-2 therapy (younger age, patients older than 50 years with normal cardiac function, no brain involvement, and normal organ function), there is potential for long-term

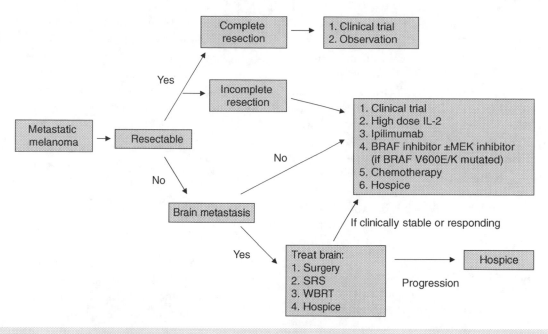

**Figure 20.3**

Workup and management algorithm for patients with metastatic (stage IV) melanoma. *Note:* All patients with unresectable or stage IV melanoma should undergo *BRAF* mutational analysis. IL, interleukin; SRS, stereotactic radiosurgery; WBRT, whole-brain radiotherapy.

control, although the likelihood is on the order of 5% (13). In 2011, 2 new agents, ipilimumab and vemurafenib, were approved by the U.S. FDA based on statistically significant overall survival advantages in large randomized clinical trials. Ipilimumab, an antibody against cytotoxic T-lymphocyte antigen 4 (CTLA-4), demonstrated a 4-month improvement in median overall survival (6.4 months for the non-ipilimumab group compared with 10.1 months for the ipilimumab group) (14). A recent pooled analysis of trials found that 22% of patients survived for >3 years, at which point, the survival curve begins to plateau. Thus, for some patients, this therapy may result in long-term control of the disease. Ipilimumab has unique side effects that mimic autoimmune disease, including colitis, hepatitis, hypophysitis, rash, and fatigue. These immune-related adverse events are treated with systemic steroids.

*BRAF* mutations occur in approximately 50% of melanomas, and therapeutic agents targeting *BRAF* V600E have now demonstrated response rates approaching 80% and improvements in survival. In a phase III trial, patients with previously untreated metastatic melanoma expressing *BRAF* V600E mutations were randomized to treatment with either the oral *BRAF* kinase inhibitor vemurafenib or dacarbazine. In an interim analysis of overall survival, vemurafenib therapy was associated with a 63% reduction in the risk of death as compared to dacarbazine therapy (15); this was confirmed in an updated analysis of overall survival. Treatment with vemurafenib can result in rash, abnormal liver function tests, and the development of secondary cutaneous neoplasms, including up to 25% incidence of

squamous cell carcinoma and keratoacanthomas. A second *BRAF* kinase inhibitor, dabrafenib, demonstrated similar activity as a single agent. Dabrafenib was tested in combination with a mitogen-activated protein kinase kinase (MEK) inhibitor, trametinib, with the intent to block the growth signal at a second step in the mitogen-activated protein kinase (MAPK) pathway. Median progression-free survival with dabrafenib and trametinib combination therapy was 9.4 months, as compared with 5.8 months in patients receiving dabrafenib alone. The response rate was 76% versus 54%, respectively (16). The impact of combination therapy on overall survival is unknown at this time.

Recently, antibodies against another immune checkpoint, the programmed death-1 (PD-1) and its ligand, PD-L1, have demonstrated activity in metastatic melanoma. The response rate to nivolumab as a single agent is 30%, and most of these responses are durable, consistent with the pattern of other immunotherapies. These agents remain investigational at this time, but FDA approval is expected in late 2014 or 2015. Combination first-line therapy with nivolumab and ipilimumab is being evaluated currently in a phase III trial.

Other agents (e.g., temozolomide, carboplatin/paclitaxel, and nab-paclitaxel) and multidrug combinations (e.g., biochemotherapy and the Dartmouth regimen) have demonstrated activity in clinical trials. The response rates range from 0% to 30% without an associated survival advantage when compared to dacarbazine alone. These regimens are now often reserved for disease that requires a response for palliation or if surgery might be possible with some shrinkage of a tumor that was previously considered unresectable.

A common complicating factor limiting treatment options is brain involvement. This is often associated with poorer survival. Clinical trials often require exclusion of brain metastases or documented disease control over time for consideration of enrollment. A brain MRI is thus often required in staging and periodically in follow-up, even if there was no brain involvement initially. If the brain is involved, then resection, stereotactic radiosurgery, or whole-brain radiotherapy are considered for palliative management. Ipilimumab and BRAF inhibitors have demonstrated some activity in brain metastases and can be considered in the course of treatment when there is active disease in both the brain and the body.

The patient in this case was not considered to be a candidate for high-dose IL-2 due to her advanced age, comorbidities, and the risks associated with treatment. Ipilimumab was still only available on a clinical trial and no trial was available to her at the time. She was BRAF V600E negative. She was screened for first-line protocol therapy testing combinatorial targeted agents, and at first follow-up had a partial response by Response Evaluation Criteria in Solid Tumors (RECIST) criteria. She continued on protocol therapy.

## REVIEW QUESTIONS

1. A 50-year-old woman is diagnosed with an ulcerated melanoma arising on the right arm. She underwent wide local excision and sentinel lymph node biopsy, which was remarkable for 2 positive lymph nodes. A CT scan of the chest, abdomen, and pelvis show no evidence of metastases. Which one of the following studies should be ordered at this time?

   (A) PET/CT scan
   (B) Ultrasound of right axillary lymph node basin
   (C) MRI of the brain
   (D) CT scan of the head with contrast

2. An obese 44-year-old accountant comes to a follow-up visit 3 months after completing therapy with ipilimumab for stage IV melanoma. He reports fatigue, erectile dysfunction, and headaches. Laboratory findings show sodium of 131 mmol/L (low), potassium of 4.8 mmol/L, thyroid stimulating hormone of 0.2 mIU/L (low), free T4 of 0.54 ng/dL (low), and testosterone of 1.31 ng/mL (low). On examination, blood pressure is found to be 100/54 mmHg and he looks fatigued. What is the pathophysiology of his endocrine disruption?

   (A) Obesity-related hypogonadism
   (B) Primary hypothyroidism
   (C) Autoimmune lymphocytic hypophysitis
   (D) Addison's disease

3. A 74-year-old woman notes a new pigmented lesion on her shoulder. Pathological examination of a shave biopsy specimen reveals a superficial spreading melanoma with a Breslow depth of 0.5 mm. It is not ulcerated. All margins are negative. What is the next appropriate step in management?

   (A) No further therapy
   (B) Wide local excision with a 1-cm margin
   (C) Wide local excision with a 2-cm margin
   (D) Sentinel lymph node mapping and biopsy, followed by wide local excision with a 2-cm margin
   (E) Interferon-alpha

4. A 22-year-old lifeguard has a history of stage IIIA melanoma arising on the back, diagnosed 4 years ago. On surveillance imaging, he is found to have multiple new nodules in the lungs. Biopsy of one of the larger lung nodules shows metastatic melanoma. What genetic testing should be performed on the tumor tissue at this time?

   (A) C-KIT
   (B) K-RAS
   (C) EGFR
   (D) BRAF
   (E) GNAQ

5. A 28-year-old executive is diagnosed with stage IIIA melanoma arising on the leg. She is offered adjuvant therapy with high-dose alpha interferon for 1 year. What is the expected benefit of interferon?

   (A) Improvement in disease-free survival at 7 years
   (B) Improvement in overall survival at 7 years
   (C) Decrease in the incidence of brain metastases
   (D) Decrease in the rate of a second primary melanoma

6. A 67-year-old man with a history of coronary artery disease has progressive metastatic melanoma despite therapy with ipilimumab. His tumor demonstrates an activating mutation in BRAF at the V600E position. He is offered treatment with vemurafenib. What is his risk of developing squamous cell carcinoma of the skin on this therapy?

   (A) 0–5%
   (B) 5–10%
   (C) 20–25%
   (D) 55–70%

## REFERENCES

1. Siegel, R, Ma, J, Zou, Z, et al. Cancer statistics, 2014. *CA Cancer J Clin*. 2014;64:9–29.
2. ACS. *Cancer Facts & Figures*; 2014. http://www.cancer.org. Accessed December 2014.

3. Davies H, Bignell GR, Cox C, et al. Mutations of the BRAF gene in human cancer. *Nature*. 2002;417:949–954.

4. Curtin JA, Busam K, Pinkel D, et al. Somatic activation of KIT in distinct subtypes of melanoma. *J Clin Oncol*. 2006;24: 4340–4346.

5. Balch CM, Gershenwald JE, Soong SJ, et al. Final version of 2009 AJCC melanoma staging and classification. *J Clin Oncol*. 2009;27:6199–6206.

6. Morton DL, Thompson JF, Cochran AJ, et al. Final trial report of sentinel-node biopsy versus nodal observation in melanoma. *N Engl J Med*. 2014;370:599–609.

7. Burmeister BH, Henderson MA, Ainslie J, et al. Adjuvant radiotherapy versus observation alone for patients at risk of lymph-node field relapse after therapeutic lymphadenectomy for melanoma: a randomised trial. *Lancet Oncol*. 2012;13:589–597.

8. Kirkwood JM, Strawderman MH, Ernstoff MS, et al. Interferon alpha-2b adjuvant therapy of high-risk resected cutaneous melanoma: the Eastern Cooperative Oncology Group Trial EST 1684. *J Clin Oncol*. 1996;14:7–17.

9. Kirkwood JM, Manola J, Ibrahim J, et al. A pooled analysis of Eastern Cooperative Oncology Group and intergroup trials of adjuvant high-dose interferon for melanoma. *Clin Cancer Res*. 2004;10:1670–1677.

10. Wheatley K, Ives N, Hancock B, et al. Does adjuvant interferon-alpha for high-risk melanoma provide a worthwhile benefit? A meta-analysis of the randomised trials. *Cancer Treat Rev*. 2003;29:241–252.

11. Sosman JA, Moon J, Tuthill RJ, et al. A phase 2 trial of complete resection for stage IV melanoma: results of Southwest Oncology Group Clinical Trial S9430. *Cancer*. 2011;117:4740–4746.

12. Howard JH, Thompson JF, Mozzillo N, et al. Metastasectomy for distant metastatic melanoma: analysis of data from the first multicenter selective lymphadenectomy trial (MSLT-I). *Ann Surg Oncol*. 2012;19:2547–2555.

13. Atkins MB, Lotze MT, Dutcher JP, et al. High-dose recombinant interleukin 2 therapy for patients with metastatic melanoma: analysis of 270 patients treated between 1985 and 1993. *J Clin Oncol*. 1999;17:2105–2116.

14. Hodi FS, O'Day SJ, McDermott DF, et al. Improved survival with ipilimumab in patients with metastatic melanoma. *N Engl J Med*. 2010;363:711–723.

15. Chapman PB, Hauschild A, Haanen JB, et al. Improved survival with vemurafenib in melanoma with *BRAF* V600E mutation. *N Engl J Med*. 2011;364:2507–2516.

16. Flaherty KT, Infante JR, Daud A, et al. Combined BRAF and MEK inhibition in melanoma with BRAF V600 mutations. *N Engl J Med*. 2012;367:1694–1703.

# 21

## *Bone Sarcoma*

ELIZABETH J. DAVIS AND SCOTT M. SCHUETZE

## OSTEOSARCOMA

### Epidemiology, Risk Factors, Natural History, and Pathology

Osteosarcoma is the most common nonhematopoietic bone tumor, but accounts for <1000 cases per year. There is a bimodal age distribution most frequently arising during the second and sixth decades of life. In older patients, osteosarcoma is often secondary to Paget's disease, radiation, or enchondroma. Other risk factors for development of osteosarcoma include genetic syndromes such as familial retinoblastoma (RB1 mutation) and Li–Fraumeni syndrome (*TP53* mutation). Osteosarcoma is more common in males than in females.

Patients typically present with pain and a hardened mass. The most common sites of disease are the intramedullary metaphyses of the long bones, typically the distal femur, proximal tibia, and proximal humerus. Osteosarcoma arising in the axial skeleton is more common in adults than in teenagers. Extraosseous osteosarcoma arises in the soft tissue, does not primarily involve bone, and is usually treated as a soft tissue sarcoma.

Osteosarcoma is typically composed of malignant spindle cells, osteoblasts, and bone matrix (osteoid). The common histological subtypes of osteosarcoma include osteoblastic, chondroblastic, and fibroblastic variants. Osteosarcoma can arise on the surface of the bone or within the intramedullary canal, and it can be high or low grade. Grading is based on several components including mitotic count, pleomorphism, and cellular atypia. Intramedullary tumors are usually high grade, whereas low-grade tumors are found along the bone surface. Grade is more informative than histological type because it affects prognosis and treatment decisions.

Osteosarcoma spreads hematogenously, with lung followed by bone being the most common sites of metastasis.

At diagnosis, 10–20% of patients present with metastatic disease. Skip metastases within the medullary canal can occur. Lymph node or bone marrow involvement is very rare.

### Staging

Overall staging for osteosarcoma is dependent on tumor stage, grade of tumor, and involvement of regional lymph nodes, or other sites distant from the primary involved bone. Tumor stage is based on size: T1 ≤ 8 cm, T2 > 8 cm, or T3 discontinuous tumor in the primary affected bone. Grade is dependent on pathological review of the tumor—GX: cannot be determined, G1: low grade or well differentiated, G2: low grade or moderately differentiated, G3: poorly differentiated, G4: undifferentiated. Nodes are rarely involved in osteosarcoma but are staged as either N0—no evidence of lymph node disease—or N1—regional lymph node metastases. Metastases are determined by location: M1a: lung or M1b: other distant sites.

| 2010 AJCC Staging System for Bone Sarcoma | |
|---|---|
| **Stage** | **Definition** |
| IA | ≤8 cm, no lymph node involvement, no metastases, low grade |
| IB | >8 cm or discontinuous tumors in the primary bone, no lymph node involvement or metastases, low grade |
| IIA | ≤8 cm, no lymph node involvement, no metastases, high grade |
| IIB | >8 cm, no lymph node involvement or metastases, high grade |

*(continued)*

AJCC, American Joint Committee on Cancer.
*Source*: From Ref. (1). Edge S, Byrd DR, Compton CC, et al. *American Joint Committee on Cancer Staging Manual*. 7th ed. New York, NY: Springer Science+Business Media LLC; 2010:281–287.

## CASE SUMMARIES

### Early-Stage Osteosarcoma

L.B. is a 74-year-old male who enjoyed excellent health until 2 months before diagnosis when he developed right lower quadrant abdominal pain and concomitant pain in his right testicle. He noted difficulty with urination but no change in his bowel habits. He was evaluated by an urologist who treated him with a 2-week course of antibiotics without improvement in his symptoms. He had no constitutional symptoms. His medical history included hypertension, diabetes, prostate cancer, which had been treated with surgery and radiation 15 years earlier and Parkinson's disease. Family medical history was notable only for a father with prostate cancer at an advanced age. On physical examination, there were no palpable abdominal or testicular masses and no lymphadenopathy. CT abdomen–pelvis was ordered by the patient's primary care physician and demonstrated destructive changes of the right superior pubic ramus and right pubic symphysis (see Figure 21.1). A CT-guided core needle biopsy of this lesion demonstrated high-grade osteosarcoma. MR of the pelvis demonstrated a 3.6 × 4 × 4 cm mass in the right pubic ramus. Pathological fractures of the superior and inferior pubic ramus were also noted. Serum alkaline phosphatase and lactate dehydrogenase (LDH) were within normal range. Chest CT was normal. Bone scan showed increased technetium uptake in the right pubic symphysis, but no other foci to suggest metastatic disease. Baseline renal function and multigated acquisition scan (MUGA) were normal. Audiology testing demonstrated moderate high-frequency hearing loss.

### Evidence-Based Case Discussion

This is an elderly adult man presenting with a stage IIA (<8 cm, high grade) radiation-associated osteosarcoma of the right pubic ramus. This case reminds us of the bimodal incidence of osteosarcoma. Older patients typically do not present with de novo disease. They instead present with osteosarcoma secondary to another cause such as prior radiation exposure. Baseline studies showed normal levels

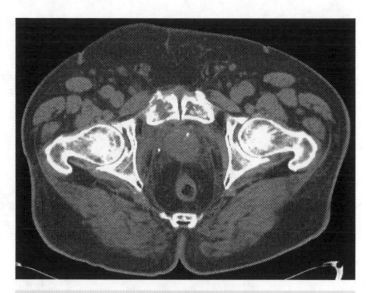

**Figure 21.1**

CT abdomen/pelvis without contrast demonstrating intraosseous mass in the right pubic ramus. MRI (T2, STIR sequence; coronal image) of knee demonstrating intraosseous mass in distal femur.

of serum alkaline phosphatase and LDH, portending a favorable prognosis. There was also normal cardiac function, renal function, and hearing; if abnormal, these issues could impact the choice of chemotherapy. There were no skip metastases or distant disease noted. The presence of either of these factors would increase stage of disease and change sarcoma management.

With localized disease, the treatment paradigm is dependent on grade (see Figure 21.2). Low-grade lesions are treated with surgery alone, and high-grade lesions are treated with chemotherapy and surgery.

Osteosarcoma tends to be radiation resistant, and radiation has not been shown to be beneficial in the adjuvant setting. Radiation may be useful when the primary is unresectable or for palliation. The role of radiation in management of low-grade lesions is not defined but may be considered for treatment of unresectable disease.

Doxorubicin-based combinations make up the current backbone of chemotherapy, which is part of the standard of care for localized osteosarcoma. In early studies, adjuvant chemotherapy with single-agent doxorubicin or methotrexate improved 5-year survival rates to about 50% from 20% following amputation alone (2). Investigators at Memorial Sloan Kettering Cancer Center developed a T10 protocol using methotrexate, doxorubicin, cyclophosphamide, dactinomycin, bleomycin, with or without cisplatin started prior to surgical resection that has demonstrated a 76% disease-free survival at 5 years from diagnosis in young adults with extremity primary osteosarcoma. There was a correlation between lower disease-free survival rate and elevated serum LDH or alkaline phosphatase levels at diagnosis (3).

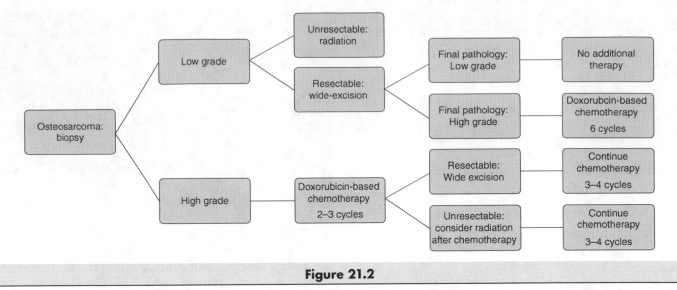

**Figure 21.2**

Treatment algorithm for localized osteosarcoma.

The T10 regimen was the standard treatment for osteosarcoma for much of the 1970s and 1980s. It was not until the pivotal randomized trial performed by the European Osteosarcoma Intergroup (EOI) that a new standard was determined in the 1990s (4). This study compared 18 weeks (6 cycles) of doxorubicin and cisplatin versus 44 weeks (20 cycles) of the T10 multidrug regimen in nearly 400 patients with high-grade osteosarcoma. Surgery occurred during weeks 9 and 7 for the doublet and the multidrug regimens, respectively, with the remainder of chemotherapy being initiated 2 weeks postoperatively. Not surprisingly, more patients were able to complete the doublet treatment (94%) compared to the multidrug regimen (51%). Both overall survival and progression-free survival were similar in the treatment groups, 55% and 44%, respectively, at 5 years.

High-dose methotrexate is routinely used in the pediatric population and in young adults with osteosarcoma. The use of methotrexate in adults older than 40 years is problematic because of decreased renal clearance and significantly increased risk of severe toxicity. Another study by the EOI compared doxorubicin and cisplatin for 6 cycles versus doxorubicin, cisplatin, and methotrexate for 4 cycles (5). Approximately 200 patients younger than 40 years were randomized between the 2 treatments. Twice as many patients in the methotrexate arm were unable to complete treatment compared to those in the study arm. Overall survival was the same in both groups, and disease-free survival was better in the group without methotrexate. These results garnered criticism because the methotrexate arm received lower total doses of doxorubicin and cisplatin, which may have compromised the results. Two randomized studies comparing moderate-dose methotrexate to high-dose methotrexate in a doxorubicin-based regimen failed to demonstrate a

difference in survival (6,7). Based on the available evidence, patients presenting with resectable, high-grade osteosarcoma should be offered chemotherapy using 6 cycles of doxorubicin and cisplatin as side effects permit. The addition of methotrexate to the chemotherapy may be considered in patients younger than 40 years with 2 kidneys and normal renal function. Carboplatin is active in osteosarcoma and may be substituted for cisplatin in specific patients, for example, those with significant hearing impairments or neuropathy. However, to the best of our knowledge, a noninferiority comparison of carboplatin to cisplatin has not been performed in osteosarcoma, and cisplatin remains the standard drug.

The timing of chemotherapy does not seem to be critical with respect to survival. A randomized clinical study performed by the Pediatric Oncology Group (POG) compared surgery prior to the start of chemotherapy versus after 10 weeks of chemotherapy, which demonstrated equivalent 5-year event-free survival rates of 60–65% (8). Neoadjuvant chemotherapy is practically appealing because it allows time for careful surgical planning, manufacture of custom prosthetics, and collection of allograft bone used in limb-sparing surgical techniques. Tumor response to preoperative chemotherapy also provides prognostic and predictive information. Generally, in patients being considered for limb-sparing surgery, chemotherapy is given for about 10 weeks prior to surgery.

Other agents in the armamentarium to treat osteosarcoma include ifosfamide, with or without etoposide. Ifosfamide is an active agent in osteosarcoma, but its addition to standard chemotherapy does not improve survival in the frontline setting and results in more toxicity. The Italian Sarcoma group conducted a study investigating whether the addition of ifosfamide and etoposide to postoperative chemotherapy for patients with a less than good histological response to neoadjuvant chemotherapy will improve relapse-free and overall survival rates. A good histological response was defined as <10% residual viable tumor. The study enrolled 246 patients younger than 40 years with nonmetastatic osteosarcoma of the extremity. Patients were randomized to 2 arms. Arm A received preoperative methotrexate, cisplatin, and doxorubicin, and postoperative therapy depended on pathological response. If they had good pathological response, 3-drug therapy was continued. If they had poor response, ifosfamide was added to their therapy. Arm B received methotrexate, cisplatin, doxorubicin, and ifosfamide. The 5-year overall survival and event-free survival were not significantly different between treatment arms. Adding ifosfamide to preoperative chemotherapy did not improve the good responder rate, but did increase the rate of severe hematologic toxicities (9).

In summary, for localized, low-grade disease, surgical resection alone is the recommended treatment. For localized, high-grade disease, chemotherapy using 6 cycles of doxorubicin and cisplatin is recommended. Surgery may be performed prior to chemotherapy or after 2–3 cycles. The use of methotrexate and ifosfamide–etoposide doublet is more controversial. Most experts recommend that methotrexate be used in addition to cisplatin and doxorubicin for patients younger than 40 years with normal renal function and without preexisting renal disease, administered under the supervision of physicians experienced in the management of methotrexate clearance and leucovorin rescue.

In the case of L.B. with stage IIA disease, consultation with orthopedic oncology confirmed that surgical resection could be performed with acceptable morbidity and long-term functional outcome. The patient received 3 cycles of neoadjuvant chemotherapy with doxorubicin and carboplatin. Cisplatin was not used because of hearing impairment. Methotrexate was not used because of the patient's age. After his third cycle of chemotherapy, the patient underwent surgical resection and then completed 3 cycles of adjuvant carboplatin and doxorubicin. Radiation therapy was not recommended.

## Advanced-Stage Osteosarcoma

T.B. is a 38-year-old woman who developed pain in her right shoulder, which she attributed to an overuse injury. After 2 months, conservative management was unsuccessful, and she presented to the emergency department for evaluation of worsening pain. CT of the chest demonstrated a 5.5 × 4 × 4.3 cm partially calcified mass involving the right anterior chest wall including the second rib. A core needle biopsy demonstrated a high-grade osteosarcoma. Immunohistochemistry was negative for CK7, CK20, TTF-1, estrogen and progesterone receptors,

CD45, CD20, and CD79a. Cells were positive for S100. An MRI of the shoulder, brachial plexus, and chest wall revealed an 8.7 × 5 × 6.5 cm well-defined ovoid mass in the right anterior chest wall situated between the first and second rib with enhancement on post contrast images causing mild compression of the subclavian vein. There were also 3 enhancing subcentimeter pulmonary nodules.

The patient's medical history was notable for hypertension and gestational diabetes. Medications included hydrochlorothiazide, lisinopril, and ibuprofen. There was no relevant family history. On physical examination, a chest wall mass was tender to palpation. There were no other abnormalities. Labs were notable for a mildly elevated LDH. Nuclear medicine bone scan demonstrated increased radiotracer uptake in the right second rib and no other findings. Cardiac and audiology testing were normal.

### Evidence-Based Case Discussion

Here we have a young patient with osteosarcoma of the chest wall and bilateral lung nodules concerning for metastases. An elevated LDH at presentation portends a poorer prognosis. At initial presentation, it was unclear whether the subcentimeter pulmonary nodules were malignant, but at worst case, the patient had limited pulmonary-only metastases. Therefore, following the treatment paradigm for localized osteosarcoma is appropriate (see Figure 21.2).

Pulmonary metastases are the most common site of metastasis. If the lung is the only site of disease, surgical resection should be considered when feasible because this is the only potentially curative therapy in the metastatic setting. Retrospective series have demonstrated prolonged disease-free survival in 7–30% of patients who were able to undergo complete resection of osteosarcoma metastases (10). Those patients in whom osteosarcoma relapsed >2 years from diagnosis and had only 1–2 metastatic nodules were shown to have the greatest event-free survival rate following metastasectomy. There are limited data from nonrandomized, retrospective series regarding additional benefit from postmetastasectomy chemotherapy giving conflicting results, but ifosfamide with or without etoposide and methotrexate can be considered.

In patients who at presentation have a high-grade lesion with a limited number of resectable pulmonary metastases, the treatment approach should follow that of early-stage disease (i.e., neoadjuvant chemotherapy, surgery with resection of primary and metastases, and adjuvant chemotherapy).

In those patients who are unable to undergo complete resection, chemotherapy and radiation therapy are given with palliative intent. No standard approach has been established in the metastatic setting, but it is reasonable to attempt treatment with a doxorubicin-based regimen, if not used previously. If a patient was treated with doxorubicin initially, ifosfamide with or without etoposide would be an acceptable approach at the time of relapse. Ifosfamide and etoposide used in the relapsed setting have shown response rates of 50–60% (11,12).

Amputation should be considered for management of local relapse without distant disease as a potentially curative treatment. Radical surgery in the setting of distant metastasis may be considered for palliation of severe sequelae of local tumor progression.

In summary, in metastatic osteosarcoma, the treatment approach is determined by resectability. Preoperative treatment may be given for high-grade tumors, preferably using drugs not previously administered to improve the likelihood of resection of osteosarcoma with clear surgical margins. Preoperative chemotherapy also allows for detection of rapidly progressing, chemotherapy-resistant disease in which aggressive resection may not be advised. Metastatic low-grade tumors should be managed by surgery, if possible.

In the case of T.B., she was initially treated with 2 cycles of preoperative doxorubicin, cisplatin, and high-dose methotrexate with the goal of shrinking or stabilizing the lung nodules, making metastatectomy an appropriate choice. She had a good response to 2 cycles of preoperative chemotherapy and was able to have her rib lesion and right lung nodules resected. Postoperatively, she completed an additional 4 cycles of chemotherapy and then had her left lung nodules resected. She has been followed without evidence of recurrent disease.

## EWING'S SARCOMA

### Epidemiology, Risk Factors, Natural History, and Pathology

Ewing's sarcoma makes up about 10% of bone sarcomas, but is the second most common bone tumor in children and accounts for 350 cases per year in the United States. Both Ewing's sarcoma of bone and extraskeletal primitive neuroectodermal tumor (PNET) are thought to arise from ectodermal tissue and not mesoderm. Older literature treats these 2 entities, along with Askin's tumor, as distinct diseases, but now all 3 fall into the Ewing's sarcoma family of tumors (ESFT) grouping based on common molecular characteristics. The majority of patients with Ewing's sarcoma of bone are <18 years of age, and the peak incidence is at 10–15 years of age. Males are more commonly affected than females. Whites are the most common race affected. There are no known risk factors.

Patients typically present with pain and can complain of fever, weight loss, or fatigue. These "B-type" symptoms correlate with a higher chance of developing metastatic disease. Tumors arise in the diaphysis of the long or flat bones, most commonly in the femur or pelvis (20% each) followed by the fibula, tibia, or humerus (10% each).

Distal bone involvement is more favorable than proximal bone involvement and pelvic involvement carries the worst prognosis, presumably because tumor volume is often greater at the time of diagnosis when disease arises in the pelvis.

Ewing's sarcoma is classically described as highly cellular, uniform, round to ovoid, small blue cells separated by fibrous tissue (see Figure 21.3). Ewing's sarcoma can be characterized by the fusion of the *EWS* gene on chromosome 22 with *ETS* family members. More than 90% of Ewing's tumors will have either a $t(11;22)$ or $t(21;22)$ translocation involving *FLI-1* or *ERG*, respectively, and will be CD99 positive in a membranous staining pattern on immunohistochemistry (see Figure 21.4). Fluorescence in situ hybridization (FISH) and polymerase chain reaction (PCR) techniques have been developed to detect the translocation. FLI-1 can also be expressed in Ewing's sarcoma and detected by immunohistochemical stains.

Like osteosarcoma, there is a high rate of hematogenous spread, with lung followed by bone being the most commonly affected by metastasis. Ewing's sarcoma may occasionally metastasize to lymph nodes and bone marrow. About one third of patients present with gross metastatic disease at presentation. Like osteosarcoma and other small blue cell cancers, micrometastatic disease at presentation should be assumed because there is a high relapse rate following local treatment alone. Diagnosis at a younger age and tumors <8 cm are better in terms of prognosis.

### Staging

Staging for Ewing's sarcoma is not uniform. The AJCC staging schema, as detailed previously in the osteosarcoma

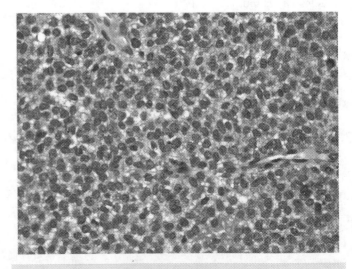

**Figure 21.3**

Photomicrograph of hematoxylin and eosin stained Ewing's sarcoma showing finely granular chromatin and cytoplasmic vacuolization caused by glycogen accumulation (400×).

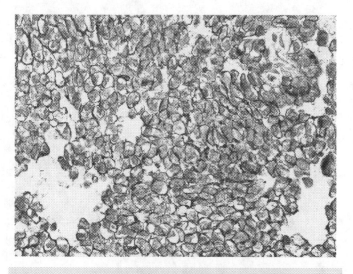

**Figure 21.4**

Photomicrograph of CD99 immunohistochemical stained Ewing's sarcoma showing intense cytoplasmic membrane staining (immunoperoxidase, 400×).

section, may be adapted to Ewing's sarcoma. However, all tumors are of high grade; so there is no stage I disease. Ewing's sarcoma can also be divided into localized and metastatic disease.

## CASE SUMMARIES

### Early-Stage (Localized) Ewing's Sarcoma

B.L. is a 19-year-old white college student who developed left ankle pain after falling down the stairs. He developed some swelling but assumed that this was due to the injury. X-rays were unremarkable. After 1 month, the swelling and pain persisted and he sought evaluation by an orthopedist. On examination, he was noted to have a calcaneal mass. Ultrasound-guided biopsy demonstrated a small, round, blue cell tumor. By immunohistochemistry, the tumor cells stained for CD99 in a membranous pattern, and vimentin, pancytokeratin, CD45, CD56, TdT, CD43, and CD79a were negative. FISH detected a translocation between chromosomes 11 and 22. He was referred to Medical Oncology. On presentation, the patient noted difficulty wearing shoes and ambulating due to his heel mass. He had pain in his ankle and his heel that worsened when standing. He denied constitutional symptoms. He had no past medical history and was taking only hydrocodone–acetaminophen 4 times a day for pain control. Family history was notable for a grandfather with lung cancer and an aunt with breast cancer. On examination, he had a large mass overlying his left calcaneus with some overlying warmth and erythema. The remainder of the examination was normal.

MRI of the left lower extremity demonstrated a 5.8 × 7.9 × 5.8 cm infiltrative lesion of the calcaneus with extraosseous soft tissue spread. Serum LDH, other chemistry values, and a complete blood count were within normal range. CT scan of the chest, abdomen, and pelvis was negative for any abnormalities. A technetium bone scan demonstrated increased uptake in the left calcaneus, but was otherwise unremarkable. A bone marrow aspirate and biopsy from the left posterior iliac crest showed normal cellular marrow and no evidence of bone marrow metastasis. Baseline cardiac evaluation was normal.

### Evidence-Based Case Discussion

This is a young patient with localized, lower extremity, Ewing's sarcoma. Diagnosis was confirmed with cytogenetic analysis. Favorable prognostic features include younger age, tumor <8 cm, and lack of constitutional symptoms.

All Ewing's sarcomas are considered to be of high grade, and early-stage localized disease receives a standard approach to treatment (see Figure 21.5). Unlike osteosarcoma or other bone sarcomas, Ewing's sarcoma is radiation sensitive.

An initial treatment decision is whether to proceed with surgical resection or definitive radiation for local treatment. Choosing the primary modality of treatment depends on several practical factors. If the tumor is in an easily resectable location that would also allow reconstruction to occur, then surgery is preferred. If the location is not amenable to surgery, or if surgery is not able to be performed for other reasons, primary radiation therapy is recommended. Furthermore, adjuvant radiation therapy is recommended for incomplete surgical resection or positive surgical margin (tumor present at the inked surface of the specimen). Careful consideration should be given to the long-term effects of radiation therapy in growing children; radiation-induced sarcomas are the most common second malignancy in children with Ewing's sarcoma. In addition, the available evidence suggests that local failure rates are higher using radiation versus complete resection to control the primary tumor.

Regardless of the selected local treatment, the cure rate from local control measures alone is no better than 15% because of the high rate of distant disease recurrence. The inclusion of chemotherapy therefore becomes an important facet in the treatment of Ewing's sarcoma and, like osteosarcoma, a combination of neoadjuvant and adjuvant treatment is preferred.

Current treatment for Ewing's sarcoma developed from the Intergroup Ewing's Sarcoma Studies (IESS) performed in the late 1970s and early 1980s. Nonrandomized trials had suggested a benefit to adjuvant chemotherapy. The first intergroup study, IESS-I, enrolled 342 children and adults with localized Ewing's sarcoma. The primary

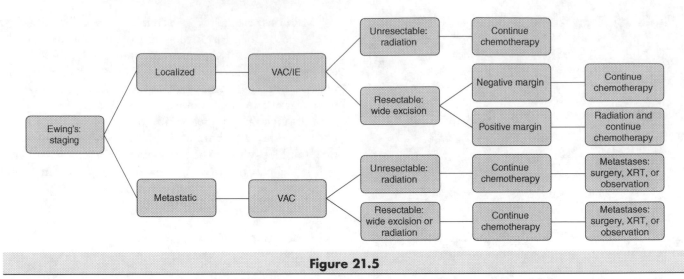

**Figure 21.5**

Treatment algorithm for Ewing's sarcoma. VAC, vincristine, doxorubicin, and cyclophosphamide; IE, ifosfamide and etoposide; XRT, radiation therapy.

tumor was in place in the majority of patients; patients treated with surgical amputation were ineligible. Patients were randomized to vincristine, actinomycin-D, and cyclophosphamide, with or without doxorubicin. All patients received radiation therapy to the primary lesion. A separate randomization was to prophylactic bilateral whole lung radiation versus no lung radiation in those not receiving doxorubicin. Patients receiving doxorubicin along with vincristine, actinomycin-D, and cyclophosphamide had improved 5-year relapse-free (60% vs. 24%) and overall (72% vs. 36%) survival rates (13). The addition of prophylactic bilateral whole lung radiation was not as beneficial as the addition of doxorubicin to the backbone of vincristine, actinomycin-D, and cyclophosphamide.

The addition of ifosfamide and etoposide was evaluated by the POG–Children's Cancer Group (CCG). Patients <30 years of age with any stage of Ewing's sarcoma were randomized to receive vincristine, actinomycin-D, cylophosphamide, and doxorubicin, with or without ifosfamide and etoposide given in alternating cycles every 3 weeks for 17 treatments. The 5-year event-free (69% vs. 54%) and overall survival (72% vs. 61%) rates favored the 6-drug regimen in the nonmetastatic patients. The addition of ifosfamide and etoposide made no significant survival difference in those with metastatic disease (14). The Children's Oncology Group conducted a follow-up prospective, randomized controlled trial for patients younger than 50 years of age with newly diagnosed localized extradural Ewing's sarcoma. Patients were assigned to either standard (chemotherapy cycles every 21 days) or intensified treatment (cycles every 14 days). Patients were treated with doxorubicin, vincristine, and cyclophosphamide alternating with ifosfamide and etoposide along with granulocyte colony-stimulating

factor (G-CSF) support. Primary tumor treatment occurred at week 13 (after 4 cycles in the standard arm and 6 cycles in the intensified arm). The 5-year event-free survival rate was improved in the group receiving chemotherapy every 2 weeks (73% vs. 65%, *P* = .048) (15).

Different regimens have been developed from these 6 core drugs, but the most commonly used regimen continues to be the POG–CCG treatment. Despite most of these studies being done in children or young adults, the same treatment is recommended for older adults if feasible.

In summary, 4–6 courses of chemotherapy are recommended for nonmetastatic disease followed by local treatment that includes surgical resection alone, radiation therapy alone, or a combination of the 2 depending on the clinical situation. On recovery from surgery, the remainder of the chemotherapy is administered to provide a total of 12–14 cycles. Cyclophosphamide, doxorubicin, and vincristine are administered together in cycles alternating with ifosfamide and etoposide. Actinomycin-D is substituted for doxorubicin after administering approximately 450 mg/m$^2$ body surface area of doxorubicin or if reduction in cardiac function occurs.

In the case of B.L. with localized disease, he was treated with neoadjuvant chemotherapy using vincristine, cyclophosphamide, doxorubicin, ifosfamide, and etoposide. After 6 cycles, options including surgery with a below the knee amputation and radiation were discussed with the patient. Given his desire to avoid amputation, definitive radiation was given. After completion of radiation, he completed the remainder of his chemotherapy for a total of 14 cycles.

## Advanced-Stage (Metastatic) Ewing's Sarcoma

T.J. is a 22-year-old white male who noted diffuse bony pain of his ribs, hips, and spine and myalgias for approximately 2 years before presentation. He had a rheumatologic workup done by his primary care physician, which was unrevealing. Three months before diagnosis, the patient's left hip pain intensified and began radiating into his left foot causing difficulty with ambulation. Due to concern for sciatica, the patient underwent physical therapy for 1 month without improvement in his symptoms. Given worsening hip pain and leg weakness, he was evaluated in the emergency department. CT abdomen and pelvis demonstrated a heterogeneous mass surrounding his left iliacus and gluteus muscles, innumerable liver lesions, lytic lesion within the left pelvis, and lytic lesions throughout the spine. CT chest demonstrated scattered lytic lesions in the spine and sternum and a compression deformity of T11.

On examination, T.J. was found to have no palpable masses over his buttocks or hips. Muscle strength was normal in bilateral lower extremities except for 4 out of 5 strength in the left hip flexors. There was mildly decreased range of motion upon hip flexion on the left. There were no palpable lymph nodes. Examination was otherwise normal. Serum LDH was elevated at 290 IU/L. Hemoglobin was decreased at 9.3 g/dL. The rest of the complete blood count and serum chemistries were within normal limits.

CT-guided core needle biopsy was performed during hospitalization. Pathology revealed a small, round, blue cell tumor. Immunohistochemical staining detected CD99 in a membranous pattern with focal S100 and synaptophysin. The tumor was negative for desmin, myogenin, CD3, CD20, CD34, melan-a, and cytokeratin. The tumor was positive for EWSR1 translocation by FISH. A technetium bone scan demonstrated heterogeneous uptake in the left parietal bone, cervical spine, right scapula, sternum, anterior right fifth and sixth ribs, L2 vertebrae, and left iliac wing. Right-sided bone marrow biopsy was consistent with metastatic Ewing's sarcoma involving 80% of the marrow space.

## Evidence-Based Case Discussion

This is a young adult with diffuse metastatic disease. Given the widespread skeletal involvement, the metastases are unresectable. Patients with visceral metastases or diffuse involvement in the bone marrow have the poorest long-term survival rates. The goal of therapy in these patients is usually palliation. Chemotherapy should be the initial treatment unless a patient is markedly symptomatic from pain, in which case palliative radiation may be considered. Chemotherapy should include vincristine, cyclophosphamide, doxorubicin, and actinomycin-D.

In approximately 20% of patients who present with metastatic Ewing's sarcoma, treatment is curative. These are generally patients with lung-only metastases. Preoperative chemotherapy should be administered as described previously in the localized Ewing's section for patients presenting de novo with metastatic Ewing's sarcoma. Then, surgical resection or definitive radiation of both the primary and metastatic lesions should be performed if feasible (see Figure 21.5).

A significant number of patients who were initially treated for localized Ewing's sarcoma experience local and distant recurrence. Several characteristics influence the prognosis following relapse. A long interval to relapse after treatment of primary disease and lung-only disease is more favorable than their counterparts. When doxorubicin was administered as part of the initial therapy for localized disease, it is not given for relapsed disease due to the potential for cardiotoxicity to develop. Ifosfamide and etoposide may be used to treat relapsed Ewing's sarcoma. When the primary disease treatment did not use these drugs, the combination in relapsed Ewing's sarcoma demonstrated response rates of 50% and 1- and 2-year overall survivals of 49% and 28%, respectively, in children and young adults (16).

Studies have also been done using topoisomerase I inhibitors. A study of 55 patients with participants aged 3–50 years, who were in first or second relapse, used cyclophosphamide with topotecan. The treatment provided an overall objective response rate (complete plus partial response) of 44%, with 25.9% of patients maintaining response after 23 months (17). A smaller study of 14 patients evaluated the combination of irinotecan and temozolomide in patients with advanced Ewing's sarcoma and noted some responses (18). Another study of 22 patients evaluated irinotecan, temozolomide, and vincristine and found an overall response rate of 68.1%. The median time to progression was 3 months, but with a median follow-up of 10.3 months, 5 patients were alive without disease (19), docetaxel and gemcitabine have been evaluated in metastatic Ewing's sarcoma. A small study of 22 patients with bone sarcomas showed a 29% overall objective response rate with this regimen; however, the median duration of response was short, at just under 5 months (20).

Antibodies to the type 1 insulin-like growth factor 1 receptor (IGFR-1) have also been investigated in patient with refractory or recurrent Ewing's sarcoma. A recent phase II study demonstrated an overall response rate of 10% with median duration of response of 29 weeks (21). Further studies are ongoing.

In summary, in advanced Ewing's sarcoma, the recommended treatment is chemotherapy followed by local therapy using radiation and/or surgery for residual disease, if possible. For treatment of widely metastatic relapsed Ewing's sarcoma, palliative care using chemotherapy, radiation, and/or surgery may be considered. Participation in clinical trials should be encouraged for patients with relapsed disease.

In the case of T.J. with advanced disease, he received 12 cycles of doxorubicin, vincristine, cyclophosphamide, and actinomycin-D with excellent response in his hepatic and osseous lesions. Ifosfamide and etoposide could have been incorporated, but are more cumbersome to administer and the 5-drug regimen would have been unlikely to improve survival. After completion of chemotherapy, control of the primary site of the disease in the pelvis was considered. Ultimately, radiation was chosen over surgery because of the lower morbidity.

## GIANT-CELL TUMOR OF BONE

### Epidemiology, Risk Factors, Natural History, and Pathology

Giant-cell tumor of bone (GCTB) is a rare osteolytic, benign tumor of bone. It accounts for 3–5% of all primary bone tumors and 15–20% of all benign bone tumors. GCTB is a locally aggressive tumor with a 20–50% chance of local recurrence. Metastases to the lung occur in <5% of cases. Transformation into an aggressive sarcoma can occur, but is rare. GCTB is most frequently found in patients who have reached skeletal maturity (20–40 years old) with a slight predilection for females. Asians have a higher incidence of GCTB than whites.

Patients often present with pain, swelling, and decreased range of motion at the location of the tumor. The most common location for GCTB is at the epiphyses of long bones. Histologically, the tumor is composed of numerous multinucleated osteoclast-like giant cells. The giant cells express receptor activator of nuclear factor κB (RANKL), which is important for the development and survival of osteoclasts. In the absence of RANKL, osteoclasts undergo apoptosis. Other giant cell containing tumors share similar histological characteristics, but must be distinguished from benign GCTB because the treatments are different. These include malignant GCTB, aneurysmal bone cyst, giant-cell rich osteosarcoma, brown tumor in hyperparathyroidism, fibrous metaphyseal defects, and chondroblastoma.

### Staging

GCTB is divided into localized and metastatic diseases.

## CASE SUMMARY

A.B. is a 21-year-old white female who noted left-sided lower back pain 6 months before diagnosis. Her primary care physician ordered an x-ray of her lumbar spine, which was unremarkable. The patient then had 3 months of chiropractic treatment without improvement in her pain. One month before diagnosis, she noted swelling over her left flank. MRI of the pelvis was ordered and demonstrated a large mass centered within the superior aspect of the left iliac wing, measuring 8 × 10 × 12.7 cm. The mass traversed the left sacroiliac joint and involved the left sacrum. CT-guided biopsy of the mass demonstrated GCTB.

At presentation to medical oncology, the patient reported ongoing left flank pain that occasionally radiated to her thigh and knee. She had difficulty with walking due to pain. She noted fatigue, but denied weight loss or night sweats.

Her medical history was only notable for attention deficit hyperactivity disorder (ADHD). Her medications included Adderall and oral contraceptive pills. There was no family history of malignancy. On physical examination, a firm, 10-cm soft tissue swelling palpable on the left flank that was mildly tender to palpation was found. There was no lymphadenopathy or other palpable masses. Sensation, strength, and range of motion were intact. CT chest demonstrated no lung nodules.

### Evidence-Based Case Discussion

This is a young patient with localized pelvic GCTB. The initial decision in localized GCTB is whether or not it is surgically resectable. If the tumor is resectable, surgery should be undertaken with curative intent. If the tumor is unresectable without significant morbidity, medical therapy with denosumab can be considered. Other local control options include serial embolization or radiation therapy. Radiation has been associated with increased risk for malignant transformation and should only be used if embolization or medical therapy is not possible. If metastatic disease is evident upon presentation, determining surgical resectability of the primary tumor and metastatic sites is again the first step in management. If disease is not surgically resectable, treatment options are the same as for localized unresectable disease.

Denosumab is a fully human monoclonal antibody against RANKL. The malignant stromal cells in GCTB express high levels of RANKL which results in recruitment and differentiation of monocytes into multinucleated, activated osteoclasts (the "giant cells" seen in the tumors) that result in bone matrix lysis and destruction. Inhibition of RANKL by denosumab leads to loss of osteoclasts and allows for new bone formation.

Denosumab received Food and Drug Administration (FDA) approval in June of 2013 after it was found to increase durable objective responses in 2 multicenter studies. In a phase II study of 37 patients with recurrent or unresectable disease, patients received 120 mg subcutaneously every 28 days except during the first cycle when they were treated on days 1, 8, and 15. Eighty-six percent of evaluable patients demonstrated response to treatment defined as elimination of at least 90% of giant cells or no radiological progression of the target lesion up to week 25. The most common toxicities reported were pain in an extremity or the back and headache (22). A subsequent larger phase II study used denosumab in 282 patients with GCTB. Patients were placed into 3 groups: patients with surgically unsalvageable GCTB, patients with salvageable GCTB whose surgery would result in serious morbidity, and patients previously treated on a study of denosumab for GCTB. Patients in the first 2 groups received denosumab 120 mg subcutaneously every 28 days except for the first cycle with additional doses on days 8 and 15. Patients in group 3 continued their denosumab regimen from their previous study. In the first group, with a median follow-up of 13 months, 96% of patients had no disease progression. In the second group, with a median follow-up of 9.6 months, 16 of 26 patients (62%) who underwent surgery were able to have a less morbid procedure than initially planned. Safety data from this trial revealed that 9% of patients had a serious adverse event. The most common grade 3–4 events were hypophosphatemia, anemia, back pain, and extremity pain (23). Other side effects include hypocalcemia, fatigue, and osteonecrosis of the jaw. The optimal duration of therapy is not known.

In the case of A.B., medical therapy with denosumab was recommended. Surgical resection would have been too morbid. With 1 year of therapy, the patient had a significant reduction in tumor volume and resolution of her pain. She was fully ambulatory and tolerating therapy without side effects.

## REVIEW QUESTIONS

*Questions 1 and 2 are coupled*

A 24-year-old man presents with right thigh pain × 4 weeks. He can ambulate without difficulty. Physical examination is notable only for a firm right thigh mass that is only mildly tender to palpation. MRI of the right lower extremity reveals an 8.1 × 5.3 × 3.4 cm mass at the midshaft of the femur. Biopsy of the mass demonstrated a small round blue cell tumor. Immunohistochemical stains were positive for CD99 and negative for desmin, myogenin, and the cytokeratins. Molecular testing reveals a translocation between chromosomes 11 and 22.

1. What additional workup should be performed?

   (A) No additional workup is needed
   (B) Bone scan and CT chest
   (C) CT of the chest, abdomen, and pelvis
   (D) Sentinel lymph node biopsy and bone scan

2. Which of the following treatment options should be recommended as the initial treatment for this patient?

   (A) Surgical resection
   (B) Chemotherapy alternating vincristine, cyclophosphamide, and doxorubicin with ifosfamide and etoposide
   (C) Chemotherapy with doxorubicin and ifosfamide
   (D) Radiation

3. A 55-year-old man presents with pelvic pain ongoing for several months. He denies any other symptoms and is otherwise enjoying his normal state of good health. Pelvic x-ray demonstrates a poorly marginated mass in the pelvis with bony destruction. MRI demonstrates a 5.0 × 9.2 × 8.4 cm mass with increased T2 signal and intermediate T1 signal with post-contrast enhancement. Biopsy demonstrates Ewing's sarcoma. Which of the following is a favorable prognosistic feature?

   (A) Pelvic location
   (B) Older age at diagnosis
   (C) Absence of constitutional symptoms
   (D) Tumor size >8 cm

4. A 29-year-old man presented for evaluation of a lump on his left chest wall that had been present × 3 years but was recently enlarging. CT chest demonstrated an 8.6 × 5.7 cm expansile mass arising from the anterior left second rib at the costochondral junction. Pathology on the resected specimen demonstrated an 11.5 × 6.2 × 5 cm high-grade tumor composed of spindle cells, osteoblasts, and osteoid. Margins were negative. Lactate dehydrogenase and kidney function were normal. Bone scan, audiology testing, and transthoracic echocardiogram were unremarkable. Which of the following treatments should be recommended?

   (A) Active surveillance
   (B) Doxorubicin and ifosfamide
   (C) Methotrexate, cisplatin, and doxorubicin
   (D) Carboplatin and doxorubicin

5. A 72-year-old man with Paget's disease involving the pelvis was noted to have a significant rise in serum alkaline phosphatase from 200 to 857 IU/L over a 2-year period. Bone scan detected abnormal uptake of technetium only in the right ilium. He had no pain in the pelvis or right leg and no constitutional symptoms. MRI of the pelvis detected a 5.2 × 4.1 × 2.8 cm enhancing area involving the right ilium adjacent to the right sacroiliac joint. Biopsy of this area demonstrated a malignant process. Which of the following is the most likely diagnosis?

   (A) Osteosarcoma
   (B) Ewing's sarcoma
   (C) Giant cell tumor of bone
   (D) Chordoma

6. An 18-year-old woman seeks evaluation for pain that developed in her right posterior thigh while playing volleyball. Since onset of the pain, she has developed a limp as well as pain and paresthesias in her right lateral leg and foot. MRI demonstrated a 5.5 × 5.1 × 4.8 cm expansile mass within the right sacrum centered at S2 extending into the right S1-S2 neural formina and into the spinal canal causing nerve root and thecal sac

compression. Biopsy demonstrated a giant cell tumor of bone. Which one the following treatment should be offered next?

(A) Surgical resection
(B) Radiation therapy
(C) Denosumab
(D) Interferon

7. A 36-year-old man developed right knee pain which he attributed to playing soccer. When it persisted, he had an MRI that demonstrated a 1.5 × 1 × 1.8 cm rounded lucent lesion within the proximal lateral tibial metadiaphysis extending to the subchondral bone. Biopsy demonstrated a giant cell tumor of bone. Patient underwent curettage and allograft placement. Two years later, he developed recurrence and underwent debridement of the area with cement removal and placement of tibial hardware. Less than 1 year later, he developed another recurrence. Given his young age, multiple surgeries and recurrences, denosumab was recommended. What is the most likely side effect from this therapy?

(A) Osteonecrosis of the jaw
(B) Hypocalcemia
(C) Myelosuppression
(D) Infertility

## REFERENCES

1. Edge S, Byrd DR, Compton CC, et al. *American Joint Committee on Cancer*. 7th ed. New York, NY: Springer Science+Business Media LLC; 2010:281–287.
2. Rosen G, Marcove RC, Huvos AG, et al. Primary osteogenic sarcoma: eight-year experience with adjuvant chemotherapy. *J Cancer Res Clin Oncol*. 1983;106(Suppl):55–67.
3. Meyers PA, Heller G, Healey J, et al. Chemotherapy for nonmetastaticosteogenic sarcoma: the Memorial Sloan-Kettering experience. *J Clin Oncol*. 1992;10(1):5–15.
4. Souhami RL, Craft AW, Van der Eijken JW, et al. Randomised trial of two regimens of chemotherapy in operable osteosarcoma: a study of the European Osteosarcoma Intergroup. *Lancet*. 1997;350(9082):911–917.
5. Bramwell VH, Burgers M, Sneath R, et al. A comparison of two short intensive adjuvant chemotherapy regimens in operable osteosarcoma of limbs in children and young adults: the first study of the European Osteosarcoma Intergroup. *J Clin Oncol*. 1992;10(10):1579–1591.
6. Bacci G, Gherlinzoni F, Picci P, et al. Adriamycin-methotrexate high dose versus adriamycin-methotrexate moderate dose as adjuvant chemotherapy for osteosarcoma of the extremities: a randomized study. *Eur J Cancer Clin Oncol*. 1986;22(11):1337–1345.
7. Krailo M, Ertel I, Makley J, et al. A randomized study comparing high-dose methotrexate with moderate-dose methotrexate as components of adjuvant chemotherapy in childhood nonmetastatic

osteosarcoma: a report from the Children's Cancer Study Group. *Med Pediatr Oncol*. 1987;15:69–75.
8. Goorin AM, Schwartzentruber DJ, Devidas M, et al. Presurgical chemotherapy compared with immediate surgery and adjuvant chemotherapy for nonmetastatic osteosarcoma: Pediatric Oncology Group Study POG-8651. *J Clin Oncol*. 2003;21(8):1574–1580.
9. Ferrari S, Ruggieri P, Cefalo G, et al. Neoadjuvant chemotherapy with methotrexate, cisplatin, and doxorubicin with or without ifosfamide in nonmetastatic osteosarcoma of the extremity: an Italian sarcoma group trial ISG/OS-1. *J Clin Oncol*. 2012;30(17):2112–2118.
10. Kempf-Bielack B, Bielack SS, Jürgens H, et al. Osteosarcoma relapse after combined modality therapy: an analysis of unselected patients in the Cooperative Osteosarcoma Study Group (COSS). *J Clin Oncol*. 2005;23(3):559–568.
11. Goorin AM, Harris MB, Bernstein M, et al. Phase II/III trial of etoposide and high-dose ifosfamide in newly diagnosed metastatic osteosarcoma: a pediatric oncology group trial. *J Clin Oncol*. 2002;20(2):426–433.
12. Gentet JC, Brunat-Mentigny M, Demaille MC, et al. Ifosfamide and etoposide in childhood osteosarcoma. A phase II study of the French Society of Paediatric Oncology. *Eur J Cancer*. 1997;33(2):232–237.
13. Nesbit ME Jr, Gehan EA, Burgert EO Jr, et al. Multimodal therapy for management of primary, nonmetastatic Ewing's sarcoma of the bone: a long-term follow-up of the first intergroup study. *J Clin Oncol*. 1990;8(10):1664–1674.
14. Grier HE, Krailo MD, Tarbell NJ, et al. Addition of ifosfamide and etoposide to standard chemotherapy for Ewing's sarcoma and primitive neuroectodermal tumor of bone. *N Engl J Med*. 2003;348(8):694–701.
15. Womer RB, West DC, Krailo MD, et al. Randomized comparison of every-two-week versus every-three-week chemotherapy in Ewing sarcoma family tumors (ESFT). *J Clin Oncol*. 2008;26: (Abstract 10504).
16. Miser JS, Kinsella TJ, Triche TJ, et al. Ifosfamide with mesnauroprotection and etoposide: an effective regimen in the treatment of recurrent sarcomas and other tumors of children and young adults. *J Clin Oncol*. 1987;5(8):1191–1198.
17. Hunold A, Weddeling N, Paulussen M, et al. Topotecan and cyclophosphamide in patients with refractory or relapsed Ewing tumors. *Pediatr Blood Cancer*. 2006;47:795–800.
18. Wagner LM, McAllister N, Goldsby RE, et al. Temozolomide and intravenous irinotecan for treatment of advanced Ewing sarcoma. *Pediatr Blood Cancer*. 2007;48:132–139.
19. Raciborska A, Bilska K, Drabko K, et al. Vincristine, irinotecan and temozolomide in patients with relapsed and refractory Ewing sarcoma. *Pediatr Blood Cancer*. 2013;60(10):1621–1625.
20. Navid F, Willert JR, McCarville MB, et al. Combination of gemcitabine and docetaxel in the treatment of children and young adults with refractory bone sarcoma. *Cancer*. 2008;113(2):419–425.
21. Pappo AS, Patel Sr, Crowley J, et al. R1507, a monoclonal antibody to the insulin-like growth factor 1 receptor, in patients with recurrent or refractory Ewing sarcoma family of tumors: results of a phase II Sarcoma Alliance for Research through Collaboration study. *J Clin Oncol*. 2011;29(34):4541–4547.
22. Thomas D, Henshaw R, Skubitz K, et al. Denosumab in patient with giant-cell tumour of bone: an open-label, phase 2 study. *Lancet Oncol*.2010;11(3):275–280.
23. Chawla S, Henshaw R, Seeger L, et al. Safety and efficacy of denosumab for adults and skeletally mature adolescents with giant cell tumour of bone: interim analysis of an open-label, parallel-group, phase 2 study. *Lancet Oncol*. 2013;14(9):901–908.

# 22

# *Soft Tissue Sarcoma*

DANA E. ANGELINI AND RASHMI CHUGH

## EPIDEMIOLOGY, RISK FACTORS, NATURAL HISTORY, AND PATHOLOGY

Soft tissue sarcomas (STS) are a rare and heterogeneous group of malignancies that arise from mesenchymal tissue and comprise approximately 1% of all adult malignancies and 12% of pediatric malignancies. The list of potential cells of origin of STS is extensive, as embryonic mesenchymal cells can differentiate into a variety of different tissues, including striated muscle, smooth muscle, cartilage, bone, and fibrous tissue. Approximately 12,020 cases of STS are diagnosed annually in the United States and there are approximately 4740 deaths each year from STS (1).

The majority of STS are sporadic, with no clearly defined cause. However, there are some established risk factors, including radiation, chemical exposure, chronic lymphedema, and certain genetic disorders such as Li Fraumeni syndrome, neurofibromatosis type 1, and Gardner's syndrome. Specific chromosomal translocations have been identified in approximately one third of all sarcomas (2). STS are classified based on morphology and tissue resemblance or origin (Table 22.1). Mesenchymal cells are present throughout the body, as such, STS can originate from various locations. A multicenter cohort study of 4508 adults showed the anatomical distribution of STS to be thigh, buttock, and groin in 46%, while the torso, upper extremity, retroperitoneum, and head and neck accounted for 18%, 13%, 13%, and 9% of cases, respectively (3).

Patients often present with a growing mass lesion with or without associated symptoms such as pain or neurologic complaints depending on the location of the tumor and surrounding structures. The work up of a suspicious mass lesion, defined as deep, enlarging, or >5 cm in diameter, should include imaging, with ultrasound or MRI. Visceral lesions are often visualized with a CT scan. If imaging confirms a mass in which sarcoma is in the differential diagnosis, referral to an orthopedic or surgical oncologist is recommended for an optimally performed biopsy with a biopsy tract that can be encompassed within a future resection. Core needle biopsy is often sufficient to make a diagnosis, but occasionally an incisional or excisional biopsy is required.

For the majority of STS, the spread of disease is hematogenous and the most common area of metastasis is the lung. Specific histological subtypes may have different patterns of spread, including nodal disease with rhabdomyosarcomas, liver and peritoneal metastases with gastrointestinal stromal tumors (GISTs), and abdominal and bony spread in myxoid liposarcomas. Thus, staging evaluation may need to be adjusted based on specific histological subtype and site of origin.

With >50 histological subtypes and a continuously evolving classification nomenclature, accurate pathological diagnosis of STS is challenging. Table 22.1 lists some of the most common histologies of STS and presumed cell of origin. Confirmation of the diagnosis of STS by a pathologist with sarcoma expertise is imperative. Access to molecular diagnostics to identify molecular abnormalities associated with STS is also instrumental in the diagnosis and treatment.

## STAGING

The most widely used staging system for STS is the Tumor, Node, and Metastasis (TNM) system developed by the International Union Against Cancer (UICC) and the American Joint Committee on Cancer (AJCC), the most recent of which is the 2010 7th edition (4). The system uses

**Table 22.1**  Common Subtypes of STS in Adults

| Subtype | Presumed Tissue of Origin |
|---|---|
| Undifferentiated pleomorphic sarcoma | Unknown |
| Liposarcoma | Adipose tissue |
| Fibrosarcoma | Fibrous connective tissue |
| Synovial sarcoma | Unknown |
| Rhabdomyosarcoma | Striated muscle |
| Leiomyosarcoma | Smooth muscle |
| Malignant peripheral nerve sheath tumor | Neural sheath/peripheral nerves |
| Angiosarcoma | Blood or lymphatic vessels |

STS, soft tissue sarcomas.

**Table 22.2**  TNM Staging for STS; AJCC, 7th Edition

**Primary Tumor**

| | |
|---|---|
| Tx | Primary tumor cannot be assessed |
| T0 | No evidence of primary tumor |
| T1 | Tumor 5 cm or less |
| T1a | Superficial tumor |
| T1b | Deep tumor |
| T2 | Tumor >5 cm |
| T2a | Superficial |
| T2b | Deep |

**Regional Lymph Nodes**

| | |
|---|---|
| Nx | Cannot be assessed |
| N0 | No regional lymph nodes |
| N1 | Regional lymph node metastasis |

**Distant Metastasis**

| | |
|---|---|
| M0 | No distant metastasis |
| M1 | Superficial tumor is located above the superficial fascia without invasion of the fascia[a] |
| | Deep tumor is located beneath the superficial fascia or superficial to fascia with invasion of the superficial fascia[b] |
| | Distant metastasis |

**Histological Grade**

| | |
|---|---|
| Gx | Cannot be assessed |
| G1 | Grade 1 |
| G2 | Grade 2 |
| G3 | Grade 3 |

AJCC, American Joint Committee on Cancer; STS, soft tissue sarcomas; TNM, tumor, node, and metastasis.

[a]Superficial tumor is located above the superficial fascia without invasion of the fascia.

[b]Deep tumor is located beneath the superficial fascia or superficial to fascia with invasion of the superficial fascia

tumor size (T), depth (superficial or deep), lymph node involvement (N), presence or absence of distant metastases (M), and histological grade (G) in determining the anatomic stage grouping for STS (Table 22.2).

**Anatomic Stage**

| Stage IA | T1a | N0 | M0 | G1, Gx |
|---|---|---|---|---|
| | T1b | N0 | M0 | G1, Gx |
| Stage IB | T2a | N0 | M0 | G1, Gx |
| | T2b | N0 | M0 | G1, Gx |
| Stage IIA | T1a | N0 | M0 | G2, G3 |
| | T1b | N0 | M0 | G2, G3 |
| Stage IIB | T2a | N0 | M0 | G2 |
| | T2b | N0 | M0 | G2 |
| Stage III | T2a, T2b | N0 | M0 | G3 |
| | Any T | N1 | M0 | Any G |
| Stage IV | Any T | Any N | M1 | Any G |

## CASE SUMMARIES

### Locally Advanced STS

D.M. is a 54-year-old male who presented with a right-arm mass in May 2013. He saw his primary care provider, who obtained an ultrasound of the mass, and was reassured that the mass was likely benign. Over the next several months, he noted that the mass was enlarging. Examination of his right upper extremity revealed a large, superficial, mobile, nontender posterior mass. MRI of his right arm showed a large subcutaneous heterogeneous mass approximately 9 cm in greatest dimension (Figure 22.1). Core biopsy was obtained in December 2013, which revealed a high-grade undifferentiated pleomorphic sarcoma. He was started on neoadjuvant chemotherapy consisting of doxorubicin/ifosfamide delivered every 21 days for 4 cycles. He tolerated chemotherapy well and had marked shrinkage of his tumor. He underwent wide-staged excision of the mass. Pathology of the surgical specimen revealed undifferentiated pleomorphic sarcoma with the greatest dimension of 7.3 cm, with extensive treatment effect and negative margins. His case was discussed at the multidisciplinary tumor board. He will undergo postoperative radiation therapy to the resected tumor bed.

### Evidence-Based Case Discussion

This is a relatively healthy patient presenting with stage III, high-grade STS of the right arm. The tumor's high grade as well as large size (>5 cm) confers a higher risk of eventual tumor recurrence. Routine staging with chest CT showed no evidence of distant metastatic disease.

In general, the management of newly diagnosed STS is complicated and ideally consists of a multidisciplinary team at a specialized treatment center. Research has shown that treatment in expert centers improves local control and translates to improved outcomes in some patients (5). As such, patients suspected of having STS should be referred to a center with expertise in sarcoma. Although many histological subtypes of sarcoma are treated similarly when localized, certain subtypes have their own characteristic behavior and response to therapy.

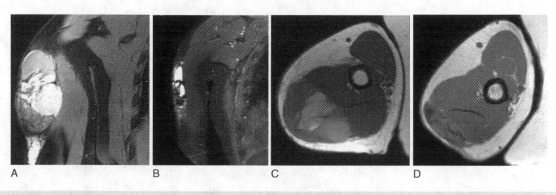

A          B          C          D

**Figure 22.1**

MRI of upper extremity before (A and C) and after (B and D) neoadjuvant chemotherapy.

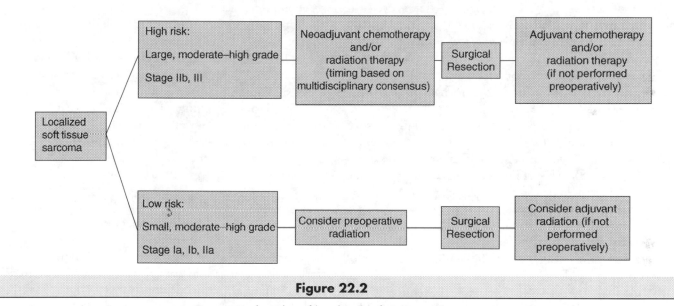

**Figure 22.2**

Treatment algorithm of localized soft tissue sarcoma.

Figure 22.2 shows a generalized treatment algorithm for STS. Current treatment modalities of surgery and radiation for extremity STS yield excellent local control, but distant failure is common and almost universally fatal in high-risk STS. The sequencing of therapy, including surgery, chemotherapy, and radiation, is best considered in the multidisciplinary setting based on histological subtype, tumor location, and patient-specific factors.

For patients with high-risk STS, which includes large (>5 cm) and moderate- to high-grade tumors, the prognosis is generally poor, with approximately 50% of patients developing metastatic disease. For this reason, neoadjuvant or adjuvant chemotherapy is used in many centers for this population, even though its role remains controversial due to the lack of properly conducted controlled clinical trials. Most published trials of adjuvant chemotherapy were inadequately powered, included a heterogeneous collection of sarcomas, and did not use full doses of the most effective cytotoxic agents, now known to be doxorubicin

and ifosfamide. Because of this, some studies show benefit to adjuvant chemotherapy, whereas others show no benefit or are inconclusive. In 1997, the Sarcoma Meta-Analysis Collaboration published a meta-analysis of 14 trials of doxorubicin-based adjuvant chemotherapy consisting of 1568 patients. This revealed a longer local, distant, and overall recurrence-free survival (RFS) with adjuvant chemotherapy (hazard ratios [HRs] = 0.73, 0.70, and 0.75; $P$ = .016, .0001, and .0001, respectively). There was no difference in overall survival (OS), although there was a trend in favor of adjuvant chemotherapy (HR = 0.89, $P$ = .12). Patients with extremity sarcomas did have a survival benefit on subgroup analysis, with a 7% absolute survival benefit at 10 years ($P$ = .029) (6). Although a statistically significant survival benefit was not seen in all groups, only 1 study included in the meta-analysis used ifosfamide in addition to doxorubicin. As with any meta-analysis, the heterogeneous patient population, tumor inclusion criteria, and drug dosing make these data difficult to interpret. However, in the correctly selected patient with a high-risk extremity sarcoma of specific histological subtypes, adjuvant chemotherapy with the most effective agents known (a combination of doxorubicin and ifosfamide) may yield some benefit.

Although most studies performed have evaluated the role of adjuvant chemotherapy, many centers prefer the use of neoadjuvant treatment when possible. Response to neoadjuvant chemotherapy may improve surgical resection options, such as allowing a limb salvage operation, when otherwise not possible. The use of neoadjuvant chemotherapy may also allow identification of a subgroup of patients likely to benefit from additional adjuvant chemotherapy.

Given our patient's high-risk features of a large, high-grade STS and his otherwise good health, he received neoadjuvant doxorubicin and ifosfamide. After 4 cycles of chemotherapy, repeat imaging showed marked decrease in tumor size and he underwent wide surgical resection with negative margins. After discussion at multidisciplinary tumor board, the consensus was to offer postoperative radiation to the tumor bed to help prevent local recurrence.

Advances in reconstructive surgical techniques, institution of multimodality therapy, and improved selection of patients for neoadjuvant and adjuvant therapy have significantly increased the role of limb-sparing surgery with adequate local control of disease. Rosenberg et al. (7) published the first prospective randomized trial comparing limb-sparing surgery plus radiation compared to amputation in 43 adult patients with STS of the extremity. This demonstrated an increased limb salvage rate with the use of radiation following surgery, with no differences in disease-free survival (DFS) and OS rates between the treatment groups. This and other randomized controlled trials have demonstrated low local recurrence rates (7–15%) with no detriment in OS when patients with extremity STS are treated with limb-sparing surgery and radiation as compared to amputation (7,8). Thus, limb-sparing surgery with or without adjuvant radiation therapy is an effective treatment option for extremity STS. Amputation, which was once considered standard, should be reserved only for cases of very large tumors involving a neurovascular bundle or where resection or re-resection with adequate margins cannot be performed without sacrificing functional outcome.

Several trials have shown the benefit of radiation in local control of STS combined with resection. In a prospective randomized trial from Memorial Sloan Kettering Cancer Center (MSKCC), 5-year local control rates in high-risk lesions were 89% with brachytherapy and 66% without (9), whereas Yang et al. (10) randomized 91 patients with high-risk extremity sarcomas to receive postoperative chemotherapy and radiation or chemotherapy alone. With a median follow-up of 9.6 years, no patients in the radiation arm had local recurrence, whereas 19% in the chemotherapy-alone arm had local recurrence. On the basis of these randomized trials and several other single-institution retrospective studies, the addition of radiation, whether delivered preoperatively, postoperatively, or as brachytherapy, has become the standard of care for large, high-risk sarcoma.

The sequencing of radiation therapy in relation to surgery is a subject of debate, each with advantages and disadvantages but similar local control and progression-free survival (PFS) rates. Preoperative radiation has an increased rate of acute wound complications, but can allow a smaller resection. When deciding between preoperative versus postoperative radiation therapy, one should consider the type of surgical procedure, extent of operative bed, likelihood of obtaining negative margins, factors of wound closure and tension, grade of the sarcoma, and surgeon preference.

For the first 2 years after completion of treatment, serial tumor bed imaging with MRI (or CT scan or ultrasound based on location) is recommended every 6 months. Chest imaging and physical examinations are performed every 3–6 months. After 2 years, follow-up evaluations are spaced to every 6 months, for a minimum of 5 years of total follow-up. As late recurrences have been commonly reported, follow-up evaluations annually are often continued beyond the 5-year mark.

## Advanced Metastatic Sarcoma

T.A. is a 50-year-old male who noticed a painless left frontal scalp lump. He underwent Moh's procedure to remove the scalp nodule. Pathology was reviewed at a tertiary cancer center and was consistent with leiomyosarcoma. Staging CT scans demonstrated a 12.5 × 9 × 13 cm right kidney mass infiltrating the inferior vena cava (IVC) and exerting mass effect on the pancreas, duodenum, and anterior margin of the liver. Multiple pulmonary nodules and liver lesions were also seen, consistent with metastatic disease. He underwent CT-guided biopsy of a liver mass and a right renal mass; both specimens returned as high-grade leiomyosarcoma.

He was treated on clinical trial with 4 cycles of doxorubicin and an analog of ifosfamide. Treatment was eventually discontinued for disease progression. He was then switched to gemcitabine and docetaxel and had stable disease after 7 cycles, but treatment was discontinued for cumulative toxicities of lower extremity edema and myositis. He was then initiated on pazopanib therapy and continues with stable disease after 5 months of therapy.

### Evidence-Based Case Discussion

Our patient is a 50-year-old man with a high-grade leiomyosarcoma who presented with metastatic disease. Unfortunately, the median survival for metastatic STS patients is approximately 12–18 months (11,12).

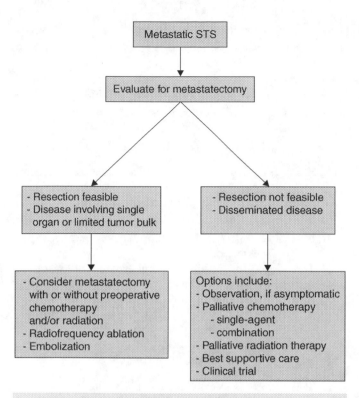

**Figure 22.3**

Treatment algorithm of metastatic soft tissue sarcoma. STS, soft tissue sarcomas.

Figure 22.3 shows a treatment algorithm for patients with metastatic disease.

For appropriately selected patients with isolated metastases from STS, surgical resection is often the treatment of choice and has been shown to be potentially curative, with long-term DFS rates of approximately 25% in retrospective studies (13–15). Commonly used criteria for selecting patients for metastasectomy include limited or no extrathoracic disease, pleural effusion, or mediastinal/hilar adenopathy; good performance status and pulmonary reserve; and technical feasibility of complete resection (16). Stereotactic radiosurgery is being increasingly used in some situations for small pulmonary metastases, but its true role is unclear.

Systemic chemotherapy is a therapeutic option for patients presenting with metastatic disease not amenable to complete surgical resection. For the majority of these patients, cytotoxic chemotherapy is regarded as palliative, although a small subset of patients experience long-term survival (11). Active cytotoxic agents in metastatic STS with a 10% or greater response rate include single-agent doxorubicin, ifosfamide, gemcitabine, and dacarbazine. Doxorubicin, which was identified as an active drug in the 1970s, continues to be the most commonly used single agent. The response rate with doxorubicin averages approximately 10–25%, depending on the era and response criteria used. It has been shown to have a dose–response relationship in sarcoma, but its use is limited by the risk of cardiotoxicity after high cumulative doses.

Ifosfamide is the first drug to demonstrate significant efficacy in doxorubicin-refractory disease. Ifosfamide does have unique potential toxicities, including hemorrhagic cystitis, renal tubular acidosis, and neurotoxicity. Ifosfamide-induced hemorrhagic cystitis can be avoided by prophylactic use of 2-mercaptoethane sulfonate sodium (Mesna).

Combination chemotherapy for metastatic STS can yield higher response rates than single-agent chemotherapy, but is generally more toxic. In 2003, the Sarcoma Disease Site Group published a meta-analysis including 2281 patients from 8 randomized controlled trials comparing single-agent doxorubicin versus doxorubicin-based combination chemotherapy. No significant differences were seen in OS, although increased response rates as well as increased toxicities were seen with combination therapy (17). A recently published randomized controlled trial by the European Organization for Research and Treatment of Cancer (EORTC) compared doxorubicin alone with doxorubicin and ifosfamide combination. Patients included in this trial had locally advanced, unresectable, or metastatic high-grade STS. This study did not find a significant difference in OS between the 2 study groups (12.8 vs. 14.3 months) in the doxorubicin group and the doxorubicin and ifosfamide group, respectively (HR = 0.83, 95.5% confidence interval [CI] [0.67–1.03], $P$ = .076). There was a statistical difference in median PFS (7.4 vs. 4.6 months, HR = 0.74, 95% CI [0.60–0.90], $P$ = .003) and the objective response (26.5% with the combination vs. 13.6% with doxorubicin) favoring combination doxorubicin plus ifosfamide (18). However, combination chemotherapy was associated with significantly increased toxicities. Other doxorubicin-based combinations such as MAID (Mesna, doxorubicin, ifosfamide, and dacarbazine), and doxorubicin/dacarbazine are still routinely used in clinical practice. It is recommended that in general, doxorubicin-based combination chemotherapy be reserved for patients with metastatic STS who may benefit from tumor shrinkage and can tolerate the potential increased toxicities, while others should be considered for single-agent doxorubicin versus clinical trials if available.

Combination chemotherapy with gemcitabine and docetaxel is also considered a standard therapy for patients with metastatic STS. A randomized phase II study compared the combination of gemcitabine and docetaxel with gemcitabine alone in patients with metastatic STS. There was improvement of response rate (16% vs. 8%), median PFS (6.2 vs. 3 months), and OS (17.9 vs. 11.5 months) favoring combination therapy (19). Given the survival benefit observed, gemcitabine-based therapies, including gemcitabine and docetaxel as well as gemcitabine and dacarbazine, are preferably given in combination in most histologies. As limited active agents exist for the treatment of metastatic STS, participation in clinical trials is an important part of patient care as well as in understanding the disease.

Pazopanib, a multitargeted tyrosine kinase inhibitor that blocks tumor growth and inhibits angiogenesis, has recently been shown to have a role in the management of metastatic STS. The phase III multicenter placebo-controlled PALETTE trial randomized 372 patients with non-adipose STS to pazopanib 800 mg daily or placebo. Median PFS was 5.6 months (95% CI [3.7–4.8]) for pazopanib compared with 1.6 months (0.9–1.8) for placebo (HR = 0.31, 95% CI [3.7–4.8]). Although there was a nonsignificant difference in OS, pazopanib was approved for use by national and international regulatory agencies as a new treatment option for patients with metastatic non-adipocytic STS after previous chemotherapy (20). There has also been much interest in less toxic ifosfamide analogs. The phase III PICASSO study of patients with metastatic STS looked at the combination of palifosfamide (the active metabolite of ifosfamide) and doxorubicin as compared to single-agent doxorubicin. Preliminary results do not demonstrate a benefit of the combination over doxorubicin and placebo.

## GASTROINTESTINAL STROMAL TUMOR

### Epidemiology, Risk Factors, Natural History, and Pathology

GIST represents a unique subtype of STS derived from the interstitial cells of Cajal, the pacemaker cells of the gastrointestinal (GI) tract. They are the most common form of STS, with an incidence of 5–10 cases/million in the United States. GISTs can occur anywhere along the GI tract, with the majority arising from the stomach (21). Patients with GIST often present with symptoms including early satiety, abdominal discomfort, palpable mass, or GI bleeding. Image-guided, endoscopic biopsy or fine needle aspiration (FNA) is usually sufficient to make the diagnosis. As opposed to other types of STS, GIST tumors spread locally within the peritoneum and to the liver, whereas lungs and other sites of distant metastases are uncommon.

The majority of GIST tumors have activating mutations in KIT (approximately 50%) or platelet-derived growth factor receptor alpha (PDGFRA; approximately 5–8%). Mutations are also rarely found in succinate dehydrogenase (SDH) subunits and the serine–threonine kinase, BRAF. The mutational status is proving to be of increasing clinical significance. For example, mutations in exon 11 of KIT have a higher chance of responding to standard dose imatinib (400 mg daily), whereas mutations in exon 9 of KIT often require a higher serum level of imatinib to effectively inhibit the mutant kinase. For such patients, a higher dose (800 mg daily) is often more efficacious. In addition, tumors with PDGFRA D842V are insensitive to imatinib, but other PDGFRA mutations can be sensitive.

## STAGING

Staging consists of a CT of the abdomen and pelvis, because peritoneal and hepatic spread occurs most commonly.

GISTs are also highly metabolically active; so PET scans are frequently used for staging or assessing response to treatment.

The staging system for GIST is different from that of other STS and is shown in the following tables (according to the *AJCC Cancer Staging Handbook, 7th Edition*).

| Stage Grouping for GIST With a Primary Site in the Stomach or the Omentum | |
|---|---|
| **Stage** | **Description** |
| Stage IA | Tumor is ≤5 cm (T1 or T2), has not spread to regional lymph nodes (N0) or distant sites (M0), low mitotic rate |
| Stage IB | Tumor is >5 cm but ≤10 cm (T3), has not spread to regional lymph nodes (N0) or distant sites (M0), low mitotic rate |
| Stage II | Tumor is ≤5 cm (T1 or T2), has not spread to regional lymph nodes (N0) or distant sites (M0), high mitotic rate[a] *or* tumor is >10 cm (T4), has not spread to regional lymph nodes (N0) or distant sites (M0), low mitotic rate |
| Stage IIIA | Tumor is >5 cm but ≤10 cm (T3), has not spread to regional lymph nodes (N0) or distant sites (M0), high mitotic rate |
| Stage IIIB | Tumor is >10 cm (T4), has not spread to regional lymph nodes (N0) or distant sites (M0), high mitotic rate |
| Stage IV | Any size tumor with regional lymph node or distant metastases, any mitotic rate |

[a]High mitotic rate = ≥5 mitoses per 50 hpf.
GIST, gastrointestinal stromal tumor.

| Stage Grouping for GIST of the Small Intestine, Esophagus, Colon, Rectum, and Peritoneum | |
|---|---|
| **Stage** | **Description** |
| Stage IA | Tumor is ≤5 cm (T1 or T2), has not spread to regional lymph nodes (N0) or distant sites (M0), low mitotic rate[a] |
| Stage II | Tumor is >5 cm but ≤10 cm (T3), has not spread to regional lymph nodes (N0) or distant sites (M0), low mitotic rate |
| Stage IIIA | Tumor is ≤2 cm (T1), has not spread to regional lymph nodes (N0) or distant sites (M0), high mitotic rate[a] *or* tumor is >10 cm (T4), has not spread to regional lymph nodes (N0) or distant sites (M0), low mitotic rate |
| Stage IIIB | Tumor is >2 cm (T2 to T4), has not spread to regional lymph nodes (N0) or distant sites (M0), high mitotic rate |
| Stage IV | Tumor of any size (any T) that has spread to regional lymph nodes (N1) with no metastases (M0) or any tumor with distant metastasis (M1), any mitotic rate |

[a]Mitotic rate: (low ≤5 mitoses/50 HPF, high >5 mitoses/50 HPF).
GIST, gastrointestinal stromal tumor.

In clinical practice, the staging system is not used frequently, because the patient's treatment course and decisions are usually based on whether the patient has localized or metastatic disease. If the patient does have localized disease, the determination of prognosis as well as consideration for adjuvant therapy is often based on whether the tumor confers a low-, intermediate-, or high-risk metastatic potential based on tumor size and pathological characteristics. The original National Institutes of Health (NIH) risk stratification includes tumor size and mitotic index of resected specimen. Tumors >5–10 cm and mitotic index >5/50 high power field (HPF) have poorer outcome. The modified NIH risk stratification also incorporates site of origin, as tumors arising from the stomach have better prognosis than those originating from other sites along the GI tract. Tumor rupture and incomplete resection also negatively impact DFS.

## CASE SUMMARY

### Metastatic GIST

G.A. is a 61-year-old male with no pertinent past medical history who presented with abdominal pain, fatigue, and a 30-pound weight loss over 6 months. Abdominopelvic CT showed a large mass, which appeared to have started in the stomach (see Figure 22.4). CT-guided biopsy demonstrated a spindle cell neoplasm that stained strongly positive for c-kit, consistent with GIST. Mutational analysis of c-kit revealed an exon 11 mutation. The large mass was deemed resectable and he underwent resection of his primary tumor. Pathology reviewed the specimen, which was 33 cm in longest dimension with negative margins and had >200 mitotic figures per 50 HPF. Given his high-risk features, adjuvant imatinib was started. The patient had no evidence of disease for approximately 3 years until new liver lesions appeared while on imatinib therapy, and biopsy was consistent with metastatic disease. Given the location and multiplicity, the patient was considered to have unresectable GIST and his imatinib dose was increased to 400-mg BID. Due to intolerable side effects of this dose, he was switched to sunitinib and had 1 year of stable disease. At the time of tumor progression, he was started on third-line regorafenib and remains on this medication to date.

### Evidence-Based Case Discussion

Our patient presented with a large GIST tumor with a high mitotic rate that originated in the stomach. He underwent resection of this mass and was subsequently treated with adjuvant therapy with imatinib. For localized or resectable GIST, surgical resection is the mainstay of treatment. However, the overall outcome of surgery is poor in certain patients due to the high risk of recurrence, and conventional chemotherapy and radiation are of limited benefit.

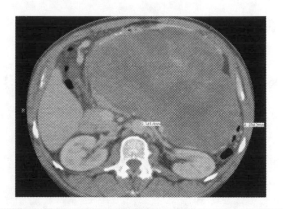

**Figure 22.4**

Primary GIST prior to resection and treatment. GIST, gastrointestinal stromal tumor.

Patients with GISTs possessing high-risk features (tumor size > 10 cm or mitotic rate > 10 per 50 HPF) have a >50% risk of recurrence within 2 years (22).

Imatinib, an oral inhibitor of the KIT, PDGFRA, and ABL tyrosine kinases, has been shown to induce durable tumor responses in metastatic disease. These encouraging results led to the rationale of initiating trials in the adjuvant setting. To date, several trials have examined the role of adjuvant imatinib. In 2009, a study was published that compared 1 year of imatinib to placebo in the adjuvant setting for patients with GIST tumors >3 cm. The estimated 1-year RFS was 98% (95% CI [0.96–1.00]) in the imatinib arm compared to 83% (95% CI [0.78–0.88]) in the placebo arm, with a corresponding 65% risk reduction of disease recurrence (HR = 0.35; 95% CI [0.22–0.53]; $P < .0001$). There was no statistical difference in OS; however, patients who progressed on placebo were able to cross over into the treatment arm (23).

This study led to the Food and Drug Administration (FDA) approval of imatinib for adjuvant treatment of GIST over 3 cm in size. However, the optimal use of imatinib in the adjuvant setting is yet to be determined. The duration of treatment in the adjuvant setting was addressed in a large randomized study that looked at 1 year versus 3 years of imatinib therapy for high-risk resected GIST. Patients assigned to 36 months of imatinib had longer RFS compared with those assigned to 12 months (HR = 0.46; 95% CI [0.32–0.65]; $P = .001$; 5-year RFS = 65.6% vs. 47.9%, respectively) and longer OS (HR = 0.45; 95% CI [0.22–0.89]; $P = .02$; 5-year survival = 92.0% vs. 81.7%) (24). This study led to the current recommendation of at least 36 months for adjuvant imatinib therapy following surgical resection for high-risk GIST. Exactly which patients need adjuvant therapy and the optimal duration of therapy (i.e., duration beyond 36 months) are currently the topics of ongoing research and debate.

Figure 22.5 shows a treatment algorithm for patients with metastatic GIST. Imatinib has been approved as

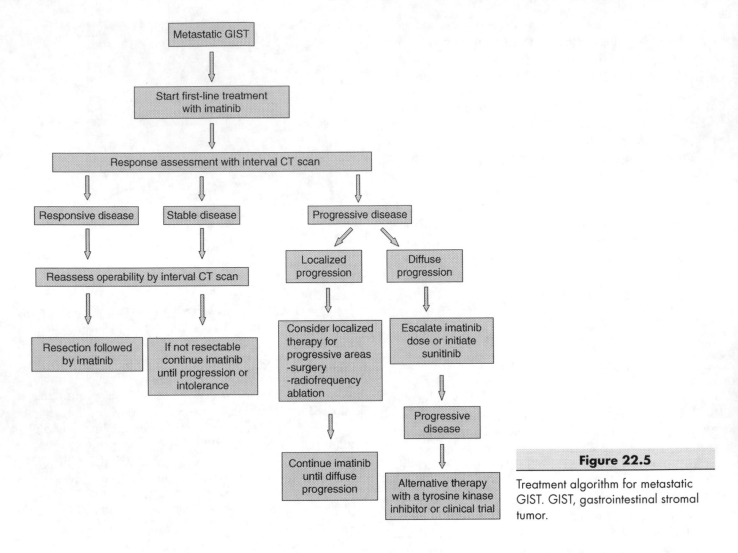

**Figure 22.5**

Treatment algorithm for metastatic GIST. GIST, gastrointestinal stromal tumor.

first-line therapy in advanced, inoperable, or metastatic GIST since 2002. Many studies have illustrated the role of imatinib in metastatic GIST. A multicenter trial of 147 patients with advanced GIST randomized patients to treatment with imatinib 400 or 600 mg once daily and showed 53.7% partial response and 27.9% stable disease, with similar outcomes at both doses (25). EORTC 62005 and SWOG 0033 also evaluated the benefit of imatinib in this same population. In both of these phase III studies, patients were randomized to receive 400 or 800 mg/d imatinib and had equivalent response rates and OS with either dose, although more toxicity was seen at the higher dose (25,26). In a later meta-analysis, patients with GISTs with an exon 9 mutation were the only subset that demonstrated a PFS benefit from the higher dose of imatinib, presumably because that mutation confers a higher MIC50 to imatinib (27).

Unfortunately, the majority of patients treated with imatinib will eventually develop resistance and progression of disease, primarily attributed to development of secondary mutations that confer resistance to imatinib. If progressing disease is localized or unifocal, surgery, or local approaches such as radiofrequency ablation should be considered to address the resistant area, and effective

systemic therapy for other areas of tumor involvement can be continued. If local control is not an option, higher dose imatinib (400 mg twice daily) can result in approximately one third of patients with stable disease or tumor shrinkage. Sunitinib is another option approved for metastatic GIST patients with imatinib resistance or intolerance. Sunitinib is a multitargeted tyrosine kinase inhibitor of KIT, vascular endothelial growth factor receptor (VEGFR), and PDGFR. A randomized placebo-controlled trial of sunitinib in patients with imatinib-resistant GIST demonstrated a median time to tumor progression of 27.3 weeks compared with 6.4 weeks in the placebo arm (28).

Regorafenib is an oral multi-kinase inhibitor that was approved by the FDA in February 2013 for the treatment of advanced GIST tumors in patients who were no longer responding to imatinib and sunitinib. Approval was based on a double-blind placebo-controlled randomized phase III trial of patients with metastatic or unresectable GIST. Patients were randomized to receive oral regorafenib 160 mg daily or placebo, plus best supportive care in both groups. Median PFS was 4.8 months for regorafenib and 0.9 months for placebo. HR = 0.27, 95% CI [0.19–0.39]; $P < .0001$ (29).

## KAPOSI'S SARCOMA

### Epidemiology, Risk Factors, Natural History, and Pathology

Kaposi's sarcoma (KS) is another entity that falls under the category of STS based on its malignant mesenchymal origin, despite fairly unique causative factors and epidemiology. KS is a multifocal angioproliferative spindle cell tumor of endothelial origin due to Kaposi's sarcoma–associated herpes virus (KSHV/HHV8) infection. On the basis of the clinical setting in which it occurs, KS is classified as classic (primarily affecting elderly men of Ashkenazi Jewish and/or Mediterranean descent); endemic (in Africa); iatrogenic (in patients with immune disorders, including following organ transplantation); and epidemic or AIDS related. Yet, histologically, all 4 are indistinguishable. KSHV is now thought to be transmitted through saliva, as the reported evidence of sexual transmission of the virus is inconclusive, with some studies not supporting a sexual transmission route. In addition, KSHV is detectable in the peripheral blood by polymerase chain reaction (PCR), suggesting blood transmission is also possible. KSHV infection is necessary but not sufficient for the development of KS, and host immunity plays a key role in pathogenesis.

In the Western world, AIDS-KS predominantly affects HIV-infected homosexual men, and patients tend to be young. Skin lesions are characterized by deep red or purple colored macules or raised lesions that may ulcerate or bleed easily. Extracutaneous involvement can include lymph nodes and mucosal surfaces. Even though no organ is consistently spared from involvement by AIDS-KS, visceral organ and bone metastasis are uncommon. Classic KS has a peak incidence of about 40–70 years with a wide range, affecting primarily people of Mediterranean or Central/Eastern European ancestry. The lesions usually occur on the distal extremities, particularly the lower legs and feet. Extracutaneous involvement is unusual and rarely is the presenting symptom. In general, oral mucosa and GI tract involvement is less common than with AIDS-KS,

affecting <10% of patients. The diagnosis requires biopsy of a lesion. To date, there is no universally accepted assay to detect KSHV in the serum. On pathological diagnosis, screening for visceral involvement with stool guaiac and chest x-ray is recommended. Additional evaluations with CT scanning of the chest–abdomen–pelvis, endoscopy, and bronchoscopy may be performed as clinically indicated.

Factors associated with the risk of developing AIDS-KS include the presence of HIV infection and its detrimental effect on the immune system, the proangiogenic effect of HIV-1 transcriptional trans-activator (Tat) protein, as well as KSHV viremia, increasing anti-KSHV antibody titers, and lack of neutralizing antibodies. KSHV-infected patients who develop KS have decreased CD4 response when compared to HIV-KSHV-infected patients without the clinical manifestations of KS. In addition to T-cell function, humoral activity also seems to play a role in pathogenesis. It is not entirely clear at present, but it appears that B cells may produce neutralizing antibodies to protect against KS (30). Unlike classic KS, which has an indolent course and rarely accounts for mortality, AIDS-KS can present as an aggressive, life-threatening disease.

### Staging

There is no widely accepted staging system accepted for KS. A staging system for patients with classic KS was proposed based on observation of subjective criteria in 300 patients with classic KS, but has not yet been validated and is not routinely used in clinical practice (31). Subjective evaluation of patient tumors results in tumor classification of maculonodular (stage 1), infiltrative (stage 2), florid (stage 3), and disseminated (stage 4).

There is also no officially accepted AIDS-related KS staging system, but when needed most physicians use the AIDS Clinical Trials Group (ACTG) system that divides patients into good- or poor-prognosis disease groups according to the extent of the tumor (T), immune status (I), and severity (S) of systemic illness (Table 22.3) (32).

**Table 22.3** AIDS Clinical Trial Group Staging of HIV Kaposi's Sarcoma

| Disease Stage | Tumor State | Immune Status | Systemic Illness |
|---|---|---|---|
| Good prognosis (T0 I0 S0) | Tumor limited to skin and/or lymph node and/or minimal oral diagnosis | CD4 count ≥200 cells/mm³ | No history of opportunistic infections or thrush<br>KPS ≥70<br>No B symptoms |
| Poor prognosis (T1 I1 S1) | Tumor-associated edema/ulceration, extensive oral KS, gastrointestinal KS, and visceral KS | CD4 count <200 cells/mm³ | History of opportunistic infections or thrush<br>KPS <70<br>B symptoms<br>Other HIV-related illness (e.g., neurological disease, lymphoma) |

KPS, Karnofsky performance status; KS, Kaposi's sarcoma.

## CASE SUMMARY

### Metastatic KS

D.C. is a 35-year-old homosexual man who presented with an enlarging lesion in his hard palate of 4 weeks' duration, resulting in progressive dysphagia and impaired speech. He was evaluated by an oral surgeon and underwent a biopsy. Pathology showed KS. Laboratory evaluation revealed a positive HIV test with a viral load of 164,000 and a CD4 count of 87. A diagnosis of AIDS-related KS was made. He was initiated on highly active antiretroviral therapy (HAART) and trimethoprim/sulfa for pneumocystis pneumonia (PCP) prophylaxis.

Shortly after starting HAART, he noted erythematous to violaceous macular and patchy skin lesions involving his face, neck, and right groin. He also developed a dry cough without associated fever or dyspnea. A CT of the chest, abdomen, and pelvis showed ill-defined bilateral pulmonary nodules as well as multiple slightly enlarged mediastinal, axillary, retroperitoneal, mesenteric, and pelvic lymph nodes.

He was referred to the Oncology Clinic for further evaluation and management. His examination was remarkable for an extensive violaceous fungating mass within the upper palate and scattered purplish cutaneous macular lesions over the face, back, extremities, and right groin, with associated right lower extremity pitting edema. More than 35 cutaneous lesions were noted in total.

The patient was initiated on liposomal doxorubicin at a dose of 20 mg/m² every 3 weeks. He experienced tolerable side effects of mild nausea and fatigue on days 2–4 of each cycle. The oral/hard palate lesions steadily decreased in size, and the cutaneous lesions faded with each treatment cycle. After 6 months of therapy, the patient had resolution of his oropharyngeal disease, dramatic improvement in his cutaneous lesions, and resolution of his lower extremity edema.

### Evidence-Based Case Discussion

Our patient illustrates progressive AIDS-related KS with possible visceral (pulmonary), lymph node, oral, and extensive cutaneous involvement. There was worsening in the setting of HAART, suggesting immune reconstitution inflammatory syndrome (IRIS). Even though the incidence of KS has decreased substantially after the introduction of HAART, it continues to be the second most common neoplasm in patients with AIDS. AIDS-related KS can range from relatively indolent in behavior to fulminant spread. The introduction and widespread use of HAART has led to a marked decline in the incidence and mortality of AIDS-KS. Although there is no cure for AIDS-related KS, there are multiple effective therapies that are given with the goal of symptom palliation. Treatment has been shown to delay disease progression, shrink visible lesions, and improve lymphedema and function of affected extremities. Figure 22.6 is a treatment algorithm for patients with AIDS-related KS. HAART can be effective as the sole modality of treatment for this disease, as approximately 80% of patients will have disease regression with HAART alone, with median time

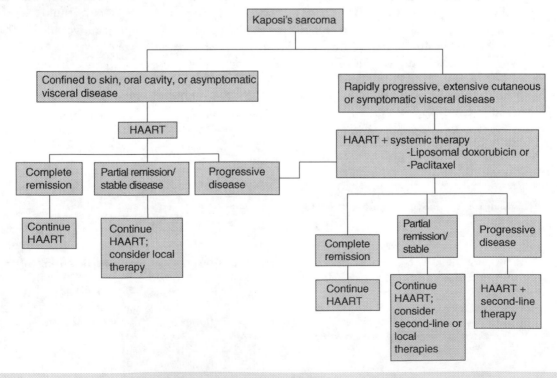

**Figure 22.6**

Treatment algorithm for metastatic Kaposi's sarcoma. HAART, highly active antiretroviral therapy.

to response ranging from 3 to 9 months. However, patients with visceral involvement, extensive cutaneous involvement (>25 skin lesions), rapidly progressive disease, or immune IRIS (worsening disease in the setting of HAART) often benefit from the use of systemic chemotherapy.

It is important to note that the immune reconstitution syndrome can result in a flare of disease prior to objective response. It typically presents as worsening of tumor burden within 12 weeks of initiation of HAART therapy. KS IRIS is generally distinguished from failure of HAART by improvements of CD4 count and decrease in viral load. The general treatment approach is to continue HAART. However, addition of systemic chemotherapy may be required based on symptoms and degree of systemic involvement.

Liposomal doxorubicin is often used as frontline therapy, with response rates in the 30–60% range. Preclinical data showed pegylated liposomes accumulate in the highly vascularized KS lesions. A randomized trial of 73 patients with AIDS-related KS showed that liposomal doxorubicin has a response rate of 46%, median PFS of 12.2 months, and 2-year survival of 78% (33). The effective dose of liposomal doxorubicin is 20 mg/m² every 3 weeks, which is substantially lower than the dose used for other malignancies. Long-term follow-up of 98 patients treated with liposomal doxorubicin combined with HAART demonstrated 78% treated with combination therapy had partial response or better, with a relapse rate of 13.5% per year. Treatment is typically well tolerated, although continuous assessment for overlapping toxicities with concomitant HAART, antibiotic, and antiemetic therapies is recommended.

Paclitaxel also induces tumor regression with acceptable toxicity, and is associated with significant improvement in quality of life. It should be considered as a second-line therapy in patients with advanced KS who progress on liposomal doxorubicin (34). However, paclitaxel requires the use of dexamethasone in this already immunocompromised population and can have interactions with HAART based on its metabolism through the cytochrome P450 (CYP450) system. Other potentially effective systemic therapies include vinorelbine, etoposide, imatinib, and interferon-alpha. For patients with symptomatic localized involvement, effective local strategies include radiation therapy and intralesional chemotherapy. Several agents are under clinical investigation including VEGF inhibitors, mammalian target of rapamycin (mTOR) inhibitors, and immune modulating agents such as lenalidomide.

## REVIEW QUESTIONS

1. A 44-year-old male presented with a slowly growing mass on his right upper thigh. CT imaging revealed a 11 × 6 × 4 cm heterogeneous mass with irregular borders. Biopsy revealed high-grade undifferentiated pleomorphic sarcoma. CT of his chest did not reveal metastatic disease. He was discussed at multidisciplinary tumor board and the consensus was neoadjuvant chemotherapy followed by resection followed by radiation to the surgical bed. Which of the following is the most appropriate chemotherapy option for the neoadjuvant setting?

   (A) Single-agent chemotherapy with liposomal doxorubicin
   (B) Single-agent chemotherapy with gemcitabine
   (C) Combination chemotherapy with doxorubicin and ifosfamide
   (D) Combination chemotherapy with carboplatin and paclitaxel

2. A 35-year-old man is undergoing cycle 6 of palliative chemotherapy with doxorubicin and high-dose ifosfamide for metastatic synovial sarcoma. He has been receiving Mesna and granulocyte colony-stimulating factor support with each cycle. His course has been complicated by nausea and vomiting, treated with prochlorperazine. He develops blood-tinged urine with dysuria but no fever or suprapubic pain. His examination reveals a fatigued-appearing male with normal vital signs, clear lungs, heart with regular rate and rhythm, and no peripheral edema. Labs are notable for a white blood cell (WBC) count of 3000 wbc/mcL with ANC = 1500 mm³, Hb = 13 g/dL, Plt = 140 × 10³/µL, BUN = 20 mg/dL, and Cr = 1.0 mg/dL. UA is negative for nitrites and leukocyte esterase, with 2+ blood. Cultures are pending. The most likely cause of his gross hematuria is

   (A) Hemorrhagic cystitis secondary to ifosfamide toxicity
   (B) Kidney injury from hypovolemia
   (C) Decreased ejection fraction from doxorubicin causing acute tubular necrosis
   (D) *Escherichia coli* urinary tract infection

3. A 58-year-old previously healthy male was recently diagnosed with an 8 × 8 cm abdominal wall mass. Biopsy of this mass revealed high-grade leiomyosarcoma. Staging CT scan of chest shows 2 pulmonary nodules in the right upper lobe, the largest of which is 3 cm in greatest diameter. He was treated with systemic chemotherapy with doxorubicin, with a good response after 4 cycles. There was shrinkage of the primary lesion and the lung nodules now measure 1.5 and 2 cm. What would be the next most appropriate management strategy?

   (A) Observation
   (B) Resection of the primary abdominal wall mass followed by ifosfamide
   (C) Radiation to the primary mass lesion followed by gemcitabine
   (D) Resection of the primary mass and evaluation for wedge resection of the right upper lobe

4. A 63-year-old female taking 400 mg of imatinib once daily for treatment of metastatic gastrointestinal stromal tumor is noted to have progression of disease throughout her peritoneum on CT scan. The patient maintains good performance status and does not complain of any side effects from imatinib. Which of the following is the next best step in treatment?

(A) Change therapy to regorafenib
(B) Change therapy to doxorubicin
(C) Increase dose of imatinib to 400-mg BID
(D) Resect all enlarging and new lesions and continue current dose of imatinib

5. A 50-year-old otherwise healthy male was recently diagnosed with gastrointestinal stromal tumor (GIST) tumor localized to his jejunum. CT imaging revealed a 7-cm tumor that was amenable to surgical resection, with no sites of distant metastatic disease. He underwent total resection of the mass. Final pathology revealed a 7-cm GIST tumor with 7 mitoses/50 high-power fields and KIT mutation in exon 11. Which of the following should be offered next?

(A) with CT scan of the abdomen and pelvis every 3 months
(B) Imatinib starting at 400-mg daily
(C) Imatinib starting at 400-mg BID
(D) Adjuvant chemotherapy with doxorubicin ± radiation

6. A 28-year-old female presents with a 12-cm enlarging mass growing on her upper outer left thigh. Core biopsy of the mass is obtained and consistent with high-grade myxoid round cell liposarcoma. Staging scans do not reveal any sites of distant metastatic disease. Her case is discussed at the multidisciplinary tumor board and the consensus is to perform preoperative radiation followed by resection with limb-sparing procedure. Which of the following is a potential complication of preoperative radiation?

(A) Increased chance of postoperative infection
(B) Decreased tumor response to adjuvant chemotherapy
(C) Difficulty analyzing margins for disease involvement
(D) Increased postsurgical mortality

7. A 32-year-old male with untreated HIV infection presents with approximately 10 purple macules and nodules on his lower extremity and a 2-cm purple macular lesion on his upper palate. Biopsy confirms Kaposi's sarcoma. His CD4 count is 20 cells/mm³ and his viral load is >1 million copies. He is started on highly active antiretroviral therapy (HAART). Eight weeks into treatment, he notes his lesions have grown slightly.

He continues to have good performance status and remains asymptomatic without any dysphagia. Which of the following is the most appropriate management option?

(A) Continue HAART therapy and continue to observe lesions
(B) Begin liposomal doxorubicin
(C) Consider surgical resection of visible lesions and continue HAART
(D) Begin paclitaxel chemotherapy

8. Which of the following is *not* an important prognostic marker for gastrointestinal stromal tumors according to the modified National Institutes of Health criteria?

(A) Tumor size
(B) Tumor location
(C) Mitotic index
(D) Age of patient

9. Which of the following statements is FALSE regarding the use of combination therapy in metastatic soft tissue sarcomas?

(A) Doxorubicin and ifosfamide each have response rates of 10–25%, and the combination of these agents is additive but not synergistic
(B) Studies have shown a higher tumor response rate with the combination of doxorubicin and ifosfamide
(C) Studies have shown improved overall survival (OS) for the combination of doxorubicin and ifosfamide compared to single-agent therapy
(D) The combination of gemcitabine and docetaxel has superior progression-free survival and OS compared to gemcitabine alone

## REFERENCES

1. Siegel R, Ma J, Zou Z, et al. Cancer statistics, 2014. *CA Cancer J Clin*. 2014;64(1):9–29.
2. Helman LJ, Meltzer P. Mechanisms of sarcoma development. *Nat Rev Cancer*. 2003;3(9):685–694.
3. Lawrence W, Jr., Donegan WL, Natarajan N, et al. Adult soft tissue sarcomas. A pattern of care survey of the American College of Surgeons. *Ann Surg*. 1987;205(4):349–359.
4. Edge SB, Byrd DR, Compton CC, et al. *AJCC Cancer Staging Manual*. 7th ed. New York, NY: Springer; 2010:175–180, 291–298.
5. Bhangu AA, Beard JA, Grimer RJ. Should soft tissue sarcomas be treated at a specialist center? *Sarcoma*. 2004;8(1):1–6.
6. Sarcoma Metaanalysis Collaboration. Adjuvant chemotherapy for localized resectable soft-tissue sarcoma of adults: meta-analysis of individual data. *Lancet*. 1997;350(9092):1647–1654.
7. Rosenberg SA, Tepper J, Glatstein E, et al. The treatment of soft-tissue sarcomas of the extremities: prospective randomized evaluations of (1) limb-sparing surgery plus radiation therapy compared with amputation and (2) the role of adjuvant chemotherapy. *Ann Surg*. 1982;196(3):305–315.
8. Baldini EH, Goldberg J, Jenner C, et al. Long-term outcomes after function-sparing surgery without radiotherapy for soft

tissue sarcoma of the extremities and trunk. *J Clin Oncol.* 1999;17(10):3252–3259.

9. Pisters PW, Harrison LB, Leung DH, et al. Long-term results of a prospective randomized trial of adjuvant brachytherapy in soft tissue sarcoma. *J Clin Oncol.* 1996;14(3):859–868.

10. Yang JC, Chang AE, Baker AR, et al. Randomized prospective study of the benefit of adjuvant radiation therapy in the treatment of soft tissue sarcomas of the extremity. *J Clin Oncol.* 1998;16(1):197–203.

11. Blay JY, van Glabbeke M, Verweij J, et al. Advanced soft-tissue sarcoma: a disease that is potentially curable for a subset of patients treated with chemotherapy. *Eur J Cancer.* 2003;39(1):64–69.

12. Van Glabbeke M, van Oosterom AT, Oosterhuis JW, et al. Prognostic factors for the outcome of chemotherapy in advanced soft tissue sarcoma: an analysis of 2,185 patients treated with anthracycline-containing first-line regimens—a European Organization for Research and Treatment of Cancer Soft Tissue and Bone Sarcoma Group Study. *J Clin Oncol.* 1999;17(1):150–157.

13. Casson AG, Putnam JB, Natarajan G, et al. Five-year survival after pulmonary metastasectomy for adult soft tissue sarcoma. *Cancer.* 1992;69(3):662–668.

14. Putnam JB Jr, Roth JA, Wesley MN, et al. Analysis of prognostic factors in patients undergoing resection of pulmonary metastases from soft tissue sarcomas. *J Thorac Cardiovasc Surg.* 1984;87(2):260–268.

15. Jablons D, Steinberg SM, Roth J, et al. Metastasectomy for soft tissue sarcoma. Further evidence for efficacy and prognostic indicators. *J Thorac Cardiovasc Surg.* 1989;97(5):695–705.

16. McCormack P. Surgical resection of pulmonary metastases. *Semin Surg Oncol.* 1990;6(5):297–302.

17. Bramwell VH, Anderson D, Charette ML. Doxorubicin-based chemotherapy for the palliative treatment of adult patients with locally advanced or metastatic soft tissue sarcoma. *Cochrane Database Syst Rev.* 2003;(3):CD003293.

18. Judson I, Verweij J, Gelderblom H, et al. Doxorubicin alone versus intensified doxorubicin plus ifosfamide for first-line treatment of advanced or metastatic soft-tissue sarcoma: a randomised controlled phase 3 trial. *Lancet Oncol.* 2014;15(4):415–423.

19. Maki RG, Wathen JK, Patel SR, et al. Randomized phase II study of gemcitabine and docetaxel compared with gemcitabine alone in patients with metastatic soft tissue sarcomas: results of sarcoma alliance for research through collaboration study 002 [corrected]. *J Clin Oncol.* 2007;25(19):2755–2763.

20. van der Graaf WT, Blay JY, Chawla SP, et al. Pazopanib for metastatic soft-tissue sarcoma (PALETTE): a randomized, double-blind, placebo-controlled phase 3 trial. *Lancet.* 2012;379(9829):1879–1886.

21. Miettinen M, Lasota J. Gastrointestinal stromal tumors: review on morphology, molecular pathology, prognosis, and differential diagnosis. *Arch Pathol Lab Med.* 2006;130(10):1466–1478.

22. Rutkowski P, Nowecki ZI, Michej W, et al. Risk criteria and prognostic factors for predicting recurrences after resection of primary gastrointestinal stromal tumor. *Ann Surg Oncol.* 2007;14(7):2018–2027.

23. Dematteo RP, Ballman KV, Antonescu CR, et al. Adjuvant imatinib mesylate after resection of localised, primary gastrointestinal stromal tumour: a randomised, double-blind, placebo-controlled trial. *Lancet.* 2009;373(9669):1097–1104.

24. Joensuu H, Eriksson M, Sundby Hall K, et al. One vs three years of adjuvant imatinib for operable gastrointestinal stromal tumor: a randomized trial. *JAMA.* 2012;307(12):1265–1272.

25. Verweij J, Casali PG, Zalcberg J, et al. Progression-free survival in gastrointestinal stromal tumours with high-dose imatinib: randomised trial. *Lancet.* 2004;364(9440):1127–1134.

26. Blanke CD, Rankin C, Demetri GD, et al. Phase III randomized, intergroup trial assessing imatinib mesylate at two dose levels in patients with unresectable or metastatic gastrointestinal stromal tumors expressing the kit receptor tyrosine kinase: S0033. *J Clin Oncol.* 2008;26(4):626–632.

27. Gastrointestinal Stromal Tumor Meta-Analysis Group. Comparison of two doses of imatinib for the treatment of unresectable or metastatic gastrointestinal stromal tumors: a meta-analysis of 1,640 patients. *J Clin Oncol.* 2010;28(7):1247–1253.

28. Demetri GD, van Oosterom AT, Garrett CR, et al. Efficacy and safety of sunitinib in patients with advanced gastrointestinal stromal tumour after failure of imatinib: a randomised controlled trial. *Lancet.* 2006;368(9544):1329–1338.

29. Demetri GD, Reichardt P, Kang YK, et al.; GRID Study Investigators. Efficacy and safety of regorafenib for advanced gastrointestinal stromal tumors after failure of imatinib and sunitinib (GRID): an international, multicenter, randomized, placebo-controlled, phase 3 trial. *Lancet.* 2013;381(9863):295–302.

30. Uldrick TS, Whitby D. Update on KSHV-epidemiology, Kaposi sarcoma pathogenesis and treatment of Kaposi sarcoma. *Cancer Lett.* 2011;305(2):150–162.

31. Brambilla L, Boneschi V, Taglioni M, et al. Staging of classic Kaposi's sarcoma: a useful tool for therapeutic choices. *Eur J Dermatol.* 2003;13(1):83–86.

32. Krown SE, Metroka C, Wernz JC. Kaposi's sarcoma in the acquired immune deficiency syndrome: a proposal for uniform evaluation, response, and staging criteria. AIDS Clinical Trials Group Oncology Committee. *J Clin Oncol.* 1989;7(9):1201–1207.

33. Cianfrocca M, Lee S, Von Roenn J, et al. Randomized trial of paclitaxel versus pegylated liposomal doxorubicin for advanced human immunodeficiency virus-associated Kaposi sarcoma: evidence of symptom palliation from chemotherapy. *Cancer.* 2010;116(16):3969–3977.

34. Tulpule A, Groopman J, Saville MW, et al. Multicenter trial of low-dose paclitaxel in patients with advanced AIDS-related Kaposi sarcoma. *Cancer.* 2002;95(1):147–154.

# 23

# Primary Brain Tumors

ABHISHEK MARBALLI, JANET WANG, AND PAMELA NEW

## EPIDEMIOLOGY, RISK FACTORS, NATURAL HISTORY, AND PATHOLOGY

In 2015, an estimated 68,470 cases of primary brain and central nervous system (CNS) tumors are expected to be diagnosed, of which 23,180 will be malignant and 45,300 will be nonmalignant (1). The overall average annual age-adjusted incidence rate for primary brain and CNS tumors in 2007–2011 was 23,180 per 100,000 (5.42 per 100,000 for children 0–19 years of age and 27.86 per 100,000 for adults). The median age at diagnosis is 59 years. Incidence rates are higher among females (23.26 per 100,000) than males (19.42 per 100,000). The most frequently encountered histology is nonmalignant meningioma, which comprises more than one third of all tumors followed by malignant glioblastoma, which accounts for 15.4%. Meningiomas represent 53.7% of all nonmalignant tumors and glioblastomas represent 45.6% of malignant tumors. For malignant tumors, glioblastoma has the highest incidence rate of 3.19 per 100,000 followed by diffuse astrocytoma (0.55 per 100,000) and lymphoma (0.44 per 100,000). For nonmalignant tumors, meningioma has the highest incidence rate of 7.5 per 100,000 followed by pituitary tumors (3.28 per 100,000) and nerve sheath tumors (1.69 per 100,000). The estimated mortality rate from malignant brain and CNS tumors is 4.26 per 100,000. The estimated 5- and 10-year relative survival for malignant tumors is 34.2% and 28.5%, respectively, with a large variation depending upon histology of the tumor. For example, a 5-year survival rate for pilocytic astrocytoma is 94.4% but for glioblastoma it is <5% (1).

There is no definite etiology for primary brain tumors. However, several genetic, environmental, and therapeutic factors have been implicated as risk factors. Previous exposure to ionizing radiation is an established risk factor.

Studies have verified an increased risk of gliomas associated with various doses of radiation used to treat tinea capitis, adenoid hypertrophy, childhood leukemia, and other cancers. Low-dose radiation has been linked more often to the incidence of meningioma and nerve sheath tumors. Whether exposure to electromagnetic fields and cell-phone usage are risk factors is a source of continued controversy, but as yet no direct link has yet been established. Occupational studies of airline employees with exposure to cosmic radiation, and atomic energy employees remain equivocal. A recent cohort of U.S. nuclear workers has been examined and an increased risk of developing a primary brain tumor was found to be 15%. An increase in nervous system tumors was also found in survivors of the atomic bombs in Nagasaki and Hiroshima. Exposure to low doses of diagnostic radiation does not seem to play a role, except for a slight risk of meningioma from exposure to dental x-rays. Diet and smoking have also not been associated with increase in risk, nor has occupational exposure to chemicals. Exposure to various tumor-inducing viruses remains plausible and studies continue.

Familial aggregation of brain tumors occurs in 5%, and likely reflects the result of environmental exposures to heritable genetic mutability. Certain familial syndromes (tuberous sclerosis, neurofibromatosis, Turcot's, Li-Fraumeni) may predispose to gliomas in children or young adults. These account for approximately 5–10% of all brain tumors. Inherited mutations in the *TP53* gene in some families with Li-Fraumeni syndrome have an increased incidence of many cancers including breast, soft tissues, bone, leukemia, and brain tumors, including glioma and medulloblastoma. Patients with *p53* mutations are more likely to have a first-degree relative affected with cancer (58% vs. 42%), or a previously diagnosed cancer (17% vs. 8%).

Gliomas, occurring in the support tissues of the brain, are the most common primary brain tumor, accounting for >40% of primary CNS neoplasms. Subtypes include astrocytomas, oligodendrogliomas, and ependymomas. Gliomas display a broad spectrum of histological features, and variation in their behavior most likely reflects the genes involved in their transformation. Astrocytomas are the most commonly occurring primary brain tumors in all ages. Oligodendrogliomas, arising from oligodendrocytes in the brain, account for <10% of intracranial tumors, and are less aggressive than astrocytomas. Nevertheless, they can invade and disseminate via the cerebrospinal fluid (CSF), causing swelling of the ventricles or hydrocephalus. Typically, they are located in the supratentorial hemispheres and are potentially resectable. Ependymomas arise from the ependymal cells lining the brain ventricles. Their growth can block the flow of CSF causing enlargement of the ventricles or hydrocephalus. They tend not to infiltrate the brain and therefore may be amenable to surgical treatment. When not completely resectable, radiotherapy (RT) is delivered. Chemotherapy has not been found to be effective in this tumor. Meningiomas arise from the dural sheathes surrounding the brain. Most occur near the surface of the brain and are surgically removable. Malignant variants are less frequent (25–30% of meningiomas). They are associated with deletions of loci on chromosome 1, 6p, 9q, and 17p. Medulloblastomas are primitive neuroectodermal tumors that arise in the cerebellum, replicate quickly and disseminate in the CSF. They occur most commonly in children. Chromosome 17p is a frequent site of deletion. RT is the mainstay of treatment and usually includes the entire craniospinal compartment. Gangliogliomas are low-grade tumors containing both neurons and glial cells. They have a high rate of cure with surgery alone or surgery combined with RT. Schwannomas (neurilemmomas) arise from Schwann cells that surround cranial and other nerves. These are most often benign tumors and occur near the cerebellum and around the eighth cranial nerve.

Primary CNS lymphoma (PCNSL) is a diffuse large B-cell lymphoma presenting in the brain or spinal cord in the absence of systemic lymphoma. About 1000 cases are diagnosed in the United States each year. The incidence of this tumor has been increasing steadily in the immunocompetent population since the 1970s. A reason for this may be improved methods of detection and diagnosis, rather than a true increase in the incidence of the tumor. Nevertheless, the number of patients diagnosed with PCNSL over the next decade is likely to continue to increase, particularly within the elderly population.

PCNSL most commonly presents as a contrast-enhancing lesion in the deep brain parenchyma, but may also present as a multifocal or diffuse tumor, often with involvement of the leptomeningeal space. Regardless of initial presentation, the entire cranial–spinal axis is at risk for involvement because of the tendency for PCNSL cells to spread throughout the CSF pathways. Therapy targeted to the tumor site alone is never curative and surgery is limited to a diagnostic biopsy. Treatment is generally systemic chemotherapy (including high-dose methotrexate) with RT often reserved for relapses. This chapter focuses on the major non-lymphomatous malignant brain tumors.

## STAGING

### Grading System for Primary Brain Tumors and Prognosis

There is no formal staging system such as the tumor, node, and metastasis (TNM) classification for primary brain tumors. Primary brain tumors are typically locally invasive and do not spread to lymph nodes or distant organs, therefore a TNM classification for these tumors is not relevant.

The pathological grading of primary brain tumors, however, is very important for treatment and prognosis. The international classification of tumors published by the World Health Organization (WHO) was initiated in 1956 and had been updated for the fourth time in 2007. Its objective has been to create a classification and grading system of human tumors that can be accepted worldwide thus facilitating the international collection of epidemiological data and clinical trials. This classification system is extremely important particularly for primary brain tumors because it directs prognosis and therapy. The 2007 WHO classification is focused on genetic data features that define tumor subsets, such as the 1p/19q codeletion in oligodendroglioma. Nevertheless, morphology is still the gold standard for the WHO classification. Astrocytomas that are well differentiated and low grade are classified as grade I (pilocytic)/grade II (diffuse) and comprise 15–20% of all gliomas (Table 23.1). They are characterized by slow growth but can progress to anaplastic astrocytoma or glioblastoma. Anaplastic astrocytomas are classified as grade III and account for 30–35% of gliomas. They are characterized by increased cellularity, mitoses, and proliferative activity. Glioblastomas are classified as grade IV and comprise up to 40–50% of gliomas. They display evidence of angiogenesis and/or tumor necrosis. Anaplastic astrocytomas and glioblastomas are frequently referred to as high-grade gliomas.

Low-grade gliomas have a median survival of 5–10 years with eventual risk of transformation to high-grade tumors. Prognosis worsens with increasing grade and age. Patients older than 40 years with low-grade glioma may have a much more aggressive disease with a median survival of <5 years. Even with standard treatment (surgical resection, RT, or chemotherapy), median survival for anaplastic astrocytomas is 3 years and only 1 year for glioblastoma.

Features of malignant gliomas that distinguish these tumors from other cancers and pose unique problems for treatment include the blood–brain barrier, which excludes

**Table 23.1** Astrocytoma

| Grade | Tumor Type | Glioma % | Median Survival (Years) |
|-------|-----------|----------|-------------------------|
| I/II | Low-grade astrocytoma | 15–20 | 5 |
| III | Anaplastic astrocytoma | 30–35 | 3 |
| IV | Glioblastoma | 40–50 | 1 |

**Table 23.2** Oligodendroglioma

| Grade | Tumor Type | Median Survival (Years) |
|-------|-----------|-------------------------|
| II | Oligodendroglioma | 4–10 |
| III | Anaplastic oligodendroglioma | 3–4 |

many drugs that may have otherwise been effective; angiogenic edema, which increases tumor interstitial pressure that can reduce the penetration of drugs that do cross the blood–brain barrier; diffuse infiltration of white matter tracts that makes local therapy difficult, including RT and surgery; heterogeneity of tumor microenvironments that may allow "tumor stem cells" to develop resistance to radiation and chemotherapy; genetic heterogeneity between tumors of different patients as well as within a specific tumor that limits the effectiveness of targeted therapies; and finally, the "immune sanctuary" provided by the brain that aids in tumor evasion of immune surveillance. The development of tumor immunotherapies has therefore been difficult.

Oligodendrogliomas are divided into 2 grades: grade II (well-differentiated oligodendrogliomas) and grade III (anaplastic oligodendrogliomas; Table 23.2). Oligodendrogliomas account for 2.5% of all primary brain tumors and 5% of gliomas. These percentages, however, are increasing because of new diagnostic criteria, such as the specific molecular deletion of chromosomes 1p and 19q. This tumor has long been of interest to neuropathologists because of its distinctive appearance under the microscope, including small round nuclei with perinuclear halos, which is actually a formalin fixation artifact (conveniently termed the "fried egg appearance"), a branching capillary network (described as "chicken wire"), and microscopic calcification. Some tumors may also contain neoplastic astrocytes, resulting in the classification of oligoastrocytoma or mixed glioma. Grading of oligodendrogliomas is based on cellularity, mitotic rate, nuclear atypia, and the presence or absence of vascular proliferation or necrosis. Nevertheless, over the previous 20 years, there has been a lack of agreement among neuropathologists on the histological diagnosis of this tumor, until molecular markers were discovered.

Progress in molecular diagnostics has identified a number of markers and profiles that have the potential for distinguishing subtypes of tumors and thus aid in the differential diagnosis of brain tumors that are difficult to distinguish based on histology alone. They also help in estimating outcomes of specific tumors and possibly predict benefit from certain types of treatment. Molecular markers like 1p/19q codeletion, O-methylguanine methyltransferase

(MGMT), and isocitrate dehydrogenase (IDH) 1/2 have displayed prognostic relevance in outcomes independent of therapeutic intervention and/or predictive value in estimating benefit from alkylating chemotherapy. These markers may prove beneficial in formulating personalized therapeutic approaches in neuro-oncology. The predictive value of MGMT methylation and 1p/19q codeletions are discussed in the relevant evidence-based discussion sections. IDH1 mutations are frequently seen in grade II and III astrocytomas and oligodendrogliomas, are rarely present in primary glioblastoma multiforme (GBM) and pilocytic astrocytomas, and are absent in ependymomas. IDH1 mutations may be present in combination with TP53 mutations and in 1p/19q codeleted tumors, and in several large clinical trials may be a marker for a more favorable prognosis in grade II, III, and IV gliomas.

Patients with brain tumors typically present with headache, seizures, nonspecific cognitive or personality changes, or focal neurological deficits. The precise clinical features will depend on the location, histology, and rate of growth of the tumor.

## CASE SUMMARIES

### High-Grade Astrocytoma/GBM

J.B. is a 55-year-old woman with no past medical history, who presented to the emergency department (ED) with altered mental status, progressive difficulty in walking, and imbalance slowly worsening over the prior 2 months. A CT scan performed in the ED revealed a left temporal-parietal mass with edema and midline shift. The patient was admitted to the hospital. An MRI of the brain with contrast was obtained and showed a 3.8 × 4.5 × 3.8 cm subcortical mass in the left posterior or superior temporal lobe or parietal region with surrounding vasogenic edema resulting in marked effacement of the left cerebral sulci and 8-mm left-to-right midline shift with subfalcine herniation (Figure 23.1). Her neurological examination was remarkable for mild expressive aphasia and right hemiparesis. She was placed on dexamethasone 4 mg every 6 hours, which resulted in improvement in memory and balance. The patient underwent resection of the left temporal parietal mass. Pathology was consistent with grade IV GBM. MGMT by immunohistochemistry (IHC) was methylated. She did very well postoperatively and began concurrent RT plus temozolomide chemotherapy: 6000 cGy

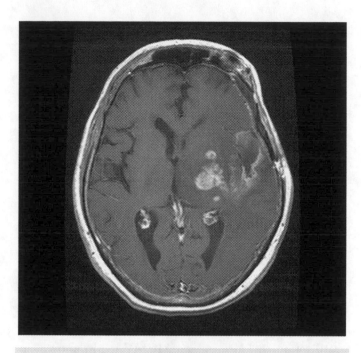

**Figure 23.1**

T1 axial contrast-enhanced MRI scan of the brain revealing a large contrast enhancing mass involving the left temporal-parietal lobes as well as the basal ganglia, with edema and midline shift.

of radiation delivered in 30 180-cGy fractions over 6 weeks, and temozolomide at a dose of 75 mg/m² was prescribed daily during this 6-week period. Two weeks after completion of RT J.B. began adjuvant temozolomide at a dose of 150 mg/m² for 5 days. The second and all subsequent doses of temozolomide were prescribed as 200 mg/m² for 5 days every 28 days. J.B. tolerated 18 cycles of temozolomide. Speech and mobility returned to normal, and she continued to perform all activities of daily living and chores. MRI scans of the brain performed every 2 months continued to reveal no recurrence of tumor.

After completion of the 18 cycles of temozolomide, MRI scans of the brain were obtained every 4–6 months for surveillance. These remained free of disease until 46 months after diagnosis, when an MRI scan revealed a 5-mm contrast-enhancing nodule in the posterior aspect of the resection cavity in the left temporal lobe. A follow-up MRI 4 weeks later revealed an increase in size of the lesion to 9 mm. During this time, J.B. remained asymptomatic, without speech problems, headaches, or seizures. She was referred to radiation oncology for consultation and it was decided that she could safely receive 3000 cGy in 5 fractions over 12 days to this 9-mm lesion.

A follow-up MRI scan 4 weeks after completion of RT revealed a much larger area of contrast enhancement with edema and necrotic areas. The patient continued to be asymptomatic at this time. The differential diagnosis for this mass included radiation effect, because this was the

site of the previous nodule and stereotactic boost versus rapid tumor regrowth of a radio-resistant lesion. A repeat MRI scan of the brain was planned in 4 weeks, but J.B. presented earlier to the ED for evaluation of a seizure. A CT scan of the brain revealed a marked increase in the size of the lesion, which now measured 4 cm with surrounding edema. For several days prior to the seizure, J.B.'s husband noted mild right-sided weakness and difficulty with expressive speech. She was admitted to the hospital and a PET scan demonstrated marked ¹⁸F-fludeoxyglucose (FDG) uptake in the region of abnormality on CT. Dexamethasone was prescribed and the patient improved in right limb strength and speech. A neurosurgical consultation was obtained, and J.B. underwent craniotomy with resection of tumor. Pathology was consistent with glioblastoma and treatment-related changes.

Postoperatively J.B. did well, with residual weakness in her right extremities and expressive speech difficulties. She underwent rehabilitation and gained the ability to transfer from bed to chair with assistance, and speech therapy was provided. Treatment options at this time included reinitiation of temozolomide at either the previously tolerated 5-day schedule, or a dose-intense schedule. J.B. was also eligible for enrollment in a research trial of temozolomide plus an angiogenesis inhibitor. After discussion of these options with the patient and family, their decision was to proceed with the investigational protocol. After one 4-week cycle, an MRI scan was performed because the patient seemed to be declining further in mobility and speech. The MRI scan of the brain revealed progression of disease in the left temporal lobe, as well as new involvement of the thalamus and brainstem. At this point J.B. was taken off study and bevacizumab 10 mg/m² plus carmustine (BCNU) 200 mg/m² were administered 4 weeks after study discontinuation. After 1 course of both agents, neurological functions continued to deteriorate and hospice care was offered. The patient expired 4 months after the surgical resection of her recurrent glioblastoma.

## Evidence-Based Case Discussion

J.B.'s case is a very typical clinical presentation of a high-grade GBM. The patient received standard of care treatment that included gross total resection. Pathology was consistent with GBM. J.B. received postoperative RT concurrently with temozolomide followed by adjuvant temozolomide that has been shown to improve overall survival (OS) compared to RT alone (see the following). J.B. responded very well to standard treatment but relapsed 4 years after her initial diagnosis. As will be described, her initial durable response to treatment might have been predicted by the methylation status of MGMT promoter in her tumor cells.

High-grade gliomas represent the largest percentage of primary brain tumors and, unfortunately, median survival for high-grade gliomas continues to be very poor. Elderly patients with GBM have an especially poor prognosis, with a median survival of 4–6 months. Malignant gliomas have high recurrence rates due to the infiltrative nature of the tumor. Most glioblastomas recur within 18 months of original diagnosis. Recurrent tumors often respond poorly to treatment and survival is often <6 months. Most recurrences are local, occurring within 2 cm of the original lesion.

Maximal total resection continues to be the overall goal. Resection of >98% of tumor volume has been shown to prolong OS in GBM and high-grade astrocytomas (13 vs. 8.8 months) (2). More recent studies have shown that even 89% reduction of tumor burden can have a positive impact on survival.

External brain RT is standard of care postoperatively. Alternative dose fractionation schedules have been employed but without additional benefit in malignant gliomas. Other techniques for dose intensification such as hyperfractionation, brachytherapy, and stereotactic radiation boosts have been evaluated but are not superior to external beam radiation therapy (XRT). There is a small benefit in median survival of 29.1 weeks when compared to supportive care alone, 16.9 weeks ($P$ = .002) (3). In about 20–30% of patients who have completed their radiation, the first MRI may show increased contrast enhancement that eventually subsides without any intervention. This phenomenon is termed "pseudoprogression" and is difficult to differentiate from true tumor progression (4). This occurs due to increased permeability of the vasculature from the radiation and may be enhanced by temozolamide (TMZ).

Early trials in high-grade gliomas employing concurrent chemotherapy/RT were disappointing. Walker et al. (5) randomized patients to RT in combination with nitrosourea compared with RT alone. There was a slight improvement in OS; however, this was not statistically significant. In 2001, the largest adjuvant chemotherapy randomized controlled trial was conducted by the Medical Research Council (MRC) for high-grade astrocytomas. Six hundred seventy-four patients were assigned to RT plus PCV (procarbazine, lomustine [CCNU], and vincristine) chemotherapy versus RT alone. Unfortunately, no survival benefit was seen even with the addition of PCV ($P$ = .50; HR = 0.95) nor was there improvement in progression-free survival (PFS; $P$ = .46, HR = 0.93) (6).

The European Organization for Research and Treatment of Cancer (EORTC) and the National Cancer Institute of Canada (NCIC) then conducted a phase III randomized controlled trial comparing RT alone (60 Gy over 6 weeks) versus RT/temozolomide followed by adjuvant temozolomide in 573 newly diagnosed GBM patients. The median survival was increased from 12.1 to 14.6 months, $P$ < .0001, and the survival rate at 2 years was also improved from 10.4% to 26.5% (7). Temozolomide

concurrent with XRT followed by adjuvant temozolomide has since become the new standard postoperative treatment of GBM.

Post hoc subgroup analysis of these patients showed that patients with O$^6$-methylguanine-DNA methyltransferase (*MGMT*) gene promoter methylation had a significantly improved median survival as compared with patients whose tumors had unmethylated *MGMT* promoters (23.4 vs. 15.3 months) (7). The cytotoxic effects of temozolomide were found to be mediated mainly through the methylation of the O6 position of guanine. Epigenetic silencing of *MGMT* via methylation prevented DNA damage caused by temozolomide from being rapidly repaired, which improved efficacy of the medication. The prognostic value of tumor MGMT methylation has been supported by the results of several prospective, randomized clinical trials. In Radiation Therapy Oncology Group (RTOG) 0525, 833 patients diagnosed with GBM were randomized to standard TMZ or dose dense (DD) TMZ. Stratification included tumor MGMT methylation. The primary endpoint was OS, and secondary analyses evaluated the impact of MGMT status. Whereas there was no statistically significant difference in terms of OS between the standard TMZ and DD TMZ arms, patients with methylated MGMT had a significantly better OS of 21.2 months compared to 14 months in patients with unmethylated tumors (8). The predictive impact of MGMT methylation has been demonstrated in elderly patients with GBM (9). Out of 233 GBM patients >70 years of age who were prospectively enrolled in the German Glioma Network, MGMT promoter methylation was detected by methylation-specific polymerase chain reaction (PCR) (MSP) in 134. The patients in whom pyrosequencing revealed >25% MGMT methylated alleles, had a longer OS with RT plus chemotherapy or chemotherapy alone compared to RT alone. Patients with unmethylated MGMT had no survival benefit from chemotherapy, irrespective of whether it was given concurrently with RT or as a salvage treatment. Similarly, in the NOA-08 trial, 331 patients with GBM and 40 patients with anaplastic astrocytoma aged >66 years were randomized to RT alone versus TMZ alone. The patients with MGMT promoter methylation benefited with TMZ alone in terms of PFS (8.4 vs. 4.6 months) compared to RT alone, whereas patients with unmethylated MGMT had longer PFS with RT alone (4.6 vs. 3.3 months) when compared to TMZ alone (10). Finally, in the Nordic trial, patients with GBM aged >60 years were randomized to standard RT versus hypofractionated RT versus TMZ (11). Among patients receiving TMZ, patients with MGMT methylation had significantly better OS when compared to unmethylated patients (9.7 vs. 6.8 months; HR = 0.56; $P$ = .03). Conversely, in patients receiving RT, MGMT methylation had no significant survival impact over unmethylated MGMT (8.2 vs. 7.0 months; HR = 0.97; $P$ = .88) (11). These trials demonstrate that MGMT methylation

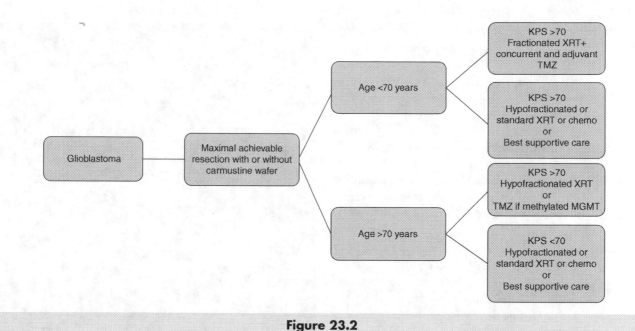

**Figure 23.2**

Algorithm for the initial management of glioblastomas. XRT, external beam radiation therapy; KPS, Karnofsky performance status; MGMT, O-methylguanine methyltransferase; TMZ, temozolamide.

is predictive of response to alkylating chemotherapy in the elderly population with high-grade astrocytomas and indicate that MGMT testing could be helpful in personalizing therapy in this patient population. However, the MGMT methylation status does not have predictive value in patients younger than 70 years because they benefit from TMZ irrespective of the MGMT promoter methylation status.

Carmustine or BCNU impregnated wafers have also been found to provide benefit in the treatment of malignant gliomas. A phase III randomized, placebo-controlled trial evaluated 240 patients by implanting biodegradable polymers (either containing carmustine or placebo) into the tumor bed after resection followed by RT (12). These wafers contained 3.85% carmustine and were designed to release the drug slowly over a 2- to 3-week period after implantation. Median survival was improved from 11.6 to 13.9 months ($P = .03$). Adverse effects were comparable between the 2 groups, with a higher incidence of intracranial hypertension noted in the BCNU wafer group.

As shown in Figure 23.2, temozolomide remains the first-line chemotherapy in patients with malignant gliomas. Unfortunately, chemotherapy is not curative and despite treatment, all malignant gliomas eventually recur. Patients may benefit from evaluation for re-resection. National Comprehensive Cancer Network (NCCN) guidelines recommend resection, BCNU wafer, bevacizumab, systemic chemotherapy, clinical trials, or supportive care as reasonable options for recurrent high grade gliomas.

Data for second-line chemotherapy using systemic agents such as irinotecan, cisplatin, and etoposide agents have been disappointing with low response rates. There

is a growing popularity for the use of targeted agents in recurrent GBM.

A high percentage of GBM tumors have been found to express vascular endothelial growth factor (VEGF), which stimulates tumor angiogenesis and is associated with a poor prognosis. Bevacizumab is a humanized immunoglobulin IgG1 monoclonal antibody that inhibits the activity of VEGF. An initial phase II study (13) enrolled 35 patients who had experienced disease progression after RT/concurrent temozolomide to receive bevacizumab/irinotecan. The 6-month PFS was 46% with a median PFS of 24 weeks. The 6-month OS was 77% and the median OS was 42 weeks. Out of the 35 patients, 20 (i.e., 57%) had at least a partial response, whereas 11 patients had to discontinue therapy due to toxicity. Only 1 patient developed CNS hemorrhage (in the tenth cycle), whereas 4 patients had thromboembolic events (13). In another phase II study, patients with recurrent GBM were randomly assigned to bevacizumab alone or bevacizumab in combination with irinotecan. The 6-month PFS was 42.6% in the bevacizumab group and 50.3% in the combination group, results which were significantly better than the historical control of 15% with salvage treatment or with irinotecan alone. Similarly, the objective response (OR) rate was 28% in the bevacizumab group and 37.8% in the combination group, which was also significantly higher than the 10% OR rate observed in the historical control where patients received irinotecan alone (14). In 2010, the Food and Drug Administration (FDA) approved the use of bevacizumab in patients with recurrent GBM. Two recent phase III randomized trials have evaluated the role of bevacizumab in the upfront setting. In one trial reported by Gilbert et al., 978 patients were randomized to the standard of care consisting of TMZ plus RT, or the same therapy with bevacizumab (15). In the experimental arm, bevacizumab was started during week 4 of RT and continued every 4 weeks for up to 12 cycles. The PFS was longer in the bevacizumab group (10.7 vs. 7.3 months; HR = 0.79) but did not achieve the prespecified target of 30% reduction in the risk of progression, and there was no significant difference in OS (15.7 vs. 16.1 months; HR = 1.13). Rates of hypertension, thrombotic events, neutropenia, and intestinal perforation were higher in the bevacizumab group, and patients in the bevacizumab group had comparitively more decline in neurocognitive function and a worse quality of life (15).

Another approved therapy for recurrent glioblastoma is the NovoTTF-100Af, which received approval by the FDA on April 15, 2011. This device is a novel, noninvasive alternative to chemotherapy that in clinical trials has been shown to be safe and effective. It is a portable, wearable device that delivers low intensity, intermediate frequency electric fields (tumor treatment fields [TTF]), which inhibit the replication of tumor cells. Nonproliferating cells and tissues are not affected. These electrical treatment fields disrupt the normal polymerization-depolymerization process of microtubules during mitosis. A 237-patient randomized pivotal trial demonstrated that patients who failed standard radiation and chemotherapy had a comparable median OS with fewer side effects and improved quality-of-life scores (16). The rate of PFS at 6 months was 21% in the NovoTTF group and 15% in the chemotherapy group. The device, which weighs 6 pounds, is worn throughout the day by the patient.

Enrollment in clinical trials is also an option for patients with newly diagnosed glioblastoma or recurrent tumor. The roles of targeted therapy and immunotherapy are being explored in this venue.

## Anaplastic Astrocytoma

M.F. is a 47-year-old man who had been noting increasing occurrence of left-sided headaches over a 4-month period of time. They gradually worsened in severity to the point of not responding to over-the-counter medications. The patient's family noted that he had difficulty with speech and word finding. His memory had also declined. The patient presented to the ED where an MRI scan of the brain revealed a left temporal lobe mass (Figure 23.3). Family history was negative for brain tumors, but positive for an uncle with prostate cancer. Review of systems was entirely negative. He was admitted to the hospital and treatment with dexamethasone 4 mg every 6 hours was begun. M.F. was then noted to have improvement in speech and memory. The patient underwent craniotomy and resection of tumor. Pathology revealed an anaplastic

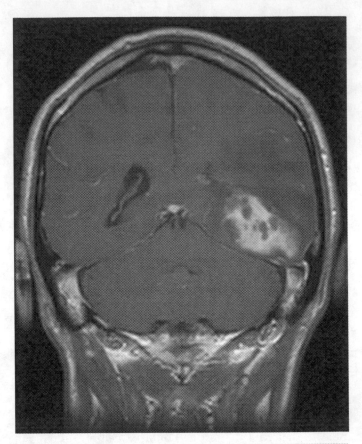

**Figure 23.3**

T1 coronal enhanced MRI scan of the brain depicting a left temporal lobe cystic enhancing mass with surrounding edema.

(grade III) astrocytoma. The patient recovered fluent speech and mentation improved postoperatively.

Two weeks after surgery M.F. began intensity modulated RT (IMRT), to the tumor bed. He also began chemotherapy with temozolomide daily at a dose of 75 mg/m². These treatments were completed in 42 days, and a total of 6000 cGy was delivered. Two weeks following completion of radiation, M.F. began treatment with temozolomide on the fifth day of every 28-day regimen. He tolerated treatment very well, with minimal nausea, and no myelosuppression. MRI scans of the brain with and without gadolinium were obtained 4 weeks after the completion of RT and every 2 months thereafter. Subtle changes were noted approximately 6 months postoperatively that were worrisome for tumor progression. A perfusion sequence was added to his MRI study and this revealed no increase in blood volume in the region. Meanwhile M.F. continued to feel well, his speech returned to normal, and he continued to work full time. After 18 months of temozolomide treatments, and continued stable MRI scans, chemotherapy was stopped. Surveillance MRI scans then were scheduled for every 3–4 months and ultimately every 6 months. The patient continues to work full time and has a normal neurological examination 5 years after the original diagnosis.

## Evidence-Based Case Discussion

M.F. presents as a typical case of dominant hemisphere tumor involvement with deterioration in expressive language on a background of several months of increasing headache. Anaplastic astrocytoma constitutes 8.3% of all CNS gliomas. The 5-year survival rate is poor at 28%. The mean age at the time of diagnosis is 41 years with a slight male predominance of 1.8–1.0 females. MRI is the diagnostic imaging tool of choice and usually presents a T1 hypointense and T2 hyperintense mass. Partial or heterogeneous enhancement may occur, lacking the ring enhancement/necrotic pattern seen often in glioblastoma. Anaplastic astrocytoma is characterized by increased cellularity, nuclear atypia, and increased mitotic activity.

M.F. received standard of care surgery with maximal resection as could safely be performed in the left temporal lobe. Maximal surgical resection is important, when possible, for bulk reduction of tumor mass and improvement in neurological function, adequate tissue sampling for pathological assessment, and cytoreduction to improve outcome. Intraoperative ultrasonography and image-guided systems have influenced the safety with which maximal tumor volume can be resected without damaging important brain structures. Awake craniotomies and cortical mapping with somatosensory-evoked potentials are also useful tools for aggressive removal of tumor involving eloquent brain tissue. This technique highlights the area of cerebral cortex involved in speech, and the entire speech pathway can be outlined to aid the surgeon in his resection. Maximal surgical resection is important also for histological grading, because these tumors may present low-grade features in one portion and high-grade features in another portion of the same mass, therefore risking an inaccurate diagnosis with biopsy alone.

After surgery, M.F. went on to receive RT. In the history of treatment for high-grade gliomas, XRT has been a cornerstone. Randomized trials in the 1970s and 1980s using whole brain radiation revealed an increase in survival from 5 to 9 months. Involved field RT involving the T2 weighted imaging abnormality and an additional 1- to 2-cm margin has replaced whole-brain RT because it carries equivalent efficacy and less neurotoxicity. Conformal radiation fields have been estimated to reduce the dose of radiation to normal brain by 50%. Standard practice is to deliver 58–60 Gy in 1.8–2.0 Gy fractions administered 5 days per week for 30–35 fractions. Trials of radiosensitizers, such as hydroxyurea, misonidazole, carboplatin, and etoposide have added no benefit to survival. Brachytherapy (the implantation of radioactive sources, such as I-125, iridium-192, and gold-198) and stereotactic RT are other options for patients with recurrent anaplastic astrocytoma. However, there have been no randomized controlled trials to evaluate these techniques. A small trial of patients with recurrent anaplastic astrocytoma found that with stereotactic radiosurgery, time to progression averaged 4–7 months and median survival was 31 months. Other complications of both of these procedures include corticosteroid dependence and risk of symptomatic radiation-induced necrosis requiring further surgery. The risk of radiation-induced necrosis for recurrent malignant gliomas is reported as 6–14%, and following brachytherapy it is as high as 26–64% (17).

The first study to address the effect of chemotherapy in anaplastic astrocytoma was reported in 1978 and included 222 subjects in a 4-arm randomized trial. Patients received radiation at doses of 50–60 Gy. The arms of the study consisted of best supportive care, RT alone, BCNU alone, and the combination of BCNU plus radiation. In each arm, patients received maximal surgical debulking. The combined group had an OS of 34.5 weeks, whereas the radiation-alone group had an OS of 35 weeks with less toxicity. From then on, radiation alone has been the standard treatment for anaplastic astrocytoma (18). Nevertheless, chemotherapy continued to be evaluated, and a phase III trial reported by Levin et al., in 1990, randomized patients with anaplastic astrocytoma and glioblastoma to receive either procarbazine, CCNU, and vincristine (PCV) or BCNU after standard RT. OS was improved in both groups, but statistically so in the anaplastic astrocytoma cohort treated with PCV; 82 versus 57 weeks in the BCNU arm (19). PCV then became the standard therapy for anaplastic astrocytoma.

Other investigators have explored the potential benefit of concomitant radiosensitizers such as BUdR (bromodeoxyuridine), an analog of thymidine, or hydroxyurea in the treatment of newly diagnosed anaplastic astrocytomas. RTOG 94–04 was a randomized phase III study published in 1999, comparing radiation therapy with or without BUdR followed by adjuvant PCV (20). There was no added benefit in OS with the addition of BUdR to radiation therapy. Another RTOG trial (RTOG 98–13) randomized patients to RT (59.4 Gy in 33 fractions) concurrently with BCNU or CCNU versus temozolomide. The trial did not meet accrual goals and closed early.

Given the conflicting results of individual clinical trials, the impact of chemotherapy on outcomes in anaplastic astrocytoma has been evaluated in several meta-analyses. One such meta-analysis retrospectively reviewed 432 patients who had been treated on 4 RTOG protocols comparing BCNU versus PCV as adjuvant chemotherapy (21). There was no added benefit to OS, again questioning the results of the earlier phase III trial (20). Another meta-analysis reviewed 16 randomized control studies and revealed an estimated OS increase of 10% at 1 year and 9% at 2 years (22). For these reasons, the addition of adjuvant chemotherapy in the treatment of anaplastic astrocytoma remains controversial.

Temozolomide has been evaluated in the setting of recurrent anaplastic astrocytoma and in fact the drug was

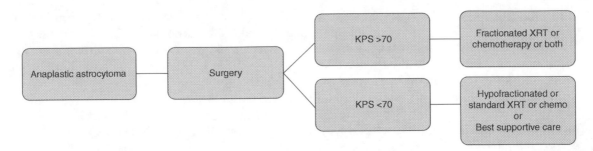

**Figure 23.4**

Algorithm for the management of anaplastic astrocytomas. XRT, external beam radiation therapy; KPS, Karnofsky performance status.

first approved by the FDA for this indication. A multi-center phase II trial enrolled 162 patients, of whom 111 were eligible. The primary endpoint for this trial, PFS at 6 months, was 46%. Median PFS was 5.4 months and median OS was 13.6 months (23). Because of a favorable toxicity profile as compared to PCV, temozolomide became the standard of care for recurrent anaplastic astrocytoma. Over the years following this study, trials in glioblastoma began to report the efficacy of temozolomide, and neuro-oncologists became familiar with its side-effect profile. Because of the toxicity of the PCV regimen, temozolomide became a more attractive alternative for use in *newly* diagnosed anaplastic astrocytoma. See Figure 23.4 for an algorithm for the management of patients with anaplastic astrocytoma.

A current ongoing trial, RTOG 0834, has been designed to shed light on these important issues. This study will determine whether concurrent and adjuvant temozolomide improves the outcome of patients with intact 1p/19q anaplastic gliomas. Patients are randomized to RT, RT with concomitant temozolomide, RT followed by adjuvant temozolomide, and RT with concurrent temozolomide followed by adjuvant temozolomide. Patients will be stratified for MGMT status as well. The primary objectives of this trial are to determine whether concomitant daily temozolomide with RT improves PFS in this tumor compared to RT alone and to determine whether adjuvant temozolomide improves OS as compared to RT alone. Secondary objectives will assess whether the addition of temozolomide prolongs PFS in patients with intact 1p, 19q anaplastic astrocytoma, as well as assess safety including long-term effects on cognition as well as quality of life.

## Oligodendroglioma

N.H. is a 34-year-old woman who presented with a sensation of transient numbness in the left toe, which gradually progressed over 2 months to involve her left foot and entire left leg. These symptoms developed during her exercise routine in the sport of kickboxing and would then dissipate. At first, she felt that it was a pinched nerve. Finally, the spells occurred while cleaning at home and

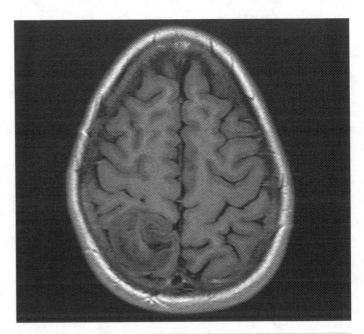

**Figure 23.5**

T1 axial contrast-enhanced MRI scan revealing a large right posterior parietal nonenhancing mass with mild associated edema.

involved shaking of her left leg. The patient presented to the ED where a CT scan was performed and revealed a right posterior parietal mass. Otherwise, her physical examination was entirely normal as was her neurological examination. An MRI scan with contrast revealed the mass to be nonenhancing (Figure 23.5). With initiation of the anticonvulsant, levetiracetam, the spells of lower extremity numbness resolved. Because of the location of the mass, the patient underwent biopsy, which revealed a low-grade oligodendroglioma. The genetic test for 1p/19q heterozygocity was performed on the sample and codeletion was reported.

N.H. went on to treatment with temozolomide at 200 mg/m$^2$ daily for 5 days every 28 days. She completed a total of 18 courses of treatment. Treatment was well tolerated with an occasional delay of 1 week for myelosuppression. MRI scans performed every 3 months revealed stable disease. N.H. is working full time and has no neurological symptoms or signs at 3.5 years postdiagnosis. She has had several sensory symptoms reminiscent of her original presentation over the years when engaged in vigorous workout. She remains on an anticonvulsant. Neurological evaluation remains normal and Karnofsky performance status (KPS) is 100%.

## Evidence-Based Case Discussion

N.H.'s case is a very typical clinical presentation of a low-grade oligodendroglioma, presenting with focal seizures, which were sensory in nature. Because of the location of the tumor, the surgeon chose to biopsy only. Surgical excision is the first line of therapy when this can be done without causing neurological deficit. The decision to proceed with RT versus chemotherapy may depend on the size of the tumor and the patient's performance status.

RT was the mainstay of treatment for this tumor until the late 1980s, when investigators noted that patients with anaplastic oligodendrogliomas responded to the multidrug regimen PCV (procarbazine, lomustine, or CCNU, and vincristine). During the next decade, researchers acquired data on survival time when this drug regimen was added to RT. Interest peaked again when certain molecular subtypes were discovered, with different natural histories and responses to treatment. Durable responses to PCV and longer OS were found to correlate with simultaneous loss of the entire short arm of chromosome 1 (1p) and the entire long arm of chromosome 19 (19q) (24). This combined deletion is usually mediated by an unbalanced translocation t(1;19)(q10;p10). 1p and 19q deletions are associated with tumors that have oligodendroglial features. In addition to its diagnostic role, 1p/19q codeletion is associated with improved survival in anaplastic oligodendroglioma and oligoastrocytomas and, as observed in 2 randomized clinical trials, predicts the benefit of combined radiation and chemotherapy as compared to radiation alone. In RTOG 9402, 289 patients with anaplastic oligodendroglioma or anaplastic oligoastrocytoma were randomized to neoadjuvant PCV (procarbazine/CCNU/vincristine) followed by RT versus RT alone (25). The primary endpoint was OS. For the entire cohort, there was no difference in survival by treatment. However, patients with 1p/19q codeleted tumors had a significantly better survival compared to those with noncodeleted tumors (median OS was 14.7 versus 2.6 years, $P < .001$ in PCV plus RT arm and 7.3 versus 2.7 years, $P < .001$ in RT alone arm). The median survival of codeleted patients receiving PCV plus RT was twice that of patients who received RT alone (14.7 vs. 7.3 years; $P = .03$), whereas patients with noncodeleted tumors did not benefit by addition of PCV to RT: median survival was 2.6 years in the PCV plus RT arm versus 2.7 years in RT alone arm ($P = .39$). In EORTC 26951, 368

patients with anaplastic oligodendroglioma were randomized to receive RT versus RT followed by 6 cycles of adjuvant PCV (26). The primary endpoints were OS and PFS based on intent to treat analysis. The OS in the RT/PCV arm was significantly better than that in the RT-alone arm (42.3 vs. 30.6 months). In 80 patients with 1p/19q codeleted tumors, OS was not reached in the RT/PCV arm versus 112 months in the RT arm. In patients with noncodeleted tumors the OS was 25 months in RT/PCV arm versus 21 months in RT alone arm. Although a trend toward improved OS was observed in noncodeleted patients receiving RT/PCV, there is a larger risk reduction in 1p/19q codeleted patients (HR = 0.56; $P = .0594$). The results of these 2 studies confirmed that tumor 1p/19q codeletion predicts for a survival benefit resulting from neoadjuvant or adjuvant PCV.

The original correlation between 1p/19q codeletion and treatment response was observed in patients treated with PCV. Further studies have shown that this susceptibility also includes temozolomide (81% response rate) that causes less toxicity than PCV (27). The NCCN recommends that in completely resected low-grade oligodendrogliomas, postoperative RT can be administered upfront or delayed. The use of front-line chemotherapy is still not definitive in low-grade oligodendrogliomas. Chemotherapy is recommended as a NCCN Category 2B recommendation in patients with stable controlled symptoms and good performance status.

Accordingly, after total gross surgical resection, the management of newly diagnosed low-grade oligodendrogliomas with codeletion of 1p/19q would involve observation versus treatment with temozolomide for 1 year (Figure 23.6). If partially resected, treatment with temozolomide versus RT is acceptable. In the recurrent setting, resection is recommended if possible, followed by chemotherapy (temozolomide or PCV) or RT if not previously delivered. In patients with intact 1p, 19q status, a gross total resection would again allow for observation or chemotherapy/radiation. If partially resected, chemotherapy or RT and close observation are warranted. As in all patients with malignant primary brain tumors, decisions for therapy will rely on patient's age, performance status, location of tumor, as well as the molecular characteristics.

The chemosensitivity of oligodendroglial tumors has made upfront chemotherapy strategies popular, with the rationale to defer RT with its known impact on cognitive skills. The molecular characteristic of 1p/19q codeletion and the mechanisms by which these tumors are sensitive to chemotherapy and RT is unknown. Nevertheless, molecular signature tends to be the most important prognostic factor for survival and will direct therapy and impact all future trials of this tumor.

In recurrent low-grade oligodendroglioma, the 1p/19q status is usually retained. However, in the salvage setting, response to temozolomide falls to 10–20%, even in the

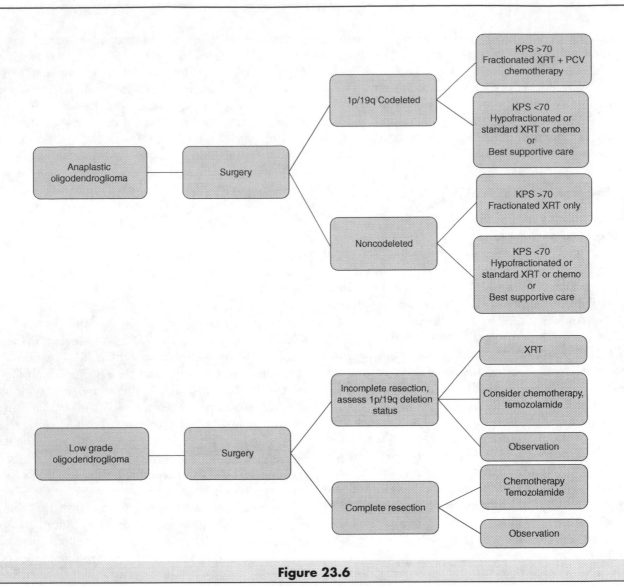

**Figure 23.6**

Algorithm for the management of anaplastic and low-grade oligodendrogliomas. KPS, Karnofsky performance status; MGMT, O-methylguanine methyltransferase; PCV, procarbazine, CCNU (lomustine), and vincristine; TMZ, temozolamide; XRT, external beam radiation therapy.

group with 1p/19q deletions. Twenty percent of low-grade oligodendroglioma tumors may recur as the anaplastic variant. In the setting of recurrent oligodendrogliomas, NCCN guidelines recommend surgery for possible resection. In unresectable lesions, RT can be administered if none was administered previously. Chemotherapy would be a reasonable option if patients previously had RT alone. Options include temozolomide if not recently prescribed, PCV, carboplatin, or etoposide.

As previously described, anaplastic (grade III) oligodendrogliomas with losses of chromosome 1p and 19q are particularly responsive to chemotherapy. Whereas the results of the 2 trials previously outlined verified that the upfront combination of PCV plus RT improved survival in patients with anaplastic oligodendroglial tumors with 1p/19q codeletion, the optimal treatment sequence has not yet been established. Accordingly, after total gross surgical resection, the management of newly diagnosed anaplastic oligodendroglioma, with codeletion of 1p/19q, would involve chemotherapy plus RT (Figure 23.6). It is unknown whether chemotherapy should precede or follow RT, or whether PCV or TMZ should be used. There are ongoing trials, which may help answer these unanswered questions.

## REVIEW QUESTIONS

1. A 52-year-old man with no significant past medical history presented with 2 days of bifrontal headache without any motor or sensory deficits. A brain MRI revealed 3.1 × 4.8 × 3.4 cm heterogeneous T2 hyperintense, heterogeneously enhancing necrotic lesion in the left inferior temporal gyrus with confluent T2 FLAIR hyperintensities extending to surrounding temporal

lobe. He underwent left craniotomy and resection of the mass. Pathology revealed a glioblastoma (World Health Organization 2007 grade IV). A postoperative MRI brain revealed no residual disease. He went on to receive concurrent chemoradiation with 60 Gy and temozolomide 75 mg/m² daily. On completion of chemoradiation, at the 2-month mark, an MRI brain was done that revealed increased enhancement along the margin of surgical cavity. The patient was asymptomatic without any neurological deficits. What is the next best step?

(A) Craniotomy and biopsy
(B) Start bevacizumab because this is disease progression
(C) After a 4-week break from end of chemoradiation, start temozolomide 150 mg/m² daily for 5 days per 28-day cycle
(D) Initiate palliative care

2. A 48-year-old man presented with new onset seizures. A brain MRI revealed a 4.3 × 4.0 × 3.4 cm mass in right frontal lobe. He underwent a craniotomy and partial resection of mass. Pathology demonstrated an anaplastic oligodendroglioma (World Health Organization 2007 grade III). Tumor 1p/19q codeletion is detected. What is the best management for this patient?

(A) 60 Gy radiation therapy
(B) 60 Gy radiation therapy followed by adjuvant procarbazine, CCNU, and vincristine (PCV) chemotherapy
(C) Serial brain MRI
(D) Start temozolomide postoperative 150 mg/m² for 5 days in 28-day cycle

3. A 42-year-old woman with history of 2.4 × 2.5 × 2 cm right paramedial parietal lobe glioblastoma multiforme was initially treated with resection and concurrent temozolomide and 60 Gy radiation. She is currently on cycle 3, day 21, of adjuvant temozolomide 200 mg/m². She presents with left arm twitching and loss of consciousness. The brain MRI revealed a new 2.2 × 2.6 cm mass centered in right paracentral lobule. She underwent resection of mass and pathology was consistent with a glioblastoma (World Health Organization grade IV). She has no neurological deficits and has a good Karnofsky performance status >70. What is the next step in terms of treatment?

(A) Continue temozolomide
(B) Start irinotecan
(C) Start bevacizumab
(D) Palliative care

4. A 45-year-old man presented with new onset seizures and a brain MRI revealed a 3.4 × 2.6 cm mass in the left temporal lobe. Craniotomy and resection of the mass was performed and the pathology was consistent with glioblastoma (World Health Organization

grade IV). Additional studies revealed methylated O-methylguanine methyltransferase (MGMT) promoter. The patient questions you about the significance of this test. Explain that:

(A) Status of MGMT methylation needs to be determined before starting treatment because it helps decide whether or not temozolamide should be used
(B) Patients with MGMT methylation have an improved survival but knowledge of its status will not change management for this patient
(C) Methylation of MGMT is marker for poor prognosis
(D) MGMT promoter methylation status provides no additional information regarding the patient's prognosis

5. A 59-year-old man presented with altered mental status. Brain imaging revealed a 3.1 × 2.8 × 3.3 cm mass in the right temporal region. Craniotomy and resection revealed grade IV glioblastoma. What is the best course of management of this patient?

(A) Radiation 60 Gy followed by temozolomide 200 mg/m² for 5 days every 28 days
(B) Temozolomide 75 mg/m² daily followed by radiation 60 Gy
(C) Concurrent chemoradiation with temozolomide 75 mg/m² daily with radiation 60 Gy followed by temozolomide 150–200 mg/m² for 5 days every 28 days for at least 6 cycles
(D) Concurrent chemoradiation with temozolomide 75 mg/m² daily with radiation 60 Gy only

6. A 76-year-old woman is seen in the emergency department complaining of a severe headache. Imaging revealed a 3 × 3.2 cm mass in left temporal lobe. Maximal safe resection was performed and path revealed glioblastoma multiforme. The patient does not have any neurological deficits and has Karnofsky performance status >60. What would constitute best management for this patient?

(A) Concurrent temozolomide and radiation followed by adjuvant temozolomide
(B) Hypofractionated radiotherapy or temozolomide alone
(C) Standard radiotherapy
(D) Bevacizumab alone

7. A 35-year-old man presented to the emergency department following a generalized seizure at home. A CT revealed a calcified left frontal mass measuring 3.1 × 2.4 × 1.5 cm. He underwent gross total removal of the lesion. The pathology was consistent with anaplastic astrocytoma. Chromosome studies revealed an intact 1p, but deleted 19q. IDH1 was wild type. The

patient was treated with radiotherapy, 6000 cGy, to the involved field followed by 6 months of temozolomide as adjuvant therapy, at 150–200 mg daily × 5 every 28 days. He was then followed with brain MRI every 3 months. He did well for 2 years, but then a local recurrence was noted on routine follow-up MRI. What is the best course of action at this time?

(A) Consider stereotactic radiotherapy
(B) Treatment with bevacizumab
(C) Reoperation to verify pathology, and reinitiate treatment with temozolomide
(D) Re-resection and stereotactic radiotherapy

8. A 40-year-old woman has a recent history of focal motor seizures involving the left arm and leg. She presents for neurological evaluation and an MRI is ordered. It reveals a 2.5 × 3.0 × 3.2 cm mass in the right frontal lobe, infiltrating into the motor strip. A subtotal resection is performed and the pathology is read as low-grade oligodendroglioma. Chromosome studies revealed codeletion of 1p/19q. Which of the following is the best treatment option for this patient?

(A) Observation alone
(B) Stereotactic radiotherapy
(C) Radiotherapy and concomitant temozolomide followed by temozolomide as adjuvant chemotherapy
(D) Treatment with temozolomide, on the 5-day regimen every 28 days

9. A 58-year-old man is diagnosed with a glioblastoma of the left occipital lobe. He undergoes gross total resection. Molecular studies demonstrate that the tumor is O-methylguanine methyltransferase unmethylated. His performance status is 90%. He has a right visual field defect. What would be the recommended treatment for this patient?

(A) Radiation with concomitant temozolomide followed by adjuvant temozolomide (Stupp regimen)
(B) Radiation alone
(C) Radiation plus temozolomide plus bevacizumab
(D) Hypofractionated radiotherapy plus temozolomide

## REFERENCES

1. Ostrom QT, Gittleman H, Liao P, et al. CBTRUS statistical report: primary brain and central nervous system tumors diagnosed in the United States in 2007–2011. *Neuro Oncol.* 2014;16(suppl 4):ii1–ii63.

2. Lacroix M, Abi-Said D, Fourney DR, et al. A multivariate analysis of 416 patients with glioblastoma multiforme: prognosis, extent of resection, and survival. *J Neurosurg.* 2001;95(2):190–198.

3. Keime-Guibert F, Chinot O, Taillandier L, et al.; Association of French-Speaking Neuro-Oncologists. Radiotherapy for glioblastoma in the elderly. *N Engl J Med.* 2007;356(15):1527–1535.

4. Wen PY, Macdonald DR, Reardon DA, et al. Updated response assessment criteria for high-grade gliomas: response assessment in neuro-oncology working group. *J Clin Oncol.* 2010;28(11):1963–1972.

5. Walker MD, Green SB, Byar DP, et al. Randomized comparisons of radiotherapy and nitrosoureas for the treatment of malignant glioma after surgery. *N Engl J Med.* 1980;303(23):1323–1329.

6. Medical Research Council Brain Tumor Working Party. Randomized trial of procarbazine, lomustine, and vincristine in the adjuvant treatment of high-grade astrocytoma: a Medical Research Council Trial. *J Clin Oncol.* 2001;(19):509–518.

7. Stupp R, Hegi ME, Mason WP, et al.; European Organisation for Research and Treatment of Cancer Brain Tumour and Radiation Oncology Groups; National Cancer Institute of Canada Clinical Trials Group. Effects of radiotherapy with concomitant and adjuvant temozolomide versus radiotherapy alone on survival in glioblastoma in a randomised phase III study: 5-year analysis of the EORTC-NCIC trial. *Lancet Oncol.* 2009;10(5):459–466.

8. Gilbert MR, Wang M, Aldape KD, et al. RTOG 0525: A randomized phase III trial comparing standard adjuvant temozolomide (TMZ) with a dose-dense (dd) schedule in newly diagnosed glioblastoma (GBM) *J Clin Oncol.* 2011;29(abstract 2006).

9. Reifenberger G, Hentschel B, Felsberg J, et al.; German Glioma Network. Predictive impact of MGMT promoter methylation in glioblastoma of the elderly. *Int J Cancer.* 2012;131(6):1342–1350.

10. Wick W, Platten M, Meisner C, et al.; NOA-08 Study Group of Neuro-oncology Working Group (NOA) of German Cancer Society. Temozolomide chemotherapy alone versus radiotherapy alone for malignant astrocytoma in the elderly: the NOA-08 randomised, phase 3 trial. *Lancet Oncol.* 2012;13(7):707–715.

11. Malmstrom A, Grønberg BH, Marosi C, et al. Temozolomide versus standard 6-week radiotherapy versus hypofractionated radiotherapy for patients aged over 60 years with glioblastoma: the Nordic randomized phase 3 trial. *Lancet Oncol.* 2012;13(9):916–926.

12. Westphal M, Hilt DC, Bortey E, et al. A phase 3 trial of local chemotherapy with biodegradable carmustine (BCNU) wafers (Gliadel wafers) in patients with primary malignant glioma. *Neuro-oncology.* 2003;5(2):79–88.

13. Vredenburgh JJ, Desjardins A, Herndon JE 2nd, et al. Bevacizumab plus irinotecan in recurrent glioblastoma multiforme. *J Clin Oncol.* 2007;25(30):4722–4729.

14. Friedman HS, Prados MD, Wen PY, et al. Bevacizumab alone and in combination with irinotecan in recurrent glioblastoma. *J Clin Oncol.* 2009;27(28):4733–4740.

15. Gilbert MR, Dignam JJ, Armstrong TS, et al. A randomized trial of bevacizumab for newly diagnosed glioblastoma. *N Engl J Med.* 2014;370(8):699–708.

16. Stupp R, Kanner A, Engelhard H, et al. A prospective, randomized, open-label, phase III clinical trial of NovoTTF-100A versus best standard of care chemotherapy in patients with recurrent glioblastoma [abstract]. *Proc ASCO. J Clin Oncol.* 2010;(28): LBA2007.

17. Laperriere NJ, Leung PM, McKenzie S, et al. Randomized study of brachytherapy in the initial management of patients with malignant astrocytoma. *Int J Radiat Oncol Biol Phys.* 1998;41(5): 1005–1011.

18. Walker MD, Alexander E Jr, Hunt WE, et al. Evaluation of BCNU and/or radiotherapy in the treatment of anaplastic gliomas. A cooperative clinical trial. *J Neurosurg.* 1978;49(3):333–343.

19. Levin VA, Silver P, Hannigan J, et al. Superiority of post-radiotherapy adjuvant chemotherapy with CCNU, procarbazine, and vincristine (PCV) over BCNU for anaplastic gliomas: NCOG 6G61 final report. *Int J Radiat Oncol Biol Phys.* 1990;18(2):321–324.

20. Prados MD, Scott C, Sandler H, et al. A phase 3 randomized study of radiotherapy plus procarbazine, CCNU, and vincristine (PCV) with or without BUdR for the treatment of anaplastic astrocytoma: a preliminary report of RTOG 9404. *Int J Radiat Oncol Biol Phys.* 1999;45(5):1109–1115.

21. Prados MD, Scott C, Curran WJ Jr, et al. Procarbazine, lomustine, and vincristine (PCV) chemotherapy for anaplastic astrocytoma: a retrospective review of radiation therapy oncology group

protocols comparing survival with carmustine or PCV adjuvant chemotherapy. *J Clin Oncol.* 1999;17(11):3389–3395.

22. Fine HA, Dear KB, Loeffler JS, et al. Meta-analysis of radiation therapy with and without adjuvant chemotherapy for malignant gliomas in adults. *Cancer.* 1993;71(8):2585–2597.

23. Yung WK, Prados MD, Yaya-Tur R, et al. Multicenter phase II trial of temozolomide in patients with anaplastic astrocytoma or anaplastic oligoastrocytoma at first relapse. Temodal Brain Tumor Group. *J Clin Oncol.* 1999;17(9):2762–2771.

24. Jenkins RB, Curran W, Scott CB, et al. Pilot evaluation of 1p and 19q deletions in anaplastic oligodendrogliomas collected by a national cooperative cancer treatment group. *Am J Clin Oncol.* 2001;24(5):506–508.

25. Cairncross G, Berkey B, Shaw E, et al. Phase III trial of chemotherapy plus radiotherapy compared with radiotherapy alone for pure and mixed anaplastic oligodendroglioma: Intergroup Radiation Therapy Oncology Group Trial 9401. *J Clin Oncol.* 2008;24:2707–2714.

26. van den Bent MJ, Brandes AA, Taphoorn MJ, et al. Adjuvant procarbazine, lomustine, and vincristine chemotherapy in newly diagnosed anaplastic oligodendroglioma: long-term follow-up of EORTC brain tumor group study 26951. *J Clin Oncol.* 2013;31(3):344–350.

27. Kouwenhoven MC, Kros JM, French PJ, et al. 1p/19q loss within oligodendroglioma is predictive for response to first line temozolomide but not to salvage treatment. *Eur J Cancer.* 2006;42(15):2499–2503.

# 24

# Cancer of Unknown Primary

MIHO TERUYA, YUVAL RAIZEN, AND GERALD S. CYPRUS

## EPIDEMIOLOGY, RISK FACTORS, NATURAL HISTORY, AND PATHOLOGY

The overall incidence of patients with cancer of unknown primary (CUP) is difficult to predict accurately because of the variability in patient presentation as well as frequent classification of tumors as specific to other diagnoses. On the basis of the statistics reported by the Surveillance, Epidemiology, and End Results (SEER) registries between 1973 and 1987, CUPs account for about 2% of all cancer diagnoses. Siegel et al. reported an incidence of 31,860 new cases of "other and unspecified primary sites" in the United States in 2013. This accounts for 1.9% of all cancers diagnosed during this year, with a very slight predominance in females. In this report, 7.8% of all cancer deaths were attributed to CUP (1). In other studies, the incidence was as high as 7%. This entity has been reported to be among the top 10 most common cancer diagnoses worldwide. Based on epidemiological data from the World Health Organization (WHO) and International Agency for Research on Cancer summarized by Ferlay et al., SEER, and local registries from Australia, there was a 1.2–3.9% incidence, as shown in Table 24.1 (2,3).

The median age at presentation is approximately 60 years. It is infrequently seen in children, accounting for <1% of cancer diagnoses, with those rare cases being mostly embryonal malignancies (such as small round blue cell tumors). There have not been any risk factors identified as an etiology for the development of CUP. The median overall survival in patients with carcinoma of unknown primary is reported to be between 4 and 9 months.

These tumors are often characterized by an aggressive nature and poor overall prognosis. Multiple metastatic sites are frequently observed due to early dissemination. As opposed to common metastatic patterns seen in known primary solid tumors, the pattern of metastasis is frequently unpredictable. An example of this difference is the frequency of bone metastases in patients with lung cancer presenting as CUP (4%) compared with those presenting as a known lung cancer primary (30–50%) (4). Almost 30% of patients with CUP present with metastases in >1 location. Metastases are seen in the liver in 24%, lung or pleura in 12%, lymph nodes in 11%, peritoneum in 9%, bone in 8%, brain in 2%, and other sites in 8%.

Evaluation of the tumor using light microscopy with hematoxylin and eosin (H&E) staining is often not sufficient to classify the histological subtype. Use of specialized pathological studies including immunohistochemical (IHC) markers, tumor markers, and specific cytogenetic alterations may assist in further classification. Various imaging modalities are also being used with increased frequency to narrow the differential diagnosis. According to a 1982 study by Neumann and Nystrom, the primary site may not be identified even in a postmortem examination in up to 20–50% of cases (5). In a more recent review of previously published autopsy studies (as well as studies using microarray technology), a primary site was identified in 73% of the cases. Among the sites identified, the reported relative frequencies by Pentheroudakis et al. were 27% lung, 19% pancreas, 11% bowel, 6% kidney/adrenals, 6% hepatobiliary, 5% gastric, 3% ovary/uterus, 2% prostate, and 21% "other," as seen in Figure 24.1 (6). Notably breast was found to be the primary site with an incidence of <1%.

There is no clear evidence suggesting that CUPs are distinct phenomena with unique alterations in genetics and phenotypic expression. Thus far, no consistent abnormalities have been identified that are common between different CUPs. There is also no evidence that there are genetic differences between these tumors, which tend to have an atypical metastatic pattern, and those tumors with

**Table 24.1** Epidemiology of Cancer of Unknown Primary

| Geographical Area | Source | Incidence (%) | Period |
|---|---|---|---|
| USA | SEER | 1.9 | 2013 |
| Australia | AACR | 2.5 | 2009 |
| The Netherlands | IARC | 3.9 | 2012 |
| Finland | IARC | 2.5 | 2012 |
| Germany | IARC | 2.0 | 2012 |
| Russian Federation | IARC | 1.2 | 2012 |
| Switzerland | IARC | 1.6 | 2012 |

AACR, Australian Association of Cancer Registries; IARC, International Agency for Research Into Cancer; SEER, Surveillance, Epidemiology, and End Results.
*Source:* Adapted with permission from Ref. (4). Pavlidis N, Briasoulis E, Hainsworth J, et al. Diagnostic and therapeutic management of cancer of an unknown primary. *Eur J Cancer.* 2003;39(14):1990–2005.

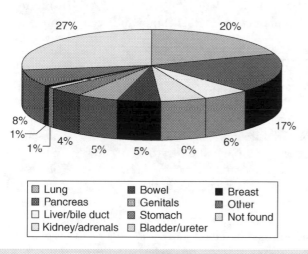

27% 20% 8% 1% 1% 4% 5% 5% 6% 6% 17%

| | | |
|---|---|---|
| ☒ Lung | ▨ Bowel | ■ Breast |
| ▨ Pancreas | ▨ Genitals | ▨ Other |
| ☐ Liver/bile duct | ▨ Stomach | ▨ Not found |
| ☐ Kidney/adrenals | ▨ Bladder/ureter | |

**Figure 24.1**

Distribution of sites of origin in cancer of unknown primary. *Source:* Used with permission from Ref. (6). Pentheroudakis G, Golfinopoulos V, Pavlidis N. Switching benchmarks in cancer of unknown primary: from autopsy to microarray. *Eur J Cancer.* 2007;43(14):2026–2036.

metastases from a known primary site. An area of interest is in the explanation of why the primary is not identifiable and several hypotheses have been proposed to explain why the primary site is not identifiable (7). These include involution or regression of the primary after the metastasis occurs. Some tumors may have arisen from fully differentiated embryonic epithelial cells that did not complete their migration in utero, thus presenting as a "metastatic" lesion. Alternatively, the primary neoplasm remains unrecognized because of its small size or location (obscured by surrounding tissue). A sequence of genetic events during carcinogenesis supports metastatic but not local growth (8). Finally, CUPs may arise from yet undifferentiated pluripotent cells, which remain present in postnatal life, and display an ability to differentiate into multiple lineages (7).

## STAGING

Although other tumors are customarily staged using systems such as the WHO, CUPs are by definition metastatic and are therefore not assigned a staging system. The challenge in assigning a staging system to CUPs lies in the previously mentioned heterogeneity of the diseases with wide range of histopathology. For purposes of this chapter as well as clinical practice, CUPs are considered metastatic by definition.

## CASE SUMMARIES

### Pathological Evaluation and Role of IHC

J.H., a 52-year-old man with a history of hypertension, presented to his primary care physician with a 3-month history of vague abdominal pain associated with a 15-pound weight loss. Prior to this, he had been healthy, only taking antihypertensive medication. He complained of early satiety with occasional nausea and nonbilious, nonbloody emesis, but normal bowel movements. He had an unremarkable colonoscopy at age 50 years. J.H.'s mother had breast cancer in her 60s, but his family was otherwise healthy. He denied smoking or drug use, and drank alcohol socially. His lifestyle had been active and he worked as a restaurant manager. His physical examination revealed a soft but tender abdomen, mostly in the right upper quadrant, with palpable hepatomegaly of 17 cm. Laboratory studies showed a mild normocytic anemia, moderate hypoalbuminemia, and elevated aspartate aminotransferase (AST) and alanine transaminase (ALT). HIV and hepatitis tests were negative. A chest x-ray was unremarkable. Right upper quadrant ultrasound showed a number of masses in the liver with hepatomegaly. A CT of the chest, abdomen, and pelvis revealed 6 discrete masses in the enlarged liver, the largest measuring 3.3 cm. A number of enlarged retroperitoneal and perihepatic nodes were noted as well. Percutaneous CT-guided biopsy of one of the hepatic masses was performed, with pathology showing adenocarcinoma, with no further characterization or site of origin. Upper endoscopy and colonoscopy did not reveal any masses and were mostly unremarkable. An IHC panel showed that the tumor was cytokeratin (CK)7– and CK20+, as well as CDX-2+. With this information, he was offered chemotherapy targeted at treating metastatic adenocarcinoma of colon origin.

### Evidence-Based Case Discussion

#### Initial Pathological Evaluation

The case of J.H. highlights the importance of the pathological evaluation of unknown cancer, as well as the role of IHC in determining the tissue site of origin. A stepwise approach, as described by Oien, can help direct this process (9).

CUP is classified into a number of histological groups, with about 50–60% being classified as well-to-moderately differentiated adenocarcinomas. Approximately 30% are classified as undifferentiated or poorly differentiated carcinoma, 5–15% as squamous cell carcinoma, 5% as undifferentiated neoplasm, and 1% as either well differentiated or poorly differentiated neuroendocrine carcinoma (7,10). With evolving techniques, pathologists have been able to more precisely identify not only the histology but the origin of the malignancy. A close collaboration between the pathologist and the medical oncologist is important in determining the management and optimal therapy of a CUP.

The initial pathological evaluation includes staining of the tissue with H&E with review under light microscopy, often to determine histological subtype. Light microscopy classifies 60% of cases as adenocarcinoma, 5% as squamous cell carcinoma, with the other 35% not clearly being classified, either as poorly differentiated adenocarcinoma, poorly differentiated carcinoma, or poorly differentiated neoplasm (11). Light microscopy alone infrequently identifies the site of origin in patients with CUP. After inspection by light microscopy, the tumor can then be subjected to IHC investigation, using peroxidase-labeled antibodies against specific tumor antigens, performed on paraffin-embedded, formalin-fixed tissue. To rule out lymphoma, germ cell tumor, and melanoma, antibodies against epithelial antigens (pan-CKs); lymphoid antigens (CD45, CD20, and CD3); melanotic antigens (PS100 and HMB45); and germ cell tumor antigens (alpha-fetoprotein [AFP], beta human chorionic gonadotropin [βhCG], and placental-like alkaline phosphatase [PLAP]) are employed (12). Notably none of the IHC tests is 100% specific and should thus be interpreted with caution, correlating the findings with the patient's clinical presentation.

## Electron Microscopy

As IHC markers have been identified, the use of electron microscopy has fallen out of favor. It is disadvantageous in that it is expensive, not readily available, and time consuming. The use of electron microscopy has been essentially limited to situations in which patients are found to have poorly differentiated neoplasms with inconclusive immunoperoxidase staining.

## Tumor Markers

Certain serum tumor markers may be helpful in ascertaining a primary tumor site, such as the prostate-specific antigen (PSA), βhCG, and alpha-fetoprotein (AFP). On the other hand, certain tumor markers commonly used as surrogate measures of response to therapy, such as carcinoembryonic antigen (CEA), CA125, CA19–9, and CA15–3, are not especially helpful in establishing the site of the primary cancer. This is due to the lack of specificity of these tests. Although their use in establishing the primary tumor is limited, these tumor markers play more of a prognostic role.

## Cytogenetics

Conventional cytogenetics do not offer a significant advantage in narrowing a diagnosis, as few cytogenetic abnormalities specific to particular tumors have been found. One chromosomal alteration, isochrome 12p-i, is seen in about 25% of patients with testicular carcinoma or other germ cell tumors. In addition to the predictive value of this cytogenetic abnormality, it is also prognostic in that patients with this abnormality have been noted to have a high sensitivity to chemotherapy for germ cell tumors. Other chromosomal abnormalities that have been found specific to particular tumors include t(11;22) in primitive neuroectodermal tumors (PNET), desmoplastic small round cell tumors, and Ewing's sarcoma. In some cases where the diagnosis of lymphoma is not initially evident, cytogenetics can be helpful, such as the presence of t(8;14) (q24;q32) in non-Hodgkin lymphoma, t(14;18) in follicular lymphoma, and t(11;14) in mantle cell lymphoma.

## Approaching the Diagnosis of CUP

The initial approach once a biopsy is obtained is to determine that the abnormal cells are present within that biopsy specimen. Once that is confirmed, an assessment of whether those cells are malignant is made based on the presence of a "foreign" cell population, cytologic features, and abnormal architectural features, such as invasiveness. When a biopsy shows malignant cells, a decision must be made on their general classification as representing a carcinoma, germ cell tumor, melanoma, lymphoma, or sarcoma. This can often be distinguished based on morphology as seen by light microscopy (Figure 24.2). If a morphological evaluation is not sufficient to distinguish the general tumor type, a "first-line" IHC panel is performed. This panel typically includes an epithelial marker to evaluate for carcinomas, such as pan-CK. It would also include a melanocytic marker like S100 and a lymphoid marker like common leukocyte antigen (CLA). A second-line panel is then performed based on the positivity of the first-line markers. Additional melanocyte markers to evaluate for melanoma include Melan-A and HMB45, which are less sensitive than S100 but more specific. Positive IHC staining with these antibodies in the absence of staining with other first-line IHC markers is suggestive of melanoma. See Table 24.2 for a list of commonly used IHC markers. A number of additional markers that can be used in differentiating melanoma, lymphoma, and sarcoma, as well as further subclassification can be found in Figure 24.3.

## Lymphoma

The use of CLA is both very sensitive and specific for lymphoma, thus making the broad diagnosis of lymphoma much easier. Two lymphoid neoplasms, anaplastic large cell lymphoma (ALCL) and granulocytic sarcoma (chloroma of myeloid leukemia), are typically negative for

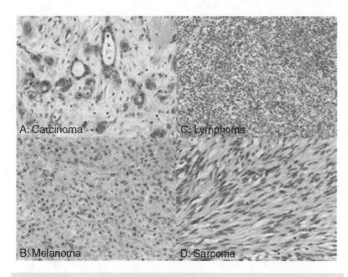

**Figure 24.2**

Microscopic appearance of cancer types. Carcinoma, as seen in (A), can be described as cohesive cells with a cuboidal or columnar shape, lying in tubules and glands. Melanoma, as seen in (B) with cohesive cells with large nuclei, prominent nucleoli, and abundant brown melanin pigment. Lymphoma (C) has uniform small round lymphoid cells with little cytoplasm. Sarcoma (D) has cells with an elongated spindle shape, lying in sheets. *Source*: The figures are used with permission from Ref. (9). Oien KA. Pathologic evaluation of cancer of unknown primary. *Semin Oncol.* 2009;36(1):8–37.

CLA. To evaluate for these lymphoid malignancies, additional IHC markers are tested. ALCL is generally positive for either anaplastic lymphoma kinase protein (ALK1) or CD30. Granulocytic sarcomas are typically positive for myeloid markers, including CD15, CD43, CD68, and others. Once a diagnosis of lymphoma is made, additional markers can be used to further subtype, including B-cell markers CD20 and CD79a, T-cell markers such as CD3; plasmacytic markers CD38 and CD138; CD30 positivity in Hodgkin lymphoma, as well as others.

## Sarcoma

Sarcoma markers are typically not included in the initial IHC panel because sarcomas are uncommon in CUP. If a general tumor type is not established with the first-line IHC panel, a second panel can be performed for evaluation of sarcoma. No single marker is used with high sensitivity for sarcoma. Vimentin is present in most sarcoma because it is present in most mesenchymal cells. It is also seen, however, in many carcinomas as well as 96% of melanomas. Other markers used in evaluating for sarcoma include smooth muscle actin (SMA), desmin, MyoD1, myogenin, S100, c-kit (CD117), CD34, and CD99.

## Carcinoma

The most frequent general tumor types presenting as a CUP are carcinomas, which can be further subcategorized

**Table 24.2** Immunohistochemical Markers Useful in the Diagnosis of Carcinoma of Unknown Primary

**Abbreviations**

| | |
|---|---|
| CK | Cytokeratins $KL_1$, CK5/6, CK7, CK19, CK20, carcinoma markers |
| CD45 | Leukocyte differentiation antigens |
| PS 100 | Protein S100 |
| CD20 | B lymphocyte |
| CD3 | T lymphocyte |
| EMA | Epithelial membrane antigen |
| CD30 | Activation antigen |
| ALK | Anaplastic lymphoma kinase |
| HMB45, melan A | Melanic markers |
| SMA | Smooth muscle actin |
| SMD | Striated muscle desmin |
| CD31, CD34 | Vascular "markers" |
| CD68 | Histiocyte "marker" |
| CD99 | Peripheral neuroectodermal tumor (PNET) "marker" |
| CD117 | c-Kit protein |
| VIM | Vimentin |
| Calretin, HBME1, WT1 | Mesothelial markers |
| PLAP | Placental alkaline phosphatase |
| AFP | Alpha-fetoprotein |
| βhCG | Beta human chorionic gonadotropin |
| CGA | Chromogranin A |
| SYN | Synaptophysin |
| NSE | Neurone-specific enolase |
| CEA | Carcinoembryonic antigen |
| Hep Par1 | Hepatocellular antigen |
| PSA | Prostate-specific antigen |
| TTF1 | Thyroid transcription factor 1 |
| GCDFP | Gross cystic disease fluid protein |
| ER | Estrogen receptor |
| PR | Progesterone receptor |
| GFAP | Glial fibrillary acidic protein |
| NF | Neurofilaments |

*Source*: Adapted with permission from Ref. (12). Bugat R, Bataillard A, Lesimple T, et al. Summary of the standards, options, and recommendations for the management of patients with carcinoma of unknown primary site (2002). *Br J Cancer.* 2003;89(suppl. 1):S59–S66.

into adenocarcinomas; squamous cell carcinomas; carcinomas arising from liver, kidney, or endocrine glands; neuroendocrine tumors; and germ cell tumors. Aside from initial evaluation based on morphology, use of IHC is valuable in further categorizing tumor types.

### Adenocarcinomas

Adenocarcinomas make up at least 60% of CUPs. The diagnosis of adenocarcinoma based on biopsy is suggested by the presence of glandular morphology. Occasionally, the specific morphology of the adenocarcinoma can be suggestive of the primary site, with morphology able to correctly identify the primary site in about 25% of cases.

**Carcinoma**

- Positive epithelial markers such as pancytokeratin
- Squamous cell carcinoma: CD 5/6, p63
- Solid organ carcinomas
  - Lung carcinoma: TTF-1, napsin A
  - Gastrointestinal carcinoma: CDX-2
  - Breast carcinoma: ER, PR, HER2, GCDFP-15, MGB1
  - Hepatocellular carcinoma: Hepar-1; AFP; polyclonal CEA, CD10, or CD 13
  - Renal clear cell carcinoma: RCC, CD10, aquaporin-1, PAX-2
  - Papillary and follicular thyroid carcinoma: TTF1, Thyroglobulin
  - Gynecologic carcinomas: CA125, WT1, mesothelin
  - Medullary thyroid carcinoma: calcitonin
- Germ cell tumor: PLAP, OCT4 (embryonal carcinoma and seminoma), AFP (yolk sac tumor), HCG (choriocarcinoma)
- Neuorendocrine carcinoma: Chromogranin, synaptophysin, PGP9.5, CD56, TTF-1 (small cell carcinomas), CDX2 (intestinal carcinoid tumors)
- Adrenocortical carcinoma: Alpha-inhibin, Melan-A

**Melanoma**

- Melanocyte markers
  - S100
  - HMB-45 and Melan-A (less sensitive, not more specific than S100)

**Sarcoma**

- Vimentin, alpha smooth muscle actin, (SMA) despin, myoD1, myogenie, CD34, ckit (CD117), and CD99
- S100 melanocyte marker positive in nerve sheath tumors

**Lymphoma**

- Positive lymphoid markers such as CLA (CD45RB)
- B-cell markers: CD20, CD79a
- T-cell marker: CD3
- Anaplastic large cell lymphoma: ALK1 and CD30
- Granulocytic sarcoma: myeloid markers; e.g., CD15, CD43, CD68, myeloperoxidase
- Hodgkin lyphoma: CD30
- Plasmacytic markers: CD38, CD138

**Figure 24.3**

Initial immunohistochemical panel for broad cancer types with additional panels for subtyping.

IHC is used to further narrow the differential diagnosis, as was done in the case of J.H., ultimately determining that his cancer was most likely of colon origin. The most frequently used IHC markers are the CK, which are cytoplasmic filaments that are specific to epithelial cells and are the key positive marker of carcinomas. Tumor sites of origin can be narrowed using monoclonal antibodies to specific subtypes of CK, most commonly 2 low-molecular-weight CKs, CK7, and CK20. A general guideline for the interpretation of the CK7/CK20 phenotype is seen in Figure 24.4 (5). CK7 is normally expressed in simple glandular epithelium, and is seen in tumors of the lung, breast, pancreas, biliary tract, ovary, endometrium, and transitional epithelium. Expression of CK7 is notably absent in lower gastrointestinal tract tumors. CK20 is expressed in gastrointestinal epithelium (especially colon), urothelium, and Merkel neuroendocrine cells of the skin. CK5 is expressed in the basal cells of squamous epithelium, as well as mesothelium. Analysis of the expression pattern of CK7 and CK20 can give the clinician a suggestion of the origin of the tumor, especially detailed subtyping of adenocarcinomas. A tumor that stains CK20−/CK7+ suggests that the tumor is most likely of lung (adenocarcinoma), breast, hepatobiliary, pancreatic, ovarian, endometrium, or transitional cell in origin. Upto 85% of carcinomas of lung origin stain positive for CK7, whereas only up to 15% stain positive for CK20. A tumor that stains CK20+/CK7− favors a lower gastrointestinal origin, such as colorectal or less likely, Merkel cell carcinoma. Positive staining for both CK7 and CK20 favors an upper gastrointestinal or urothelial–transitional cell carcinoma, whereas negative staining for both favors prostatic, renal, or liver carcinomas. Notably, expression of CK20 is mostly absent in lung adenocarcinoma, as well as

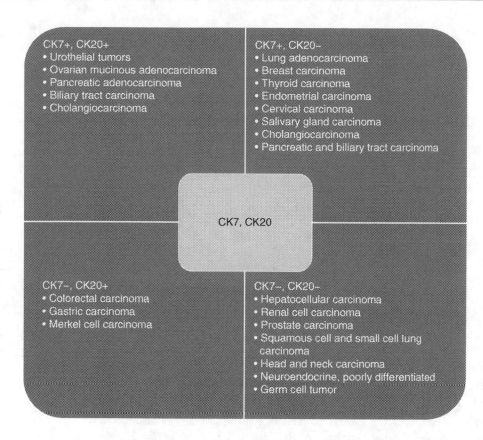

**Figure 24.4**

The use of cytokeratin markers.
*Source*: Adapted with permission from
Ref. (11). Varadhachary GR, Abbruzzese
JL, Lenzi R. Diagnostic strategies for
unknown primary cancer. *Cancer*.
2004;100(9):1776–1785.

carcinomas of the breast and prostate. A high false-positive and false-negative rate exists for these studies and care should be used when using these staining phenotypes alone in making a diagnosis of a primary site. A schematic approach to evaluating CK7 and CK20 phenotype can be found in Figure 24.4.

Other IHC markers used to distinguish CUPs include thyroid transcription factor-1 (TTF-1), thyroglobulin, gross cystic fibrous protein-15 (GCDFP-15), uroplakin III (UROIII), CDX-2, Wilm's tumor-1 (WT-1), and hep par 1. TTF-1 is a nuclear protein that is important in transcriptional activation during embryogenesis in the thyroid diencephalon and respiratory epithelium, and is thus positive frequently in carcinomas of the lung and thyroid. Thyroglobulin is a very specific marker for both papillary and follicular thyroid carcinoma. GCDFP-15 is a marker of apocrine differentiation, specifically seen with high frequency (62–72%) in patients with carcinoma of the breast. It is also found in the skin, salivary gland, bronchial gland, prostate, and seminal vesicle. UROIII positivity suggests urothelial origin because the monoclonal antibody to UROIII is positive in up to 60% of primary urothelial cancers and 50% of metastatic urothelial cancers. This coexpressed with CK20, which is present in almost 50% of urothelial carcinomas, is strongly suggestive of urothelial origin. Caudal-type homeobox transcription factor-2, that is, CDX-2, is normally found in the nucleus of intestinal epithelial cells from the proximal duodenum to the rectum. It is present in up to 90%

of adenocarcinomas of the colon. A phenotype of CK7−/ CK20+/CDX-2+ is highly suggestive of colon primary. It is also present in up to 30% of gastroesophageal adenocarcinomas, but rarely seen in pancreaticobiliary tumors. In addition to gastrointestinal tumors, all primary bladder adenocarcinomas express CDX-2, as do about 65% of ovarian mucinous adenocarcinomas. WT1 is a marker for epithelioid mesothelioma, and it is also found to be positive in most cases of ovarian serous carcinoma. Hep par 1 expression is seen almost exclusively in hepatocytes, both benign and malignant. In patients presenting with liver-only metastases, diagnosis of hepatocellular carcinoma is supported by hep par 1 positivity, and cholangiocarcinoma is mostly excluded.

Lung is the most common primary site for adenocarcinomas, representing 27% of CUPs. The majority of lung adenocarcinomas are CK7+/CK20−/TTF1+, although infrequently atypical expression is seen. For example, bronchoalveolar carcinomas are often CK20+ and mucinous carcinomas may be both CK20+ and TTF-1 negative. Of note, squamous cell carcinomas of the lung are typically TTF-1 negative and malignant mesotheliomas are always TTF-1 negative. Napsin A, a proteinase involved in surfactant B maturation, is an emerging marker thought to be more sensitive than TTF-1 for lung adenocarcinoma. It is expressed in up to 89% of cases.

Colorectal carcinomas are characterized by the phenotype CK7−/CK20+. This diagnosis can be further supported with CDX-2 staining, as described. CDX-2, in

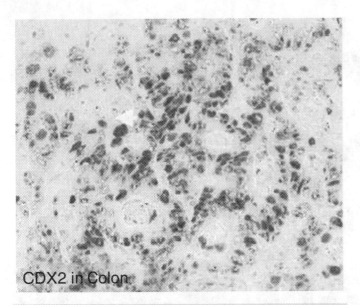

**Figure 24.5**

CDX-2 positivity in colon cancer. *Source:* Used with permission from Ref. (9). Oien KA. Pathologic evaluation of cancer of unknown primary. *Semin Oncol.* 2009;36(1):8–37.

contrast to many other markers that are either "positive" or "negative," is variably expressed. Most colorectal adenocarcinomas show strong and diffuse CDX-2 expression, as demonstrated in Figure 24.5, as do duodenal adenocarcinomas. Expression is low in gastroesophageal adenocarcinomas.

Villin is another colonic marker, which is expressed in almost all adenocarcinomas of colorectal origin. However, it is also expressed in 90% of lung adenocarcinomas. Pancreaticobiliary and upper gastrointestinal tumors present a diagnostic dilemma. They account for a large percentage of CUPs; however, a lack of sensitive and specific markers make their diagnosis challenging. CK and CDX-2 staining can be difficult to interpret because it relates to upper gastrointestinal tumors, and can be seen with any combination of phenotypes of CK7 and CK20, as well as any level of expression of CDX-2. Pancreaticobiliary cancers are CK7+ in 96% of cases, with two thirds CK20–. CA19–9 is a tumor marker expressed in up to 90% of pancreaticobiliary tumors; however it lacks specificity. Another marker that lacks specificity, but can be helpful in differentiating pancreaticobiliary and upper gastrointestinal cancers from breast cancers is lysozyme, a secreted antibacterial enzyme.

Breast cancer infrequently presents as CUP, accounting for <1% of the cases. The majority of breast carcinomas are CK7+/CK20–. Other markers used in diagnosis of breast cancer as CUP are the estrogen receptor (ER) and GCDFP-15. ER expression is up to 85% specific to carcinomas of the breast and gynecologic tract, with 60–80% of breast cancers being ER positive. As mentioned previously, GCDFP-15 is expressed frequently in breast cancers,

often in ER-negative tumors, and is noted to have a specificity of up to 96% for breast cancer. Mammaglobin-1 (MGB1) is a marker that is often expressed in otherwise diagnostically difficult breast cancers and can be useful in cases of suspected breast primary.

Gynecologic cancers, including ovarian and endometrial cancer, can often be easily differentiated from breast cancers because they are typically positive for other markers, such as CA125, WT1, and mesothelin. CA125, a membrane glycoprotein, is expressed in most gynecological malignancies, but infrequently in adenocarcinomas of other sites, with the exception of 50–60% of pancreaticobiliary carcinomas and 25–40% of lung adenocarcinomas. The use of CA125 in combination with ER staining assists in differentiating gynecological primaries from breast primaries. Mesothelin is another membrane glycoprotein with a frequency of distribution similar to CA125. WT1 is frequently expressed in ovarian serous tumors, though negative in mucinous and endometrioid tumors. Positive staining for WT1 can be used to distinguish an ovarian primary from a pancreaticobiliary, gastrointestinal, and breast primary because WT1 is typically negative in these tumor types. Absent WT1 staining can be useful as well in the setting of an ovarian mucinous or endometrioid cancer in combination with CEA to distinguish an ovarian primary from a gastrointestinal or pancreaticobiliary primary. They would all most likely be negative for WT1, but ovarian serous and endometrioid tumors do not express CEA.

Two percent of CUPs are prostate adenocarcinomas. The typical CK phenotype is CK7–/CK20–. Use of PSA has an extremely high sensitivity and specificity for prostate adenocarcinoma in the setting of CUP because PSA is expressed in 95–100% of these tumors and rarely in other sites. Other prostate markers include prostatic acid phosphatase (PAP), NKX3.1, and prostein (p501s).

### Squamous Cell Carcinomas

Squamous cell carcinomas account for about 5% of all cases of CUP. Squamous histology can usually be assessed by light microscopy, but as with adenocarcinomas, IHC can be used in cases where the histology is nondiagnostic. CK5 and p63 are the 2 markers most commonly used for squamous cell carcinoma. Unlike adenocarcinoma, there are not any markers that consistently help to further narrow the primary to a specific site of origin. CK5 is expressed in up to 90% of squamous cell carcinomas as is p63, giving these tests a high sensitivity. Individually, CK5 and p63 have a lower specificity because expression is observed in a number of adenocarcinomas. Coexpression increases specificity of these tests for squamous cell carcinomas to 96%. Use of CK7 and CK20 can be useful in squamous cell carcinoma, which typically have a CK7–/CK20– phenotype, in contrast to adenocarcinomas that are mostly

CK7+. Transitional cell carcinomas are typically positive for both CK7 and CK20, as well as UROIII, unlike squamous cell carcinomas.

### Germ Cell Tumors

Germ cell tumors are typically very chemosensitive and potentially curable, making accurate diagnosis extremely important. These are classified as either seminomatous or nonseminomatous tumors. Nonseminomatous tumors are further classified into embryonal carcinoma, teratoma, yolk sac tumor, and choriocarcinoma. IHC is very helpful in confirming germ cell origin of a tumor. PLAP is very sensitive, but not completely specific for germ cell tumors. Nonseminomatous germ cell tumors stain with pan-CK, whereas the seminomatous germ cell tumors do not. Octamer-binding transcription factor-4 (OCT4) is 100% specific for germ cell tumors because it is not expressed in any other tumor types. It is notably negative in yolk sac tumors and choriocarcinomas. Yolk sac tumors are positive for AFP and choriocarcinomas are positive for βhCG.

### Neuroendocrine Tumors

Neuroendocrine tumors are a heterogeneous group accounting for 5% of CUPs. Recognition of neuroendocrine tumors is prognostically important because they respond favorably to therapy. These are often easily recognized based on morphology alone; however, IHC is very useful when this is not the case, given the existence of very sensitive and specific markers. Neuroendocrine markers include chromogranin A, synaptophysin, protein gene product 9.5 (PGP9.5), and CD56. The site of origin of carcinoid tumors (well-differentiated neuroendocrine tumors) can be determined using TTF1 and CDX-2. This is not the case with poorly differentiated tumors, although the site of origin is less important in neuroendocrine tumors than the degree of differentiation.

### Solid Organ Carcinomas

Carcinomas arising in solid organs are occasionally considered in the realm of CUP in situations where primary tumors need to be distinguished from metastases—such as in liver or adrenal cancers, or in tumors that are commonly present as metastatic disease, such as thyroid or kidney cancer. The morphology of carcinomas arising from solid organs is mostly distinctive and the tumors are generally well differentiated. Specific considerations include hepatocellular carcinoma, renal cell carcinoma, thyroid carcinoma, and adrenocortical carcinoma. The liver and biliary tracts are the primary sites of origin in up to 10% of CUPs. Hepatocellular carcinomas are mostly CK7+/CK20−. A number of other useful markers for hepatocellular carcinoma are Hepar1, AFP, CD10, and CD13. Renal carcinomas account for 6% of CUP, 85% of which are renal clear cell carcinomas. Coexpression of vimentin and pan-CK is 1 characteristic of renal cell carcinoma; however, it is not absolutely specific. CK10 is often expressed in renal cell carcinomas, but CD10 has a low specificity. The antibody RCC, which reacts against a brush border protein of the proximal convoluted tubule in the kidney, appears to have a very high specificity for renal cell carcinoma. Aquaporin-1 and PAX-2 are additional markers that are frequently positive in renal cell carcinoma. Thyroid carcinomas, both follicular and papillary, are typically CK7+/CK20−, and use of TTF-1 and thyroglobulin yields high sensitivity. Medullary thyroid carcinoma can be distinguished by expression of calcitonin. Adrenocortical carcinomas are very uncommon as CUPs, though adrenal metastases are quite common. Alpha-inhibin and Melan-A are very sensitive and highly specific for adrenocortical carcinomas.

## Prognostic Clinical Scenarios in CUP

R.L., a 56-year-old man with a history of hypertension and dyslipidemia, presented to his primary care physician complaining of generalized fatigue and a 15-pound weight loss over 3 months. Prior to the onset of these symptoms, he had been in good health, although he had not seen a doctor in many years. Other than the fatigue and weight loss, he had felt well but did notice a nontender lump on his neck that had developed over the same time period. He had a mild chronic cough, which he attributed to being a "smoker's cough." Notably, he had smoked 1 pack per day for 25 years. He drank a moderate amount of alcohol at least twice a week. His family history was significant: his father died of lung cancer at age 67 years and his mother has breast cancer. His physical examination was remarkable for a 4-cm firm, nontender, nonmobile lymph node in the right anterior cervical chain with no overlying skin changes. Laboratory analysis did not show any abnormalities and a chest x-ray was also unremarkable. A fine-needle aspiration of the lymph node showed squamous cell carcinoma, negative for both CK7 and CK20. R.L. was referred to an otolaryngologist, who on extensive oropharyngeal examination and direct laryngoscopy, did not note any significant abnormalities. A CT of the neck revealed a 4.5 × 3.7 cm necrotic right cervical lymph node, with no other abnormalities. Panendoscopy did not show any visible lesions. Given the presentation and distribution of his adenopathy, R.L. was given therapy guided toward locally advanced squamous cell carcinoma of the head and neck: high-dose radiation therapy including the bilateral neck and the mucosa in the entire pharyngeal axis and larynx.

## Evidence-Based Case Discussion

The case of R.L. illustrates the importance of clinical scenarios in CUP. As can be seen with R.L., who was found

**Table 24.3**  Favorable Prognostic Factors Identified by Clinical and Pathological Features

| Histology | Clinical Subset | Therapy | Prognosis |
|---|---|---|---|
| Adenocarcinoma | Women, peritoneal carcinomatosis (usually serous) | Treat as stage III ovarian cancer | Survival improved |
| | Women, axillary node involvement | Treat as primary breast cancer | Survival improved |
| | Men, blastic bone metastases or high serum PSA/tumor PSA staining | Treat as metastatic prostate cancer | Survival improved |
| | Colon cancer profile (IHC and/or molecular assay) | Treat as metastatic colon cancer | Survival improved |
| | Single metastasis | Surgical resection and/or radiotherapy ± chemotherapy | Survival improved |
| Squamous cell carcinoma | Inguinal adenopathy | Inguinal node dissection, radiation therapy, ± chemotherapy | 15–20% 5-yr survival |
| | Cervical adenopathy | Treat as locally advanced head/neck primary | 25–40% 5-yr survival |
| Poorly differentiated carcinoma | Extragonadal germ cell syndrome | Treat as poor prognosis germ cell tumor | 10–20% cured |
| Neuroendocrine carcinoma | Low grade | Treat as advanced carcinoid/islet cell tumor | Indolent biology/long survival |
| | Aggressive (small cell/large cell poorly differentiated) | Treat like extensive-stage small cell lung cancer | High response rate/ survival improved |

*Source*: Used with permission from Ref. (17). Greco FA. Cancer of unknown primary site: evolving understanding and management of patients. *Clin Adv Hematol Oncol.* 2012;10(8):518–524.

to have squamous cell carcinoma within a solitary cervical lymph node, certain presentations can dictate not only prognosis but also management. Clinical presentations in CUP can represent either a good or poor prognosis.

Because of the difficulty of determining the primary source of the metastatic malignancy, using specific disease-targeted therapy is often not possible. Many patients with CUP have tumors that are resistant to systemic treatments and chemotherapy, and the use of these therapies is often palliative. Median overall survival has been reported to range from 3 to 9 months depending on the publication (13,14), and the 5-year overall survival was <10%. Despite the overall poor prognosis, when considering this group as a whole, there are various factors that portend a better prognosis. A multivariate analysis by Abbruzzese et al. identified numerous variables with prognostic importance (8). A favorable prognosis was observed in patients with isolated neuroendocrine liver metastases and those with lymphadenopathy, excluding supraclavicular nodes. The presence of lymphadenopathy in and of itself was a favorable feature, although supraclavicular lymphadenopathy was associated with worse outcomes. The diagnoses of carcinoma, squamous cell carcinoma, and neuroendocrine carcinoma were all positive prognostic indicators. Male sex, identification of adenocarcinoma as the histological subtype, hepatic involvement, and greater number of involved organs were some of the variables associated with poorer outcomes. Specifically, metastatic involvement of the liver (non-neuroendocrine), lung, bone, pleura, or brain was associated with a poorer prognosis, as described by Greco and Pavlidis (15). Hainsworth and Fizazi identified additional subsets

**Table 24.4**  Unfavorable Prognostic Factor Patients With Carcinoma of Unknown Primary

**Male Gender**

Adenocarcinoma with multiple metastases involving other organs (liver, lung, or bone)

Nonpapillary malignant ascites (adenocarcinoma)

Multiple cerebral metastases (adenocarcinoma or squamous cell carcinoma)

Adenocarcinoma with multiple lung/pleural or multiple osseous metastases

of patients with desirable features, associated with specific clinical scenarios (16). These include women with isolated axillary lymph nodes, women with papillary serous peritoneal adenocarcinoma, young men with extragonadal germ cell syndrome, men with blastic bone metastases and elevated serum level PSA, and squamous cell carcinoma with either isolated cervical or inguinal lymph nodes. Tables 24.3 and 24.4 summarize the clinical scenarios with favorable and unfavorable prognoses.

## CUPs With Favorable Prognostic Factors: Neuroendocrine Carcinoma

Neuroendocrine carcinomas uncommonly present as CUPs, accounting for 5% of unknown primary diagnoses. Presenting as CUPs, neuroendocrine carcinomas represent a group with a favorable prognosis, regardless of grade. Categorization of these tumors is based on pathological grade and degree of differentiation, which can predict the clinical behavior and response to therapy.

Low-grade, well-differentiated neuroendocrine tumors appear similar to typical carcinoid tumors, islet cell tumors, paragangliomas, pheochromocytomas, and medullary thyroid carcinomas. When presenting as CUP, they typically present in the liver, bone, or lymph nodes. It is more uncommon for low-grade neuroendocrine tumors to present as CUPs than for the higher grade tumors, representing only 10% of neuroendocrine CUPs. Typical primary sites for these tumors should be investigated, which include the stomach, small intestine, colon, rectum, pancreas, and bronchus. This should be done with imaging including CT scanning, as well as invasive investigations including bronchoscopy, upper endoscopy, and colonoscopy. Other imaging modalities, such as octreotide scan, PET scanning, and/or MRI can be implemented, which will be discussed in a later section (Imaging in CUP and Future Directions). These tumors have an indolent behavior, with a median overall survival of 120 months. Management should be similar to that of metastatic typical carcinoid with either local therapy or therapy aimed at symptomatic control. Systemic chemotherapy does not play a significant role in treatment of low-grade neuroendocrine tumors because they tend to be relatively unresponsive. Local therapeutic options include resection, radiation, chemoembolization, or ablation. Octreotide, a somatostatin analog, is often used as a monthly depot injection as first-line therapy in low-grade neuroendocrine tumors. It is well tolerated and has a significant impact on control of symptoms due to hormone excess.

The high-grade or anaplastic, poorly differentiated neuroendocrine tumors include atypical carcinoids, small cell carcinomas, and poorly differentiated large cell neuroendocrine tumors. Although still considered to have a "favorable prognosis" when presenting as CUP, high-grade neuroendocrine tumors are significantly more aggressive than low-grade tumors. The median overall survival is 10 months. Large cell carcinomas are the most common high-grade neuroendocrine tumors, accounting for 75% of neuroendocrine carcinomas of unknown primary. These have a very heterogeneous presentation, and can involve a variety of sites, often >1. Small cell carcinomas represent 15% of neuroendocrine carcinomas of unknown primary. A number of more rare tumors are often mistaken for small cell carcinomas due to similar morphology, such as germ cell tumors with neuroendocrine differentiation, peripheral neuroectodermal tumors, Ewing's sarcoma, and desmoplastic small round cell tumors. Both small cell and large cell carcinomas are highly aggressive, though they tend to be sensitive to systemic chemotherapy. Treatment of large cell carcinoma of unknown primary mirrors that of small cell carcinoma of unknown primary. Surgical resection or radiation therapy is considered in cases where the disease is localized to a limited region. Systemic chemotherapy with a platinum-based combination regimen, most commonly

cisplatin and etoposide, is the recommended treatment, following guidelines of therapy for treating small cell lung cancer. Addition of paclitaxel has not been shown to have advantage over 2-drug platinum-based therapy, and carries additional toxicity. Compared to low-grade neuroendocrine tumors, overall response rates to chemotherapy are high, approaching 70% in some studies. This is in contrast to the very low overall response rates of <10% seen in the use of chemotherapy in low-grade neuroendocrine tumors (see Chapter 9: Neuroendocrine Cancer).

### Women With Axillary Lymph Node Metastases

A woman who is found to have a CUP presenting as adenocarcinoma with isolated axillary lymph node metastases should raise a suspicion in the clinician for breast cancer. Imaging should be directed toward investigating a possible breast primary. If mammography is unrevealing, breast MRI should be obtained with consideration of PET scanning as well to look for an occult breast primary. IHC staining of the biopsy should include ER, progesterone receptor (PR), and HER2 testing—their presence is highly suggestive of breast cancer. Occasionally, despite this workup, no definitive breast primary can be identified. In that situation treatment should be initiated following guidelines for management of stage II breast cancer. This should include a surgical approach with either a modified radical mastectomy or an axillary lymph node dissection. If an axillary lymph node dissection is performed, it should be followed by radiation therapy and should not be done as stand-alone therapy. Mastectomy is often very effective in identifying the occult primary, with reports of up to 82% of primaries found on pathological evaluation of the resected breast. Identified primaries are typically <2 cm, and occasionally only noninvasive tumor is discovered. Following surgical management, adjuvant therapy is indicated as administered to patients with node-positive breast cancer. As in known primary breast cancer, selection of adjuvant therapy depends on hormone receptor status, HER2 status, menopausal status, and the number of involved lymph nodes. Prognosis for these patients is similar to that of women with stage II breast cancer. Of note, men may present in this manner as well, although rarely, and should be managed in the same way.

In the setting of axillary lymph nodes identified as adenocarcinoma with metastases in a distribution typical of metastatic breast cancer, such as multiple bone metastases or pleural metastases, breast cancer should remain the primary consideration. These patients should be managed based on guidelines for metastatic breast cancer, with careful attention to ER, PR, and HER2 status.

### Women With Peritoneal Carcinomatosis

Peritoneal carcinomatosis is often seen in women with carcinoma of the ovary, but it is also seen less commonly in the setting of gastrointestinal, lung, or breast cancer. It can also be seen in women with no clear intra-abdominal primary and normal ovaries, presenting as a CUP or in primary peritoneal carcinomatosis. This is a situation with a favorable prognosis, given the effectiveness of chemotherapy directed against ovarian cancer. One clinical scenario in which this is seen is in women at high risk for ovarian cancer due to genetic predisposition (such as in BRCA1 families) who have undergone prophylactic oophorectomy. The histologic appearance of the malignant cells in the peritoneal fluid frequently resembles ovarian carcinoma, but can be variable and is occasionally poorly differentiated. Treatment of women with isolated peritoneal carcinomatosis should follow guidelines for the management of advanced ovarian cancer, including initial maximal surgical debulking, followed by combination chemotherapy. Chemotherapy should include taxane and a platinum agent, with the combination of cisplatin and paclitaxel being the most commonly used. The presence of minimal residual disease following debulking surgery has been associated with better outcomes, including increased frequency of complete response as well as prolonged overall survival. Up to 15% of patients receiving such therapy may experience prolonged survival.

## Young Men With Features of Extragonadal Germ Cell Tumor

In young men with poorly differentiated carcinoma with midline distribution in either the mediastinum or retroperitoneum, a diagnosis of extragonadal germ cell tumor should be suspected. This diagnosis would be supported by elevation in either HCG or AFP, and can also be supported by cytogenetic evaluation with an isochrome 12p abnormality. If these tests are equivocal or there is limited availability of cytogenetic analysis, young men with poorly differentiated carcinoma in either of these locations should be treated based on guidelines for poor-prognosis germ cell tumor. This should include combination chemotherapy with a platinum-containing regimen, such as cisplatin, etoposide, and bleomycin. If after a partial response to 4 cycles of chemotherapy, residual tumor is noted on follow-up imaging, surgical resection should be considered.

The "extragonadal germ cell tumor syndrome" was described in 1979 in men younger than 50 years, with midline tumors (mediastinum or peritoneum) or multiple pulmonary nodules, short symptom interval with rapid tumor growth, elevated levels of serum AFP and/or HCG, and a good response to chemotherapy or radiation (7). Patients rarely are seen to have all of these clinical features, but the presence of any 2 suggests the possibility of a germ cell tumor.

## Men With Adenocarcinoma and Osteoblastic Bone Metastases

Men with predominant bone metastases with adenocarcinoma should be suspected to have prostate cancer, especially if the bone metastases are osteoblastic. IHC staining of the biopsy should include PSA and PAP. Serum PSA levels should be measured for confirmation of the diagnosis and the patients should be treated based on guidelines for metastatic prostate cancer. In the presence of multiple osteoblastic bone metastases with unknown primary, androgen deprivation therapy should be given as a trial empirically, irrespective of PSA level. Response to androgen deprivation therapy has also been noted in men with PSA levels suggestive of prostate cancer but who have atypical metastatic patterns. These patients should thus also be managed using guidelines for metastatic prostate cancer.

## Adenocarcinoma Presenting as a Single Metastatic Lesion

In some cases (such as R.L.'s), only 1 metastatic lesion can be identified. Additional metastatic lesions frequently become evident in a short period of time in those who present with a single metastatic lesion. Local treatment with radiation therapy or definitive resection, if feasible, should be considered in this subset of patients. Adjuvant radiation therapy after resection to improve chances of local control may be considered as well. A significant number of these patients have a prolonged disease-free survival with local therapy. The role of adjuvant chemotherapy in combination with local therapy has not been strictly defined. It is reasonable to offer a short course of adjuvant chemotherapy using an empiric chemotherapy regimen for CUP.

## Squamous Carcinoma

Squamous cell carcinoma of unknown primary is an uncommon entity, representing about 5% of all patients with CUP. Effective therapies exist for certain clinical syndromes including squamous carcinoma of either cervical or inguinal lymph nodes.

## Squamous Cell Carcinoma Involving Cervical Lymph Nodes

The cervical lymph nodes are the most common site for metastatic squamous cell carcinoma of unknown primary and the presence of these metastases is suggestive of a head and neck cancer, as is described in the case of R.L. This is especially true if the lymph nodes are in the middle or upper cervical lymph node region. Many of the patients with these isolated nodes have risk factors for head and neck cancer, such as smoking, alcohol use, and exposure to human papillomavirus (HPV). When this situation is identified, further investigation should be performed in search of the occult primary with panendoscopy. This should include examination of the head and neck by an experienced otolaryngologist, examining the oropharynx, nasopharynx, hypopharynx, larynx, and upper esophagus with direct endoscopy. Bronchoscopy should be included in this evaluation as well if chest imaging and examination of the head and neck are unrevealing. Biopsies should be taken of any suspicious areas. Tonsillectomy should be performed empirically in patients with subdigastric, submandibular, or mid-jugular carotid adenopathy because these patients have a high likelihood of having a tonsillar primary. Ipsilateral tonsillectomy can be performed in patients with a single node in this distribution. Bilateral tonsillectomy should be performed in those patients who present with bilateral adenopathy as described. Tonsillectomy can identify a primary site in about 25% of cases. Imaging in this scenario should include plain radiographs of the chest and CT of the neck. PET scanning is recommended because it identifies primary site in up to 25% of patients with this presentation. The biopsy sample should be evaluated for the presence of Epstein–Barr virus genome, the presence of which would be suggestive of a nasopharyngeal primary site. The tumor tissue should also be examined for the presence of HPV-16 and 18, which is specific for an oropharyngeal primary site, seen increasingly in nonsmokers and nondrinkers.

If no primary is located, treatment should follow guidelines for management of locally advanced squamous cell carcinoma of the head and neck. This should involve local therapy with high-dose radiation therapy, radical neck dissection, or a combination of these approaches. Responses to these treatments have been similar, with 30–60% of patients achieving long-term, disease-free survival. Surgery is typically not offered alone except in select patients, such as those with pN1 neck disease with no extracapsular extension. Radiation therapy should include the bilateral neck and the mucosa in the entire pharyngeal axis and larynx. This approach is superior to radiation to ipsilateral cervical lymph nodes alone. Although concurrent chemotherapy and radiation therapy are standard in locally advanced head and neck cancer, the role of chemotherapy in metastatic squamous cell carcinoma in cervical lymph nodes with unknown primary is controversial. Platinum-based chemotherapy given concurrently with radiation appears to be beneficial, especially in patients with N2 or N3 lymph node involvement.

Poorer prognosis is seen in patients with extensive lymphadenopathy or those with poorly differentiated tumors. Those patients with lower cervical or supraclavicular lymph nodes also do not do as well as those with higher cervical nodes. These patients are more likely to have an occult primary lung cancer. Despite the poorer prognosis, the recommended therapy is similar to that for patients with higher cervical nodes. They should receive aggressive local therapy and should be considered for concurrent chemotherapy.

### Squamous Cell Carcinoma Involving Inguinal Lymph Nodes

Patients with inguinal lymphadenopathy with squamous histology should undergo thorough genitourinary examination,

with careful attention paid to the penis, scrotum, vulva, vagina, and cervix. Any suspicious lesion should be biopsied. The anorectal area should be examined as well with digital rectal examination and anoscopy. If the primary cannot be identified, treatment should be offered with definitive local therapy, including inguinal lymph node dissection, with or without radiation therapy. Long-term survival can result from local therapy, especially in patients found to have squamous cell carcinoma of the anus, vulva, vagina, or cervix. Combined therapy with concurrent radiation and chemotherapy improves prognosis for a number of primary cancers originating in the inguinal region. Systemic therapy with concurrent platinum-based chemotherapy and radiation should be considered in patients without an identified primary site.

### CUP With a Single Small Metastasis

Patients with a single small site of metastasis with an unidentified primary are a group with a favorable prognosis, often with a long-term disease-free survival, independent of the pathology. These patients should be offered aggressive local therapy with radiation, resection, or both.

### Poorly Differentiated Carcinoma

Approximately 20% of patients with CUP site are identified to have poorly differentiated carcinoma. Despite the heterogeneity of this group, there is a subset of these patients who have chemotherapy-sensitive tumors. Occasionally, specific diagnoses can be made using specialized pathological studies, allowing for more disease-guided therapy. In cases of poorly differentiated carcinoma with unknown primary site, a trial of empiric combination chemotherapy should be offered. Use of platinum-based chemotherapy (with or without combination taxane chemotherapy) has produced relatively high response rates, with the substitution of carboplatin for cisplatin being equally effective with less toxicity.

## CUPs With Unfavorable Prognostic Factors

While approximately 20% of patients with CUP are considered to have a favorable prognosis as detailed in the previous section, the majority of patients continue to have a poor prognosis. No chemotherapeutic regimen has been found to be effective convincingly in this subset of patients and treatment is empiric, with aim at palliation. The historical data for survival in patients with CUP are described by Greco and Pavlidis (15). In a retrospective review of an extensive series of almost 45,000 patients, the combined median overall survival was noted to be 4.5 months, with 20% 1-year survival, 4.7% 5-year or greater survival. Of note, the patients in this series with long-term survival were mostly those with favorable prognostic factors. When excluding 3871 of those patients who either had squamous or epidermoid carcinoma or well-differentiated neuroendocrine carcinoma, 1-year survival dropped to 12% in the remaining 40,828 patients. Initial chemotherapeutic trials throughout the 1970s involved mostly single-agent regimens with very low response rates and very rare long-term survival. Platinum-based combination chemotherapy was evaluated starting in the 1980s. A review of 38 phase II trials performed between 1964 and 1996 showed a response rate of about 20% and median overall survival of 6 months. Some of the larger trials showed longer survival and increased response; however, these trials included many patients with previously unrecognized favorable prognostic factors. It is important to note when discussing older data in CUP that all of the trials were small, with no large randomized phase III data. Long-term follow-up results were rarely published due to either patient death or rapid publishing of results.

In the last decade, with the development of new drugs with broad activity and new targeted agents, a number of larger prospective phase II trials have been conducted. Nine sequential studies were reported by the Minnie Pearl Cancer Research Network (MPCRN) since 1997, including 692 patients with CUP. These studies used various combinations of paclitaxel, docetaxel, cisplatin, carboplatin, gemictabine, irinotecan, capecitabine, oxaliplatin, bevacizumab, and erlotinib, either as front-line therapy or salvage therapy, as seen in Figure 24.6. Only those patients not identified to have favorable features were included in first-line therapy trials. Among the 396 patients included in the first 5 studies done by the MPCRN, there was an objective response rate of 30% with 24% partial response and 6% complete response. The median overall survival was 9.1 months with 38% 1-year, 10% 5-year, and 8% 10-year survival. There was a 5-month median progression-free

survival with 17% 1-year, 4% 5-year, and 3% 10-year progression-free survival. In comparing the various regimens there was no significant difference in survival between the groups.

The phase III multicenter Sarah Cannon Oncology Research Consortium Trial randomized 198 patients to receive paclitaxel, carboplatin, and etoposide (PCE) versus gemcitabine and irinotecan first line, both followed by gefitinib (18). In this trial, which is one of the largest phase III trials of CUP to date, patients were given between 4 and 6 cycles of chemotherapy, after which those with no progression of disease were maintained on gefitinib until disease progression. Notably, this trial was stopped early due to slow accrual and did not meet the primary end point of showing a 10% difference in overall survival (increasing the 2-year overall survival to 30%). The 2 regimens were not statistically different in median overall survival, median progression-free survival, and response rate: In comparing PCE with gemcitabine/irinotecan, median 2-year survival was 15% versus 18%, median overall survival was 7.4 versus 8.5 months, median progression-free survival was 3.3 versus 5.3 months, respectively, and the response rate was 18% in both arms. The authors concluded that the gemcitibine–irinotecan combination is favorable due to its lower toxicity profile. The trial was not powered to detect a difference in efficacy with the addition of gefitinib, and its inclusion was intended to assess the possible activity of this agent. Based on the available data from this trial, gefitinib did not appear to have significant activity as a single-agent therapy in maintenance.

The use of targeted agents, which have been approved for use in advanced cancers of known primary such as colorectal, breast, and non-small cell lung cancer, has been studied in CUP. A phase II trial was conducted by the MPCRN combining bevacizumab (inhibitor of vascular endothelial growth factor) and erlotinib (inhibitor of epidermal growth factor receptor [EGFR]) in 51 patients with CUP. Most of the patients were previously untreated, with the untreated patients all having poor prognostic features. Twenty-nine of the patients (61%) had stable disease and 5 of the patients (10%) had a partial response, with the majority of patients receiving at least 8 weeks of therapy. The median overall survival was 7.4 months, with a 33% 1-year survival. In a retrospective comparison to second-line chemotherapeutic agents, these responses were superior. Based on the positive results with these targeted agents, a recent MPCRN phase II trial evaluated use of targeted agents in the front-line setting. Patients received paclitaxel–carboplatin–bevacizumab every 21 days with daily erlotinib for a total of 4 cycles, followed by up to 1 year of maintenance therapy with bevacizumab and erlotinib. Only the 56 patients who were not known to be in a favorable subset were included in the trial. An objective response rate of 38% was noted with 19 patients (34%)

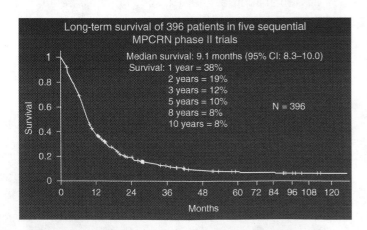

**Figure 24.6**

Survival curve for 396 patients treated on the first 5 sequential prospective phase II trials by the Minnie Pearl Cancer Research Network (MPCRN). *Source:* Used with permission from Ref. (15). Greco FA, Pavlidis N. Treatment for patients with unknown primary carcinoma and unfavorable prognostic factors. *Semin Oncol.* 2009;36(1):65–74.

having stable disease. Median progression-free survival was 10.4 months, with median overall survival of 11.6 months, 1-year survival of 46.5%, and a tolerable toxicity profile. Targeted agents may have a beneficial role in the management of CUP with unfavorable prognostic factors and their utility may be directed by the results of gene expression profiling (see the Gene Expression Assays section).

Analysis of all patients in the MPCRN showed that in patients with CUP with poor prognostic factors, there is no difference in survival for adenocarcinoma over poorly differentiated carcinomas. Men have a shorter survival than women in this category, as do patients with an Eastern Cooperative Oncology Group (ECOG) performance status of 2 or greater compared to those with and ECOG performance status of 0 or 1. Other identified poor prognostic variables included elevated lactate dehydrogenase level, low serum albumin, and the presence of liver metastases.

In addition to the MPCRN trials, 12 other trials have reported long-term follow-up with 1-year survival data, and 8 of those 12 trials reported a 2-year survival data. These phase II trials used multiple regimens, mostly platinum, paclitaxel, docetaxel, gemcitabine, irinotecan, or vinorelbine based. Inclusive of the MPCRN trials, the mean 1-year survival was 34.6%, mean 2-year survival was 13%, mean 3-year survival was 12%, and median overall survival was 8.9 months, as can be seen in Table 24.5.

Despite the fact that no phase III studies have clearly shown a benefit of systemic chemotherapy over best supportive care in survival of patients with CUP with poor prognostic features, aggregate data of numerous phase II studies do appear to suggest such a benefit.

## Imaging in CUP and Future Directions

A.W., a healthy 41-year-old woman, presented to her primary care physician with a slowly growing nontender nodule in her right axilla that was noted during a self-breast examination at home. She had been up to date on her health maintenance and had her first mammogram the previous year, which was normal. Her only previous hospitalization was for a cesarian section, and she did not have any pertinent family history. She was previously a smoker with 14 pack-years, although she quit smoking 5 years earlier. Her physical examination showed a 3-cm firm, nontender, mobile nodule in the right axilla. Laboratory studies including a complete blood count, serum chemistries, and liver function tests, which were normal, as was a chest x-ray. A bilateral mammogram did not reveal any abnormalities in the breast tissue, but a breast ultrasound showed a hypoechoic nodule in the right axilla measuring $3.4 \times 2.7$ cm. A fine needle aspiration showed adenocarcinoma, though tissue site of origin was indeterminate. An IHC panel showed that the tumor was CK20−, CK7+, ER+, PR−, and HER2−. A CT scan of the chest, abdomen, and pelvis was otherwise unremarkable, as was a breast MRI and bone scan. An axillary lymph node dissection was performed, identifying only the 1 positive lymph node. Because of these findings, A.W. was treated as if she had node-positive breast cancer.

**Table 24.5** Long-Term Survival in Patients With Unknown Primary Carcinoma and Unfavorable Prognostic Factors

| Greco and Pavlidis (15) | No. of Patients | Regimen | Median Survival (mo) | 1-Yr Survival (%) | 2-Yr Survival (%) | 3-Yr Survival (%) |
|---|---|---|---|---|---|---|
| Briasoulis et al., 2000 | 33 | PCb | 10 | 25 | 5 | NR |
| Dowell et al., 2001 | 34 | P5FUL (17) | 8.3 | 26 | NR | NR |
| | | CbE (17) | 6.4 | | | |
| Balana et al., 2003 | 30 | GCE | 7.2 | 36 | 14 | NR |
| Park et al., 2004 | 37 | PC | 11 | 38 | 11 | NR |
| Piga et al., 2004 | 102 | CbDoxE | 9 | 35.3 | 18 | 11 |
| Pouessel et al., 2004 | 35 | GD | 10 | 43 | 7 | NR |
| El-Rayes et al., 2005 | 22 | PCb | 6.5 | 27 | NR | NR |
| Pittman et al., 2006 | 51 | GCb | 7.8 | 26 | 12 | NR |
| Palmeri et al., 2006 | 66 | GPC (33) | 9.6 | 30 | NR | NR |
| | | GVC (33) | 13.6 | 52 | NR | NR |
| Berry et al., 2007 | 42 | PCb | 8.5 | 33 | 17 | NR |
| Briasoulis et al., 2007 | 47 | OxIr | 9.5 | 40 | NR | NR |
| Schneider et al., 2007 | 33 | GCaCb | 7.6 | 35.6 | 14.2 | NR |
| MPCRN (5 trials) 1997–2008 | 396 | Multiple regimens (see text) | 9.1 | 38 | 19 | 12 |
| Total | 928 | | 8.9[a] | 34.6[a] | 13[a] | 12[a] |

[a] Mean survivals of all studies.

5-FUL, 5-fluorouracil/leucovorin; C, cisplatin; Ca, capecitibine; Cb, carboplatin; D, docetaxel; Dox, doxorubicin; E, etoposide; G, gemcitabine; Ir, irinotecan; NR, not reported; Ox, oxaliplatin; P, paclitaxel; V, vinorelbine.
*Source*: Used with permission from Ref. (15). Greco FA, Pavlidis N. Treatment for patients with unknown primary carcinoma and unfavorable prognostic factors. *Semin Oncol*. 2009;36(1):65–74.

## Evidence-Based Case Discussion

### The Role of Imaging in CUP

A.W.'s case provides another example in which the clinical scenario points to a good prognosis in CUP, as well as dictating therapy. It also shows the importance of imaging in the management of CUP.

### *Chest X-Ray and CT*

Routine radiographs of the chest are included as part of the initial evaluation in all patients with CUP. Autopsy studies suggest that chest x-ray alone is able to differentiate a primary and secondary malignancy in only one third of cases. The routine use of CT of the chest is somewhat more debatable. An argument could be made to only obtain a CT of the chest in those patients with chest x-ray abnormalities. However, a chest CT is often included in the initial evaluation due to frequent involvement of the mediastinum in CUP. If a patient is a smoker or a former smoker, it may be reasonable to order a CT scan. A major study published in 2011 called the National Lung Screening Trial, compared mortality from lung cancer among patients screened with CT scans and chest x-rays (19). It found a 20% relative reduction in mortality from lung cancer with low-dose CT screening. Another factor supporting the use of initial CT scanning of the chest is the frequency of identifying lung carcinoma as the primary tumor. If pathological testing is suggestive of a lung primary, a CT of the chest should certainly be performed. CT of the abdomen and pelvis in patients with CUP has a well-studied benefit and detects a primary site in 30–35% of patients. This is routinely performed in the initial evaluation and is often useful in determining the extent of disease, as well as localizing the most favorable site for biopsy.

### *Mammography and Other Breast Imaging Tests*

A mammogram should be routinely performed in all women who are found to have adenocarcinoma of unknown primary, regardless of the pathological evaluation. This, along with a breast ultrasound, should especially be done in women with adenocarcinoma with positive supraclavicular, axillary, or mediastinal nodes. In cases where a breast primary is strongly suspected and mammography and ultrasound are noncontributory, bilateral MRI of the breast should be considered, as was done for A.W. MRI scanning is very sensitive for the detection of occult breast cancers in women with malignant axillary lymphadenopathy. Although not included in the routine initial evaluation, MRI of the breast should be used when mammography and ultrasound are inadequate in assessing the extent of the disease, particularly in women with dense breast tissue, malignant axillary adenopathy, and an occult primary breast tumor. It is also helpful in evaluation of the chest wall.

### *¹⁸F-Fludeoxyglucose PET Scan*

The use of PET scan in CUP is not yet a clearly proven diagnostic modality, but it does have various indications for which it is very valuable. Most of the trials that have been performed using PET scans in the diagnostic evaluation of patients with CUP have involved patients with squamous cell carcinoma with cervical lymphadenopathy. A number of both prospective and retrospective studies have been performed in this subset, with mostly small sample sizes (no more than 50) (11). In these trials, a primary tumor was identified through the use of PET scanning in up to 30% of patients with metastatic cervical lymph nodes. In these patients, PET scan appears to have a clear benefit, allowing for guidance of biopsy, determining extent of disease, guiding therapy such as narrowing radiation fields to limit toxicity, and surveillance after treatment.

Aside from patients with cervical adenopathy on presentation, the use of PET is not recommended as part of a standard evaluation in patients with CUP. Small retrospective studies have suggested that PET studies are able to detect a primary tumor in about 20% of cancer cases of unknown primary in patients not presenting with neck adenopathy.

One limitation of PET studies is the absence of significant accumulation of the ¹⁸F-fludeoxyglucose (FDG) tracer in some neoplastic tissues, leading to limited accuracy of anatomic localization. Combination of PET with CT using intravenous contrast has become increasingly routine, improving localization. Combination PET-CT has been noted to identify primary tumors in 33–35% of patients with CUP, and up to 57% in smaller studies. To date, there have not been any large prospective trials comparing PET or PET-CT with conventional imaging modalities. Larger clinical studies with long-term follow-up need to be performed using PET scanning before it can be routinely recommended as a diagnostic tool in CUP. In addition to efficacy, cost-effectiveness should be evaluated as well, given the expense of this imaging, which thus far has not been studied.

In addition to the evaluation of patients with cervical adenopathy, there are a number of situations where PET appears to be a valuable imaging modality. One example is the use of PET when there is a single site of metastasis, and therapy with curative intent is planned. This allows for the possible identification of disease beyond the single metastatic site, if it is present. Assessment of residual cancer in patients who are candidates for postsurgical adjuvant therapy can be achieved with PET. When surgical resection or radiation therapy is being considered for residual tumor following systemic therapy, PET can be useful in localization of the residual disease. Another situation in which PET scanning would be useful is in patients with an iodine dye allergy who would be unable to undergo conventional CT scanning.

*MRI*

The role of MRI in the diagnosis of CUP, outside of its use in the diagnosis of occult breast cancers, is unclear. Those patients who are unable to have CT scans due to contraindications may have MRI as an alternative. Otherwise, there have not been large studies comparing the accuracy of MRI versus CT scanning in the diagnostic evaluation of CUP. Used as an adjunct to CT scanning, it does not appear that MRI significantly alters the treatment plan in most cases. Also due to high costs, routine use of MRI in the initial evaluation of CUP is not recommended. As discussed, MRI is accepted in patients with isolated axillary lymph node metastases and suspected occult breast cancer. A number of small studies suggest that a negative MRI is predictive of low yield of mastectomy in patients with suspected breast cancer. It is also beneficial in identifying and localizing the site of the primary tumor in up to 70–75% of women with isolated axillary lymphadenopathy and suspected occult breast cancer. This provides the advantage of improved surgical planning and the possibility of breast-conserving surgery.

## FUTURE DIRECTIONS

Treatment of CUP often requires the use of empiric therapies. However, improvements in IHC and molecular profiling have improved our ability to define tissue of origin and have allowed tissue-specific treatment in some tumor types. Although it is still only available to limited tumor types, more people are benefiting from site-specific therapy. In the absence of a specific diagnosis or suggestive clinical scenario, this creates the possibility of choosing a suboptimal treatment for an individual patient. There is ongoing research to shift from empirically treating all patients with CUP as a single entity to specifically tailored therapy using targeted agents and novel therapies. The expression profile of a primary tumor should be mostly the same as that of a metastasis. This allows for comparison of a pattern of gene expression of a CUP to known patterns of different tumor types (which can be very useful in identification of the primary site), or it allows for further classification. This pattern of gene expression can be identified using microarray or by reverse transcription polymerase chain reaction (RT-PCR).

### Gene Expression Profiling: Microarray

Measurement of mRNA, and thereby measurement of gene expression, has been used to guide prognostication as well as therapeutics in known primary malignancies, most notably in breast cancer. The use of gene expression profiling in breast cancer creates a genomic taxonomy of the tumor, which stratifies patients according to the likelihood of recurrence. This allows the physician to assess the benefit of adding chemotherapy to the treatment regimen, which individually tailors therapy based on various characteristics of the tumor. The process of gene expression profiling involves extraction of mRNA from tissue, amplifying the mRNA, fluorescently labeling it, and hybridizing it to a microarray. The microarray contains a variety of DNA spots, which code for a unique sequence of a specific gene. After hybridization of the amplified mRNA to the microarray, the fluorescent signal is quantitated at a particular DNA spot. Microarray allows for measurement of thousands of genes simultaneously; however, as such, it is not highly sensitive and is often difficult to reproduce.

### Real-Time Polymerase Chain Reaction

Real-time polymerase chain reaction (RT-PCR) allows for quantitation of a specific desired amount of mRNA. RT-PCR is notably more sensitive than gene expression using microarray and unlike microarray allows for quantitative measurement of mRNA. However, unlike microarray, only tens to hundreds of genes can be measured simultaneously. It is also a more time-intensive and expensive test, which needs to be highly sensitive to be compatible with most tumor biopsies that are formalin-fixed, paraffin-embedded (FFPE).

### Gene Expression Assays

A number of gene expression assays to determine primary tumor origin have been developed (20). Five of these are currently commercially available in the United States and Europe or are in development. Two of the assays are compatible with FFPE samples. These assays have been validated using mostly samples from primary tumors or known metastatic sites. Metastases from CUP represent a minority of those tested. In a prospective trial with 252 patients, molecular tumor profiling was able to predict a tissue of origin in 98% of patients. This allowed for assay-directed site-specific therapy with median survival time of 12.5 months, which compared favorably with previous results using epiric therapy (21). In a retrospective study of patients with CUP, 42 patients with tissue of origin were predicted to be colorectal site of origin by a 92-gene RT-PCR molecular profiling assay. When 32 of these patients were treated with site-specific regimens, they had median survival similar to survival in patients with known metastatic colon cancer. The median survival was substantially better than the historical median survival for patients with CUP treated with empirical CUP regimens (22). A follow-up prospective trial in which molecular gene expression profiling was used to detect the tissue of origin and to determine site-directed specific therapy led to an improved overall survival (23). Another study by the same group showed that prognosis is improved when site-directed therapy is chosen over empiric chemotherapy (24).

## REVIEW QUESTIONS

1. A 51-year-old man has multiple hepatic lesions but no evidence of a primary tumor. A biopsy of one of the liver lesions reveals an adenocarcinoma with an immunohistochemistry profile that is CK7–; CK20+; and CDX-2+. Which of the following is the most likely primary site of origin?

   (A) Prostate carcinoma
   (B) Colon carcinoma
   (C) Lung carcinoma
   (D) Hepatocellular carcinoma

2. A 35-year-old man presents with neck and facial swelling with a CT of the chest showing a large mediastinal mass with no other abnormalities seen on a CT of the chest, abdomen, and pelvis; his physical examination is otherwise normal. Interventional radiology-guided biopsy of the mass shows a poorly differentiated neoplasm with an immunohistochemical profile of CK7–; CK20–; PLAP+; and AFP+. Which of the following is the most likely site of origin:

   (A) Lung adenocarcinoma
   (B) Lung squamous carcinoma
   (C) Thymoma
   (D) Extragonadal germ cell tumor

3. A 47-year-old woman is found to have a painless 4 × 4 cm right axillary lymph node mass. She has no other lymphadenopathy and her physical examination, including a breast examination, is otherwise normal. A core biopsy of the lymph node demonstrates a high-grade tumor with an immunohistochemical profile of CK7+; CK20–; GCDFP-15+; and MGB1+; HER2–. Among the following, which is the most likely primary tumor:

   (A) Non-Hodgkin lymphoma
   (B) Hodgkin lymphoma
   (C) Melanoma
   (D) Breast carcinoma

4. A 48-year-old woman complains of diffuse abdominal pain and an increase in her abdominal girth. Her physical examination demonstrates moderate ascites and a CT of the abdomen and pelvis shows abdominal carcinomatosis with diffuse omental masses. A diagnostic pericentesis reveals malignant cells with an immunohistochemical profile of CK7+; CK20+; WT1+; CDX-2–; and CA125+. Which of the following represents the most likely primary tumor type:

   (A) Colon carcinoma
   (B) Peritoneal mesothelioma
   (C) Pancreatic carcinoma
   (D) Mucinous ovarian carcinoma

5. A 70-year-old man presents with a painless 3-cm right supraclavicular lymph node that has been growing over the past 2 months. His physical examination is otherwise unremarkable and he has no other lymphadenopathy. He reports a 60-pack-year history of smoking, has a chronic cough, and carries a diagnosis of chronic obstructive pulmonary disease. A chest x-ray is unremarkable apart from hyperexpanded lungs with depressed diaphragms. A core biopsy of the lymph node demonstrates a poorly differentiated tumor with an immunohistochemical profile of CK7–, CK20–; synaptophysin-positive; chromogranin-positive; and TTF-1-negative. Which of the following is most likely to be the primary site of origin:

   (A) Squamous cell carcinoma of the lung
   (B) Adenocarcinoma of the lung
   (C) Small cell carcinoma of the lung
   (D) Squamous cell carcinoma of the larynx

6. Among the following patients with carcinoma of unknown primary, who is considered to have an unfavorable prognosis?

   (A) 66-year-old man with adenocarcinoa with multiple blastic bone metastases and an elevated prostate-specific antigen
   (B) 55-year-old man with adenocarcinoma with multiple metastases involving liver, lung, and bone
   (C) 47-year-old woman with poorly differentiated neuroendocrine carcinoma
   (D) 34-year-old woman with papillary adenocarcinoma of the peritoneal cavity

7. A 64-year-old man is found to have a single 3-cm chest wall mass. A biopsy demonstrates an adenocarcinoma and a PET-CT scan shows no $^{18}$F-fludeoxyglucose-avid lesions apart from the chest mass. What is the best course of management?

   (A) Chemotherapy
   (B) Observation
   (C) Surgery–radiotherapy
   (D) Radiotherapy alone

8. A 49-year-old, previously healthy woman is found to have a poorly differentiated carcinoma involving retroperitoneal lymph nodes, liver, and lungs, with no primary site identified. She has an excellent performance status and is interested in treatment. Which of the following should be included in her initial empiric therapy?

   (A) Platinum-based chemotherapy
   (B) Doxorubicin
   (C) Cyclophosphamide
   (D) Bevacizumab

9. A 67-year-old woman with a new persistent cough is found to have a suspicious fullness in the right hilar region

by chest x-ray. Her physical examination is unremarkable. Which of the following diagnostic tests are most appropriate for the initial evaluation of her condition?

(A) A PET scan
(B) An MRI of the chest
(C) A CT of the chest
(D) A mammogram

10. A 25-year-old man presents with a 4-cm painless lump in his left groin that has been slowly growing over the course of several months. A core biopsy demonstrates adenocarcinoma. Among the following serum biomarkers, which one is the most selective in pointing to a specific tumor type:

(A) Carcinoembryonic antigen
(B) CA125
(C) Beta human chorionic gonadotropin (βhCG)
(D) CA19–9

11. A 52-year-old woman presents with multiple enlarged right axillary lymph nodes, which on biopsy test positive for GCDFP-15 and HER2, but are negative for estrogen receptor and progesterone receptor. She has no palpable breast masses. Which among the following would represent the next best step in her diagnostic evaluation?

(A) Colonoscopy
(B) Pelvic–intravaginal ultrasound
(C) Breast MRI
(D) Bronchoscopy

12. A 75-year-old man presents with a 2-month history of back pain and diffuse body aches and a bone scan reveals technetium uptake in multiple thoracic vertebrae, sacrum, and ribs. Among the following serum biomarkers, which is the most likely to lead to a specific cancer diagnosis?

(A) Carcinoembryonic antigen
(B) Alpha-fetoprotein
(C) Prostate-specific antigen (PSA)
(D) Chromogranin

## REFERENCES

1. Siegel R, Naishadham D, Jemal A. Cancer statistics, 2013. *CA Cancer J Clin.* 2013;63(1):11–30.
2. Ferlay J, Steliarova-Foucher E, Lortet-Tieulent J, et al. Cancer incidence and mortality patterns in Europe: estimates for 40 countries in 2012. *Eur J Cancer.* 2013;49(6):1374–1403.
3. Australian Institute of Health and Welfare, 2012. *Cancer in Australia: An Overview 2012.* Australian Institute of Health and Welfare, catalog number 70.
4. Pavlidis N, Briasoulis E, Hainsworth J, et al. Diagnostic and therapeutic management of cancer of an unknown primary. *Eur J Cancer.* 2003;39(14):1990–2005.
5. Neumann KH, Nystrom JS. Metastatic cancer of unknown origin: nonsquamous cell type. *Semin Oncol.* 1982;9(4):427–434.
6. Pentheroudakis G, Golfinopoulos V, Pavlidis N. Switching benchmarks in cancer of unknown primary: from autopsy to microarray. *Eur J Cancer.* 2007;43(14):2026–2036.
7. Greco GA, Hainsworth JD. Cancer of unknown primary site. In: DeVita Jr. VT, Hellman S, Rosenberg SA, eds. *Cancer: Principles and Practice of Oncology.* 8th ed. Philadelphia, PA: Lippincott Williams & Wilkins; 2008:2363–2387.
8. Abbruzzese JL, Abbruzzese MC, Hess KR, et al. Unknown primary carcinoma: natural history and prognostic factors in 657 consecutive patients. *J Clin Oncol.* 1994;12(6):1272–1280.
9. Oien KA. Pathologic evaluation of cancer of unknown primary. *Semin Oncol.* 2009;36(1):8–37.
10. Pavlidis N, Fizazi K. Carcinoma of unknown primary (CUP). *Crit Rev Oncol Hematol.* 2009;69(3):271–278.
11. Varadhachary GR, Abbruzzese JL, Lenzi R. Diagnostic strategies for unknown primary cancer. *Cancer.* 2004;100(9):1776–1785.
12. Bugat R, Bataillard A, Lesimple T, et al. Summary of the standards, options, and recommendations for the management of patients with carcinoma of unknown primary site (2002). *Br J Cancer.* 2003;89 (suppl. 1):S59–S66.
13. *National Cancer Institute: PDQ® Carcinoma of Unknown Primary Treatment.* Bethesda, MD: National Cancer Institute, 2014. http://cancer.gov/cancertopics/pdq/treatment/unknownprimary/HealthProfessional. Accessed July 5, 2014.
14. National Comprehensive Cancer Network (NCCN). *NCCN Clinical Practice Guidelines in Oncology. Occult Primary (Cancer of Unknown Primary [CUP]) Version 3.2014.* 2014 April 15; National Comprehensive Cancer Network.
15. Greco FA, Pavlidis N. Treatment for patients with unknown primary carcinoma and unfavorable prognostic factors. *Semin Oncol.* 2009;36(1):65–74.
16. Hainsworth JD, Fizazi K. Treatment for patients with unknown primary cancer and favorable prognostic factors. *Semin Oncol.* 2009;36(1):44–51.
17. Greco FA. Cancer of unknown primary site: evolving understanding and management of patients. *Clin Adv Hematol Oncol.* 2012;10(8):518–524.
18. Hainsworth JD, Spigel DR, Clark BL, et al. Paclitaxel/carboplatin/etoposide versus gemcitabine/irinotecan in the first-line treatment of patients with carcinoma of unknown primary site: a randomized, phase III Sarah Cannon Oncology Research Consortium Trial. *Cancer J.* 2010;16(1):70–75.
19. The National Lung Screening Trial Research Team. Reduced lung-cancer mortality with low-dose computed tomographic screening. *N Engl J Med.* 2011;365:395–409.
20. Bender RA, Erlander MG. Molecular classification of unknown primary cancer. *Semin Oncol.* 2009;36(1):38–43.
21. Hainsworth JD, Rubin MS, Spigel DR, et al. Molecular gene expression profiling to predict the tissue of origin and direct site-specific therapy in patients with carcinoma of unknown primary site: a prospective trial of the Sarah Cannon research institute. *J Clin Oncol.* 2013;31(2):217–223.
22. Hainsworth JD, Schnabel CA, Erlander MG, et al. A retrospective study of treatment outcomes in patients with carcinoma of unknown primary site and a colorectal cancer molecular profile. *Clin Colorectal Cancer.* 2012;11(2):112–118.
23. Greco FA, Rubin MS, Boccia RV, et al. Molecular gene expression profiling to predict the tissue of origin and direct site-specific therapy in patients with carcinoma of unknown primary site (CUP): results of a prospective Sarah Cannon Research Institute (SCRI) trial. *J Clin Oncol.* 2012;30:abstract 10530.
24. Greco FA, Lennington WJ, Spigel DR, et al. Carcinoma of unknown primary site: outcomes in patients with a colorectal molecular profile treated with site-specific chemotherapy. *J Cancer Ther.* 2012;3:37–42.

# 25

# *Hodgkin Lymphoma*

JESUS H. HERMOSILLO-RODRIGUEZ, POLLY A. NIRAVATH,
CATHERINE M. BOLLARD, AND CARLOS A. RAMOS

Hodgkin lymphoma (HL) is a lymphoid tumor that comprises about 10% of all lymphomas and 0.6% of all cancers diagnosed in the developed world each year (1). HL is divided into 2 main types by the 2008 World Health Organization (WHO) classification: classical Hodgkin lymphoma (CHL) and nodular lymphocyte-predominant Hodgkin lymphoma (NLPHL) (2).

## CHL: EPIDEMIOLOGY, RISK FACTORS, NATURAL HISTORY, AND PATHOLOGY

CHL accounts for 95% of cases of HL and is further divided into 4 subtypes: nodular sclerosis (approximately 70% of cases), mixed cellularity (20–25%), lymphocyte rich (5%), and lymphocyte depleted (1%). A hallmark feature of CHL is its bimodal age incidence, with 1 peak at 15–34 years of age, and a second peak after 55 years. There is a slight male predominance (1.4:1) and a 2- to 5-fold increased incidence in siblings.

Individuals with a history of infectious mononucleosis have 2–3 times increased risk of developing CHL. Although this association has been known for many years, it was only in 1987 that the presence of Epstein–Barr virus (EBV) was demonstrated in malignant Hodgkin Reed–Sternberg (HRS) cells. One EBV protein in particular, known as latent membrane protein 1 (LMP1), is thought to be key in the oncogenic process, as it is known to elicit B-lymphocyte transformation in vitro. Approximately half of all CHL cases in economically developed countries harbor EBV in HRS cells in contrast to up to 90% of patients in developing countries. EBV is infrequently found in nodular sclerosis CHL but is seen with increasing frequency in lymphocyte-rich, mixed-cellularity, and in almost all cases of lymphocyte-depleted CHL. Partly

related to these epidemiological differences, the nodular sclerosis CHL subtype is associated with factors that are linked to higher socioeconomic status, such as single-family homes, smaller family sizes, and higher level of maternal education. In contrast, mixed-cellularity CHL is inversely related to socioeconomic status.

There is clearly a relationship between immune dysfunction and higher incidence of CHL, as seen in patients with HIV, common variable immune deficiency, and solid organ or hematopoietic stem cell transplantation. On the other hand, patients with history of autoimmune disorders also have a higher incidence of CHL. Some CHL subtypes (mixed-cellularity and lymphocyte-depleted) appear to occur more frequently in the setting of HIV infection. Although CHL is included among the WHO HIV-associated lymphomas and there has been an increased incidence of CHL in HIV patients since the use of antiretroviral therapy (ART), the exact nature of this association remains unclear. There is a 10-fold increased risk of CHL among HIV-positive individuals, but this risk seems to decline with lower CD4 counts. More than 80% of HIV-associated CHL is connected to EBV infection, presumably related to impaired T-cell activity, which normally limits EBV proliferation (3). Even without another underlying disease, CHL patients typically have T-cell dysfunction and/or lymphopenia, having higher rates of bacterial, fungal, and viral infections even before starting treatment. Transfusion-related graft-versus-host disease has also been described in these patients.

CHL is generally considered to be a slow-growing lymphoma. Some cases of CHL may be preceded by a condition called "progressive transformation of the germinal center," a type of follicular lymphoid hyperplasia containing many small B cells of mantle zone type. This pathological entity is also seen in about one fifth of lymph nodes in NLPHL. However, there are many cases of patients with this condition who never develop HL. Thus, its significance is not totally clear. In contrast to most non-HLs, a notable feature of CHL is its tendency for contiguous, instead of distant, spread. However, with more advanced disease, the lymphoma can eventually invade blood vessels and spread to more distant organs (1). In the past several decades, significant advances have been made in the treatment of CHL, with the current 5-year overall survival (OS) rate from 2003 to 2009 being 88%. Even for those with stage III and IV disease at diagnosis, 5-year OS has been approximately 82% (4).

Pathologically, CHL is notable for its characteristic, sparse neoplastic HRS cells, which are clonal B cells of follicular center origin, in a background of inflammatory cells (T lymphocytes, macrophages, eosinophils, and plasma cells) (2). Fibrosis is common. The relative predominance of these elements defines each histological subtype. Immunophenotypically, CHL HRS cells will express CD15 in 70–85% of cases, and CD30 and fascin in nearly all cases. CD20 is positive in 30–40% of cases, more commonly in lymphocyte-rich CHL. The B-cell marker CD79a may be expressed (10% of CHL). Expression of T-cell antigens is rare, and has been associated with decreased event-free and OS.

## NLPHL: EPIDEMIOLOGY, RISK FACTORS, NATURAL HISTORY, AND PATHOLOGY

NLPHL comprises 5% of all HL cases. As with CHL, there is a slight male predominance (1). One of the main risk factors identified so far is family history of NLPHL, with first-degree family members having 19 times the risk of having this disease (5), and also a higher incidence of CHL and non-HL in relatives. The main difference between CHL and NLPHL is the neoplastic cell immunophenotype. In NLPHL, there is a lymphohistiocytic (L&H) Reed–Sternberg (RS) cell variant, or "popcorn" cell, which represents a clonal population of germinal center-derived tumor B cells (4). NLPHL is more commonly CD15 and CD30 negative, with strong CD20 and CD45 positivity. Also in contrast with CHL, NLPHL has not been associated with EBV infection. Staining for CD3 may further support the diagnosis because T cells characteristically form rosettes around the L&H cells. The remaining background cells in NLPHL are usually CD20 and CD79a positive B cells, and macrophages (1).

NLPHL usually presents at an early stage without B symptoms, and has a more indolent course, with delayed relapses compared to CHL. Estimating prognosis is challenging because of the paucity of data, but in a retrospective analysis complete remission (CR) with first-line treatment was achieved in 91.6% versus 85.9% of patients with favorable early-stage NLPHL compared to CHL, and

in 76.8% versus 77.8% of patients with advanced stages. Early-stage patients with NLPHL also seem to have better survival outcomes than early-stage CHL, with OS at 50 months of 96% and 92%, respectively (4).

## HL: STAGING

HL is staged using the Ann Arbor Staging System.

| Hodgkin Lymphoma Staging System | |
|---|---|
| Stage | Definition |
| I | Involvement of a single lymph node region (I), or localized involvement of a single extralymphatic organ or site (IE) |
| II | Involvement of 2 or more lymph node regions on the same side of the diaphragm (II), or localized involvement of a single associated extralymphatic organ or site and its regional lymph node/nodes, with or without involvement of other lymph node regions on the same side of the diaphragm (IIE) |
| III | Involvement of lymph node regions on both sides of the diaphragm (III), which may also be accompanied by localized involvement of an associated extralymphatic organ or site (IIIE), by involvement of the spleen (IIIS), or by both (IIIES) |
| IV | Disseminated (multifocal) involvement of 1 or more extralymphatic organs, with or without associated lymph node involvement, or isolated extralymphatic organ involvement with distant (nonregional) nodal involvement |
| **Further Classification Applicable to Any Stage** | |
| A | No systemic symptoms present |
| B | Unexplained fever > 38°C, drenching night sweats, or weight loss > 10% of body weight in the previous 6 months |
| X | Bulky disease: mediastinal widening > 1/3 the diameter of the chest at T5–T6 interspace in a posteroanterior chest radiograph, or nodal mass ≥ 10 cm |
| E | Involvement of single extranodal site contiguous or proximal to the known nodal site |

## CASE SUMMARIES

### Early-Stage Classical HL

N.P. is a 23-year-old white woman with no significant past medical history who presented with 4 months of a slowly enlarging right neck mass. She denied fever, chills, night sweats, pruritus, and weight loss. Physical examination revealed only right-sided cervical lymphadenopathy, although CT scans showed right-sided cervical and mediastinal lymphadenopathy measuring 4 cm in greatest dimension. Laboratory results included normal complete blood count (CBC), albumin, and erythrocyte sedimentation rate (ESR). Pregnancy test was negative. Excisional biopsy of the right cervical lymph node revealed nodules separated by fibrous bands, with classic RS cells, which were CD15 and CD30 positive, and CD20 negative. Bone marrow biopsy was unremarkable.

## Evidence-Based Case Discussion

In summary, N.P. is a 23-year-old woman with stage IIA CHL, nodular sclerosis subtype. Stages I and II are considered early-stage disease, which is further classified as favorable and unfavorable prognosis. This has been defined slightly differently in various clinical trials. The European Organization for the Research and Treatment of Cancer (EORTC) trials considers patients with any 1 of the following factors to have unfavorable prognosis (6):

- Age > 50 years at diagnosis
- Bulky mediastinal adenopathy
- Involvement of 4 or more lymph node regions
- B symptoms and ESR > 30 mm/hr, or ESR > 50 mm/hr without B symptoms

The German Hodgkin's Study Group (GHSG) does not regard age as an unfavorable risk factor, and considers involvement of 3, instead of 4, or more lymph node regions an adverse risk factor (4).

Our patient has early-stage favorable disease. Her age brings to consideration the issue of HL in pregnancy. Even though this particular patient was not pregnant, HL is the fourth most common malignancy among pregnant women (1). In staging a pregnant woman, MRI or ultrasound is usually chosen over CT scan in order to avoid radiation exposure to the fetus. Likewise, PET scanning should also not be used because the radioactive tracer crosses the placenta and is associated with higher radiation exposure than CT scan. Regarding treatment, chemotherapy should not be given in the first trimester when the fetus is particularly susceptible to teratogenic effects. Therapy can usually be delayed until the second or third trimester, when it has not been associated with higher rates of malformations, although it has been linked to higher rates of intrauterine death, growth retardation, preterm delivery, and low birth weight. Generally, though, most pregnant women can be offered chemotherapy with doxorubicin (Adriamycin), bleomycin, vinblastine, and dacarbazine (ABVD) (see the next case for description of specific drugs) in the second or third trimester with little risk to the fetus, because several case series and case reports have shown little adverse effects. Radiation to the fetus results in significantly higher risk of developing leukemia or a solid malignancy in the first decade of life, and thus should be avoided. Also, radiation to the chest in a pregnant or lactating woman confers a higher risk of breast cancer in the future.

For N.P., treatment should be tailored to optimize therapy while minimizing toxicity. Long-term toxicities of HL therapy typically include cardiac and pulmonary damage,

infertility, and secondary malignancies. Among patients with early-stage favorable CHL, mortality from these other causes increases over time, eventually overtaking HL-related mortality after 12–15 years (7). In an attempt to achieve high cure rates while decreasing side effects, many earlier studies have asked whether radiation alone is sufficient in early disease. The Southwest Oncology Group (SWOG) 9133/Cancer and Leukemia Group B (CALGB) 9391 trial enrolled 348 patients with stage IA and IIA disease, excluding patients with adverse prognostic features. Patients were randomized to receive 2 cycles of chemotherapy (adriamycin and vinblastine) followed by subtotal lymphoid irradiation (STLI), or STLI only. The trial was closed early because of the clearly superior failure-free survival (FFS) of 94% versus 81% in the combined modality therapy (CMT) arm versus the STLI-only arm, although there was no demonstrable difference in OS. However, hematologic toxicity was higher with CMT (8). Similar findings were seen in the GHSG HD 7 trial comparing extended-field radiotherapy (EFRT) following ABVD versus EFRT alone (relapse rate 3% vs. 22%, respectively) (9). Finally, in the H8-F trial, which enrolled early-stage patients with EORTC favorable risk factors, there was a significantly higher rate of CR and improved 10-year OS in patients who received 3 cycles of mechlorethamine, vincristine, procarbazine, and prednisone (MOPP)–doxorubicin, bleomycin and vinblastin (ABV) followed by involved field radiotherapy (IFRT) compared to STLI alone (10).

Although it became apparent that CMT is superior to radiotherapy alone, the question of how much radiation is necessary remained unanswered. The HD8 study analyzed 1064 early-stage GHSG unfavorable risk patients (and stage IIIA with no risk factors), who were randomized to 4 cycles of chemotherapy (2 of cyclophosphamide, vincristine, procarbazine, and prednisone [COPP] and 2 of ABVD) followed by either 30-Gy EFRT or 30-Gy IFRT (both arms adding 10 Gy to initial bulky disease). There was no difference in freedom from treatment failure (FFTF) or OS. However, EFRT had significantly higher rates of gastrointestinal and hematologic toxicity. After a median time of 55 months, there was a 4.6% rate of secondary malignancies in the EFRT arm versus 2.8% in the IFRT arm ($P = .191$) (11). Although patients treated in this trial had unfavorable disease, the data suggest that chemotherapy and IFRT should also be sufficient for favorable disease. The next question to be asked was whether the amount of chemotherapy and radiation could be further reduced. The HD10 trial randomized patients with early-stage GHSG favorable-risk disease in a 2 × 2 design to 4 versus 2 cycles of ABVD, and 30 versus 20-Gy IFRT. Four-year follow-up data showed no difference in FFTF (93% vs. 91.1%) or OS (97.1% and 96.6%) (12).

As an alternative, the abbreviated (8-week) Stanford V regimen (see the next case for description of the regimen) combined with IFRT has been studied in early-stage CHL

(4), in a study that excluded HIV-positive patients and patients with bulky disease. Of the patients treated, 48% had GHSG unfavorable risk factors and 33% had EORTC unfavorable risk factors. After 10 years, the estimated freedom from progression (FFP), disease-specific survival, and OS were 94%, 99%, and 94%, respectively. None of the patients developed secondary hematologic malignancies.

Two major trials have looked at the question of whether chemotherapy alone is a reasonable alternative for early-stage CHL. The first trial, conducted at Memorial Sloan-Kettering Cancer Center, randomized 152 patients with early-stage or stage IIIA HL without bulky disease (but who could have other unfavorable risk factors) to either 6 cycles of ABVD alone or 6 cycles of ABVD and radiotherapy (36 Gy). There was no significant difference in FFP (91% vs. 87%) at 60 months from CR. Although there was a trend for improved OS with CMT versus ABVD alone (97% vs. 90%), this was not statistically significant ($P = .08$). There were 5 secondary malignancies with CMT and 3 with chemotherapy alone, but study size precluded detection of differences of <20% (13). The other major study, HD.6 trial, randomized 399 patients with early-stage disease to 4–6 cycles of ABVD alone versus CMT using subtotal nodal irradiation (STNI). Highly unfavorable (bulky or intra-abdominal) disease was excluded. A significantly higher FFP at 5 years was observed with CMT initially (93% vs. 87%, $P = .006$). However, updated results at 12 years showed lower OS with CMT than with ABVD alone (87% vs. 94%, $P = .04$), owing to an increased number of deaths from causes other than HL, including second cancers (14).

The role of interim $^{18}$F-fludeoxyglucose (FDG)-PET/CT in the management of early-stage CHL has also been examined. In an Italian study, 304 patients underwent PET/CT before chemotherapy, after 2 cycles and at the end of treatment. Patients with interim positive uptake had worse outcomes (21% vs. 97.6% CR rate) (15). In the RAPID trial, 571 patients with early-stage CHL (62% having favorable prognosis by EORTC) received 3 cycles of ABVD followed by interim FDG-PET/CT (16). Patients with a positive PET/CT received a fourth cycle of ABVD followed by IFRT. If the PET/CT was negative, patients were randomized to IFRT versus no IFRT. One fourth of patients had a positive interim PET/CT, with PFS and OS at 3 years after CMT being 85% and 94%, respectively. In those with negative interim PET/CT, PFS at 49 months after IFRT was 95% versus 91% without IFRT ($P = .23$ in intention-to-treat analysis, although per protocol this difference became significant, as 26 patients allocated to IFRT did not receive it). At 3 years, OS was 97% versus 99% in the IFRT versus no IFRT groups, respectively. Longer follow-up results are still needed for this strategy before drawing definitive conclusions.

The concept and use of IFRT are currently evolving to involved site radiation therapy, or ISRT. This technique allows the radiation oncologist to reduce the field of treatment even in cases when pre-chemotherapy gross tumor volume is not amenable to therapy or accurate calculation (4). It also attempts to spare radiation exposure of adjacent uninvolved organs after tumor shrinkage.

Currently, based on the aforementioned data, a reasonable recommendation is to treat favorable stage I and II CHL patients with CMT, usually 4 cycles of ABVD followed by 30-Gy ISRT. If patients fulfill the GHSG favorable-risk definition, 2 cycles of ABVD followed by 20 Gy ISRT is an option, as shown by the HD10 trial. Patients with relative contraindications to radiation therapy (RT), such as females of childbearing age, as our patient N.P., in whom irradiation of mammary tissue is associated with an increased risk of breast cancer, should probably receive 4–6 cycles of ABVD alone, particularly if a PET/CT is negative after 2 cycles (see Figure 25.1). The abbreviated Stanford V regimen with 30-Gy ISRT would also be a possible alternative, although this may still be associated with a high rate of late radiation-related mortality. ISRT should ideally start within 3 weeks of completion of chemotherapy.

If our patient had unfavorable disease, the recommendation would be slightly different. Besides the HD8 trial discussed previously, which established that IFRT is less toxic than EFRT in these patients, other trials have addressed management in this setting. The GHSG HD11 trial analyzed data from 1395 patients randomized in a 2 × 2 factorial design to 4 cycles of ABVD versus 4 cycles of baseline (standard-dose) bleomycin, etoposide, doxorubicin, cyclophosphamide, vincristine, procarbazine, and prednisone (BEACOPP) (see the next case for description of the regimen) and 30 versus 20-Gy IFRT. BEACOPP conferred 5-year FFTF of 86.8% versus 81% for ABVD, when 20-Gy IFRT was used, but there was no difference when 30-Gy IFRT was used (87% vs. 85%) (4). The HD14 trial used radiation plus 4 cycles ABVD versus 2 cycles of escalated-dose BEACOPP followed by 2 cycles ABVD, with similar findings (higher FFTF but similar OS, 97% at 5 years) (17). Thus, ABVD is still more frequently used in the United States.

The standard (12-week) Stanford V regimen with radiotherapy (36 Gy) to bulky sites (≥5 cm) and to macroscopic splenic disease has also been evaluated in bulky early-stage disease. In a non-randomized trial of 142 patients with bulky early-stage or advanced-stage CHL, the FFP and OS at 5 years were 89% and 96%, respectively (18). In a later, randomized controlled trial of 520 patients with unfavorable early-stage or advanced stage, Stanford V plus radiotherapy had similar overall response rate (ORR) to ABVD plus radiotherapy (91% vs. 92%, respectively) and no difference in projected 5-year PFS (74% vs. 76%) and OS (92% vs. 90%). Although CR rate was higher with ABVD versus Stanford V (55% vs. 36%, $P < .001$), this came at the expense of more pulmonary toxicity (10% vs.

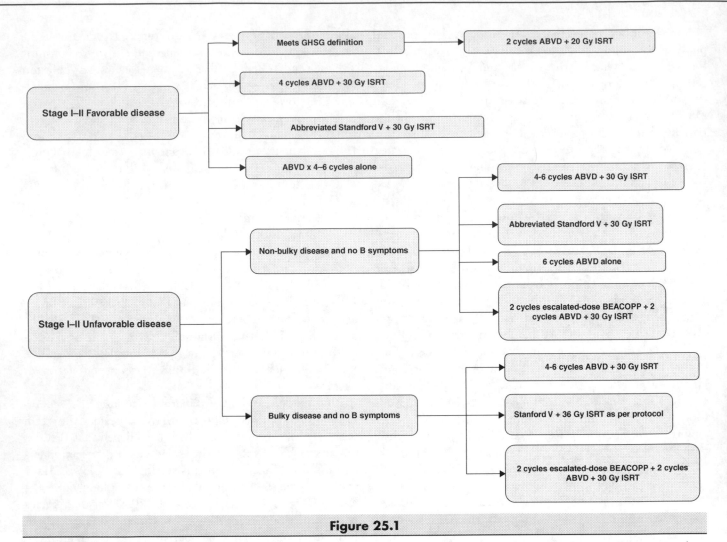

**Figure 25.1**

First-line treatment options for early-stage disease classical Hodgkin lymphoma. ABVD, doxorubicin, bleomycin, vinblastine, and dacarbazine; BEACOPP, bleomycin, etoposide, doxorubicin, cyclophosphamide, vincristine, procarbazine, and prednisone; GHSG, German Hodgkin's Study Group; ISRT, involved site radiation therapy.

2%) and higher probability of needing G-CSF (75% vs. 41%). Thus, the efficacies of Stanford V and ABVD are comparable when combined with appropriate radiotherapy (4). The advantages of the shorter duration and lower doses of chemotherapy with Stanford V may, however, be offset by the potential higher radiation exposure and its long-term toxicity. Therefore, patient selection is important.

Thus, patients with unfavorable early-stage CHL have different treatment alternatives, which may depend on the presence of bulky disease and/or B symptoms. For non-bulky disease without B symptoms, 4–6 cycles of ABVD plus 30-Gy ISRT are often used. These patients can also receive the abbreviated Stanford V followed by ISRT. In select cases, chemotherapy alone (6 cycles of ABVD) may be reasonable, especially if there are relative contraindications to radiation. Finally, 2 cycles of escalated-dose BEACOPP followed by 2 cycles of ABVD and ISRT are an alternative that has shown some evidence of improved FFTF, albeit at a higher risk of toxicity. For patients with bulky disease and/or B symptoms, treatment options are similar. However, RT is more often recommended, and

these patients would not be candidates for the abbreviated Stanford V regimen (see Figure 25.1).

## Advanced-Stage Classical HL

L.Z., a 46-year-old Hispanic woman with no past medical history, presented to the emergency department complaining of a left neck mass enlarging over the previous 6 months, fever to 101°F, night sweats, and a 30-pound weight loss. Her physical examination revealed a 6-cm firm left neck mass, along with other palpable lymphadenopathy in the right cervical, left axillary, and bilateral inguinal regions. Laboratory values were significant for anemia (hemoglobin = 10.5 g/dL), a platelet count of 125,000/µL, an albumin of 2.9 g/dL, and an ESR of 78 mm/hr. A CT scan revealed hepatosplenomegaly and diffuse bulky lymphadenopathy, including enlargement of mediastinal, bilateral cervical, left axillary, retroperitoneal, pelvic, and bilateral inguinal lymph nodes. Biopsy of a left cervical lymph node was positive for nodular sclerosis CHL, and bone marrow biopsy was positive for CHL involvement as well. She was treated

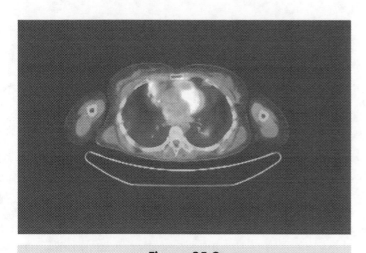

**Figure 25.2**

PET scan showing residual FDG-avid disease in the mediastinum. FDG, [18]F-fludeoxyglucose.

with 2 cycles of ABVD chemotherapy, and subsequent PET scan showed partial response (Figure 25.2).

## Evidence-Based Case Discussion

L.Z. has stage IVB CHL with several poor prognostic features, including B symptoms and bulky lymphadenopathy. Furthermore, the lack of CR on PET scan following 2 cycles of ABVD is a very poor prognostic indicator and this has generated interest in risk-adapted strategies. For instance, a retrospective study analyzed 165 patients with advanced HL who initially received 2 cycles of ABVD followed by PET scan. Those with negative PET scan were given 4 more cycles of ABVD and radiation, and those with positive PET scan were given 4 cycles of dose-escalated BEACOPP followed by 4 cycles of standard-dose BEACOPP and radiation. The 2-year FFS was 65% for the PET-positive patients and 92% for the PET-negative patients ($P = .0004$). When compared to historical controls whose treatment did not change based on interim PET scan, the 2-year PFS for PET-positive patients was improved from 12% to 62% (19). Although these results do document a prognostic role for PET scan, randomized controlled trials are still ongoing to support the role of PET in adjusting treatment in CHL.

For advanced-stage CHL, chemotherapy with MOPP was once the standard treatment. However, this was associated with high risk of acute leukemia, sterility, and myelosuppression. Randomized, prospective trials showed that, although the OS was not significantly different, the CR rate was higher in ABVD-containing regimens compared to MOPP, with fewer hematologic adverse events and sterility.

Although ABVD has emerged as the most accepted standard therapy for CHL, the Stanford V regimen is still used by some. By decreasing the total dose of alkylating

agents, doxorubicin and bleomycin, while increasing the dose density and intensity, it aims to decrease the risk of toxicities. This regimen consists of prednisone and doxorubicin, vinblastine, and mechlorethamine, alternating with vincristine, bleomycin, and etoposide, given for a period of 12 weeks (standard regimen), followed by consolidative radiotherapy (4). As mentioned in the previous case, the Stanford V regimen has been directly compared to ABVD in a randomized trial that included patients with bulky and/or advanced stage disease, which suggested these regimens are comparable, provided RT is used after Stanford V. More recently, the Intergroup E2496 trial analyzed 794 patients with stage III or IV HL or bulky mediastinal adenopathy, who were randomized to 6–8 cycles of ABVD or standard Stanford V. RT (36 Gy) was given to all patients with bulky mediastinal adenopathy 2–3 weeks after chemotherapy. Patients who were given the Stanford V regimen received in addition RT (36 Gy) to any pretreatment site ≥5 cm and for macroscopic splenic disease by CT. There was no significant difference in ORR (73% ABVD vs. 69% Stanford V) and in FFS (74% vs. 71%, $P = .32$) or OS (88% for both) (20).

Advanced HL might justify even more aggressive regimens based on potentially higher cure rates. However, these are usually associated with increased toxicity. In the GHSG HD9 study, 1196 patients with unfavorable stage IIB disease or stages III–IV were randomized to 1 of 3 arms: 8 cycles of COPP alternating with ABVD; 8 cycles of standard-dose baseline BEACOPP; or 8 cycles of increased-dose (escalated) BEACOPP. Patients received radiation after chemotherapy to initial sites >5 cm. The rate of CR was higher with dose-escalated BEACOPP (96% vs. 85% for COPP–ABVD and 88% for standard BEACOPP), and early progression was significantly lower as well (2% vs. 10% for COPP–ABVD and 8% for standard BEACOPP). In an updated report, the 10-year OS rate remained significantly higher with dose-escalated BEACOPP (86% vs. 75% for COPP–ABVD and 80% for standard BEACOPP). However, the rate of secondary acute leukemia at 5 years was 0.4% in the COPP–ABVD, 0.6% in the baseline BEACOPP, and 2.5% in the escalated BEACOPP groups ($P = .03$). Also, even with the use of G-CSF, there was a 98% incidence of grade 3–4 leukopenia, 47% grade 4 thrombocytopenia, and 22% grade 3–4 infections in the dose-escalated BEACOPP arm (21). ABVD and BEACOPP were also compared in an Italian trial of 307 patients with stages IIB, III, or IV CHL. Although BEACOPP demonstrated improved progression-free survival compared to ABVD (81% vs. 69% at a median of 41 months, $P = .038$), this did not translate into a significantly higher OS rate (4).

In the HD15 trial, 2182 patients with bulky or extranodal stage IIB disease or stages III or IV were randomized to 8 cycles of escalated-dose BEACOPP, 6 cycles of escalated-dose BEACOPP, or 8 cycles of time-intensified standard-dose BEACOPP (every 2 weeks). After chemotherapy, patients underwent FDG PET/CT and patients with PET-positive residual sites ≥2.5 cm received 30-Gy RT. The 5-year FFTF was similar in all groups (84.4%, 89.3%, and 85.4%, respectively). However, OS was higher with 6 cycles than with 8 cycles (95.3% vs. 91.9%, $P = .019$). In addition, treatment-related mortality (4.6% vs. 7.5%) and incidence of secondary cancers (2.4% vs. 4.7%) were lower with 6 cycles. These data suggest that, if BEACOPP is used for advanced CHL, 6 cycles of the escalated regimen may be optimal (22).

Overall, these studies suggest that intensifying initial chemotherapy with dose-escalated BEACOPP is a double-edged sword improving disease control but increasing toxicity. Furthermore, except for a meta-analysis suggesting that 6 cycles of escalated BEACOPP has a 10% OS advantage over ABVD at 5 years (23), a clear improvement in OS has not been demonstrated for this regimen.

Another major question for advanced HL is whether patients should receive stem cell transplant as first-line treatment. In a study of 163 adults with advanced-stage CHL and adverse prognostic features, patients who achieved a CR after 4 courses of chemotherapy were randomized to receive either 4 more courses, or high-dose therapy (HDT) followed by autologous stem cell transplant (ASCT). There was no difference between the 2 arms in CR, 5-year FFS, or 5-year OS rates (24). Similar findings were found in another randomized study (25). Thus, patients who respond well to initial chemotherapy for advanced-stage HL are unlikely to derive added benefit from early HDT/ASCT.

A final question for the treatment of advanced-stage HL is whether to irradiate radiologically eradicated disease because 80% of relapsed HL cases recur in sites of previous lymphadenopathy (1). A large meta-analysis examined data on 1740 patients with all stages of disease across 14 trials. The trials were divided into those that evaluated chemotherapy alone versus the same chemotherapy plus RT (additional RT design), and those that tested whether radiotherapy as part of CMT can be replaced with chemotherapy (parallel RT/CT design). There was a significantly more durable CR at 10 years in the additional RT design trials for those patients who received radiotherapy ($P \leq .001$). However, in the parallel RT/CT design, continuous CR rates were similar whether additional radiotherapy or additional chemotherapy was given. Interestingly, there was an 8% improvement in OS at 10 years in patients who received no radiotherapy in the parallel RT/CT design, which was due to a significantly increased rate of deaths unrelated to CHL in the CMT groups (26). This seems to suggest that additional chemotherapy can substitute for radiotherapy, possibly with less long-term toxicity and increased OS, as reported in the late analysis of the HD.6 trial (14). However, the other trials that included an additional RT component used 6–8 cycles of MOPP or BCVPP (carmustine, cyclophosphamide, vinblastine, procarbazine, and prednisone), which are not as efficacious as ABVD. Thus, it is still debatable whether these results are truly applicable in the present day. More recently, an EORTC trial of patients with advanced-stage CHL who underwent 6–8 cycles of MOPP/ABV randomized those who attained CR to no further treatment or IFRT. OS was not significantly different between patients who received or did not receive IFRT, suggesting that consolidation radiotherapy does not benefit those in CR after chemotherapy (27).

In summary, there are several treatment options for advanced-stage CHL. An effective treatment is 6–8 cycles of ABVD. As per the Intergroup E2496 trial, ISRT can be given after to initial sites of bulky mediastinal disease, especially if they remain PET-positive. Another choice is Stanford V, with radiotherapy per protocol, with careful patient selection. If a patient is considered higher risk, escalated-dose BEACOPP is an option as there is a suggestion of higher CR and OS rates in a meta-analysis compared to ABVD. Six cycles of escalated-dose BEACOPP with or without RT can be given instead of 8 cycles to decrease toxicity (see Figure 25.3).

## Relapsed and Refractory Classical HL

M.M. is a 54-year-old white woman with stage IV CHL, manifested by cervical, axillary, and bulky mediastinal lymphadenopathy as well as bone marrow involvement. She was treated with 8 cycles of ABVD and mediastinal radiation. A PET scan performed 2 months after treatment still shows residual FDG-avid disease in the mediastinum that is biopsy proven to be HL.

## Evidence-Based Case Discussion

M.M. has highly aggressive, refractory HL. Although initial CR rates are quite high in CHL, approximately 20–30% of patients relapse, presenting a complicated treatment decision. Factors associated with relapse include advanced stage, B symptoms, and extranodal disease. At relapse, all patients should be biopsied because of the relatively high risk for secondary tumors. Once CHL is confirmed, the type of relapse should be ascertained because of the marked difference in prognosis and response to treatment. Patients with primary progressive HL (who never achieve a CR, or relapse within 3 months of completing treatment) have a markedly poorer prognosis than those patients who have early relapse (3–12 months after treatment) or late relapse (>12 months after treatment). The projected 20-year OS for primary progressive CHL is approximately 0%, compared to 11% for early and 22% for late relapse (1).

In a small percentage of patients with relapsed disease who have very limited areas of involvement and in whom

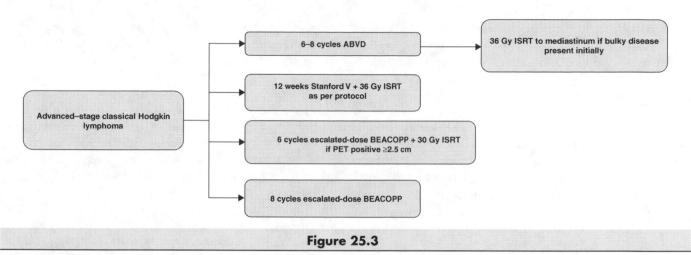

**Figure 25.3**

Treatment options for advanced-stage classical Hodgkin lymphoma. ABVD, doxorubicin, bleomycin, vinblastine, and dacarbazine; BEACOPP, bleomycin, etoposide, doxorubicin, cyclophosphamide, vincristine, procarbazine, and prednisone; ISRT, involved site radiation therapy.

radiotherapy was not used, radiotherapy alone may be very effective. Moreover, due to their overall favorable prognosis, patients with late relapses who also have very limited areas of involvement may achieve long remissions with chemotherapy alone (with or without radiotherapy, as appropriate). However, for the majority of patients with relapsed or refractory disease, the favored treatment is chemotherapy followed by HDT and ASCT. Achieving a CR prior to HDT/ASCT is prognostic, as a retrospective analysis of PET/CT after 2 cycles of salvage chemotherapy was predictive of survival after ASCT (2-year PFS of 93% vs. 10% for patients with negative and positive PET/CT, respectively) (28).

Two randomized controlled trials have established the role of ASCT in relapsed CHL. The first of these trials enrolled 40 patients, 20 of whom received HDT with BEAM (carmustine, etoposide, cytarabine, and melphalan) followed by ASCT, while the remaining 20 patients received mini-BEAM (the same drugs at lower doses) alone. The ASCT arm had improved 3-year event-free survival (53% vs. 10%, $P$ = .025), but the OS difference was not statistically significant. The second trial, which enrolled 161 relapsed patients, showed similar results, with FFTF at 3 years significantly higher in the ASCT arm (55% vs. 34%, $P$ = .019), but OS was not significantly different (29).

Allogeneic transplant has also been studied in relapsed–refractory CHL; however, its toxicities generally seem to outweigh its benefits. For instance, a retrospective study of 45 allogeneic transplants versus 45 matched autologous transplant controls found a significantly improved 4-year survival with ASCT versus allogeneic transplant (64% vs. 30%, $P$ = .007). Transplant-related mortality (65% after allogeneic vs. 12% after ASCT) was felt to be the primary culprit for this difference (30). At present, ASCT remains the widely accepted standard of care for chemosensitive relapsed or refractory CHL.

The best salvage regimen for relapsed–refractory CHL is not entirely clear, as there are many available options

and no randomized controlled trials. Usually, the treatment selected is a regimen different from the initial one, although responses have been seen when repeating the same regimen, particularly in late relapses. Typically, 2–3 cycles are given followed by HDT and ASCT, if there is a response by imaging studies. Regimens that have shown effectiveness prior to ASCT include ICE (ifosfamide, carboplatin, etoposide); DHAP (dexamethasone, cytarabine, and cisplatin); ESHAP (etoposide, steroid [methylprednisolone], high-dose cytarabine, and cisplatin), 1 of several gemcitabine-based regimens; or mini-BEAM (4). For patients who are not candidates for ASCT (or whose disease has relapsed after ASCT), options include brentuximab vedotin, bendamustine, lenalidomide, or everolimus (4). Brentuximab vedotin is a CD30 antibody–drug conjugate that has shown significant activity, with an overall response rate of 75% and CR rate of 34%, and minimal toxicity (31), although follow-up is limited. It is currently being investigated in combination as first-line therapy.

## Nodular Lymphocyte-Predominant Hodgkin Lymphoma

R.T. is an otherwise healthy 35-year-old male with a 6-month history of an enlarging right axillary mass. He denied fatigue, fevers, chills, sweats, and weight loss. On physical examination, he was noted to have bilateral axillary lymphadenopathy. Laboratory tests were unremarkable. ESR was 56 mm/hr. A CT scan showed only bilateral axillary lymphadenopathy. Lymph node biopsy showed NLPHL, positive for CD20 and negative for CD15 and CD30.

### Evidence-Based Case Discussion

This young man has stage II NLPHL, which behaves quite differently from CHL. NLPHL generally is less aggressive, carries a better prognosis, and tends to be identified at earlier stages (typically without B symptoms) with 53% of patients diagnosed in stage I disease, and only 6% in stage IV. However, NLPHL has a higher rate of transformation to aggressive non-HL and tends to relapse multiple times compared to CHL (1).

It is now widely held that NLPHL should be treated differently from CHL due to its unique behavior, as well as its CD20 positivity. For limited disease, RT alone seems to be a viable option. In a single-center study of long-term outcomes of 113 patients with stage I or II NLPHL, 93 received RT alone, 13 received chemotherapy and radiation, and 7 received chemotherapy alone. Ten-year PFS was 85% for stage I and 61% for stage II. Interestingly, those who received chemotherapy alone had worse PFS than those who received radiation alone. Moreover, the addition of chemotherapy to RT did not improve PFS or OS compared to RT alone. The extent of RT (limited field, extended field, or regional field) also did not appear to affect PFS or OS. Another review examined 131 cases of stage IA NLPHL in the GHSG, finding no significant difference in CR or OS with radiation versus CMT (5). These results indicate that IFRT alone (typically 30–36 Gy) may be sufficient for early-stage NLPHL.

Nonetheless, CMT with ABVD has been shown advantageous in at least 1 study. A long-term study of 88 patients in British Columbia compared radiation-alone treatment era (32 patients) versus ABVD treatment era (56 patients) outcomes. Patients had mostly stage IA and IIA and all but 14 patients in the ABVD treatment era also received RT. The 10-year PFS was 91% versus 65%, and OS 93% versus 84%, favoring patients treated in the CMT era (32).

Observation after excisional biopsy may also be an acceptable option for early-stage disease. A report analyzed 164 patients with NLPHL (mostly stages IA and IIA) (33), who received radiation in 27% of cases, CMT in 29%, and chemotherapy alone in 9%. The remaining 35% were observed after excisional biopsy without additional initial treatment. At 10 years, PFS was 41% versus 66% in the untreated compared to the treated patients, but the OS rate was similar (91% vs. 93%). Half of the observed patients were in CR at a median follow-up of 3 years.

Given NLPHL CD20 positivity, there has also been much interest in using rituximab in this disease. A phase II GHSG study examined 4 weekly treatments of rituximab alone in 28 patients with stage IA disease. ORR was 100% and CR rate was 86%. Three-year PFS was 81%, which is inferior to results of studies with RT or CMT (5).

In summary, radiotherapy alone is probably sufficient for most patients with early-stage NLPHL. A minority of patients with completely excised lymph nodes may be suitable for observation. On the other hand, bulkier disease (which is rare) or patients with B symptoms may benefit from CMT (see Figure 25.4).

As advanced-stage disease is rare, there are not many studies analyzing this issue. Although ABVD has been used, there are some concerns raised by data combined from CALGB trials and the Dana–Farber Cancer Institute and Joint Center for Radiation Therapy studies that reported outcomes in patients treated with non-alkylating (ABVD-based) versus alkylating (MOPP-based) regimens (5). The analysis of 37 patients showed that there were more treatment failures in the ABVD group compared to the MOPP-based group, suggesting that alkylating regimens may be more effective in this setting. On the other hand, rituximab has also shown very good response rate (4), although with similar concerns of lower PFS when used as a single agent. In light of this findings, a retrospective analysis of 63 patients with NLPHL (24 with advanced stage) receiving rituximab, cyclophosphamide, doxorubicin (hydroxydaunorubicin), and prednisone (R-CHOP) or ABVD ± rituximab from 1995 to 2010 was done in the University of Texas M. D. Anderson Cancer Center. ORR to R-CHOP was 100% and CR rate was 90%, without

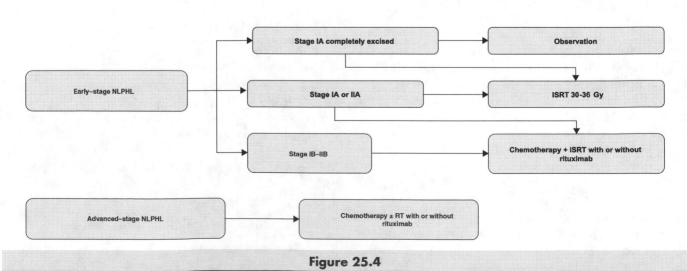

**Figure 25.4**

Treatment options for nodular lymphocyte–predominant Hodgkin lymphoma. ISRT, involved site radiation therapy; NLPHL, nodular lymphocyte-predominant Hodgkin lymphoma.

relapses or transformation at a median follow-up of 42 months. However, with other therapies, 19% patients had relapsed after median remissions of 38 months (5).

For relapsed or refractory disease, rituximab has been examined as a single agent. In a phase II trial, 22 patients (10 of whom had relapsed disease) received 4 doses of weekly rituximab. All patients responded, with a CR rate of 41%. At 13 months, 9 of the 22 patients had disease relapse, but responses were seen in 3 patients after retreatment with rituximab. This protocol was modified to allow patients to receive additional 4 weekly doses of rituximab every 6 months for 2 years. This extended regimen was associated with higher CR rate (88% vs. 56%) and FFP at 30 months (88% vs. 52%) compared to 4 doses of rituximab alone. Finally, another phase II trial conducted by the GHSG examined 15 patients with confirmed relapsed or refractory NLPHL, of whom 40% had advanced disease. Treatment with 4 weekly doses of rituximab resulted in 94% ORR, with a 53% CR rate. Median time to progression was 33 months, and median OS had not been yet reached at 7 years (5).

Although there are limited data supporting ASCT, a single-center experience of 26 patients with relapsed or transformed NLPHL who were treated with HDT and ASCT from 1990 to 2008 showed that, after median follow-up of 50 months, 5-year OS and event-free survival were 76% and 69%, respectively (5). This suggests that this modality is an option to consider in these patients.

In summary, options for advanced-stage NLPHL include chemotherapy with or without rituximab plus RT. Alkylating regimens, such as R-CHOP, are a promising alternative to ABVD that need further evaluation. In the relapsed setting, single-agent rituximab has activity, and ASCT is another treatment option that can be considered.

## REVIEW QUESTIONS

1. A 30-year-old male with no significant medical history presents with right cervical lymphadenopathy that he noticed a few months ago and has been persistent. He complains of night sweats that started recently. On physical examination, he exhibits 2-cm right cervical and supraclavicular lymphadenopathy but no other palpable lymph nodes or organomegaly. CT scan of the chest, abdomen, and pelvis does not show any other lymphadenopathy or concerning lesions. Lab work shows erythrocyte sedimentation rate of 22 mm/hr. Lymph node biopsy shows abnormal cells, which are CD15+, CD30+, CD20+, and EBV-encoded RNA+ (EBER). Which of following is an epidemiological feature of this disease?

   (A) It comprises 5% of all Hodgkin lymphoma cases
   (B) It has a female predominance
   (C) Its age incidence has a bimodal pattern of distribution
   (D) It is not associated with immunodeficiency

2. Which of the following would be the most appropriate treatment for this patient?

   (A) Two cycles ABVD + 20-Gy ISRT
   (B) Four cycles ABVD + 30-Gy ISRT
   (C) Stanford V regimen
   (D) Two cycles escalated-dose BEACOPP + 2 cycles ABVD + 30 Gy ISRT

3. A 56-year-old male with hypertension and diabetes mellitus presents with subjective fever, night sweats, and 15% weight loss in the past 3 months. CT scan of the chest, abdomen, and pelvis showed multiple mediastinal lymph nodes, the largest measuring 10.5 cm. No lymphadenopathy is seen below the diaphragm. Erythrocyte sedimentation rate 47 mm/hr. Biopsy of a lymph node showed classic Reed–Sternberg cells. Bone marrow biopsy is negative for malignancy. Which of the following would be the most appropriate treatment recommended for this patient?

   (A) Abbreviated Standford V regimen + 30-Gy ISRT
   (B) Four to six cycles ABVD + 30-Gy ISRT
   (C) Two cycles ABVD + 20-Gy ISRT
   (D) Four cycles ABVD alone

4. A 32-year-old female who is 18 weeks pregnant presented with fever, chills, night sweats, and palpable lymph nodes. Imaging shows diffuse lymphadenopathy in both sides of the diaphragm with a splenic lesion. Biopsy is consistent with classic Hodgkin lymphoma. Bone marrow biopsy is negative for malignancy. What is the most recommended management for this patient?

   (A) Twelve weeks' Standford V + 36-Gy ISRT to bulky sites and splenic disease
   (B) Six cycles of escalated-dose BEACOPP + 30-Gy ISRT to PET positive ≥2.5-cm sites
   (C) Wait to start therapy until after delivery
   (D) Eight cycles of ABVD alone

5. A 35-year-old man finished treatment with 8 cycles of ABVD for stage IIIA mixed-cellularity classical Hodgkin lymphoma (HL) 18 months ago. CT and PET scans done after completion of therapy were consistent with a complete response. Restaging studies done 3 months ago showed a mediastinal lymph node conglomerate measuring 8 cm in greatest diameter. A PET scan showed $^{18}$F-fludeoxyglucose-avid disease in the same area of the mediastinum only. Core needle biopsy confirmed relapsed HL. He was started on ifosfamide, carboplatin, etoposide (ICE) chemotherapy, which he tolerated well, having finished his second cycle approximately 3 weeks ago. A new CT of the chest showed reduction in the size of the mediastinal mass to 2 cm. He comes to your clinic for an opinion

regarding management at this point. Which of the following strategies should you recommend?

(A) Allogeneic stem cell transplant following conditioning with BEAM

(B) Change chemotherapy to etoposide, steroid (methylprednisolone), high-dose cytarabine, and cisplatin

(C) Four more cycles of ICE

(D) High-dose chemotherapy followed by autologous stem cell transplant (ASCT)

(E) Radiation therapy to the mediastinum

(F) No further treatment

6. Which of the following is an epidemiologic feature of nodular lymphocyte-predominant Hodgkin lymphoma (NLPHL)?

(A) It has worse prognosis than classical Hodgkin lymphoma (CHL)

(B) It has a higher risk of transformation to non-Hodgkin lymphoma compared to CHL

(C) It has been associated with Epstein–Barr virus infection

(D) There is a lower familial component in the development of NLPHL than in the development of CHL

7. A 34-year-old female presents to your office with a left axillary mass that she felt in the shower 5 months ago and is bothersome. She denies fever, chills, night sweats, or weight loss and is otherwise feeling well. CT scan shows several 1–2 cm lymph nodes in the left axilla and does not show any other lymphadenopathy. Erythrocyte sedimentation rate is 39 mm/hr. Excisional biopsy of 1 of the lymph nodes shows abnormal "popcorn" cells, which are positive for CD45 and CD20, and negative for CD15 and CD30. Which of the following is the most appropriate treatment recommendation?

(A) 30-Gy ISRT alone

(B) ABVD + ISRT

(C) R-CHOP + ISRT

(D) Observation

## REFERENCES

1. Engert A, Eichenauer DA, Harris NL, et al. Hodgkin lymphoma. In: DeVita VT, Lawrence TS, Rosenberg SA, eds. *Cancer: Principles and Practice of Oncology.* 9th ed. Philadelphia, PA: Lippincott Williams & Wilkins; 2011:1819–1854.

2. Swerdlow SH, Campo E, Harris NL, et al., eds. *WHO Classification of Tumours of Haematopoietic and Lymphoid Tissues.* Lyon: International Agency for Research on Cancer, 2008.

3. Carbone A, Gloghini A, Serraino D, et al. HIV-associated Hodgkin lymphoma. *Curr Opin HIV AIDS.* 2009;4(1):3–10.

4. Hoppe RT, Advani RH, Ai WZ, et al. Hodgkin lymphoma. *J Natl Compr Canc Netw.* 2011;9(9):1020–1058.

5. Fanale M. Lymphocyte-predominant Hodgkin lymphoma: what is the optimal treatment? *Hematol Am Soc Hematol Educ Program.* 2010;2013(21):406–413.

6. Cosset JM, Henry-Amar M, Meerwaldt JH, et al. The EORTC trials for limited stage Hodgkin's disease. The EORTC Lymphoma Cooperative Group. *Eur J Cancer.* 1992;28A(11):1847–1850.

7. Ng AK, Bernardo MP, Weller E, et al. Long-term survival and competing causes of death in patients with early-stage Hodgkin's disease treated at age 50 or younger. *J Clin Oncol.* 2002;20(8):2101–2108.

8. Press OW, LeBlanc M, Lichter AS, et al. Phase III randomized intergroup trial of subtotal lymphoid irradiation versus doxorubicin, vinblastine, and subtotal lymphoid irradiation for stage IA to IIA Hodgkin's disease. *J Clin Oncol.* 2001;19(22):4238–4244.

9. Engert A, Franklin J, Eich HT, et al. Two cycles of doxorubicin, bleomycin, vinblastine, and dacarbazine plus extended-field radiotherapy is superior to radiotherapy alone in early favorable Hodgkin's lymphoma: final results of the GHSG HD7 trial. *J Clin Oncol.* 2007;25(23):3495–3502.

10. Fermé C, Eghbali H, Meerwaldt JH, et al. Chemotherapy plus involved-field radiation in early-stage Hodgkin's disease. *N Engl J Med.* 2007;357(19):1916–1927.

11. Engert A, Schiller P, Josting A, et al. Involved-field radiotherapy is equally effective and less toxic compared with extended-field radiotherapy after four cycles of chemotherapy in patients with early-stage unfavorable Hodgkin's lymphoma: results of the HD8 trial of the German Hodgkin's Lymphoma Study Group. *J Clin Oncol.* 2003;21(19):3601–3608.

12. Diehl V, Brillant C, Engert A, et al. HD10: investigating reduction of combined modality treatment intensity in early stage Hodgkin's lymphoma. Interim analysis of a randomized trial of the German Hodgkin Study Group (GHSG). *ASCO Annual Meeting Proceedings.* 2005;23(16S):6506.

13. Straus DJ, Portlock CS, Qin J, et al. Results of a prospective randomized clinical trial of doxorubicin, bleomycin, vinblastine, and dacarbazine (ABVD) followed by radiation therapy (RT) versus ABVD alone for stages I, II, and IIIA nonbulky Hodgkin disease. *Blood.* 2004;104(12):3483–3489.

14. Meyer RM, Gospodarowicz MK, Connors JM, et al. ABVD alone versus radiation-based therapy in limited-stage Hodgkin's lymphoma. *N Engl J Med.* 2012;366(5):399–408.

15. Zinzani PL, Rigacci L, Stefoni V, et al. Early interim 18F-FDG PET in Hodgkin's lymphoma: evaluation on 304 patients. *Eur J Nucl Med Mol Imaging.* 2012;39(1):4–12.

16. Radford J, Barrington S, Counsell N, et al. Involved field radiotherapy versus no further treatment in patients with clinical stages IA and IIA Hodgkin lymphoma and a "negative" PET scan after 3 cycles ABVD. Results of the UK NCRI RAPID trial. *ASH Annual Meeting Abstracts.* 2012120(21):547.

17. von Tresckow B, Plütschow A, Fuchs M, et al. Dose-intensification in early unfavorable Hodgkin's lymphoma: final analysis of the German Hodgkin Study Group HD14 trial. *J Clin Oncol.* 2012;30(9):907–913.

18. Horning SJ, Hoppe RT, Breslin S, et al. Stanford V and radiotherapy for locally extensive and advanced Hodgkin's disease: mature results of a prospective clinical trial. *J Clin Oncol.* 2002;20(3):630–637.

19. Gallamini A, Patti C, Viviani S, et al. Early chemotherapy intensification with BEACOPP in advanced-stage Hodgkin lymphoma patients with a interim-PET positive after two ABVD courses. *Br J Haematol.* 2011;152(5):551–560.

20. Gordon LI, Hong F, Fisher RI, et al. Randomized phase III trial of ABVD versus Stanford V with or without radiation therapy in locally extensive and advanced-stage Hodgkin lymphoma: an intergroup study coordinated by the Eastern Cooperative Oncology Group (E2496). *J Clin Oncol.* 2013;31(6):684–691.

21. Engert A, Diehl V, Franklin J, et al. Escalated-dose BEACOPP in the treatment of patients with advanced-stage Hodgkin's

lymphoma: 10 years of follow-up of the GHSG HD9 study. *J Clin Oncol.* 2009;27(27):4548–4554.

22. Engert A, Haverkamp H, Kobe C, et al. Reduced-intensity chemotherapy and PET-guided radiotherapy in patients with advanced stage Hodgkin's lymphoma (HD15 trial): a randomised, open-label, phase 3 non-inferiority trial. *Lancet.* 2012;379(9828):1791–1799.

23. Skoetz N, Trelle S, Rancea M, et al. Effect of initial treatment strategy on survival of patients with advanced-stage Hodgkin's lymphoma: a systematic review and network meta-analysis. *Lancet Oncol.* 2013;14(10):943–952.

24. Federico M, Bellei M, Brice P, et al. High-dose therapy and autologous stem-cell transplantation versus conventional therapy for patients with advanced Hodgkin's lymphoma responding to front-line therapy. *J Clin Oncol.* 2003;21(12):2320–2325.

25. Proctor SJ, Mackie M, Dawson A, et al. A population-based study of intensive multi-agent chemotherapy with or without auto-transplant for the highest risk Hodgkin's disease patients identified by the Scotland and Newcastle Lymphoma Group (SNLG) prognostic index. A Scotland and Newcastle Lymphoma Group study (SNLG HD III). *Eur J Cancer.* 2002;38(6):795–806.

26. Loeffler M, Brosteanu O, Hasenclever D, et al. Meta-analysis of chemotherapy versus combined modality treatment trials in Hodgkin's disease. International Database on Hodgkin's Disease Overview Study Group. *J Clin Oncol.* 1998;16(3):818–829.

27. Aleman BM, Raemaekers JM, Tirelli U, et al. Involved-field radiotherapy for advanced Hodgkin's lymphoma. *N Engl J Med.* 2003;348(24):2396–2406.

28. Castagna L, Bramanti S, Balzarotti M, et al. Predictive value of early 18F-fluorodeoxyglucose positron emission tomography (FDG-PET) during salvage chemotherapy in relapsing/refractory Hodgkin lymphoma (HL) treated with high-dose chemotherapy. *Br J Haematol.* 2009;145(3):369–372.

29. Schmitz N, Pfistner B, Sextro M, et al. Aggressive conventional chemotherapy compared with high-dose chemotherapy with autologous haemopoietic stem-cell transplantation for relapsed chemosensitive Hodgkin's disease: a randomised trial. *Lancet.* 2002;359(9323):2065–2071.

30. Milpied N, Fielding AK, Pearce RM, et al. Allogeneic bone marrow transplant is not better than autologous transplant for patients with relapsed Hodgkin's disease. European Group for Blood and Bone Marrow Transplantation. *J Clin Oncol.* 1996;14(4):1291–1296.

31. Younes A, Gopal AK, Smith SE, et al. Results of a pivotal phase II study of brentuximab vedotin for patients with relapsed or refractory Hodgkin's lymphoma. *J Clin Oncol.* 2012;30(18):2183–2189.

32. Savage KJ, Skinnider B, Al-Mansour M, et al. Treating limited-stage nodular lymphocyte predominant Hodgkin lymphoma similarly to classical Hodgkin lymphoma with ABVD may improve outcome. *Blood.* 2011;118(17):4585–4590.

33. Biasoli I, Stamatoullas A, Meignin V, et al. Nodular, lymphocyte-predominant Hodgkin lymphoma: a long-term study and analysis of transformation to diffuse large B-cell lymphoma in a cohort of 164 patients from the Adult Lymphoma Study Group. *Cancer.* 2010;116(3):631–639.

# 26

# Non-Hodgkin Lymphoma

PREMAL LULLA AND SARVARI YELLAPRAGADA

## EPIDEMIOLOGY, RISK FACTORS, AND NATURAL HISTORY

In 2014, approximately 70,800 individuals in the United States developed non-Hodgkin lymphoma (NHL) and 18,990 died from this disorder (Surveillance Epidemiology and End Results [SEER] website, http://seer.cancer.gov). NHL represents the seventh most common malignancy in United States among men and women with a median age of 66 years at diagnosis. Several viruses including HIV, hepatitis B and C, Epstein–Barr virus (EBV), human T lymphotropic virus 1 (HTLV1), and human herpesvirus-8 (HHV8) are implicated in the pathogenesis of NHL subtypes as are other infectious agents like *Helicobacter pylori*, *Chlamydia psittaci*, and *Campylobacter jejuni*. These bacteria typically cause low-grade mucosa-associated lymphoid tissue lymphomas (MALToma) of the gastrointestinal tract. Treating the infectious organism can sometimes be curative. For example, *H. pylori* related limited stage MALToma of the stomach can be treated with quadruple antibiotic therapy. Thus, it is important to confirm *H. pylori* infection with the urease breath test. Other risk factors for developing lymphoma include autoimmune and immune deficiency disorders, toxin exposure, and genetic disorders like Li–Fraumeni syndrome. Presentation can range from the incidental finding of an enlarged lymph node to classic B symptoms (fevers, chills, night sweats, and weight loss), symptomatic cytopenias, or organ-specific dysfunction due to lymphoma involvement.

## PATHOGENESIS

Lymphomas develop following aberrant somatic hypermutation or chromosome translocations that may reflect errors in antigen receptor gene rearrangements involving the immunoglobulin or T-cell receptor (TCR) gene loci. Rearrangement of the IgH (heavy chain) and IgL (light chain) genes leads to expression of a B-cell receptor (BCR) in normal B lymphocytes. Active BCR signaling occurs when the corresponding antigen binds to this receptor resulting in phosphorylation and activation of intracellular kinases including Bruton's tyrosine kinase (BTK), spleen tyrosine kinase (SYK), and phosphoinositide-3 (PI3) kinase. Downstream signaling drives cell survival and proliferation through nuclear factor-kappa-B (NF-kB), protein kinase (AKT), mammalian target of rapamycin (mTOR), or mitogen-activated protein kinase (MAPK) pathways. Abnormalities in BCR signaling as a consequence of aberrant IgH and IgL gene rearrangement (e.g., translocations involving the *myc* gene) have been studied as a model for the transformation and growth of B-cell lymphomas. The downstream pathways are fast becoming potential therapeutic targets (1). T-cell lymphomas constitute <10% of all lymphomas. Molecular tests for TCR rearrangement are often used to demonstrate clonality and diagnose these disorders. T-cell lymphomas can be derived from clonal expansion of T αβ receptor or T γδ receptors of the adaptive or innate immune system. Little is known about the molecular pathogenesis, however T-cell lymphomas appear to occur more frequently in areas endemic for HTLV-1 and 2 infections.

Genomic studies of lymphomas have revealed much about disease biology. Genomic expression profiling (GEP) using microarrays has delineated the role of chromosomal translocations, aberrant signaling pathways, and dysregulation of molecules involved in abnormal proliferation and apoptosis in the pathogenesis of NHL and led to stratification based upon genetic differences (2). For example, diffuse large B-cell lymphoma (DLBCL) can be classified into "germinal center" or "activated"

322

B-cell types with the former having better overall survival than the latter (2). GEP studies have also emphasized the importance of interactions between the tumor cells and the microenvironment including both stromal elements and infiltrating lymphocytes in lymphoma biology and prognosis (3). While GEP analysis is confined to clinical trials, surrogate immunohistochemistry markers such as CD10, B cell lymphoma-6 (BCL-6) protein and multiple myeloma oncogene-1 (MUM-1) have been identified to differentiate germinal center and activated B-cell DLBCL subtypes using algorithms such as that developed by Hans (Figure 26.1) (4).

## DIAGNOSIS

When making a diagnosis of lymphoma, an excisional biopsy is preferred over a fine needle aspirate (FNA) to ensure sufficient material for immunophenotypic and cytogenetic analyses. End-organ evaluation may be indicated in tumors with predilection for certain organ systems, such as cerebrospinal fluid (CSF) analysis for Burkitt lymphoma. Determination of NHL type is extremely important as management can vary from watchful monitoring of disease for indolent types to aggressive chemotherapy and bone marrow transplant for highly aggressive types. NHLs are classified by morphology, histology, immunophenotype, extent of nodal involvement, and genetics.

## CLASSIFICATION

NHLs belong to a heterogeneous group of lymphoproliferative malignancies involving B, T, or natural killer (NK) lymphocytes, ranging from indolent to aggressive types and currently categorized by the World Health Organization (WHO) classification of lymphoma (Tables 26.1 and 26.2). B-cell lymphoma cases far outweigh T-cell and NK-cell types.

## STAGING AND RISK STRATIFICATION

Patients with NHL are assigned an anatomic stage using the Ann Arbor system based on imaging, and in some lymphomas, on the results of bone marrow biopsy. An

exception to this rule is small lymphocytic lymphoma that is staged by the Rai or the Binet system taking into account cytopenias as well as anatomic sites of disease. For staging purposes, PET-CT scans are more sensitive and specific for NHL than CT scans. Their role in monitoring disease while on treatment is being actively studied. DLBCLs are also evaluated using the International Prognostic Index (IPI), which assigns a risk category. The original IPI index remains the best prognostic assessment for patients with DLBCL, but modifications (outlined in the pertinent sections) have proved more

**Table 26.1** WHO Classification of B-Cell Neoplasms

| Neoplasm |
| --- |
| Chronic lymphocytic leukemia/small lymphocytic lymphoma |
| B-cell prolymphocytic leukemia |
| Splenic marginal zone lymphoma |
| Hairy cell leukemia |
| Splenic lymphoma/leukemia, unclassifiable |
|    Splenic diffuse red pulp small B-cell lymphoma |
|    Hairy cell leukemia variant |
| Lymphoplasmacytic lymphoma |
| Waldenström macroglobulinemia |
| Heavy chain diseases |
|    Alpha heavy chain disease |
|    Gamma heavy chain disease |
|    Mu heavy chain disease |
| Extranodal marginal zone B-cell lymphoma of mucosa-associated lymphoid tissue (MALT lymphoma) |
| Nodal marginal zone B-cell lymphoma (MZL) |
|    *Pediatric type nodal MZL* |
| Follicular lymphoma |
|    *Pediatric-type follicular lymphoma* |
| Primary cutaneous follicle center lymphoma |
| Mantle cell lymphoma |
| Diffuse large B-cell lymphoma (DLBCL), not otherwise specified |
|    T-cell/histiocyte-rich large B-cell lymphoma |
| Primary DLBCL of the CNS |
| Primary cutaneous DLBCL, leg type |
|    *Epstein–Barr virus (EBV) + DLBCL of the elderly* |
| *DLBCL associated with chronic inflammation* |
| Lymphomatoid granulomatosis |
| Primary mediastinal (thymic) large B-cell lymphoma |
| Intravascular large B-cell lymphoma |
| ALK-positive large B-cell lymphoma |
| Plasmablastic lymphoma |
| Primary effusion lymphoma |
| Large B-cell lymphoma arising in HHV8-associated multicentric Castleman disease |
| Burkitt lymphoma |
| B-cell lymphoma, unclassifiable, with features intermediate between DLBCL and Burkitt lymphoma |
| B-cell lymphoma, unclassifiable, with features intermediate between DLBCL and classical Hodgkin lymphoma |

Italicized text represent provisional entities into the 2008 WHO classification.
CNS, central nervous system.
*Source:* Adapted from Swerdlow SH, Campo E, Harris NL, et al. IARC WHO Classification Tumors. (2008); 1–439.

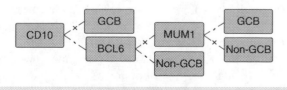

**Figure 26.1**

Hans algorithm devised to predict GCB or non-GCB subtype based on immunohistochemistry. GCB, germinal center B-cell like.

**Table 26.2** WHO Classification of Mature T- and NK-Cell Neoplasms

**Neoplasm**

T-cell prolymphocytic leukemia
T-cell large granular lymphocytic leukemia
*Chronic lymphoproliferative disorder of NK-cells*
Aggressive NK cell leukemia
Systemic EBV+ T-cell lymphoproliferative disease of childhood
Hydroa vacciniforme-like lymphoma
Adult T-cell leukemia/lymphoma
Extranodal NK/T-cell lymphoma, nasal type
Enteropathy-associated T-cell lymphoma
Hepatosplenic T-cell lymphoma
Subcutaneous panniculitis-like T-cell lymphoma
Mycosis fungoides
Sézary syndrome
Primary cutaneous CD30+ T-cell lymphoproliferative disorder
  Lymphomatoid papulosis
  Primary cutaneous anaplastic large-cell lymphoma
*Primary cutaneous aggressive epidermotropic CD8+ cytotoxic T-cell lymphoma*
Primary cutaneous gamma–delta T-cell lymphoma
*Primary cutaneous small–medium CD4+ T-cell lymphoma*
Peripheral T-cell lymphoma, not otherwise specified
Angioimmunoblastic T-cell lymphoma
Anaplastic large-cell lymphoma (ALCL), ALK+
*ALCL, ALK–*
Posttransplant lymphoproliferative disorders (PTLD)
Early lesions
  Plasmacytic hyperplasia
  Infectious mononucleosis-like PTLD
Polymorphic PTLD
Monomorphic PTLD (B- and T/NK-cell types)
Classical Hodgkin lymphoma-type PTLD

The italicized types represent provisional entities or provisional subtypes of other neoplasms. Diseases shown in italics are newly included in the 2008 WHO classification.
EBV, Epstein–Barr virus; WHO, World Health Organization.
*Source:* Adapted from Swerdlow SH, Campo E, Harris NL, et al. IARC WHO Classification Tumors. (2008); 1–439.

predictive for patients with follicular lymphoma (FL) as well as mantle cell lymphoma (MCL).

## CASE SUMMARIES

### Advanced DLBCL

B.B., a 68-year-old white man, was in good health until he noticed difficulty in swallowing solids. Physical examination demonstrated cervical, axillary, and supraclavicular lymphadenopathy, and a CT scan revealed a posterior pharyngeal mass. He denied fever, night sweats, or weight loss. Biopsy of the posterior pharyngeal mass revealed large B-cells with prominent nucleoli. Immunohistochemical stains were positive for MUM1 and Bcl-6. Ki-67 was 80%. Flow cytometry showed the cells to be CD19+, CD20+, CD22+, surface IgM+, and CD10–. A PET-CT

**Ann Arbor Classification of Non-Hodgkin Lymphoma**

| Stage | Description |
|-------|-------------|
| I | Involvement of a single lymph node region or lymphoid structure (e.g., spleen, thymus, Waldeyer's ring) |
| II | Involvement of 2 or more lymph node regions on the same side of the diaphragm |
| III | Involvement of lymph regions or structures on both sides of the diaphragm |
| IV | Involvement of extranodal site/sites beyond that designated E |
| X | Bulk >10 cm |
| *For all stages* | |
| A | No symptoms |
| B | Fever (>38°C), drenching sweats, weight loss (10% body weight over 6 mo) |
| *For stages I–III* | |
| E | Involvement of a single, extranodal site contiguous or proximal to known nodal site |

**International Prognostic Index—for Non-Hodgkin Lymphoma**

**Prognostic Factors**

| | |
|---|---|
| Age | >60 yr |
| Performance status | >1 |
| Lactate dehydrogenase | >1 × normal |
| Extranodal sites | >1 |
| Stage | III or IV |

| Risk Category | Number of Factors | 5-Yr Overall Survival (%) |
|---------------|-------------------|---------------------------|
| Low | 0 or 1 | 73 |
| Low–intermediate | 2 | 51 |
| High–intermediate | 3 | 43 |
| High | 4 or 5 | 26 |

scan revealed diffuse disease, involving the tonsillar lymph nodes, bilateral cervical lymph nodes, submental, supraclavicular, inguinal lymph nodes, and an intra-abdominal mesenteric mass. Basic laboratory studies were within normal range except the lactate dehydrogenase (LDH), which was elevated. Tests for infection with hepatitis B, C, and HIV were negative. Cardiac evaluation with multi-gated acquisition scan (MUGA) demonstrated that the patient had a normal ejection fraction. A bone marrow biopsy showed no evidence of lymphoma.

### Evidence-Based Case Discussion

This patient with DLBCL was classified as Ann Arbor stage IIIA because PET-CT scan showed lymphadenopathy on both sides of the diaphragm. A lumbar puncture was not performed as part of the staging because the patient did not present with central nervous system (CNS) symptoms or testicular, bone marrow, breast, or sinus involvement. Currently, gene expression profiling is not routinely used in the diagnosis of DLBCL, but immunohistochemistry showed positivity for the markers MUM1 and BCL6 (see Figure 26.2), suggesting that he did not fall into the better prognosis "germinal center" type (5). Patients may also be stratified into prognosis groups with the IPI. The IPI was revised in the post-rituximab era (R-IPI) and patients were stratified into 3 groups. Applying the R-IPI, based on the information provided (elevated LDH, stage III, age > 60 years), this patient would be considered at "poor risk." The prognosis for 5-year survival using R-IPI would be 55% (6) compared with 43% using the age-adjusted IPI from the pre-rituximab era. Favorable features include his performance status of 1 and the absence of extra-nodal disease. Because anthracyclines have been associated with cardiac dysfunction, it is important to verify the ejection fraction prior to using an anthracycline-containing regimen. It is also important to ascertain his hepatitis status because hepatitis B viral reactivation has been reported with the use of rituximab in combination with chemotherapy. HIV testing is essential as DLBCL occurs in HIV+ patients with a higher frequency compared to the general population and is associated with a higher risk of disease in the CNS.

The paradigm-shifting Groupe d'Étude des Lymphomes de l'Adulte (GELA) study of DLBCL in the elderly comparing CHOP (cyclophosphamide, doxorubicin, vincristine, and prednisone) with CHOP plus rituximab (R-CHOP) showed a highly significant advantage in response rate, failure-free survival, and overall survival in the rituximab-containing arm (5). Several other studies confirmed these results and R-CHOP has become the standard of care for this disease in all age groups. Clinicians must take care as the addition of rituximab increases the risk for reactivation of hepatitis B (which can progress to fulminant hepatitis) and for progressive multifocal leukoencephalopathy (PML) caused by the JC virus. All patients should be screened for hepatitis B before initiation of therapy, those with a latent or active infection should receive prophylactic entecavir, which has been proven to be superior to lamivudine in reducing rates of reactivation and resistance. Repeat imaging may be performed after 3–4 cycles of R-CHOP with the intention of assessing response and treating for 2 cycles past complete response (CR) for a total of 6 cycles. If CR has not been achieved by 6 cycles, histologic confirmation of residual disease and alternative therapy may be considered. Several other first-line approaches with increased dose density or alternative dose schedules have been the focus of clinical studies. For example, dose-adjusted R-EPOCH (rituximab, etoposide, prednisone, vincristine, cyclophosphamide, and doxorubicin) is an alternative regimen that has similar activity for carefully selected younger patients (7). If there is a bulky (>10 cm) mass at any site, radiotherapy may be considered. Figure 26.3 represents a management algorithm for the treatment of patients with DLBCL. CNS, testicular, and breast DLBCL are special subtypes that can frequently involve the leptomeninges. Studies for CNS DLBCL have shown better overall survival with agents that reliably penetrate the CNS and leptomeninges. Current protocols include high-dose methotrexate (>3 g/m$^2$ body surface area) and cytarabine for "fit" patients.

B.B. received 6 cycles of R-CHOP-21. A PET-CT scan after completion of therapy demonstrated CR. When PET-CT scanning is used for restaging, it is advisable to wait 6–8 weeks post-chemotherapy to avoid a false-positive result. This patient's PET-CT showed no evidence of disease 8 weeks after treatment and he entered surveillance. PET-CT scans are not recommended for surveillance of disease after a posttreatment scan because of an unacceptably high false-positive rate. More than 60% of relapsed DLBCL cases present with new symptoms and the majority of the others are discovered on routine physical assessments. Less than 15% of relapsed disease is initially detected on CT scans or labs (8). This has led to some experts preferring not to perform routine surveillance CT scans after CR is achieved with first-line chemotherapy.

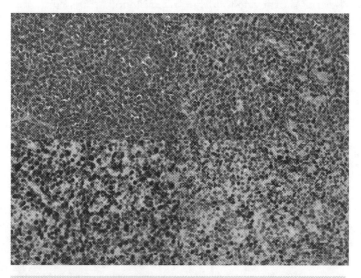

**Figure 26.2**

Diffuse large B-cell lymphoma. Upper left—H&E, 200× magnification; upper right—bcl-6 positive, 200× magnification; bottom left—MIB1 80% positive, 200× magnification; bottom right—MUM1 positive, 200× magnification.

## Advanced DLBCL in Relapse

Eight months after diagnosis and 4 months after completing therapy, B.B. noted a 1-cm node in the left posterior auricular area. Three months later, the posterior auricular lymph node, which had been quiescent, doubled in size over a few days. A biopsy revealed DLBCL with Ki-67 > 90%.

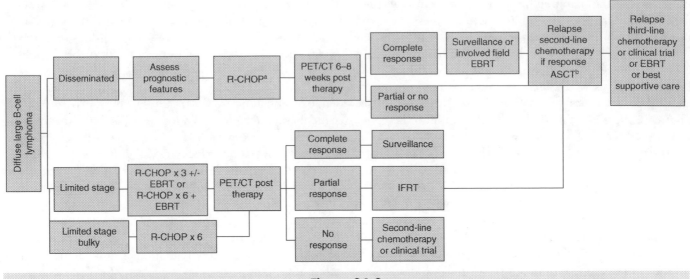

**Figure 26.3**

Suggested algorithm for the treatment of diffuse large B-cell lymphoma. ªR-CHOP refers to rituximab, cyclophosphamide, doxorubicin, vincristine, and prednisone. Those patients with depressed cardiac function should receive an alternative to doxorubicin. Those patients with adverse prognostic features may consider clinical trial. ᵇSecond-line chemotherapy options include R-ICE, R-ESHAP, R-DHAP among others. Avoid severely myelotoxic chemotherapy for transplant-eligible patients. Those unfit to proceed to autologous stem cell transplant (ASCT) may be treated according to their fitness and physician preference. Carefully selected patients may be eligible for allogeneic stem cell transplant. CHOP, cyclophosphamide, doxorubucin, vincristine, and prednisone; SCT, stem cell transplant; EBRT, external beam radiation therapy; IFRT, involved field radiation therapy.

Restaging PET-CT scan revealed disease in the neck and posterior auricular area.

## Evidence-Based Case Discussion

Approximately 30% of all patients treated with R-CHOP relapse, usually within the first 2–3 years. Careful assessment of new symptoms and repeat biopsy of suspicious lesions are indicated. Because autologous stem cell transplant (ASCT) provides significant survival benefit in relapsed patients, it is important to establish that the tumor is sensitive to chemotherapy (9). Thus, a salvage regimen is usually administered. An ideal salvage regimen should have a high response rate, low hematologic and non-hematologic toxicities, and should not impair mobilization of stem cells. The Collaborative Trial in Relapsed Aggressive Lymphoma (CORAL) study randomized relapsed and refractory lymphoma patients to 1 of the 2 platinum-containing regimens, DHAP (dexamethasone, cytarabine, and cisplatin) or ICE (ifosfamide, mesna, carboplatin, and etoposide) with rituximab. No difference in response rate (63% vs. 63.5%), event-free survival or overall survival was observed between the 2 regimens (10). A subset analysis of the CORAL study suggested that patients with a germinal center B-cell subtype have better outcomes with R-DHAP chemotherapy. For patients who are not candidates for high-dose chemotherapy with stem cell transplant, several palliative approaches have been attempted. To limit toxicities, chemotherapy agents such as etoposide or gemcitabine have been combined with rituximab and utilized sequentially.

Additionally, novel agents, like lenalidomide have shown promise in phase II studies and are currently under investigation. B.B. was treated with rituximab–etoposide, cisplatin, cytarabine and methylprednisolone (ESHAP; similar to DHAP, with the addition of etoposide and substitution of methylprednisolone for dexamethasone) with a very good partial response after 2 cycles. Stem cells were collected after the third cycle followed by autologous transplant. He remains in remission 1 year posttransplant.

## Burkitt Lymphoma

A.Y. is a 52-year-old Hispanic man with a 20-year history of HIV infection on ART therapy. Recent CD4 count was 300/μL and viral load was undetectable. He presented to the clinic with complaints of difficulty in swallowing, numbness and tingling in his hands and feet, blurry vision, headache, and neck pain. Physical examination confirmed the presence of a large pharyngeal mass and right neck swelling. His gaze was mildly disconjugate. A biopsy of the right tonsillar mass demonstrated a high-grade B-cell lymphoma with Ki67 > 99% and a "starry-sky" pattern consistent with Burkitt lymphoma. Immunophenotyping showed the cells to be positive for CD19, CD20, CD22, CD10, bcl-6, and human leukocyte antigen-DR (HLA-DR), and negative for EBV-encoded RNA (EBER), CD5, and bcl-2. Cytogenetic testing confirmed a t(8;14) translocation. On a staging CT, masses were found in both orbits surrounding the optic nerve, the left maxillary antrum, and the right tonsil. There were no parenchymal brain abnormalities. A large mass of lymph nodes encased

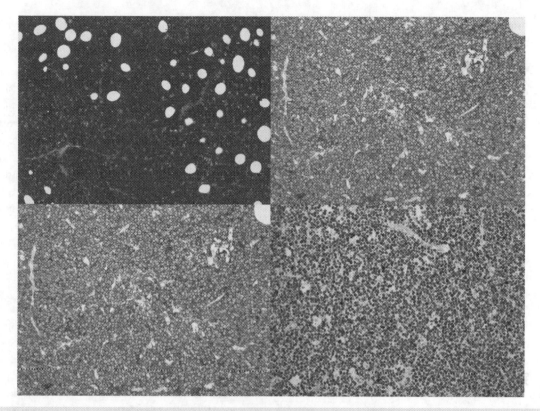

**Figure 26.4**

Burkitt lymphoma. Upper left—H&E, 40× magnification; upper right—CD20, 100× magnification; bottom left—CD10, 100× magnification; bottom right—MIB1 with >95% positivity, 100× magnification.

the celiac axis and there was a large abdominal soft tissue mass and a soft tissue mass anterior to the sacrum. A bone marrow biopsy was negative for lymphomatous involvement. A lumbar puncture was performed as part of the staging and no malignant cells were found in the CSF.

## Evidence-Based Case Discussion

Burkitt lymphoma is a highly aggressive B-cell malignancy characterized by a high proliferation index and translocations of the c-*myc* oncogene on chromosome 8 to the Ig heavy chain gene on chromosome 14 [t(8;14)], the kappa light chain gene on chromosome 2 [t(2;8)] or the lambda light chain gene on chromosome 22 [t(8;22)]. In this patient, the Ki-67 index was >99%, and the most common translocation between c-*myc* and immunoglobulin heavy chain was present. The characteristic "starry sky" appearance under the microscope was also noted (Figure 26.4). Up to 5% of patients lack c-*myc* rearrangements. Despite this, a diagnosis may be made if there is a high proliferation index and if morphology and immunophenotyping are consistent with Burkitt lymphoma. Burkitt lymphoma has both an endemic form, seen in Africa, and a sporadic form that is more commonly seen in children and adolescents and also in patients with immunodeficiency. If an adult Burkitt lymphoma patient is not known to be HIV

positive, then HIV should be tested. Type 1 latency EBV infection can be detected in tumor cells in almost all endemic Burkitt lymphoma and in 30–40% of sporadic and immunodeficiency-associated cases.

The staging evaluation for Burkitt lymphoma includes imaging from brain to pelvis, bone marrow biopsy, and lumbar puncture as described previously. PET scanning is not used because it does not provide additional information that would influence management. Despite neurological symptoms, this patient's CSF sample did not show lymphoma cells by cytology. Nevertheless, CNS involvement is so common in Burkitt lymphoma that intrathecal chemotherapy should be given with or without symptoms or signs of CNS involvement. Additional laboratory studies include chemistries, renal function tests, lactate dehydrogenase, and uric acid levels. This tumor is very sensitive to chemotherapy and highly intensive combination chemotherapy regimens with CNS prophylaxis are employed, including hyper-CVAD (which includes cyclophosphamide, vincristine, doxorubincin, dexamethasone, methotrexate, and cytarabine); DA-EPOCH (dose-adjusted etoposide, vincristine, doxorubicin, cyclophosphamide, and prednisone); CODOX-M (cyclophosphamide, vincristine, doxorubicin, and cytarabine); and CALGB 9251 (which includes cyclophosphamide, ifosfamide, methotrexate, vincristine, doxorubicin, cytarabine, and etoposide). Overall, intensive multidrug chemotherapy results in remission rates of 65–100% and long-term survival of 40–80%. Recent studies suggest the incorporation of rituximab is beneficial in reducing relapses (11). Regardless of which chemotherapy regimen is chosen, a brisk tumoricidal response is expected placing the patients at high risk of developing tumor lysis syndrome. Aggressive prophylaxis for this complication is required and, at a minimum, allopurinol and IV hydration should be instituted. In cases where uric acid is already elevated or the tumor burden is particularly substantial, uric acid blocking drugs such as rasburicase may be used. Although there is concern in HIV-positive patients that chemotherapy may exacerbate immunodeficiency, patients who remain on highly active antiretroviral therapy (HAART), as well as patients without HIV infection, generally tolerate these chemotherapy regimens. A recent study from the National Institutes of Health evaluated 30 patients with 2 different EPOCH-R regimens. A dose-adjusted regimen (DA-EPOCH-R) for sporadic cases and a low-intensity short course with double dose rituximab for HIV-related cases (SC-EPOCH-RR). Freedom from progression was 95% and 100%, respectively, at a median follow-up of 7 years. This offers a relatively less toxic and highly effective treatment approach (12). Figure 26.5 shows a suggested algorithm for the management of patients with Burkitt lymphoma.

Hyper-CVAD with rituximab was chosen for A.Y. He tolerated his full first course of the chemotherapy with very limited side effects including nausea, decreased appetite, and shaking chills on day 1, which resolved. He received intensive hydration, urine alkalinization, and allopurinol and his uric acid, which was in the normal range prior to initiation of chemotherapy, remained stable. He received intrathecal chemotherapy with methotrexate and cytarabine. During the admission for the first cycle of chemotherapy, the patient's chest mass and neck mass both decreased in size and his vision improved. His first cycle and several subsequent cycles of chemotherapy were complicated by neutropenic fever that resolved along with improvement in his neutrophil count. Despite concern that rituximab might worsen his immunodeficiency, he did not develop any opportunistic infections. Restaging at the completion of chemotherapy confirmed complete remission. Five years later, the patient remains in remission with no recurrence of Burkitt lymphoma and remains on HAART therapy.

## Posttransplant Lymphoproliferative Disorder

C.M. is a 30-year-old African American woman who received a cadaveric kidney transplant for end-stage renal disease 3 months ago. Her transplant course was complicated by multiple urinary tract infections and a rejection episode requiring additional immunosuppression. She presented to her transplant physician complaining of daily fever to 102°F and suprapubic pain and fullness. As part of her evaluation for fever of unknown origin, a CT revealed a suspicious 4 × 5 × 5 cm mass inferior to the transplanted kidney. A PET-CT showed a standardized uptake value (SUV) of 18 in the mass. A biopsy showed diffuse large-cell lymphoma that tested positive for EBER and latent

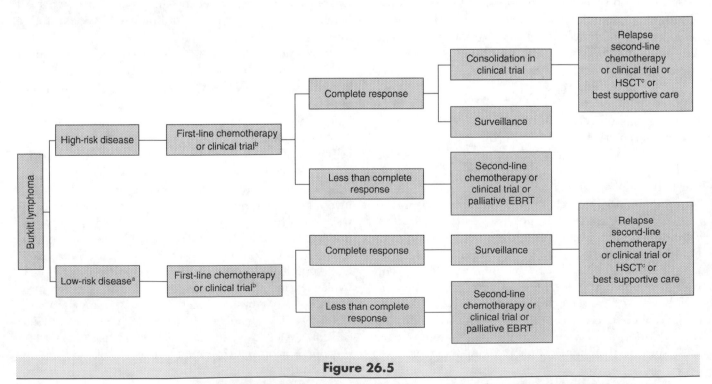

**Figure 26.5**

Suggested algorithm for the treatment of Burkitt lymphoma. ᵃLow-risk disease is marked by low LDH and excised abdominal mass <10 cm. ᵇFirst-line chemotherapy may be hyper-CVAD, CODOX-M, or other regimens as discussed in the text with CNS prophylaxis or treatment as appropriate. ᶜHSCT refers to hematopoietic stem cell transplant. EBRT, external beam radiation therapy.

membrane protein 1 (LMP1). Her peripheral EBV viral load was elevated at 1202 (normal < 200). A bone marrow aspirate and biopsy were negative for lymphoma.

## Evidence-Based Case Discussion

EBV is a latent herpes virus that infects nearly 90% of the world's population. After primary infection, reactivation in latently infected B cells is controlled by a strong EBV-specific T-cell response, but in severely immunocompromised hosts, such as patients on immunosuppression after solid organ transplant (where T-cell immunity is impaired), B-cell proliferation can occur (13). Risk factors for posttransplant lymphoproliferative disease (PTLD) include the degree of immunosuppression, with this complication most commonly occurring within 6 months of solid organ or hematopoietic stem cell transplantation (HSCT). A rise in serum EBV viral load can predict the development of PTLD, and regular surveillance has been recommended by European consensus guidelines in high-risk HSCT recipients (13). While this assay is sensitive, it is not specific, and <50% of solid organ transplant recipients with an elevated EBV DNA will develop PTLD. Consequently,

the decision of when to intervene depends on the clinical scenario. When a patient is symptomatic with fever and a mass, as in the case of C.M., the decision is clear. The evaluation includes biopsy and full-body imaging.

Treatment options for PTLD include restoring immunity to EBV or directly targeting the B-cells. Reducing the immunosuppression, in consultation with the transplant team, is often the first step, and in some patients with early lesions will result in sufficient immune recovery to obtain disease control. Second-line therapy involves direct targeting of the B-cells with monoclonal antibodies such as rituximab and/or cytotoxic chemotherapy. This strategy is used typically for those with monomorphic PTLD. Rituximab is often used as monotherapy with reported response rates of 44–100% (13). Chemotherapy with regimens such as CHOP can be reserved for patients who fail to respond or who have more extensive or progressive disease. Pneumocystis jiroveci (PJP) prophylaxis should be considered for all patients treated with chemotherapy. Radiation therapy and surgical resection may have a role in limited disease or in organ-threatening disease. Clinical trials are exploring means of reconstituting the EBV-specific response with antigen-specific T cells. For PTLD occurring post-HSCT,

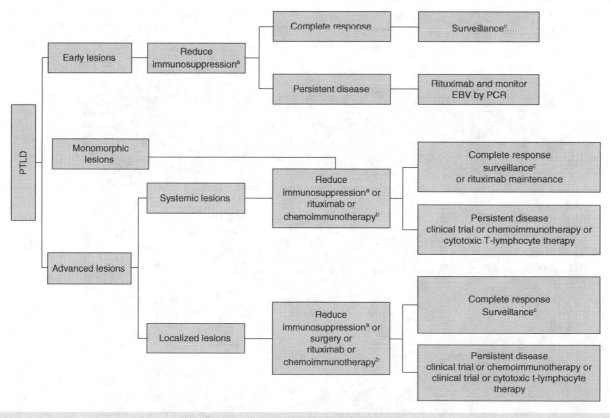

**Figure 26.6**

Suggested algorithm for the treatment of posttransplant lymphoproliferative disorder. ªDecrease or withdraw immunosuppressive agents to the degree possible without endangering the transplanted organ or marrow and always in consultation with the transplant service. ᵇChoice of therapy depends on patient factors such as performance status, presence or absence of graft versus host disease, and function of critical organs as well as tumor factors such as burden and location of disease. Common regimens include R-CHOP, RCHOEP, RCVP. ᶜContinue reduction of immunosuppression and monitor EBV by PCR. EBV, Epstein–Barr virus; PCR, polymerase chain reaction; PTLD, posttransplant lymphoproliferative disease.

infusion of donor lymphocytes is an option when the donor is EBV seropositive although this therapy carries the risk of graft versus host disease (GVHD). Figure 26.6 is a suggested management algorithm for PTLD.

C.M. initially had a trial of reduction of immunosuppression, but had persistent disease so received 4 doses of rituximab. Her mass regressed and serum EBV DNA fell to 0; she is currently being monitored for recurrence.

## Mantle Cell Lymphoma

H.R. is a 66-year-old woman who was noted to be anemic at a routine office examination. Her physical examination revealed scattered small cervical lymph nodes, 4 × 5 cm left axillary lymphadenopathy, and two 1-cm inguinal lymph nodes. She reported fatigue and unintentional weight loss over the previous 3 months and night sweats over the previous 2 months. Fecal occult blood test was positive and colonoscopy was normal. An esophagogastroduodenoscopy (EGD) revealed several solid nodules in the stomach and small intestine. Pathologic examination of these nodules demonstrated medium-sized lymphoid cells with notched nuclei consistent with mantle cells. Immunohistochemistry was positive for CD20, bcl-2, CD43, CD5, and cyclin D1+. The t(11;14) translocation was detected by fluorescence in situ hybridization (FISH). Proliferation was assessed by Ki-67 staining (MIB stain) and was intermediate. Bone marrow biopsy and aspirate were positive for disease with 3% MCL cells on flow cytometry. A staging PET-CT showed metabolically active nodes on both sides of the diaphragm. A hepatitis panel was negative and her LDH and β-2 microglobulin were both elevated. Her Eastern Cooperative Oncology Group (ECOG) performance status was 0.

## Evidence-Based Case Discussion

Many patients with MCL present with advanced disease and frequently have extranodal involvement in the spleen, liver, or gastrointestinal tract where lymphomatous lesions may be asymptomatic at presentation. The typical immunophenotypes are surface IgM+ and IgD+, CD5+, CD20+, CD43+, CD23±, cyclin D1+, and CD10± (Figure 26.7). Most MCLs contain t(11;14), which involves translocation of the immunoglobulin heavy chain promoter and the proto-oncogene cyclin D1 gene (*CCND1*) that encodes cyclin D1. FISH may be required to detect the translocation. Some MCLs have a Ki-67 index <10% and may have an indolent course, but the majority behave as an aggressive lymphoma. Four independent prognostic factors (age, performance status, lactic dehydrogenase, and leukocyte count) can be used to stratify patients into risk groups (14). The high-risk group has overall survival of 2 years, intermediate-risk group has an overall survival of 4 years, and the low-risk group has an overall survival of 6 years.

**Figure 26.7**

Mantle cell lymphoma. Top left—H&E, 100× magnification; top right—CD5, 100× magnification; bottom left—CD10, 100× magnification; bottom right—Cyclin D1, 100× magnification.

Standard staging procedures include CT of the chest, abdomen, and pelvis. A PET/CT may be used, but is not required. MCL often presents with extranodal disease in the gastrointestinal tract, and endoscopy is included in staging if it will change stage and management. MCL frequently presents at stage III or IV, and chemotherapy is indicated unless patient performance status dictates, otherwise The European MCL Network reported results of the first randomized phase III trial in MCL. They compared the use of R-CHOP followed by ASCT to alternating courses of R-CHOP/R-DHAP followed by cytarabine-containing myeloablative regimen and ASCT. The progression-free survival (PFS) was significantly better for the cytarabine-containing arm (75% vs. 60%) as was the overall survival (not reached vs. 82%). Based on this trial, most induction approaches for MCL should include cytarabine (15). The most common treatment approaches use cytarabine or methotrexate early in treatment such as Hyper-CVAD and the Nordic regimen or the CALGB 59909 regimen. The combination of rituximab plus hyper-CVAD alternating with methotrexate and cytarabine was studied in a phase II randomized single-institution clinical trial of 99 patients and resulted in 3-year overall failure-free survival of 73% (16). An alternative regimen is the Nordic regimen using "maxi"-CHOP alternating with cytarabine followed by ASCT in first complete remission. The 6-year progression-free survival was 66% with this approach (17).

Approximately 50% of MCL patients are not candidates for aggressive chemotherapy because of age or comorbidities. Less aggressive alternatives such as R-CHOP followed by R maintenance, R-CVP (cyclophosphamide, vincristine, and prednisone), bendamustine plus rituximab (BR), or dose-adjusted EPOCH may be considered. A subgroup analysis of a randomized trial comparing BR to R-CHOP in indolent lymphomas noted a superior PFS favoring BR (35 vs. 22 months) in the 70 randomized patients with MCL (18).

Although most patients will achieve remission with intensive therapy, the majority will subsequently relapse. If the patient has a good performance status at the first relapse, aggressive salvage regimens can be used with the goal of proceeding to allogeneic stem cell transplant if the disease is "chemosensitive." However, many patients with relapsed MCL will not be transplant candidates. Alternative options include standard lymphoma salvage regimens or monotherapy if the goal is palliative. Maintenance therapy with rituximab prolongs the duration of response to salvage therapy (19). For palliative therapy, both bortezomib and lenalidomide have activity as single agents. The Food and Drug Administration (FDA) has approved the use of the BTK inhibitor ibrutinib for the treatment of relapsed or refractory MCL based on a phase-II study that noted an overall response rate of 68%, 21% of which were complete remissions and a PFS estimated at 13.9 months (20). Figure 26.8 shows a suggested management algorithm for patients with MCL.

H.R. had renal dysfunction at baseline. This abnormality combined with her age led her physicians to give a more moderate regimen and she received 6 cycles of a modified Nordic regimen (R-CHOP alternating with cytarabine). Hyper-CVAD was not given because methotrexate could further compromise her renal function. She gained weight after the first cycle and maintained her baseline renal function throughout therapy. A PET/CT scan performed 8 weeks after completion of chemotherapy revealed a CR. The patient was referred for consideration of ASCT in first remission, but the potential benefit was not judged to be positive enough, given her age

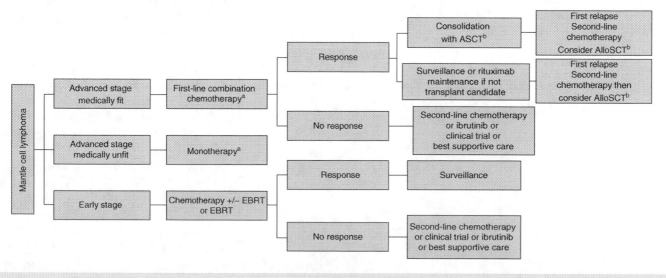

**Figure 26.8**

Suggested algorithm for the treatment of mantle cell lymphoma. [a]First-line combination chemotherapy, monotherapy, second-line chemotherapy options and indications for autologous stem cell transplant are discussed in greater detail in the evidence-based case discussion. [b]Patients appropriate for ASCT (autologous stem cell transplant) and AlloSCT (allogeneic stem cell transplant) must be carefully selected. SCT, stem cell transplant; EBRT, external beam radiation therapy.

and comorbidities. The patient was placed on rituximab maintenance every 2 months and remains recurrence-free 7 months after achieving remission.

## Follicular Lymphoma

S.S. is a 60-year-old Hispanic woman who presented with a right-sided neck mass. She reported no fevers, chills, or night sweats; her weight had been stable; and she had good appetite and energy. Examination of her neck confirmed multiple 1- to 2-cm enlarged lymph nodes limiting her range of motion. Complete blood count and chemistries including LDH were normal and HIV and hepatitis serologies were negative. A CT scan identified bilateral jugular, supraclavicular, hepatogastric, and para-aortic lymph nodes. An excisional biopsy of a right cervical lymph node showed a nodular growth pattern with centrocytes mixed with centroblasts, 11 per high-powered field (HPF), consistent with lymphoma. Flow cytometry confirmed the diagnosis of lymphoma, showing a monoclonal B-cell population positive for CD 10, CD19, CD20, CD22 HLA-DR, CD5 (partial dim), CD23 (partial), CD11c (partial), and negative for kappa, lambda, and CD2–. Cytoplasmic staining for *bcl*-2 was strongly positive. A bone marrow biopsy showed no lymphomatous involvement.

## Evidence-Based Case Discussion

S.S. has grade 2 FL stage IIIA based on the Ann Arbor system. In deciding treatment options, it is important to determine the pathologic grade, which depends on the number of centroblasts in an HPF.

Grade 1—0–5 centroblasts/HPF
Grade 2—6–15 centroblasts/HPF
Grade 3A—>15 centroblasts/HPF
Grade 3B—solid sheets of centroblasts only, no centrocytes seen

The distinction has clinical relevance because grade 1, 2, and 3A FL are categorized and treated like indolent NHL, while grade 3B FL is treated like large-cell lymphoma with more aggressive chemotherapy regimens.

The Follicular Lymphoma International Prognostic Index (FLIPI) score, comprised of the following 5 features, is a useful tool in predicting the survival of patients with FL.

- Age > 60 years
- Ann Arbor stage III or IV
- Four or more involved nodal sites
- Elevated LDH
- Serum hemoglobin <12

The FLIPI score subdivides FL into low- (0–1 factors), intermediate- (2 factors), or high (3 or more factors)-risk groups. The relative 10-year overall survival for each group is 70.7%, 50.9%, and 35.5%, respectively, with

nonoverlapping confidence intervals. S.S. falls into the intermediate-risk category with 2 factors (Ann Arbor stage III and 4 involved nodal sites).

FL is an indolent, heterogeneous disease that is generally responsive to treatment, but associated with high relapse rates. Eighty-five percent of patients with FL have t(14;18), which results in the overexpression of B-cell leukemia/lymphoma 2 (*bcl*-2) protein. One of the hallmarks of the disease is transformation to an aggressive histology. Higher grade and more extensive disease not only carry a higher risk of relapse but also a higher risk of transformation to large-cell lymphoma. Because FL typically affects an older population, the functional status and comorbidities of the patient may affect treatment decisions.

For low-grade FL, early-stage disease can be treated with involved-field radiation alone or in some cases, a period of observation. For patients with more advanced disease (stage 3 or 4), a period of observation may be appropriate if the patient is asymptomatic, but most will eventually require rituximab-containing chemotherapy regimens. The addition of rituximab to cyclophosphamide-, anthracycline-, and fludarabine-based regimens has improved response rates and response duration with time to progression and overall survival both significantly extended (20). A randomized comparison of R-CVP, R-CHOP, and R-FM (fludarabine and mitoxantrone) noted no OS difference between the groups but a higher time to treatment failure (TTF) for R-CHOP (57%) and R-FM (60%) compared with R-CVP (47%). A randomized trial, compared first-line R-CHOP versus R-bendamustine in the treatment of indolent lymphomas, the majority of which were cases of FL. The results noted a higher CR rate, longer PFS, and lesser toxicity in the bendamustine arm (21). Single-agent rituximab may also be used in the frontline setting for patients who are unable to tolerate treatment with alkylating agents.

The primary rituximab and maintenance (PRIMA) trial studied the utility of maintenance rituximab after initial treatment with R-chemotherapy. Patients were randomized to once every 2 months rituximab maintenance for 2 years or observation. The PFS in the R-containing arm was superior to observation (75% to 58%), and has become common practice; however, there was no improvement in OS (22). The use of HSCT in FL is reserved for second-line therapy. Allogeneic HSCT should be considered in younger patients with good performance status because a 5-year progression-free survival rate of 83% has been reported using a reduced intensity regimen of fludarabine, cyclophosphamide, and rituximab (23). Figure 26.9 shows a suggested treatment algorithm for low-grade FL.

S.S. was treated with 6 cycles of R-CHOP with a CR and remained in remission for 2 years when she developed recurrence of cervical lymphadenopathy. Biopsy confirmed recurrence of grade II FL with no evidence of transforma-

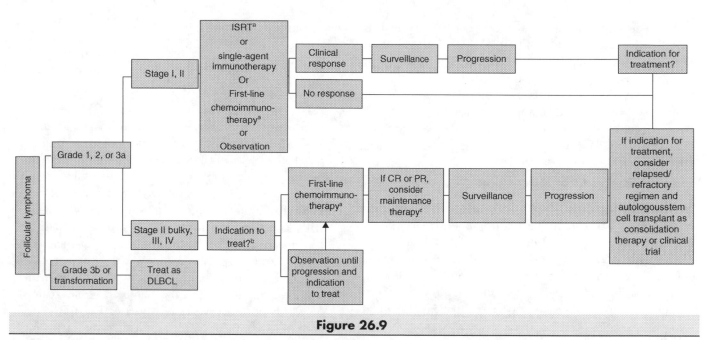

**Figure 26.9**

Suggested algorithm for the treatment of low-grade follicular lymphoma. [a]Involved site radiation therapy, avoid severely myelotoxic chemotherapy for transplant-eligible patients. First-line chemoimmunotherapy refers to fludarabine-, cyclophosphamide-, doxorubicin-, or bendamustine-based regimens with rituximab. [b]Indications include clinical trial, end-organ dysfunction, cytopenias due to lymphoma, bulky disease, steady progression, or patient preference. [c]Maintenance therapy refers to rituximab up to 2 years. CR, complete response; DLBCL, diffuse large B-cell lymphoma. ISRT, involved site radiation therapy; PR, partial remission.

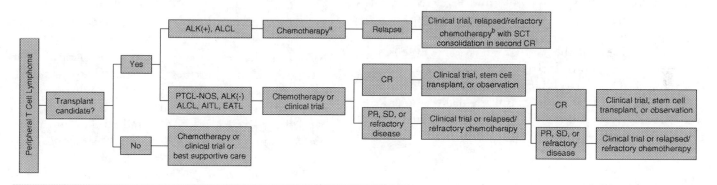

**Figure 26.10**

Suggested treatment algorithm for PTCL. [a]Combination chemotherapy with CHOP in ALK+ ALCL has shown improved survival compared to other subtypes. [b]Salvage chemotherapy with platinum and ifosfamide or cytarabine-based regimens. AITL, angioimmunoblastic T cell lymphoma; ALCL, anaplastic large-cell lymphoma; CR, complete response; EATL, enteropathy-associated T cell lymphoma; PTCL-NOS, peripheral T-cell lymphoma not otherwise specified.

tion. Because she has no other symptoms, she is currently being observed.

## Peripheral T-Cell Lymphoma

Y.A., a previously healthy 33-year-old man, was transferred to the emergency department by his primary care doctor for increasing somnolence, worsening appetite, and new visual hallucinations. He had lost 50 pounds over the last 10 months, and reported recurrent fevers and sweating at night. In the emergency department, Y.A. was found to be hyponatremic and pancytopenic with elevated liver function tests. His mental status acutely declined and he was transferred to the intensive care unit. On examination, he was noted to have a rash and inguinal lymphadenopathy. An MRI of his brain showed no masses, bleeding, or demyelination. His sodium was carefully corrected and the confusion improved. Peripheral blood flow cytometry, FNA of the lymph node, and bone marrow biopsy were nondiagnostic. An excisional biopsy of the inguinal node was performed and showed a monoclonal population of large, atypical, pleomorphic lymphoid cells. Flow cytometry revealed a population of CD3+T cells with aberrant loss of CD2, CD5, CD7, CD4, and a high Ki-67 proliferation index of 80–90%. CD57, TdT, and CD34 were all negative as were anaplastic lymphoma kinase (ALK), pancytokeratin, and EBV-LMP1. CSF cytology was negative for lymphoma. Serum uric acid and LDH were normal. A CT scan showed additional retroperitoneal lymphadenopathy and an enlarged spleen.

## Evidence-Based Case Discussion

The immunophenotype of the monoclonal lymphocyte population is consistent with a peripheral T-cell lymphoma not otherwise specified (PTCL-NOS) REAL-WHO classification because it does not meet criteria for other subtypes of T-cell lymphoma. Compared to B-cell lymphomas, peripheral T-cell lymphomas respond less well to chemotherapy and have a poorer survival. National Comprehensive Cancer Network (NCCN) guidelines recommend participation in a clinical trial if one is available and intensive chemotherapy with a regimen such as CHOP if no trial is available. More intensive regimens such as Hyper-CVAD have been used, but they do not result in improved outcome. Because 3-year overall survival rates are only 40–50% for patients with *ALK*-negative disease, autologous transplant should be considered as consolidation in first remission (24). *ALK*-positive anaplastic large-cell lymphoma is typically associated with a better prognosis and surveillance in first remission is the current standard of care. Figure 26.10 represents a treatment algorithm for peripheral T-cell lymphoma.

Y.A. was treated with CHOP, which he tolerated well. Because he is young with a high IPI score and ALK-negative disease, he has been referred for ASCT.

## REVIEW QUESTIONS

1. A 59-year-old man was referred for a new diagnosis of diffuse large B-cell lymphoma. He presented with a left-sided neck mass and night sweats. A staging PET-CT scan noted a 10.4-cm left anterior cervical adenopathy with a standardized uptake value of 12 and several [18]F-fludeoxyglucose avid mesenteric nodes. A biopsy revealed CD20+, CD19+, CD22+ large cells with a Ki-67 of 70%. Hepatitis surface antigen (HbsAg) and core antibody (HbcAb) were positive. Hepatitis B viral DNA was undetectable. Rituximab-cyclophosphamide, doxorubicin, vincristine, and prednisone (R-CHOP) chemotherapy is planned. Prior to treatment, what additional management should be considered?

   (A) Interferon plus lamivudine to treat hepatitis B prior to rituximab, proceed with cyclophosphamide, doxorubicin, vincristine, and prednisone (CHOP)
   (B) Lamivudine prophylaxis

   (C) Entecavir prophylaxis
   (D) Ribavirin prophylaxis
   (E) Avoid use of rituximab completely but proceed with CHOP

2. A 61-year-old woman presents for consideration of a clinical trial. She was diagnosed with stage IV diffuse large B-cell lymphoma 1 year prior. At that time, she received 6 cycles of rituximab-cyclophosphamide, doxorubicin, vincristine, and prednisone (R-CHOP) with no response. This was followed by 2 cycles of rituximab-ifosfamide, carboplatin, and etoposide (R-ICE) with a partial response and an autologous stem cell transplant (ASCT) with BEAM-R (carmustine, etoposide, cytarabine, and melphalan with rituximab) conditioning 3 months ago. She now presents with new lymphadenopathy involving bilateral axilla, a biopsy of which confirms relapsed disease. The tumor cells are CD45+, CD20+, CD19+, CD22+, and stain positive for bcl-2. Cytogenetics are sent and are pending. Translocations involving which gene with or without other abnormalities have been associated with a poor response to standard treatments?

   (A) histone lysine-N-methyltransferase 2 (EZH2)
   (B) *myc*
   (C) bcl3
   (D) p16

3. A 56-year-old man presented with a 60-pound weight loss, fatigue, and shortness of breath. He was noted to be anemic and thrombocytopenic. A bone marrow examination revealed a population of large T lymphocytes that were CD3+, CD4+, and CD30+ and reactive to staining for the *ALK* protein. A diagnosis of anaplastic large-cell lymphoma was made. A staging PET-CT scan noted [18]F-fludeoxyglucose avid lymph nodes above and below the diaphragm. He was treated with 6 cycles of CHOP (cyclophosphamide, doxorubicin, vincristine, and prednisone). He was in complete remission based on a PET-CT scan and a repeat bone marrow examination 2 months after his last chemotherapy cycle. What would be the next best step?

   (A) Surveillance only
   (B) Brentuximab vedotin maintenance therapy
   (C) Referral for autologous stem cell transplant
   (D) Referral for allogeneic stem cell transplant
   (E) Two more cycles with methotrexate-based chemotherapy

4. A 52-year-old man was diagnosed with World Health Organization grade 1–2 follicular lymphoma from a left axillary lymph node biopsy 4 years ago. At that time, he was noted to have [18]F-fludeoxyglucose (FDG) avid lymph nodes above and below the diaphragm. Because he had no symptoms besides lymph node swelling, a

decision was made to observe clinically. He now presents to the office for a 3-month visit, complaining of 3 weeks of left arm pain and swelling, 20-pound weight loss, nightly drenching sweats, and a rapidly enlarging left axillary mass. A PET-CT scan obtained now shows a larger more intensely FDG-avid (standardized uptake value = 14) 11-cm left axillary mass. All other lymph nodes appear stable. What is the next best step in management?

(A) Radiation therapy to the left axillary mass
(B) Rituximab in combination with chemotherapy
(C) Rituximab alone
(D) Biopsy of the axillary mass
(E) Continue surveillance

5. A 64-year-old otherwise healthy woman presented to the emergency department with a history of 2 weeks of generalized tonic–clonic seizures. An MRI of the brain showed ring-enhancing lesions in the left parietal, left frontal, and right occipital lobe. The patient's family notes that she has had vision problems for the past 1 month, which she thought was from old age. Neurosurgery performs a stereotactic brain biopsy that shows large cells. Flow cytometry of the aspirated fluid shows a population of cells which were CD19+, CD20+, CD22+, and CD79a+. Immunostains are positive for bcl6 and MUM1. Her seizures are controlled with levetiracetam. There is no evidence of such lesions elsewhere on staging scans. An ophthalmology consult is obtained. Which treatment modality has been shown to have superior outcomes for the management of this disease?

(A) Systemic treatment with high-dose methotrexate 3.5 g/m$^2$ body surface area backbone
(B) Systemic treatment with intermediate-dose methotrexate 1 g/m$^2$ body surface area backbone
(C) Intrathecal treatment with biweekly alternating 12 mg of methotrexate, 100 mg of cytarabine, and 100 mcg of hydrocortisone
(D) Systemic treatment with rituximab with cyclophosphamide, doxorubicin, vincristine, and prednisone along with intrathecal methotrexate alternating with cytarabine.
(E) Systemic corticosteroids in combination with rituximab
(F) Whole-brain radiation alone

6. A 48-year-old man presents with an enlarging neck mass 1 year after achieving complete remission with chemotherapy rituximab-cyclophosphamide, doxorubicin, vincristine, and prednisone (R-CHOP) for stage III diffuse large B-cell lymphoma transformed from a follicular lymphoma. A biopsy of the neck node reveals a CD10+, CD20+, and CD19+ large B-cell lymphoma with a Ki-67 of 90%. He has a performance status of Eastern Cooperative Oncology Group 1. Staging

studies note several enlarged lymph nodes above and below the diaphragm. What is the next best management approach?

(A) Two more cycles of R-CHOP, if in remission then 2 years of maintenance rituximab
(B) Six cycles of rituximab with bendamustine, if in remission then 2 years of maintenance rituximab
(C) Two more cycles of R-CHOP if in remission then proceed with high-dose chemotherapy with autologous stem cell rescue
(D) Two cycles of R-ICE chemotherapy, if in remission then proceed with high-dose chemotherapy with autologous stem cell rescue

7. An 80-year-old man presented to the emergency department with a 60-pound weight loss over 3 months, fevers, and night sweats over the same period. He was noted on examination to have a large spleen, 8 cm below the costal margin. A peripheral blood smear showed several intermediate-sized lymphocytes with loose chromatin. A flow cytometry study on the blood and bone marrow aspirate revealed B lymphocytes that are CD5+ and CD20+; CD23–, and CD10–. Immunostaining is positive for cyclin D1. Cytogenetics reveal t(11;14) in 90% of the cells. He also suffers from New York Heart Association class II congestive heart failure and insulin-dependent diabetes mellitus with a history of leg ulcers. He has a performance status of Eastern Cooperative Oncology Group (ECOG-2). What would be the best-suited treatment strategy for his lymphoma?

(A) Hyper-cyclophosphamide, vincristine, adriamycin and dexamethasone (CVAD) chemotherapy with rituximab followed by autologous stem cell transplant (ASCT)
(B) Cyclophosphamide, doxorubicin, vincristine, and prednisone (CHOP) chemotherapy with rituximab followed by ASCT
(C) CHOP chemotherapy with rituximab followed by rituximab maintenance therapy
(D) Bendamustine chemotherapy with rituximab followed by ASCT
(E) Bendamustine with rituximab therapy only followed by observation

8. A 40-year-old man was noted to be HIV positive 2 years ago during an insurance screening. He refused to be treated then. He presents to the emergency department with a 2-week history of a rapidly enlarging left jaw mass. He is now unable to chew or open his mouth. In addition, he has noted enlarging groin and bilateral axillary masses. His current CD4 count is 74 mm$^3$. A biopsy reveals small- to intermediate-sized cells with cleaved nuclei that have a starry sky

appearance under low power. What will be the most likely cytogenetic abnormality?

(A) t(8;14)
(B) t(14;18)
(C) t(9;22)
(D) t(8;21)

9. A 32-year-old woman of Japanese descent is referred for a new diagnosis of a lymphoma. She presented to her primary care doctor with hematemesis 2 weeks ago. An esophagogastroduodenoscopy showed gastric erosions in the pylorus associated with a 2-cm tan-colored polypoid mass. Staging CT scans reveal no other sites of disease. A biopsy of the mass confirms stage I extranodal marginal zone lymphoma that is t(11;18) negative. Staining for *Helicobacter pylori* on the biopsy is negative. What is the next best management step?

(A) Rituximab therapy for 2 years
(B) Radiation therapy to the stomach
(C) Rituximab with cyclophosphamide, doxorubicin, vincristine, and prednisone chemotherapy for 6 cycles
(D) Urease breath test or stool antigen for *H. pylori*
(E) Empiric quadruple therapy for *H. pylori* eradication

## REFERENCES

1. Young RM, Staudt LM. Targeting pathological B cell receptor signalling in lymphoid malignancies. *Nat Rev Drug Discov.* 12(3):229–243.
2. Lenz G, Staudt LM. Aggressive lymphomas. *N Engl J Med.* 2010;362(15):1417–1429.
3. Dave SS, Wright G, Tan B, et al. Prediction of survival in follicular lymphoma based on molecular features of tumor-infiltrating immune cells. *N Engl J Med.* 2004;351(21):2159–2169.
4. Meyer, PN, Fu, K, Greiner TC, et al. Immunohistochemical methods for predicting cell of origin and survival in patients with diffuse large B-cell lymphoma treated with rituximab. *J Clin Oncol.* 2011:200–207; published online on December 6, 2010.
5. Coiffier B, Lepage E, Briere J, et al. CHOP chemotherapy plus rituximab compared with CHOP alone in elderly patients with diffuse large-B-cell lymphoma. *N Engl J Med.* 2002;346(4):235–242.
6. Sehn H, Berry B, Chhanabhai M, et al. The revised International Prognostic Index (R-IPI) is a better predictor of outcome than the standard IPI for patients with diffuse large B-cell lymphoma treated with R-CHOP. *Blood.* 2007;109:1857–1861.
7. Wilson W, Dunleavy K, Pittaluga S, et al. Phase II study of dose adjusted EPOCH plus rituximab (DA-EPOCH-R) in untreated patients with poor risk B-cell lymphoma with analysis of germinal center and post-germinal center biomarkers. *J Clin.Oncol.* 2008;26: 2717–2724.
8. Thompson, CA, Maurer MJ, Ghesquireres H. Utility of pot-therapy surveillance scans in DLBCL. *J Clin Oncol.* 2013;31(suppl; abstr 8504).
9. Philip T, Guglielmi C, Hagenbeek A, et al. Autologous bone marrow transplantation as compared with salvage chemotherapy in relapses of chemotherapy-sensitive non-Hodgkin's lymphoma. *N Engl J Med.* 1995;333:1540–1545.
10. Gisselbrecht C, Glass B, Mounier N, et al. Salvage regimens with autologous transplantation for relapsed large B-cell lymphoma in the rituximab era. *J Clin Oncol.* 2010;28(27):4184–4190.
11. Ribrag, V., Koscielny, S., Bouabdallah, K, et al. Addition of rituximab improves outcome of HIV negative patients with Burkitt lymphoma treated with the LMBA protocol: results of the Randomized Intergroup (GRAALL-Lysa) LMBA02 Protocol. *Blood* (ASH Annual Meeting Abstracts). 2012;120:685a.
12. Dunleavy K, Pittaluga S, Shovlin M, et al. Low-intensity therapy in adults with Burkitt's lymphoma. *N Engl J Med.* 2013;369:1915–1925.
13. Heslop HE. How I treat EBV lymphoproliferation. *Blood.* 2009;114(19):4002–4008.
14. Hoster E, Dreyling M, Klapper W, et al. A new prognostic index (MIPI) for patients with advanced-stage mantle cell lymphoma. *Blood.* 2008;111(2):558–565.
15. Hermine O, Hoster E, Walewski J, et al. Alternating courses of 3x CHOP and 3x DHAP plus rituximab followed by a high dose ARA-C containing myeloablative regimen and autologous stem cell transplantation (ASCT) increases overall survival when compared to 6 courses of CHOP plus rituximab [abstract] *Blood* (ASH Annual Meeting Abstracts). 2012;120(21):151.
16. Romaguera JE, Fayad L, Rodriguez MA, et al. High rate of durable remissions after treatment of newly diagnosed aggressive mantle-cell lymphoma with rituximab plus hyper-CVAD alternating with rituximab plus high-dose methotrexate and cytarabine. *J Clin Oncol.* 2005;23(28):7013–7023.
17. Geisler CH, Kolstad A, Laurell A, et al. Long-term progression-free survival of mantle cell lymphoma after intensive front-line immunochemotherapy with in vivo-purged stem cell rescue: a non-randomized phase 2 multicenter study by the Nordic Lymphoma Group. *Blood.* 2008;112(7):2687–2693.
18. Flinn IW, van der Jagt R, Kahl BS, et al. Open-label, randomized, noninferiority study of bendamustine-rituximab or R-CHOP/R-CVP in first-line treatment of advanced indolent NHL or MCL: the BRIGHT study. *Blood.* 2014;123(19):2944–2952.
19. Forstpointner R, Unterhalt M, Dreyling M, et al. Maintenance therapy with rituximab leads to a significant prolongation of response duration after salvage therapy with a combination of rituximab, fludarabine, cyclophosphamide, and mitoxantrone (R-FCM) in patients with recurring and refractory follicular and mantle cell lymphomas: results of a prospective randomized study of the German Low Grade Lymphoma Study Group (GLSG). *Blood.* 2006;108(13):4003–4008.
20. Wang ML, Rule S, Martin P, et al. Targeting BTK with ibrutinib in relapsed or refractory mantle-cell lymphoma. *N Engl J Med.* 2013;369(6):507–516.
21. Rummel MJ, Niederle N, Maschmeyer G, et al. Bendamustine plus rituximab (BR) versus CHOP plus rituximab (CHOP-R) as first line treatment in patients with indolent and mantle cell lymphomas (MCL): updated results form the Stil NHL1 study. *Proc ASCO.* 2012;30:3a.
22. Salles G, Seymour JF, Offner F, et al. Rituximab maintenance for 2 years in patients with high tumour burden follicular lymphoma responding to rituximab plus chemotherapy (PRIMA): a phase 3, randomised controlled trial. *Lancet.* 2011;377(9759):42–51.
23. Khouri IF, McLaughlin P, Saliba RM, et al. Eight-year experience with allogeneic stem cell transplantation for relapsed follicular lymphoma after nonmyeloablative conditioning with fludarabine, cyclophosphamide, and rituximab. *Blood.* 2008;111(12):5530–5536.
24. Vose JM. Peripheral T-cell non-Hodgkin's lymphoma. *Hematol Oncol Clin North Am.* 2008;22(5):997–1005.

# 27

# Multiple Myeloma

VEDRAN RADOJCIC, ERLENE K. SEYMOUR, AND DANIEL LEBOVIC

## EPIDEMIOLOGY, RISK FACTORS, NATURAL HISTORY, AND PATHOLOGY

Multiple myeloma is a malignant hematological disorder characterized by the clonal proliferation of a terminally differentiated malignant plasma cell. There were an estimated 22,350 new cases of, and 10,710 deaths secondary to, multiple myeloma in 2013. The median age at diagnosis was around 65 years. There is an approximate 1.5:1 male to female predominance; the incidence is highest among patients of African descent with >2-fold increased risk compared with whites.

There exist few established risk factors associated with the development of multiple myeloma. Among the recognized risk factors are exposure to radiation, a family history of multiple myeloma, occupational exposures to petroleum products and agricultural pesticides, as well as obesity.

Pathological expansion of the malignant plasma cell clone within the bone marrow compartment results in hematological dysfunction including anemia and recurrent infection. Clonal B-cell immunoglobulin (Ig) overproduction may result in renal compromise secondary to renal tubular light chain deposition. Furthermore, increased release of pro-osteoclastic mediators such as macrophage-inflammatory factor-1α and receptor activator of nuclear factor-κB ligand (RANKL) may lead to hypercalcemia and the development of lytic bone lesions.

Multiple myeloma evolves from the premalignant state of monoclonal gammopathy of undetermined significance (MGUS). Clinicians define MGUS as the presence of a serum monoclonal protein without significant bone marrow involvement or end-organ damage (Table 27.1). The precise molecular and cellular evolution of MGUS has not yet been established; however, it has been proposed to originate with antigenic stimulation of the B cell accompanied by the activation of toll-like receptors and augmented interleukin-6 expression. These events lead to B-cell proliferation and predispose to genetic mutations permitting progression of the disease.

An intermediate state of myeloma, termed asymptomatic or smoldering myeloma, may precede the symptomatic state, and is defined as an increased serum monoclonal protein >3.0 g/dL and/or bone marrow clonal plasma cells ≥10%, with no related organ damage (Table 27.1). The final stage of multiple myeloma progression is symptomatic myeloma characterized by myeloma with end-organ dysfunction with either hyperCalcemia, Renal impairment, Anemia or Bony lesions (the CRAB criteria; Table 27.1). The emergence of these clinical symptoms has become the key diagnostic criterion determining when to initiate treatment (1).

A plasma cell disorder that shares a common etiology with multiple myeloma is the solitary plasmacytoma. It is similarly derived from a single B-cell clone but distinguishes itself from multiple myeloma as a solitary lesion, most frequently in bone. In addition, with the solitary plasmacytoma there is noted to be a normal bone marrow without evidence of a B-cell clone, no bony disease apart from the plasmacytoma itself, and no evidence of end-organ damage (Table 27.1).

Progression of multiple myeloma occurs secondary to intrinsic genetic mutations that accrue within the myeloma cell, per se, and additionally by virtue of alterations to the bone marrow microenvironment that result in increased angiogenesis and myelomagenesis.

Several clinical, laboratory, and molecular variables associated with multiple myeloma define the pathological state and prognosis of the disease. Historically, variables intrinsic to the patient have included the performance status, age, β2-microglobulin level, C-reactive protein level, lactate dehydrogenase (LDH), serum creatinine, and platelet count. Molecular and cytogenetic assessments of the myelomatous plasma cells provide key additional prognostic information.

Gene expression profiling (GEP) has recently been demonstrated to be a valuable prognostic tool to identify patients with high-risk multiple myeloma (2). In addition to clarifying prognosis, GEP has also been used to define the complex molecular pathways involved with the role of the bone marrow microenvironment in multiple myeloma progression and the identification of fundamental molecular alterations, such as aberrant cyclin D expression, underlying the development of multiple myeloma (2).

Cytogenetic assessment of multiple myeloma is achieved by both metaphase cytogenetic analysis and interphase fluorescent in-situ hybridization (FISH). Both modalities are important for accurately establishing patient prognosis.

Approximately 60% of multiple myeloma cases demonstrate hyperdiploidy (defined as chromosome number between and including 48 and 74) and consists of cells with trisomies of chromosomes 3, 5, 7, 9, 11, 19, and 21. This may be associated with a favorable prognosis. In non-hyperdiploid patients, it is believed that early in the evolution of the disease, translocations involving the Ig heavy chain (IgH) occur. Involved partner chromosomes may include chromosomes 11 (*cyclin D1*), chromosome 4 (*FGFR-3*), chromosome 6 (*cyclin D3*), chromosome 16 (*C-maf*), or chromosome 20 (*mafB*). Following these primary mutational events, secondary mutations may occur, leading to progression of the multiple myeloma and resulting in a worsening prognosis. These secondary mutations include deletion of 17p13 (the p53 tumor suppressor gene locus), chromosome 1 abnormalities, activation of NF-κB, K-ras mutations, 12p deletions, methylation of p16, inactivation of p18, microRNA dysregulation and 16q defects, among others.

Recently, a schema has been developed that stratifies multiple myeloma into high-, intermediate-, and standard-risk disease (Table 27.2).

In addition, the presence of plasma cell leukemia (>20% circulating plasma cells) and increased tumor growth rate (as indicated by the plasma cell labeling index [PCLI]) have been associated with a worse prognosis.

## STAGING

The most current staging system for multiple myeloma is the International Staging System (ISS) (4) and has largely

**Table 27.1** Diagnostic Criteria for Monoclonal Gammopathies

| Monoclonal Gammopathy | Criteria |
|---|---|
| Monoclonal gammopathy of undetermined significance | (A) M-protein in serum <3.0 g/dL<br>(B) Bone marrow clonal plasma cells <10%<br>(C) No evidence of B-cell proliferation<br>(D) No end-organ damage |
| Asymptomatic (smoldering) myeloma | (A) M-protein in serum ≥3.0 g/dL and/or bone marrow clonal plasma cells ≥10%<br>(B) No end-organ damage |
| Multiple myeloma requiring treatment | (A) M-protein in serum and/or urine<br>(B) Clonal plasma cells in the bone marrow<br>(C) End-organ damage including one of the following CRAB (creatinine, renal, anemia, bone) criteria:<br>• Calcium >11.5 g/dL<br>• Renal impairment with creatinine >2 mg/dL<br>• Anemia with hemoglobin <10 g/dL or 2 g < normal<br>• Bony disease (lytic lesions or osteoporosis with compression fracture) |
| Solitary plasmacytoma | (A) Solitary lesion of bone or soft tissue as demonstrated by biopsy<br>(B) Normal bone marrow without evidence of clonal plasma cells<br>(C) Except for primary plasmacytoma, normal skeletal survey and MRI of spine and pelvis<br>(D) Absence of end-organ damage |

*Source:* Adapted from Ref. (1). Durie BG, Harousseau JL, Miguel JS, et al.; International Myeloma Working Group. International uniform response criteria for multiple myeloma. *Leukemia.* 2006;20(9):1467–1473.

**Table 27.2** Multiple Myeloma Risk Stratification Based on Cytogenetic Changes

| High Risk | Intermediate Risk | Standard Risk |
|---|---|---|
| del17p | t(4;14) | t(11;14) |
| t(14;16) | 1q gain | t(6;14) |
| t(14;20) | Metaphase del13 | Trisomies |
| | Hypodyploidy | |
| | Complex karyotype | |

*Source:* Adapted from Ref. (3). National Comprehensive Cancer Network. Multiple Myeloma (Version 2.2014); 2014.

**Table 27.3** ISS for Multiple Myeloma

| Stage | Definition |
|---|---|
| I | Serum β2-microglobulin <3.5 mg/L<br>Serum albumin ≥3.5 g/dL |
| II | Neither stage I nor III |
| III | Serum β2-microglobulin ≥5.5 mg/L |

ISS, International Staging System.
*Source:* Adapted from Ref. (4). Greipp PR, San Miguel J, Durie BG, et al. International staging system for multiple myeloma. *J Clin Oncol.* 2005;23(15):3412–3420.

**Table 27.4** Response Criteria for Multiple Myeloma

| Response | Criteria |
| --- | --- |
| Stringent complete response (sCR) | CR with a normal free light chain ratio and with an absence of clonal cells in the bone marrow by immunohistochemistry or immunofluorescence. |
| Complete response (CR) | Negative immunofixation on the serum and urine, disappearance of any soft tissue plasmacytomas and ≤5% plasma cells in the bone marrow. |
| Very good partial response (VGPR) | Serum and urine M-protein detectable by immunofixation but not on electrophoresis or 90% or greater reduction in serum M-protein plus urine M-protein level <100 mg/24 hr. |
| Partial response (PR) | ≥50% reduction of serum M-protein and reduction in 24-hr urine M-protein ≥90% or to <200 mg/24 hr. If the serum and urine M-protein are unmeasurable, a ≥50% decrease in the difference between involved and uninvolved free light chain (FLC) levels is required in place of the M-protein criteria. If the serum and urine M-protein are unmeasurable and serum-free light assay is also unmeasurable, ≥50% reduction in plasma cells is required in place of M-protein, provided baseline bone marrow plasma cell percentage was ≥30%. In addition to the previously listed criteria, if present at baseline, a ≥50% reduction in the size of soft tissue plasmacytomas is also required. |
| Stable disease (SD) | Not meeting the criteria for CR, VGPR, PR, or progressive disease. |
| Progressive disease (PD) | Occurs when 1 or more of the following has occurred: increase of ≥25% from baseline in: <br>1. Serum M-component and/or (the absolute increase must be ≥0.5 g/dL). <br>2. Urine M-component and/or (the absolute increase must be ≥200 mg/24 hr). <br>3. Only in patients without measurable serum and urine M-protein levels: the difference between involved and uninvolved FLC levels. The absolute increase must be >10 mg/dL. <br>4. Bone marrow plasma cell percentage: the absolute % must be ≥10%. <br>5. Definite development of new bone lesions or soft tissue plasmacytomas or definite increase in the size of existing bone lesions or soft tissue plasmacytomas. <br>6. Development of hypercalcemia (corrected serum calcium >11.5 mg/dL or 2.65 mmol/L) that can be attributed solely to the plasma cell proliferative disorder. |
| Clinical relapse | Requires 1 or more of: direct indicators of increasing disease and/or end-organ dysfunction (CRAB features). It is not used in calculation of time to progression or progression-free survival but is listed here as something that can be reported optionally for use in clinical practice. <br>1. Development of new soft tissue plasmacytoma or bone lesions. <br>2. Definite increase in the size of existing plasmacytomas or bone lesions. A definite increase is defined as a 50% (and at least 1 cm) increase as measured serially by the sum of the products of the cross-diameters of the measurable lesion. <br>3. Hypercalcemia (>11.5 mg/dL) (2.65 mmol/L). <br>4. Decrease in hemoglobin of ≥2 g/dL (1.25 mmol/L). <br>5. Rise in serum creatinine by 2 mg/dL or more (177 µmol/L or more). |
| Relapse from CR | Any 1 of the following: <br>Reappearance of serum or urine M-protein by immunofixation or electrophoresis. <br>Development of ≥5% plasma cells in the bone marrow. <br>Appearance of any other sign of progression (i.e., new plasmacytoma, lytic bone lesion, or hypercalcemia). |

*Source:* Adapted from Ref. (1). Durie BG, Harousseau JL, Miguel JS, et al.; International Myeloma Working Group. International uniform response criteria for multiple myeloma. *Leukemia.* 2006;20(9):1467–1473.

replaced the older Durie–Salmon staging system. The ISS is summarized subsequently (Table 27.3). More recently, the International Myeloma Working Group (IMWG) has categorized myeloma into 2 stages: asymptomatic and symptomatic myeloma. This distinction is based on the presence or absence of organ damage. Myeloma-related organ damage (i.e., CRAB) identifies a subset of patients with symptomatic myeloma requiring treatment (Table 27.1) (1).

Response to treatment in multiple myeloma is defined by the International Uniform Response Criteria defined by the IMWG (1). These criteria are summarized in

Table 27.4. These categories are important for evaluating response to therapy, identifying disease progression, and guiding future treatment recommendations.

## CASE SUMMARIES

### Intermediate-Stage Multiple Myeloma Asymptomatic (Smoldering Myeloma)

A.B. is a 55-year-old man who on routine physical examination was noted to have an elevated serum protein level of 9.4 g/dL. This abnormal protein level then prompted an evaluation of multiple myeloma. The following laboratory results were obtained:

| | |
|---|---|
| White blood count | 6700/µL |
| Hemoglobin | 14.2 g/dL |
| Platelets | 218,000/µL |
| Calcium | 9.4 mg/dL |
| Creatinine | 1.0 mg/dL |
| Albumin | 3.9 g/dL |
| LDH | 149 IU/L |
| β2-Microglobulin | 2.2 mg/L |

The urine protein electrophoresis and Bence–Jones protein quantitation demonstrated trace amounts of intact monoclonal IgG monoclonal protein. The serum protein electrophoresis and immunofixation demonstrated an elevated total protein of 8.9 g/dL and an IgA kappa monoclonal gammopathy of 2.6 g/dL. A serum-free light chain assay was obtained and showed a kappa-free light value of 0.78 mg/dL, a lambda-free light chain value of 22.20 mg/dL, and a kappa/lambda-free light chain ratio of 0.04. Serum quantitative Igs were performed that demonstrated an elevated IgA level of 2990, a normal IgG level of 51, and a low IgM level of 20. A skeletal survey revealed mild degenerative changes but otherwise no evidence of lytic lesions. The bone marrow biopsy demonstrated a normocellular marrow with 23% plasma cells; flow cytometry did not reveal any definite evidence of a monoclonal B-cell population. Cytogenetics and FISH were performed that revealed a normal male karyotype; the del(13q), del(17p), t(4;14), t(11;14), and t(14;16) mutations were absent.

### Evidence-Based Case Discussion

The patient in the present case meets the diagnostic criteria for asymptomatic (smoldering) multiple myeloma (Table 27.1). Although the patient's monoclonal protein does not exceed 3.0 g/dL, we do note that his bone marrow plasma cells are >10%. We also observe that his calcium, creatinine, and hemoglobin remain within normal limits, and his skeletal survey does not reveal any lytic lesions. Based on these parameters, the patient has asymptomatic or smoldering multiple myeloma.

Clinically, asymptomatic myeloma is distinguished both from MGUS and symptomatic myeloma. Asymptomatic myeloma has an increased risk of progressing to symptomatic myeloma relative to MGUS, with the risk of progression 10% for each year during the initial 5 years, 3% per year during the next 5 years, and 1% each year thereafter (5). National Comprehensive Cancer Network (NCCN) guidelines recommend monitoring asymptomatic multiple myeloma at 3- to 6-month intervals with laboratory evaluation including a complete blood count (CBC), serum laboratories to assess creatinine, albumin, LDH, calcium,

β2-microglobulin and quantitative Igs, serum protein electrophoresis, serum immunofixation/electrophoresis, serum-free light chain assay, urine protein electrophoresis, and urine immunofixation/electrophoresis. A skeletal survey may be included annually in the assessment and a bone marrow biopsy may be considered as clinically indicated. However, once the patient meets the criteria for symptomatic myeloma, treatment should be initiated. Currently, a number of trials are ongoing with immunomodulatory drugs, proteasome inhibitors, and newer agents to investigate whether these treatments retard progression from the asymptomatic to the symptomatic phase of multiple myeloma.

## Symptomatic Myeloma in a Patient Eligible for Autologous Stem Cell Transplant

R.B. is a healthy 64-year-old man diagnosed with multiple myeloma after skeletal lytic lesions were noted incidentally on CT imaging. Laboratory evaluation was remarkable for mild normochromic, normocytic anemia (hemoglobin = 11.9 g/dL), and leukopenia (white blood cells [WBC] = 3600/mL). A comprehensive metabolic panel showed only mildly decreased albumin at 3.4 g/dL. IgA level was elevated at 3.3 g/dL, with immunofixation revealing a 2.2 g/dL monoclonal component. Serum-free light chain analysis was positive for elevated monoclonal lambda light chain, with no urine Bence–Jones protein detected. β2-Microglobulin level was 3.9 mg/L. A bone marrow biopsy revealed 20–30% involvement with plasma cells. Cytogenetic analysis was unremarkable, and FISH showed t(11;14). Skeletal survey showed several lytic lesions.

### Evidence-Based Case Discussion

Due to the presence of lytic skeletal lesions, our patient is diagnosed with a symptomatic ISS stage II, IgA lambda multiple myeloma. When considering treatment options for his disease, just like in any other oncologic condition, host factors, disease burden, and disease biology must be considered, as they impact therapy selection. While improved outcomes with novel myeloma therapies have called into question the role of autologous stem cell transplant (ASCT) (6,7), the latter remains a standard treatment option for patients with very good performance status and preserved organ function. While in the past, the age of 65 years represented the upper limit for ASCT, advances in supportive care measures and modifications of conditioning regimen intensity have now allowed for ASCT to be safely performed at age of 70 years or beyond.

### Primary and Adjunctive Therapy

Standard treatment for symptomatic multiple myeloma (in an ASCT-eligible patient) entails induction therapy with subsequent consolidative high-dose chemotherapy and ASCT. Adjunctive therapy targeting the complications of myeloma and its treatment should span all phases of disease management.

Historically, alkylating agents such as melphalan, anthracyclines, vincristine, and high-dose steroids have been a backbone of myeloma regimens for decades. Some of these combinations damaged stem cells; compromising feasibility of collection for ASCT. In the past decade, dramatic advancements in understanding of multiple myeloma biology were accompanied by introduction of novel immunomodulatory agents (IMiDs)—thalidomide, lenalidomide, and pomalidomide—and proteasome inhibitors (bortezomib and carfilzomib), which have altered the myeloma treatment landscape. These drugs have not only led significant improvement in response to therapy, but also accompanied by reduced toxicities, and greater feasibility of successful ASCT pursuit. For transplant-eligible candidates, a number of preferred regimens are recognized by the NCCN (3):

- Bortezomib/dexamethasone (Category 1)
- Lenalidomide/dexamethasone (Category 1)
- Bortezomib/doxorubicin/dexamethasone (PAD/VDD) (Category 1)
- Bortezomib/thalidomide/dexamethasone (VTD) (Category 1)
- Cyclophosphamide/bortezomib/dexamethasone (CyBorD) (Category 2A)
- Bortezomib/lenalidomide/dexamethasone (RVD) (Category 2A)

These regimens are associated with superior response rates (partial response [PR] or better in 90–100% patients,

very good partial response [VGPR] in 50–60% patients) when compared to those observed with traditional chemotherapy regimens, such as vincristine/doxorubicin/dexamethasone (VAD; VGPR in 10–20%, PR or better in 60–70%) (8,9). While 3-drug regimens tend to induce superior responses to those seen with 2-drug combinations, it is clear that not every patient derives added benefit from therapy intensification that is associated with higher incidence of side effects and increased costs. Thus, improved understanding of multiple myeloma biology has led to development of risk-adapted strategies for myeloma treatment. Mayo Stratification of Myeloma and Risk-Adapted Therapy (mSMART) represents one of the most widely used therapeutic algorithms, where risk stratification into high-, intermediate-, and standard-risk cohorts (Table 27.2) occurs on finalization of diagnostic workup, which includes conventional cytogenetic analysis, FISH analysis, cell cycle analysis, and increasingly GEP (10). While mSMART and alternate guidelines emphasize preference for treatment within the context of clinical trials, they, nevertheless, provide a solid framework for selection of risk-appropriate routine clinical care for multiple myeloma patients when clinical trials are not available or patients opt against participation (Figure 27.1).

The benefit of bortezomib inclusion in the primary treatment of intermediate-risk myeloma has been well documented in several clinical trials. Use of bortezomib-containing induction regimens followed by tandem ASCT was shown to almost fully eliminate poor prognostic effect of t(4;14) (11). While a similar response improvement has not been as well defined in high-risk patients, bortezomib remains a standard part of triplet therapies used in this group. After therapy selection and initiation,

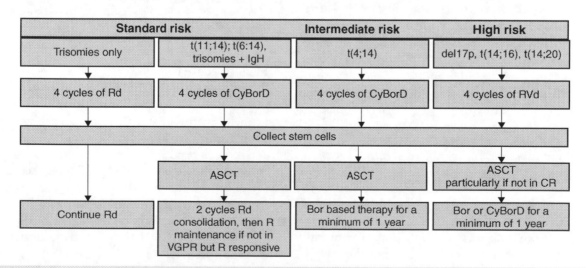

**Figure 27.1**

mSMART treatment algorithm: symptomatic multiple myeloma in transplant-eligible candidates. ASCT, autologous stem cell transplant; Bor, bortezomib; CR, complete response; CyBorD, cyclophosphamide/bortezomib/dexamethasone; Rd, lenalidomide/ low dose dexamethasone; VGPR, very good partial response. *Source*: Modified from Ref. (10). Mikhael JR, Dingli D, Roy V, et al.; Mayo Clinic. Management of newly diagnosed symptomatic multiple myeloma: updated Mayo Stratification of Myeloma and Risk-Adapted Therapy (mSMART) consensus guidelines 2013. *Mayo Clin Proc.* 2013;88(4):360–376.

response assessment should be performed after completion of 2 therapy cycles, using IMWG criteria and treatment adjusted as indicated. If lenalidomide-containing regimen is used for >4 cycles, particularly in patients older than 65 years, stem cell collection should occur with use of stem cell mobilization agents (cyclophosphamide with filgrastim or plerixafor) (12).

While novel therapies have significantly improved the outlook of myeloma patients, they also come with unique side effects and therapy risks. IMiDs, particularly when used together with high-dose dexamethasone significantly elevate risk of venous thromboembolism (VTE) and appropriate prophylaxis is recommended (Table 27.5) (13). IMiDs are known teratogens and contraception is mandated. Bortezomib, particularly when used intravenously, can lead to peripheral neuropathy, the risk of which is increased in patients with preexisting nerve damage. Increased risk of Varicella zoster reactivation has been noted in patients using bortezomib, while risk of herpes simplex virus (HSV), *Pneumocystis carinii* pneumonia (PCP), and fungal infections is increased with high-dose dexamethasone use and appropriate prophylaxis is needed. In patients with recurrent or life-threatening bacterial infections, intravenous Ig should be considered, as should pneumococcal and influenza vaccinations (14).

Profound impact of active multiple myeloma on skeletal metabolism and health is well documented and osteopenia and lytic lesions are major complications of the disease, affecting 85% of patients. These changes lead to significant morbidity and decline in quality of life and functional status, and can be ameliorated with use of bisphosphonates. Efficacy of approved bisphosphonates appears similar, with zoledronic acid having higher rates of jaw osteonecrosis, albeit extremely low. Bisphosphonates are recommended for treatment of symptomatic myeloma regardless of the skeletal involvement (3). Hyperviscosity is another major complication of multiple myeloma occurring in selective patients and often presenting as a medical emergency. Plasmapheresis is a well-established therapeutic intervention in cases of hyperviscosity, though its role in treatment of renal dysfunction caused by paraprotein is debatable. In patients with myeloma-related renal dysfunction, bortezomib-containing regimens have been proven particularly useful.

## Consolidation Therapy/ASCT

As depth of myeloma response predicts improved overall survival, additional therapies following completion of primary treatment are pursued in selective patients. ASCT represents a standard consolidative treatment option; however, its utility in the current day of novel therapeutic options is being increasingly questioned. Clinical trials addressing this question and optimal timing of ASCT are ongoing; however, the role of ASCT remains undisputed in consolidation of patients with high-risk disease,

**Table 27.5** Risk Assessment Model for the Management of Thromboprophylaxis in Myeloma Patients Treated With Thalidomide or Lenalidomide

| Risk Factor | Recommended Action |
|---|---|
| Individual risk factor<br>• Obesity (BMI ≥30)<br>• Previous VTE<br>• Central venous catheter or pacemaker<br>• Associated disease<br>  – Cardiac disease<br>  – Chronic renal disease<br>  – Diabetes<br>  – Acute infection<br>  – Immobilization<br>• Surgery<br>  – General surgery<br>  – Any anesthesia<br>  – Trauma<br>• Erythropoietin<br>• Blood clotting disorders | If no risk factor or any 1 risk factor is present:<br>• Aspirin 81–325 mg once daily<br>If 2 or more risk factors are present:<br>• LMWH (equivalent of enoxaparin 40 mg daily)<br>• Full-dose warfarin (target INR 2–3) |
| Myeloma-related risk factors<br>• Diagnosis, per se<br>• Hyperviscosity | |
| Myeloma therapy (in addition to thalidomide/lenalidomide)<br>• High-dose dexamethasone (480 mg/month)<br>• Doxorubicin<br>• Multiagent chemotherapy | • LMWH (equivalent of enoxaparin 40 mg daily)<br>• Full-dose warfarin (target INR 2–3) |

BMI, body mass index; INR, international normalized ratio; LMWH, low molecular weight heparin; VTE, venous thromboembolism.
*Source*: Adapted from Ref. (13). Palumbo A, Rajkumar SV, Dimopoulos MA, et al.; International Myeloma Working Group. Prevention of thalidomide- and lenalidomide-associated thrombosis in myeloma. *Leukemia*. 2008;22(2):414–423.

particularly those with poor responses to primary therapy (15). High-dose melphalan conditioning precedes ASCT infusion, with the entire procedure being increasingly performed on an outpatient basis due to low toxicity and resulting low transplant-related morbidity and mortality.

The role of tandem ASCT (planned sequential ASCT) has been investigated in several randomized control trials, showing benefit dominantly in the select population of patients failing to achieve VGPR/complete response (CR) before or after the first transplant. Tandem ASCT remains in the most recent NCCN guidelines as an option available to all ASCT patient candidates, with ongoing trials focusing on its role evaluation in patients in CR/VGPR versus those achieving less than VGPR with the first transplantation.

Second ASCT has shown its benefits as a salvage therapy for relapsed multiple myeloma, with benefits confined to the group of younger patients, achieving more PR with the first ASCT and maintaining the response for >9 months (16). In the newest iteration of NCCN myeloma treatment guidelines, second ASCT is therefore reserved as the therapeutic option for patients with 2–3 years of maintained disease response following ASCT.

## Allogeneic Stem Cell Transplantation

Given the paucity of data demonstrating significant graft-versus-myeloma effect, the toxicity of allogeneic SCT (AlloSCT), and myeloma-patient-specific age and comorbidity issues, AlloSCT remains primarily investigational treatment in myeloma treatment. Limited data supporting use of ASCT followed by reduced-intensity conditioning AlloSCT from matched related sibling leave this approach as a possible first-line consolidative treatment in eligible patients with an appropriate sibling donor.

### *Maintenance Therapy*

Additional therapeutic interventions following consolidative ASCT have been evaluated, and use of both thalidomide and lenalidomide led to the deepening of the myeloma response to the treatment and improved progression-free survival (PFS); however, no unequivocal improvement in overall survival occurred (17,18). Both can be recommended for post-ASCT maintenance, with notable finding of increase in secondary cancers with lenalidomide, but not thalidomide (19). While the design of clinical trials utilizing bortezomib maintenance after ASCT does not allow for evaluation of its specific maintenance efficacy, the drug was shown to deepen the post-ASCT responses and represents an alternative to thalidomide and lenalidomide, particularly in patients with t(4;14) or high-risk cytogenetics. The question of maintenance therapy duration remains unanswered.

## Advanced Myeloma in a Patient Not Eligible for ASCT

E.H. is a 76-year-old woman recently diagnosed with symptomatic IgG kappa multiple myeloma, evolving from antecedent MGUS diagnosed at age 65 years. Evolution to symptomatic multiple myeloma was accompanied by development of anemia (hemoglobin = 9.9), osteopenic bony disease, and mild worsening of stage III chronic kidney disease (CKD). On laboratory evaluation, IgG kappa was elevated at 3.6 g/dL, serum-free kappa light chain at 66.3 mg/dL, lambda at 0.76 mg/dL, with a ratio of 87.24. A total of 0.12 g of monoclonal-free kappa light chain was identified on 24-hour urine electrophoresis. $\beta2$-Microglobulin was elevated at 6, with albumin at 3.2. A bone marrow biopsy revealed plasma cell neoplasm involving up to 80% of the marrow space. Myeloma FISH showed trisomies 7, 11, 15, 17, and trisomy/tetrasomy 9, indicating a hyperdyploid clone.

## Evidence-Based Case Discussion

Ms. E.H. now has ISS stage III IgG kappa multiple myeloma, and due to her age and underlying comorbidities she is not a candidate for high-dose chemotherapy followed by ASCT.

## Primary Therapy for Transplant-Ineligible Patients

For ASCT-ineligible patients, stem cell toxicity limitations of primary therapy do not apply and alkylating agents remain at a core of regimens used in this group. The landscape of treatment options, however, has changed significantly in this subset of patients with introduction and success of IMiDs and proteasome inhibitors, replicating survival benefits demonstrated in the ASCT-eligible group. Currently, NCCN-preferred regimens include:

- Lenalidomide/low-dose dexamethasone (Rd) (Category 1)
- Melphalan/prednisone/bortezomib (MPB) (Category 1)
- Melphalan/prednisone/lenalidomide (MPL) (Category 1)
- Melphalan/prednisone/thalidomide (MPT) (Category 1)
- Bortezomib/dexamethasone (Category 2A)

While melphalan use does not feature prominently in the mSMART guidelines (Figure 27.2), due to significantly increased toxicities over cyclophosphamide, it remains as a broadly used backbone of the regimens outlined previously. Multiple randomized clinical trials have established benefit of the referenced triplet regimens over the prior standard melphalan/prednisone combination, though direct head-to-head comparisons of advanced regimens are lacking. A single meta-analysis did establish MPB as the most efficacious regimen among MP, MPT, and MPB combinations (20). Lenalidomide with low-dose dexamethasone represents another well-tolerated and highly effective treatment alternative in a group of standard-risk patients aged 65 years or older (21). The optimal duration of primary therapy after achieving maximal response is unknown, therefore, maintenance therapy or observation can be considered beyond maximal response.

## Maintenance Therapy for Transplant-Ineligible Patients

Various regimens of maintenance therapy following primary treatment completion have been investigated in the transplant-ineligible patients. Lenalidomide maintenance was shown to significantly reduce risk of disease progression and improves PFS (by 66%), though at the expense of toxicities, including that of increased rate of secondary cancers (22). Lenalidomide is the only medication to be assigned Category 1 for maintenance in transplant-ineligible patients. Bortezomib maintenance has also been shown to deepen the response rates, however, to this date, no studies have shown significant survival benefit with single-agent bortezomib maintenance. Bortezomib

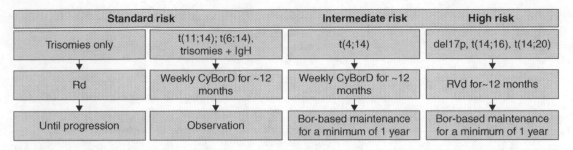

| Standard risk | | Intermediate risk | High risk |
|---|---|---|---|
| Trisomies only | t(11;14); t(6;14), trisomies + IgH | t(4;14) | del17p, t(14;16), t(14;20) |
| Rd | Weekly CyBorD for ~12 months | Weekly CyBorD for ~12 months | RVd for ~12 months |
| Until progression | Observation | Bor-based maintenance for a minimum of 1 year | Bor-based maintenance for a minimum of 1 year |

**Figure 27.2**

mSMART treatment algorithm: symptomatic multiple myeloma in transplant-ineligible patient. Bor, bortezomib; CyBorD, cyclophosphamide/bortezomib/dexamethasone; Rd, lenalidomide/low dose dexamethasone; mSMART, Mayo Stratification of Myeloma and Risk-Adapted Therapy. *Source*: Modified from Ref. (10). Mikhael JR, Dingli D, Roy V, et al.; Mayo Clinic. Management of newly diagnosed symptomatic multiple myeloma: updated Mayo Stratification of Myeloma and Risk-Adapted Therapy (mSMART) consensus guidelines 2013. *Mayo Clin Proc*. 2013;88(4):360–376.

remains an option, however, listed as a Category 2A in the most recent iteration of NCCN guidelines.

## Advanced-Stage Myeloma—Relapsed Disease

D.L. is a 62-year-old male with history of stage IIIA IgG kappa multiple myeloma, who underwent induction therapy with bortezomib, thalidomide, and dexamethasone, followed by tandem ASCT 3 years ago. He has been maintained on thalidomide since his transplant. He achieved a VGPR; however, in the last 6 months, his serum M-protein has increased from 0.1 to 0.9 g/dL. He has been having worsening fatigue and bone pain.

| White blood count | 5100/µL |
|---|---|
| Hemoglobin | 9.3 g/dL |
| Platelets | 203,000/µL |
| Calcium | 9.8 mg/dL |
| Creatinine | 1.2 mg/dL |
| Albumin | 3.4 g/dL |
| Lactate deydrogenase | 165 IU/L |
| β2-Microglobulin | 2.8 mg/L |

A follow-up serum protein electrophoresis and immunofixation assay demonstrated an IgG kappa monoclonal gammopathy of 4.2 g/dL. Quantitative Igs indicated an elevated IgG value of 3600 mg/dL, an IgA value of 96 mg/dL, and decreased IgM value of 24 mg/dL. A skeletal survey showed new osteolytic lesions in the bilateral humeri. A bone marrow biopsy revealed an increase to 17% plasma cells consistent with relapsed disease. Cytogenetics and FISH were performed on the bone marrow aspirate and demonstrated a hyperdiploid clone with trisomy 3, 7, 9, 11, and 15.

### Evidence-Based Case Discussion

This case involves a patient whose status is post-ASCT, 36 months previously on maintenance therapy, and who now has symptomatic, relapsed disease. His FISH and cytogenetic studies are consistent with standard-risk disease.

In the present clinical case, the patient is demonstrating relapse following ASCT. A number of treatment options are available. NCCN guidelines endorse participation in a clinical trial or a repetition of the original induction regimen provided that the relapse has occurred >6 months following the original induction regimen. The IMWG, on the other hand, recommends avoiding the original regimen if the duration of remission was less than the reported mean duration of remission for that particular regimen. Preferred salvage treatment regimens recognized by the NCCN include various combinations of proteasome inhibitors and immunomodulating agents.

In patients who relapse at least 1–2 years following ASCT, a second autotransplant may be considered following salvage therapy. One approach to choosing salvage therapy is the mSMART algorithm, which is outlined in Figure 27.3. In the case of our patient, he was enrolled into a clinical trial randomizing carfilzomib/lenalidomide/dexamethasone versus lenalidomide/dexamethasone.

Newer therapeutic agents have been Food and Drug Administration (FDA) approved for the treatment of relapsed multiple myeloma, including the proteasome inhibitor carfilzomib, and a novel IMiD pomalidomide; both recently were incorporated into the preferred NCCN regimens for salvage therapy. Carfilzomib showed promising clinical activity in relapsed and relapsed/refractory multiple myeloma with a substantially lower incidence of peripheral neuropathy compared to bortezomib, and when employed in a combination with lenalidomide and dexamethasone adds to the antimyeloma effects of these agents (23). Various carfilzomib-based combinations are currently being studied in several ongoing phase III trials, and the available data suggest that it produces a durable response in heavily pretreated patients. Pomalidomide is a novel IMiD approved for use in patients with heavily pretreated and refractory multiple myeloma, demonstrating efficacy even in prior recipients of bortezomib and lenalidomide (24).

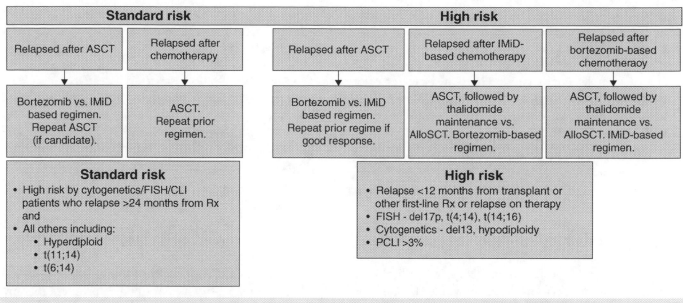

**Figure 27.3**

Treatment algorithm: refractory, progressive, or relapsed disease. AlloSCT, allogeneic stem cell transplantation; ASCT, autologous stem cell transplant; FISH, fluorescent in-situ hybridization; PCLI, plasma cell labeling index. *Source:* Modified from Ref. (25). *mSMART. Mayo Stratification for Myeloma and Risk-Adapted Therapy.* Relapsed Myeloma (v1 Jan 2008/last reviewed September 2012); 2012.

There has been an increase of promising new therapeutics in relapsed multiple myeloma. These include monoclonal antibodies such as elotuzumab (anti-CS1), which in combination with lenalidomide and dexamethasone produced a high response rate and PFS in patients with relapsed myeloma. Other monoclonal antibodies have demonstrated impressive single-agent responses including daratumumab (anti-CD38), and indatuximab ravtansine (BT062, an anti-CD138 conjugated with a cytotoxic agent). Novel proteasome inhibitors under investigation include ixazomib (MLN9708) and oprozomib. Investigation into other approaches including alkylating agents, deacetylase inhibitors, signaling transduction pathway inhibitors, and tyrosine kinase inhibitors are ongoing.

## REVIEW QUESTIONS

1. A 64-year-old man presents with hypercalcemia, acute renal failure, and anemia (Hgb = 9.0 g/dL) and multiple lytic lesions visualized on skeletal bone survey. His bone marrow is significant for 30% plasma cells. Which of the following is associated with high-risk disease in multiple myeloma?

   (A) t(11:14)
   (B) t(6;14)
   (C) del17p
   (D) del11q

2. A 50-year-old man is found to have a serum monoclonal (M) protein of 1.5 g/dL, and IgA kappa on immunofixation. He does not demonstrate any anemia, renal failure, hypercalcemia, or lytic bone lesions. Bone marrow biopsy demonstrates 2% plasma cells. What is his diagnosis?

   (A) Smoldering myeloma
   (B) Monoclonal gammopathy of undetermined significance (MGUS)
   (C) Multiple myeloma
   (D) Waldenstrom's macroglobulinemia

3. A 60-year-old man with multiple myeloma harboring t(11;14) achieved a complete remission after induction therapy with cyclophosphamide, bortezomib, and dexamethasone, then followed by autologous stem cell transplant (ASCT). He is now 3 years into maintenance therapy. He is now presenting with a significantly increasing M-protein and evidence of increased plasma cells in his bone marrow, consistent with relapse. He maintains a good performance status (Eastern Cooperative Oncology Group [ECOG] = 0) and has no additional comorbidities. Which of the following is the next appropriate step for his relapsed multiple myeloma?

   (A) Proceed directly to allogeneic bone marrow transplant
   (B) Induction therapy with lenalidomide and dexamethasone, then proceed to repeat ASCT
   (C) Induction therapy with melphalan/prednisone/thalidomide, and no bone marrow transplant
   (D) Continue maintenance therapy until he has evidence of end-organ damage (hypercalcemia, anemia, renal failure, or skeletal lytic lesions)

4. A 50-year-old man with multiple myeloma is currently undergoing induction therapy with lenalidomide, bortezomib, and dexamethasone. He is presenting to the clinic prior to his next cycle of chemotherapy. His current platelet count is 22. His platelet count prior to starting his last cycle was 56. Which of the following drugs has the lowest likelihood of causing severe thrombocytopenia?

   (A) Bortezomib
   (B) Thalidomide
   (C) Alkylating agents
   (D) Lenalidomide

5. A 67-year-old obese but generally healthy man sustained a right hip fracture in a fall. Imaging demonstrated several lytic lesions in the affected limb and concern for multiple myeloma was raised. Complete blood count with platelets and differential and comprehensive metabolic panel were remarkable only for an albumin of 3.1. Serum IgG was noted to be elevated at 4.7 g/dL, with immunofixation identifying an IgG monoclonal spike of 3.5 g/dL. Free serum lambda light chain was found to be elevated to 174.3 mg/dL and no urinary Bence–Jones protein was detected. β2-Microglobulin was 5.4 mg/L. Bone marrow biopsy showed 60% atypical plasma cells and adjunct cytogenetic studies identified presence of t(4;14). Which of the following primary therapeutic regimens are you most likely to recommend?

   (A) Lenalidomide/low-dose dexamethasone
   (B) Carfilzomib/dexamethasone
   (C) Melphalan/prednisone/bortezomib
   (D) Bortezomib/cyclophosphamide/dexamethasone
   (E) Vincristine/liposomal doxorubicin/dexamethasone

6. The same patient in Question 5 presents to the clinic to discuss treatment options. He is recovering well after surgery though remains rather immobile. After reviewing options, he opts against participation in a clinical trial, and you and patient agree to initiate lenalidomide, bortezomib, and low-dose dexamethasone induction therapy. You are discussing adjunctive therapeutic interventions and inform the patient that the following interventions should be pursued to optimally treat his disease and decrease risk of treatment-related complications:

   (A) Initiate low molecular weight heparin at doses used for venous thromboembolism treatment
   (B) Start taking 325 mg of acetylsalicylic acid daily
   (C) Bisphosphonate use should be delayed until complete recovery from hip replacement
   (D) Start acyclovir for prevention of varicella zoster reactivation
   (E) Start vitamins B6 and C for prevention of bortezomib-induced peripheral neuropathy

7. After 2 cycles of bortezomib/lenalidomide/dexamethasone (RVd) and achievement of very good partial response, plans for autologous stem cell transplant (ASCT) are finalized for the patient from Question 5. Stem cell collection is performed after 4 cycles of therapy and is uncomplicated. After 7 cycles of RVd, our patient achieves stringent complete response (sCR) and undergoes uncomplicated ASCT. Which of the following is correct regarding maintenance therapy after ASCT?

   (A) Lenalidomide maintenance yields marginally better overall survival benefit over bortezomib
   (B) Risk of secondary malignancies with maintenance therapy is equally high for patients on lenalidomide and thalidomide
   (C) Bortezomib maintenance should only be used if bortezomib was part of the primary therapy regimen
   (D) Maintenance therapy should not be pursued for >2 years after ASCT
   (E) Risk of thalidomide neuropathy increases with the duration of maintenance therapy

8. A 73-year-old woman was diagnosed with stage III International Staging System IgA kappa multiple myeloma, based on antecedent monoclonal gammopathy of undetermined significance diagnosed when she was 58 years. On initial multiple myeloma evaluation, she was found to have new acute renal failure with serum creatinine of 2.2 mg/dL (prior 0.6 mg/dL), anemia with hemoglobin of 8.5 g/dL, and mild hypercalcemia. Cytogenetic analysis performed on bone marrow biopsy specimen identified only trisomy 8. While she is activities-of-daily-living and instrumental activities of daily living independent, she has a past medical history of well-controlled non-insulin-dependent diabetes, hypertension, dyslipidemia, and osteoarthritis. What is the most appropriate initial therapy for her disease?

   (A) Lenalidomide/high-dose dexamethasone
   (B) Bortezomib/dexamethasone
   (C) Melphalan/prednisone/thalidomide
   (D) Melphalan/prednisone/lenalidomide
   (E) Dexamethasone

## REFERENCES

1. Durie BG, Harousseau JL, Miguel JS, et al.; International Myeloma Working Group. International uniform response criteria for multiple myeloma. *Leukemia*. 2006;20(9):1467–1473.
2. Zhou Y, Barlogie B, Shaughnessy JD Jr. The molecular characterization and clinical management of multiple myeloma in the post-genome era. *Leukemia*. 2009;23(11):1941–1956.
3. National Comprehensive Cancer Network. Multiple Myeloma (Version 2.2014); 2014.

4. Greipp PR, San Miguel J, Durie BG, et al. International staging system for multiple myeloma. *J Clin Oncol.* 2005;23(15): 3412–3420.

5. Kyle RA, Remstein ED, Therneau TM, et al. Clinical course and prognosis of smoldering (asymptomatic) multiple myeloma. *N Engl J Med.* 2007;356(25):2582–2590.

6. Attal M, Harousseau JL, Stoppa AM, et al. A prospective, randomized trial of autologous bone marrow transplantation and chemotherapy in multiple myeloma. Intergroupe Français du Myélome. *N Engl J Med.* 1996;335(2):91–97.

7. Barlogie B, Kyle RA, Anderson KC, et al. Standard chemotherapy compared with high-dose chemoradiotherapy for multiple myeloma: final results of phase III US Intergroup Trial S9321. *J Clin Oncol.* 2006;24(6):929–936.

8. Harousseau JL, Attal M, Avet-Loiseau H, et al. Bortezomib plus dexamethasone is superior to vincristine plus doxorubicin plus dexamethasone as induction treatment prior to autologous stem-cell transplantation in newly diagnosed multiple myeloma: results of the IFM 2005–01 phase III trial. *J Clin Oncol.* 2010;28(30):4621–4629.

9. Reeder CB, Reece DE, Kukreti V, et al. Cyclophosphamide, bortezomib and dexamethasone induction for newly diagnosed multiple myeloma: high response rates in a phase II clinical trial. *Leukemia.* 2009;23(7):1337–1341.

10. Mikhael JR, Dingli D, Roy V, et al.; Mayo Clinic. Management of newly diagnosed symptomatic multiple myeloma: updated Mayo Stratification of Myeloma and Risk-Adapted Therapy (mSMART) consensus guidelines 2013. *Mayo Clin Proc.* 2013; 88(4):360–376.

11. Barlogie B, Anaissie E, van Rhee F, et al. Incorporating bortezomib into upfront treatment for multiple myeloma: early results of total therapy 3. *Br J Haematol.* 2007;138(2):176–185.

12. Kumar S, Giralt S, Stadtmauer EA, et al.; International Myeloma Working Group. Mobilization in myeloma revisited: IMWG consensus perspectives on stem cell collection following initial therapy with thalidomide-, lenalidomide-, or bortezomib-containing regimens. *Blood.* 2009;114(9):1729–1735.

13. Palumbo A, Rajkumar SV, Dimopoulos MA, et al.; International Myeloma Working Group. Prevention of thalidomide- and lenalidomide-associated thrombosis in myeloma. *Leukemia.* 2008;22(2): 414–423.

14. Mateos MV. Management of treatment-related adverse events in patients with multiple myeloma. *Cancer Treat Rev.* 2010;36(Suppl 2):S24–S32.

15. Kumar S, Lacy MQ, Dispenzieri A, et al. High-dose therapy and autologous stem cell transplantation for multiple myeloma poorly responsive to initial therapy. *Bone Marrow Transpl.* 2004;34(2):161–167.

16. Cook G, Liakopoulou E, Pearce R, et al.; British Society of Blood & Marrow Transplantation Clinical Trials Committee. Factors influencing the outcome of a second autologous stem cell transplant (ASCT) in relapsed multiple myeloma: a study from the British Society of Blood and Marrow Transplantation Registry. *Biol Blood Marrow Transpl.* 2011;17(11):1638–1645.

17. Attal M, Lauwers-Cances V, Marit G, et al.; IFM Investigators. Lenalidomide maintenance after stem-cell transplantation for multiple myeloma. *N Engl J Med.* 2012;366(19):1782–1791.

18. McCarthy PL, Owzar K, Hofmeister CC, et al. Lenalidomide after stem-cell transplantation for multiple myeloma. *N Engl J Med.* 2012;366(19):1770–1781.

19. Usmani SZ, Sexton R, Hoering A, et al. Second malignancies in total therapy 2 and 3 for newly diagnosed multiple myeloma: influence of thalidomide and lenalidomide during maintenance. *Blood.* 2012;120(8):1597–1600.

20. Yeh Y, Chambers J, Gaugris S, et al. Indirect comparison of the efficacy of melphalan-prednisone-bortezomib relative to melphalan-prednisone-thalidomide and melphalan-prednisone for the first line treatment of multiple myeloma. *ASH Ann Meeting Abstr.* 2008;112(11):2367.

21. Rajkumar SV, Jacobus S, Callander NS, et al.; Eastern Cooperative Oncology Group. Lenalidomide plus high-dose dexamethasone versus lenalidomide plus low-dose dexamethasone as initial therapy for newly diagnosed multiple myeloma: an open-label randomised controlled trial. *Lancet Oncol.* 2010;11(1):29–37.

22. Palumbo A, Hajek R, Delforge M, et al.; MM-015 Investigators. Continuous lenalidomide treatment for newly diagnosed multiple myeloma. *N Engl J Med.* 2012;366(19):1759–1769.

23. Jakubowiak AJ, Dytfeld D, Griffith KA, et al. A phase ½ study of carfilzomib in combination with lenalidomide and low-dose dexamethasone as a frontline treatment for multiple myeloma. *Blood.* 2012;120(9):1801–1809.

24. Dimopoulos MA, Lacy MQ, Moreau P, et al. Pomalidomide in combination with low-dose dexamethasone: demonstrates a significant progression free survival and overall survival advantage, in relapsed/refractory mm: a phase 3, multicenter, randomized, open-label study. *ASH Ann Meeting Abstr.* 2012;120(21): LBA-6.

25. *mSMART. Mayo Stratification for Myeloma and Risk-Adapted Therapy.* Relapsed Myeloma (v1 Jan 2008/last reviewed September 2012); 2012. Consensus Guidelines to Management of Plasma Cell Disorders. http://www.msmart.org/Relapsed%20Myeloma .pdf

# 28

# *Acute Lymphoblastic Leukemia*

MUSA YILMAZ AND MARK M. UDDEN

## EPIDEMIOLOGY, RISK FACTORS, NATURAL HISTORY, AND PATHOLOGY

Acute lymphoblastic leukemia (ALL) is a clonal disease arising from somatic mutations in a lymphoid progenitor cell that alter regulation of cellular proliferation, differentiation, and apoptosis. Rapid accumulation of precursor lymphoid cells usually occurs in the bone marrow displacing normal hematopoiesis resulting in neutropenia, thrombocytopenia, anemia, and dissemination of leukemic cells in the peripheral blood. ALL may arise in lymph nodes or the mediastinum and may not have bone marrow or peripheral blood involvement at presentation. Such patients are said to have lymphoblastic lymphoma that is usually treated as ALL. The central nervous system (CNS) is a significant site of involvement at presentation or relapse.

ALL accounts for 12% of all leukemias diagnosed in the United States. It is estimated that 6020 new cases of ALL will be diagnosed in the United States in 2014 and approximately 1440 deaths will be attributable to ALL per American Cancer Society (1). ALL is the most common malignancy in patients younger than 15 years, accounting for 75% of all leukemia diagnosed in this age-group. Twenty percent of acute leukemia in adults is ALL. There is a bimodal age incidence, characterized by a peak between the ages of 1 and 4 years, followed by a second peak in the elderly (>60 years of age). ALL tends to affect men more often than women, although in infancy there is a slight female preponderance. ALL is more common in whites than blacks, and in the United States, there seems to be a higher incidence among Hispanic populations.

Down syndrome and ataxia-telangiectasia have been associated with a 30–70 times greater risk of developing B-cell and T-cell ALL, respectively (2). Increased incidence

has also been noted in patients with Bloom syndrome and patients with autoimmune conditions such as Sjögren syndrome. It is unknown whether the chromosomal instability or immunosuppression caused by these diseases is the driving factor in leukemogenesis. Multiple environmental factors, including nuclear, electromagnetic, and cosmic radiation, and chemical agents such as insecticides, dichlorodiphenyltrichloroethane (DDT), and vitamin K have been implicated as risk factors, but the data supporting these are inconclusive. Intrauterine exposure to radiation increases the risk of childhood leukemia.

Our understanding of the leukemogenic process has improved significantly as a result of recent progress in the field of genomic analysis. This is especially true in pediatric and young adult B- and T-cell ALL. Recent identification of novel gene fusion transcripts and altered gene expression has significantly enhanced our knowledge regarding the biology and etiopathogenesis of ALL. These markers seem to have prognostic, predictive, and possible therapeutic implications.

The best-known genetic mutation in ALL involves *BCR–ABL* gene rearrangement resulting in the formation of the "Philadelphia chromosome." The Philadelphia chromosome (Ph) is found in up to 20% of adult ALL cases (3). The resulting gene transcript in ALL patients is usually 190 kDa compared to the 210-kDa gene product expressed in patients with chronic myelogenous leukemia. Insight into the *BCR–ABL* transcript has permitted development of tyrosine kinase inhibitors (TKIs) for the treatment of both chronic myeloid leukemia (CML) and Ph+ ALL (3). Other genetic changes associated with ALL are summarized in Table 28.1.

Recent genome-wide studies in pediatric ALL have identified gene mutations in high-risk groups, such as deletion of the IKAROS family zinc finger 1 (*IKZF1*) gene

**Table 28.1** Cytogenetic Classification and Prognosis in Adult/Childhood B-Cell ALL

| Karyotype | Incidence in Adults (%) | Incidence in Children (%) | Adults Achieving CR (%) | Adults Achieving 3-Yr Survival (%) |
|---|---|---|---|---|
| Normal | 30–40 | 15–20 | 82 | 50 |
| t(9;22) | 25–30 | 3 | 78 | 18 |
| +8 | 10–12 | 2 | 87 | 17 |
| t(4;11) | 4–7 | 2 | 76 | 18 |
| +21 | 0–3 | 20–25 | 84 | 30 |
| Abnormal 9p | 6–30 | 7–10 | 89 | 43 |
| Abnormal 12p | 4–6 | 7–10 | 82 | 82 |
| t(14q11) | | | 100 | 78 |
| t(1;19) | 2–3 | 3–11 | 5–6 | |
| t(12;21) | 5 | 25–30 | 90 | 90 |
| Hyperdiploidy | 4–5 | 23–26 | 90 | 70–80 |

ALL, acute lymphoblastic leukemia; CR, complete remission.

on chromosome 9 encoding the IKAROS transcription factor. Mutation of the *JAK2* gene, resulting in replacement of valine by phenylalanine at position 617 (V617F), is well recognized in myeloproliferative diseases including polycythemia vera and myelofibrosis. However, in pediatric ALL, a group of mutations at R683 was observed in 10–15% of patients with high-risk disease. This mutation is also frequently found in Down syndrome–related ALL and is uniformly associated with overexpression of cytokine receptor-like factor 2 (CRLF2) due to gene rearrangement. It appears that *CRLF2* overexpression in combination with mutation of *JAK1* or *JAK2* genes and deletion or mutation of *IKZF* promotes leukemogenesis. The genetic signature in these cases overlaps significantly with the *BCR–ABL* signature (4).

Approximately 15% of pediatric ALL patients demonstrate gene expression profiles that match Ph+ ALL, but lack the t(9;22)/*BCR–AB-1* gene fusion (5). This "*BCR–ABL-1*-like signature" has also been shown to be an important prognostic factor that can identify patients with high relapse risk (5). Ultimately, detecting the aforementioned molecular abnormalities and *BCR–ABL-1*-like gene expression may identify high-risk patients who require alternative and/or more intensive treatment and who may respond to TKIs.

Gene expression profiling studies also enable classification of T-cell ALL into at least 4 distinct prognostic subtypes. The *TLX1* and *TLX3* subgroups are characterized by rearrangements solely of the *TLX1* or *TLX3* genes; whereas the *TAL/LMO* and *HOXA* groups are characterized by various rearrangements that affect functionally equivalent oncogenes. These genetic subgroups are associated with expression of specific immunophenotypic markers that reflect arrest at specific stages of T-cell development. In addition to these mutually exclusive "driver" mutations, other mutations have been found in >1 genetic subgroup. These additional mutations affect

various cellular processes and include *NOTCH1* activating mutations (seen in 56% of children with ALL) and *FBXWZ* inactivating mutations that are associated with favorable outcomes (6). These additional mutations may help to explain variable outcomes in different studies and may serve as therapeutic targets. Expansion of our knowledge of mutations and altered signaling pathway offers hope for new targeted therapies in T-cell ALL.

The most common presenting features of ALL in adults include fatigue, dyspnea on exertion, fever, ecchymosis, petechiae, bone pain, and headache. Bone pain is caused by the expansion of the bone marrow with leukemic cells, leukemic infiltration of the periosteum, or bone infarction. Affected bones include the long bones of the legs and arms. Renal involvement may manifest as nausea, vomiting, flank pain, or oliguria/anuria. Hepatic infiltration can cause icterus, dark urine, acholic stools, right upper quadrant fullness, or pain. Splenic involvement may be associated with left upper quadrant fullness, pain, or early satiety from splenic infiltration. Intracranial or subarachnoid hemorrhage may be a consequence of hyperleukocytosis syndrome or profound thrombocytopenia. Neutropenia may be associated with life-threatening bacterial or viral infection.

Clinical findings include nonbulky lymphadenopathy, hepatosplenomegaly, petechiae, or pallor. Hepatosplenomegaly due to organ infiltration is much more common in adults and is noted on imaging in 50–60% of adults presenting with ALL. Other presentations of ALL include CNS involvement, testicular involvement, and superior vena cava (SVC) syndrome. CNS involvement occurs in 8% of adults with ALL at presentation and should be suspected when the patient has headache, nausea, cranial nerve palsy, meningismus, or confusion. Testicular involvement may present as a firm testicular mass or hydrocele due to lymphatic stagnation. SVC syndrome occurs due to compression of the SVC or brachiocephalic vein by a mediastinal mass. Bulky mediastinal disease is more often seen with T-cell ALL with an overall incidence of 10–15%. Other rare presentations include leukemia cutis, salivary gland involvement, and spinal cord compression from epidural infiltration or paraspinal mass.

Laboratory features seen in patients presenting with ALL include varying degrees of leukocytosis. Patients with t(4;11) with *MLL* gene fusion, t(1;19) with *E2A-PBX1* fusion, t(9;22) with *BCR–ABL* fusion, and *BCR–ABL*-like disease or patients with hypodiploidy often present with higher leukocyte count, whereas those with hyperdiploidy or t(12;21) with *TEL-AML* often present with lower white blood cell (WBC) count. Thus, the adverse risk associated with high WBC counts at presentation may be a reflection of the underlying genetic mutation. ALL patients may present with eosinophilia. For example, t(5;14) results in overactivation of interleukin-3 gene on chromosome 5 that in turn supports eosinophil proliferation. This is seen in patients with specific translocations resulting in overactivation of the interleukin-3 gene on chromosome 5 and eosinophil proliferation. Anemia (Hb <8.0 g/dL) and thrombocytopenia (platelet count <50,000/µL) are seen in 25–50% of adults at presentation.

Approximately 90% of patients have circulating blasts at presentation. Typically, the B-cell precursor lymphoblasts are large with sparse cytoplasm and an enlarged nucleus, with fine chromatin and poorly defined nucleoli. Mature B-cell blasts (Burkitt lymphoma) are usually intermediate in size with intensely basophilic cytoplasm and prominent cytoplasmic vacuolation. ALL blasts do not stain with myeloperoxidase or Sudan black; however, they often stain with periodic acid-Schiff (PAS) reagent. Terminal deoxynucleotidyl transferase (TdT) staining is frequently positive in early B lymphoblasts and can also be seen in early T-ALL. Bone marrow examination is recommended in patients with suspected leukemia because 8–10% of adults with ALL do not have circulating leukemic blasts. Some of these patients have significant pancytopenia, and the clinical diagnosis may be aplastic anemia before the discovery of ALL in the bone marrow. ALL patients may present with or develop tumor lysis during treatment, resulting in hyperuricemia, hyperphosphatemia, hypocalcemia, and elevated creatinine associated with urate nephropathy.

The diagnosis of ALL was classically made by negative cytochemical staining for myeloperoxidase and Sudan black with positive TdT and PAS staining along with morphological features of the marrow lymphoblasts. Diagnosis now relies on flow cytometric determination of the immunophenotype of the marrow blasts (Immunological Classification—Table 28.2). Characteristic patterns for B-cell ALL subtypes and T-cell ALL are shown in the table. Acute myeloid leukemia (AML) blasts typically express CD34, CD13, and CD33. ALL blasts express a variety of

**Table 28.2** ALL: Immunological Classification of ALL

| Cell Lineages | CD Markers | Overall Percentage in Adults |
|---|---|---|
| *B-Cell Lineage* | CD19+, CD22+, CD79a+, HLA-DR+ | |
| Pro-B | CD10– | 11 |
| Early pre-B | CD10+ | 52 |
| Pre-B | CD10+/–, cIg+ | 9 |
| Mature-B | CD19+, CD20+ CD22+, CD79a+, cIg+, sIgλ+ or sIgκ | 4 |
| *T-Cell Lineage* | CD7+, CD3+ | |
| T cell | HLA-DR–, TdT+/–, CD2+, CD1+/–, CD4+/– | 18 |
| Pre-T cell | HLA-DR+/–, TdT+, CD2–, CD1–, CD4– | 6 |

ALL, acute lymphoblastic leukemia.

B- and T-cell markers, but may also demonstrate aberrant expression of myeloid markers. In addition to flow cytometry studies, a bone marrow cytogenetic study should also be obtained. Demonstration of the Ph, hyperdiploidy, and other translocations has prognostic significance and may determine whether patients are referred for transplantation in first or second remission. Specific genetic markers such as *BCR–ABL* are increasingly of interest as they provide prognostic information and may indicate targets for therapy.

## CASE SUMMARIES

### Adolescent Young Adult B-Cell Precursor ALL

D.N., a 19-year-old man, presented with fever, weight loss, knee pain, and petechiae. His white blood cell count at presentation was 8000/µL with 93% blasts and an absolute neutrophil count of 300/µL. His hemoglobin was 9.2 g/dL and platelet count was 120,000/µL. His uric acid was 11.6 mg/dL and serum creatinine was 1.4 mg/dL. Examination of a peripheral blood smear showed large cells with scant basophilic cytoplasm, and nuclei with fine chromatin and inconspicuous nucleoli. Flow cytometry of peripheral blood revealed a large population of cells that were CD10+, CD19+, CD22+, and CD79a+. Bone marrow examination revealed >90% leukemic blasts; chromosome analysis demonstrated hyperdiploidy (>50 chromosomes). Fluorescence in-situ hybridization (FISH) for *BCR–ABL* transcript was negative.

### Evidence-Based Case Discussion

This is a young adult with B-cell precursor ALL. The immunophenotype is consistent with CD10+ early

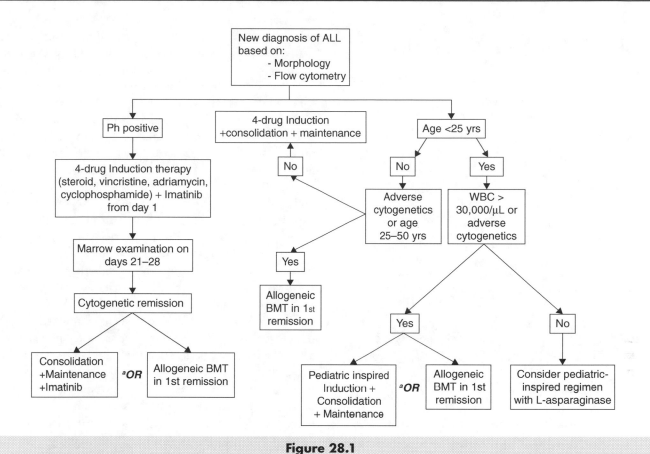

**Figure 28.1**

Treatment algorithm for the management of patients with ALL. ᵃOR is used to indicate that either treatment option is an acceptable alternative and no consensus guidelines favor one over the other. ALL, acute lymphoblastic leukemia; BMT, bone marrow transplantation; WBC, white blood cell.

pre-B-cell ALL that accounts for approximately 50% of all newly diagnosed ALL in adults. This patient has none of the usual adverse risk features in adults with B-cell precursor ALL, which include age >60 years, leukocyte count >100,000/µL, high-risk genotype (including BCR–ABL, MLL-AF4, other MLL translocations, hypodiploidy in <44 chromosomes, or complex cytogenetics with ≥5 chromosomal abnormalities). Improved treatment has negated the prognostic significance of previously identified high-risk features such as male sex, African American race, or the presence of the E2A–PBX fusion t(1;19). D.N. has hyperdiploidy, which has been associated with low leukocyte count, favorable responses to chemotherapy with >90% CR rates, and improved 5-year survival rates in the range of 70–80% (3).

Treatment strategies for B-cell precursor ALL focus on appropriate intensity antileukemic therapy, supportive care, and infection control (see Figure 28.1). Prognostic factors must be used for risk stratification of adult and pediatric patients to determine the intensity of therapy, need for reintensification, intensity and duration of CNS prophylaxis, and need for bone marrow transplant. In pediatric ALL, 3 risk groups are identified, whereas in adults, due to the poorer outcomes, only standard risk or

adverse risks are distinguished. Risk stratification tables for pediatric and adult populations are presented in Tables 28.3 and 28.4.

Standard antileukemic therapy for B-precursor-cell and T-cell ALL consists of 3 phases. Induction therapy is administered to induce a complete remission (CR) with acceptable toxicity followed by reconstitution of normal hematopoiesis, which enables administration of further intensive chemotherapy. A consolidation phase follows to weed out the drug-resistant residual leukemic cells and to eradicate minimal residual disease (MRD). This is followed by 2–3 years of maintenance therapy to reduce the risk of relapse. CNS prophylaxis is begun early during induction and given throughout the maintenance phase.

Induction regimens in adults traditionally include varying combinations and doses of corticosteroids, cyclophosphamide, vincristine, daunorubicin, asparaginase, and intrathecal methotrexate or cytarabine. The hyper-CVAD regimen developed by the MD Anderson group uses 4 alternating courses each of cyclophosphamide, vincristine, doxorubicin, and dexamethasone in conjunction with high-dose methotrexate/leucovorin and cytarabine for a total of 8 cycles of combined induction and consolidation therapy (7). Maintenance therapy consists of 2–3 years

**Table 28.3** Risk Classification in Pediatric ALL

| Risk Group | Characteristics |
|---|---|
| High risk | –*BCR–ABL*: t (9;22);<br>–Hypodiploidy (<44);<br>–*MLL-AF4*/or other *MLL*: {t(4;11); t(9;11); t(11;19)}<br>–Minimal residual disease after induction >1% |
| Standard risk | All others |
| Low risk | –B-cell precursor ALL<br>–Age 1–10 yr<br>–WBC < 50 × 10⁹/L<br>–Minimal residual disease after induction <0.01% |

ALL, acute lymphoblastic leukemia; WBC, white blood cell.

**Table 28.4** Prognostic Factors in Adult and Adolescent Young Adult (AYA) ALL

| Clinical Features | Standard Risk | Adverse Risk |
|---|---|---|
| Age (years) | <35 | >60 |
| Immunophenotype | Mid T-cell | Early T-cell, mature T-cell |
| Leukocyte count | <30,000/µL | >100,000/µL |
| Genotype | — | –Complex (≥5)<br>–Hypodiploidy (<44)<br>–*BCR–ABL1*: t(9;22)<br>–*MLL-AF4*/other *MLL*:{t(4;11); t(9;11); t(11;19)} |
| Minimal residual disease after induction | <0.01% | >0.01% |

ALL, acute lymphoblastic leukemia; WBC, white blood cell.

of 6-mercaptopurine (6-MP), methotrexate, vincristine, and steroids with intrathecal therapy. The Cancer and Leukemia Group B (CALGB) 8811 regimen developed by Larson et al. adds asparaginase to the standard induction regimen of prednisone, vincristine, anthracycline, and steroid (8). This is followed by an intensified postremission therapy comprising 6-MP, 6-thioguanine, and L-asparaginase with cyclophosphamide, cytarabine, vincristine, methotrexate, and corticosteroids. Maintenance includes only methotrexate and 6-MP. CNS irradiation is avoided because high-dose methotrexate/cytarabine penetrates the blood–brain barrier and provides CNS prophylaxis.

The goal of the maintenance therapy is to kill nascent, slow-growing ALL cells or suppress new clones that may arise. Reduction in the duration of maintenance therapy results in higher relapse rates. Most experts recommend continuing the maintenance for 2–3 years. Consensus guidelines from pediatric (but not adult literature)

recommend escalating the doses of methotrexate and 6-MP to achieve low leukocyte counts. However, if there is unexpected severe or prolonged neutropenia from 6-MP, it should be discontinued and an analysis obtained for thiopurine methyltransferase (TPMT). Patients with no TPMT activity (0.3% prevalence) demonstrate significant bone marrow suppression due to accumulation of unmetabolized drug (9). Adequate dose intensity is an important factor associated with decreased relapse in maintenance phase (10). Adult ALL protocols have not been as stringent and aggressive with maintenance dose escalation, and this may be 1 of the factors resulting in poorer outcomes in adult ALL as compared to pediatric ALL. Another treatment strategy that has shown to be of benefit is the addition of 1 or 2 reinduction cycles shortly after achieving remission. The reinduction regimens use the same drugs that were initially used to achieve induction.

An approach for the adolescent young adult (AYA) patient gaining traction is to use a more intensive pediatric-inspired regimen, including higher doses of nonmyelosuppressive "core" drugs such as L-asparaginase, vincristine, and steroids; early and frequent CNS prophylaxis with intrathecal chemotherapy, 1 or even 2 postremission reintensification cycles, and long-term maintenance for 3 years. This is based on retrospective American and European trials that showed significantly better 3- or 4-year event-free and overall survival (OS) with pediatric-inspired regimens in young adults between ages 16 and 21 years (11). The Spanish PETHEMA protocol ALL-96 was a prospective trial in which 35 adolescents (aged 15–18 years) and 46 young adults (aged 19–30 years) with standard risk ALL were treated with pediatric-inspired protocols (12). Patients received a standard 5-drug, 5-week induction, followed by 2 cycles of early consolidation, maintenance with monthly reinforcement for 1-year postremission, and standard maintenance therapy for up to 2 years. The 6-year event-free survival of 61% and OS of 69% demonstrated the efficacy and tolerability of intensive pediatric regimens in adolescent young adults up to the age of 30 years.

D.N. received aggressive IV hydration with normal saline and oral allopurinol 300-mg daily starting on the day of admission. His creatinine and uric acid came down rapidly over the ensuing 24 hours and he underwent induction with 5-drug antileukemic chemotherapy (vincristine, anthracycline, cyclophosphamide, steroids, and L-asparaginase). Intrathecal chemotherapy with methotrexate was administered on day 3 of the induction regimen. He tolerated the chemotherapy relatively well with no serious infectious or metabolic complications. Frequent monitoring of uric acid, electrolytes, liver function, and coagulation profile was performed during the first 3–4 weeks of induction. Routine antiviral and pneumocystis jiroveci prophylaxis was initiated and supportive care included packed RBC transfusions for clinically significant anemia and platelet transfusions for platelet counts <10,000/µL.

After recovering from the nadir of myelosuppression, bone marrow biopsy was performed on day 21 that revealed normocellular marrow with no identifiable blasts. Chromosome analysis revealed a normal male karyotype, confirming hematological and cytogenetic remission. Flow cytometry analysis and polymerase chain reaction (PCR) amplification were negative for MRD. The absence of high-risk features discouraged the idea of proceeding with allogeneic stem cell transplantation (SCT), and a decision was made to continue with 7 more cycles of the same chemotherapy used for induction along with intrathecal chemotherapy. This was followed by 3 years of maintenance with methotrexate, 6-MP, steroids, and monthly vincristine. D.N. received intrathecal chemotherapy at 3 monthly intervals for the duration of maintenance therapy. He tolerated therapy well, except for an episode of transaminitis during year 2 of maintenance that resolved after reducing the 6-MP dose by 25%. He is currently 4 years from initial diagnosis with no evidence of relapse. He continues to follow-up for biannual physical examinations and CBC checks.

## Adult B-Cell Precursor ALL With Adverse Features

M.R., a 48-year-old man, presented with bilateral knee and shin pain worse at night for the last 3 months. Laboratory data revealed a WBC count of >100,000/µL. Flow cytometry demonstrated a large population of cells that were CD19+, CD20+, and CD10+. Bone marrow cytogenetics revealed t(4;11) with *MLL-AF4* fusion.

## Evidence-Based Case Discussion

This is an adult patient with high-risk ALL features based on his age (>35 years) and elevated WBC count (>30,000/µL), which are poor prognostic factors. The presence of t(4;11) associated with the *MLL* gene transcript is linked with hyperleukocytosis and dismal outcome, and is more prevalent in infants and elderly patients. These features place M.R. in a high-risk group.

Although the basic approach to treatment of B-cell precursor ALL in adult patients remains the same, there are some important differences in the biology, tolerance to chemotherapy, postinduction approaches, and the role of transplant in older patients (see Figure 28.1). This patient should be treated using standard induction therapy with steroids, vincristine, anthracycline, and cyclophosphamide (7,8). High-dose methotrexate should be used with caution and may require dose reduction. Similar to pediatric patients, hypersensitivity, pancreatitis, thrombosis, and hepatic toxicity are prominent with asparaginase use. The incidence of these side effects increases with age and makes asparaginase use more difficult in adult patients (13). There is evidence that incorporation of rituximab into the hyper-CVAD regimen may improve outcome in

CD20+ Ph– B-cell precursor ALL patients <60 years old (14). Other monoclonal antibodies that are under investigation for use in ALL include inotuzumab, an anti-CD22 antibody conjugated with calicheamicin, which shows activity in relapsed/refractory B-cell ALL as a single agent (15). Blinatumomab, a bispecific T-cell engager (BITE) antibody designed to direct cytotoxic T cells to CD19-expressing leukemic cells, has also shown long-lasting remissions in relapsed/refractory B-cell ALL (16). Introduction of new monoclonal antibodies in ALL treatment may improve cure rate, in combination with conventional chemotherapy or other monoclonal antibodies.

M.R. underwent induction chemotherapy using the hyper-CVAD and rituximab regimen. He developed fever and was diagnosed with *Pseudomonas* pneumonia on day 10 of induction chemotherapy. He subsequently required ICU admission, intubation, intravenous pressors, and broad-spectrum antibiotics for a period of 5 days. His clinical course improved as his blood counts recovered. Bone marrow aspiration on day 24 revealed 40% cellularity with no discernible blasts on morphological examination. FISH revealed resolution of t(4;11). A majority of ALL patients achieve CR after induction therapy. Relapse is thought to be due to residual leukemia cells that are below the limits of detection using conventional morphological assessment. Emerging data demonstrate that patients with detectable MRD after completion of induction chemotherapy have high relapse risk (17). MRD can be detected by flow cytometry identifying B cells with aberrant immunophenotype or by PCR. Detection of MRD is 1 of the major uses for PCR in ALL diagnosis and prognostication. Flow cytometry and PCR are equally sensitive for MRD testing as long as MRD is present at a ≥0.01% level (18).

This patient should be evaluated early in his treatment for allogeneic SCT. Initial studies showed survival benefit with allogeneic SCT in high-risk patients, consequently an evidence-based review panel recommended allogeneic transplant for adults with high-risk ALL in first remission (19). Although an Eastern Cooperative Oncology Group (ECOG) trial showed a survival advantage for allotransplant in patients with standard risk (age <35 years and no adverse biological features), these patients usually receive maintenance therapy (20). M.R. had a healthy human leukocyte antigen (HLA)-matched sibling and underwent allogeneic transplantation approximately 2 months after initial diagnosis. He had mild, acute, and chronic graft versus host disease posttransplantation. Bone marrow biopsies on days 90 and 365 posttransplant showed complete donor chimerism and no evidence of ALL.

Adult patients with relapsed or refractory disease have uniformly poor outcomes. To address this issue, the MD Anderson group implemented an augmented hyper-CVAD regimen, which includes asparaginase and intensified doses of vincristine and dexamethasone (21). Forty-five percent of the relapsed/refractory ALL patients achieved CRs in this trial and some patients were bridged to transplant. Liposomal vincristine was approved by Food and Drug Administration (FDA) for treatment of Ph– ALL in second or greater relapse. In a single arm trial, 7 of 36 (19%) patients achieved CR with weekly liposomal vincristine (22). Four of the seven responding patients who achieved CR were able to undergo allogeneic SCT.

## Adult *BCR–ABL* Transcript Positive B-Cell Precursor ALL

W.L., a 46-year-old man, presented with headache, dyspnea on exertion, persistent low-grade fever with chills, and bleeding from the gums over the last 6 weeks. His WBC count on presentation was 180,000/µL and his platelet count was 8000/µL. Flow cytometry revealed a predominance of CD19+, CD79a+, CD10+ cells confirming a diagnosis of B-cell precursor ALL. Cytogenetics from the bone marrow specimen revealed t(9;22) in 6/20 metaphase cells and PCR demonstrated the p190 *BCR–ABL* variant. He has 3 siblings.

### Evidence-Based Case Discussion

W.L. is an "older" precursor B-cell ALL patient with the Ph indicating the presence of the *BCR-ABL* fusion gene. *BCR–ABL* fusion transcripts are more common in elderly patients (30%), are often associated with leukocytosis, and confer a poor prognosis and high relapse rate (3). Heretofore, allogeneic SCT in first remission was the only effective therapeutic option, with 5-year survival rates approaching 35–45%. The emergence of TKI therapy may change the approach to such patients. Currently, induction chemotherapy for ALL is used in combination with imatinib and data suggest CR rates >90% (3) (see Figure 28.1). Imatinib is continued through induction, consolidation, and maintenance phases. Newer data are emerging concerning the use of dasatinib, which may be a more potent drug as it inhibits multiple kinases and also seems to have higher CNS penetration (23). Ponatinib may be an alternative TKI in relapsed or refractory Ph+ ALL patients with unacceptable toxicities or resistance to imatinib or dasatinib or acquired *BCR–ABL* T315I mutation (24). A study combining hyper-CVAD and ponatinib in frontline setting is ongoing.

W.L. received induction chemotherapy with hyper-CVAD. Imatinib was started on day 1 of induction and continued daily through the 8 cycles of hyper-CVAD chemotherapy (25). The patient achieved hematological and cytogenetic remission after cycle 1 of induction chemotherapy. The patient had a healthy HLA-matched sibling and he underwent allogeneic SCT. He is currently at 36 months from initial diagnosis with no MRD and took 400 mg of imatinib daily for 24 months after transplant. It is questionable whether there is any benefit of receiving TKI after allogeneic SCT if no MRD is present. One recent study suggests that TKI after allogeneic SCT may improve outcome in these patients, but the duration of TKI usage still remains uncertain (23). Patients who are not candidates for transplant or who have no available donor should continue TKIs as maintenance therapy after completing combination chemotherapy (23).

## Adult T-cell ALL With Favorable Prognostic Features

A.A., a 27-year-old man, presented with fatigue, bone pain, petechiae, and recent weight loss. He had a WBC count of 65,000/µL, a hemoglobin of 8.2 g/dL, and a platelet count of 80,000/µL. His peripheral smear revealed many large cells with reduced cytoplasm, fine chromatin, and poorly defined nucleoli. Flow cytometry of peripheral blood demonstrated that the blasts were CD7+, CD3+, CD1a+, and CD13– confirming the diagnosis of T-cell ALL. No mediastinal mass was visible on chest x-ray. Cytogenetics from a bone marrow aspirate revealed a normal male karyotype.

### Evidence-Based Case Discussion

A.A. has T-cell ALL; his age <35 years and total WBC count <100,000/µL are favorable factors. The UK ALL XII/ECOG 2993 study of 1927 ALL patients contained 356 subjects with T-cell ALL. A CR rate of 94% and a 5-year OS of 48% was demonstrated for T-cell ALL patients using an aggressive chemotherapy regimen containing L-asparaginase. This study demonstrated that blast expression of CD1a and lack of expression of CD13 in T-cell disease were associated with significantly better survival. Complex cytogenetics was also associated with poor survival, but CNS involvement at diagnosis did not seem to affect survival in T-cell disease (although it did in the overall cohort). The role of allogeneic SCT in T-cell ALL is still under investigation. Nelarabine has efficacy in the relapsed setting and has been evaluated in the frontline setting (26). In a phase II trial, combination of nelarabine with hyper-CVAD induced durable CRs in adult patients with T-ALL (26). However, larger studies are needed to establish the optimal schedule of nelarabine incorporation into frontline regimens as only 20% of the cohort received all intended courses of nelarabine.

A.A received standard antileukemic therapy and CNS prophylaxis with intrathecal therapy followed by consolidation and maintenance therapy for a total of 3 years. He remains in remission and has returned to work.

## REVIEW QUESTIONS

1. A 35-year-old man presents with 1 month of increasing fatigue. A complete blood count reveals a leukocyte count of 23,000/µL, hemoglobin of 5.8 g/dL, and platelets of 12,000 /µL. The peripheral blood smear shows 40% lymphoblasts. Bone marrow is completely

replaced with CD19+, CD20+, CD22+, and CD10– cells. Which of the following is considered to be a good prognostic factor for above patient?

(A) Detection of *MLL–AF4* fusion gene
(B) Detection of *BCR–ABL1* fusion gene
(C) Translocation (9;11)
(D) Detection of *ETV6–RUNX1 (TEL–AML1)* fusion transcripts
(E) Hypodiploidy

2. A 23-year-old man presents to the hospital with abdominal distention and skin rash. He has no known medical problems and was well until now. Physical examination reveals petechial rash on the extremities and trunk. The liver is palpable 5 cm below the right costal margin and spleen is palpable 10 cm below the left costal margin. A complete blood cell count reveals a leukocyte count of 150,000/µL, hemoglobin of 8.9 g/dL, and platelets of 5,000/µL. The peripheral blood smear reveals 70% lymphoblasts. He undergoes bone marrow examination and immunophenotype reveals the blasts to be TdT+, CD3–, CD7–, CD10+, CD19+, CD20+, CD22+, CD79a+, membrane Ig–, and cytoplasmic Ig+ cells. Which one of the following is the most likely diagnosis?

(A) Pro-B acute lymphoblastic leukemia (ALL)
(B) Pre-B ALL
(C) Mature B ALL
(D) Pro-T ALL

3. A 40-year-old obese woman presented with shortness of breath. Chest x-ray revealed large mediastinal mass. Biopsy of the mass revealed T-cell lymphoblastic lymphoma. Bone marrow contained T lymphoblasts. She commenced induction with a regimen containing vincristine, peg-asparaginase, daunorubicin and prednisone. Two weeks after starting induction, she was readmitted to the hospital with severe abdominal pain, nausea, and vomiting. Her temperature was 99.5°F, heart rate was 110 bpm, blood pressure was 135/80 mmHg, and respiratory rate was 16. Her physical examination revealed epigastric tenderness without any rebound, hypoactive bowel sounds. Her laboratory testing showed the following: white blood cell count = 0.5/µL, hemoglobin = 9.5 g/dL, platelet = 75,000/µL, creatinine = 0.9 mg/dL, alanine aminotransferase = 60 IU/L, aspartate aminotransferase = 55 IU/L, total bilirubin = 1.1 mg/dL, lipase = 850 U/L, and amylase = 350 U/L. Which one of the following is the most likely etiology for above clinical presentation?

(A) Typhlitis
(B) Peptic ulcer disease
(C) Choledocholithiasis
(D) Gallstone associated pancreatitis
(E) Peg-asparaginase associated pancreatitis

4. A 71-year-old woman was diagnosed with precursor B-cell acute lymphoblastic leukemia and the karyotype demonstrated t(9;22)(q34;q11), resulting in a BCR–ABL1 fusion gene. She underwent combination chemotherapy plus dasatinib as frontline therapy. Following completion of induction and consolidation treatment, no minimal residual disease was detected by multiparameter flow cytometry. She has no sibling, and no human leukocyte antigen-matched donor is available in the bone marrow registry. Which one of the following is the best next management strategy?

(A) Cord blood transplant
(B) Autologous stem cell transplant
(C) Continue dasatinib
(D) Start monthly vincristine, prednisone, 6-mercaptopurine, and methotrexate for 2 years
(E) No further treatment needed

5. A 32-year-old man with Ph– B-acute lymphoblastic leukemia received induction and consolidation with a multiagent chemotherapy regimen. He was started on maintenance with monthly vincristine, prednisone, 6-mercaptopurine (MP) and methotrexate (POMP) 3 months ago. The 6-MP dose was reduced by 75% due to persistent neutropenia. Which of the following enzyme deficiency best explains the need for dose reduction?

(A) Adenosine deaminase
(B) Thiopurine methyltransferase (TPMT)
(C) Inosine triphosphatase
(D) Xanthine oxidase

6. A 45-year-old woman with Ph+ acute lymphoblastic leukemia was treated with combination chemotherapy and imatinib. Subsequently, she underwent allogeneic stem cell transplant from a matched sibling donor. She relapsed 6 months after transplant. Analysis of the BCR–ABL1 fusion protein reveals an amino acid substitution at position 315 in BCR–ABL1, from a threonine (T) to an isoleucine (I). Which one of the following TKI is more likely to reinduce remission in this patient?

(A) Bosutinib
(B) Nilotinib
(C) Ponatinib
(D) Dasatinib
(E) Sorafenib

## REFERENCES

1. Cancer Facts & Figures 2014. *American Cancer Society.* http://www.cancer.org/acs/groups/content/research/documents/webcontent/acspc-042151.pdf. Accessed 2014.

2.  Pui CH, Raimondi SC, Borowitz MJ, et al. Immunophenotypes and karyotypes of leukemic cells in children with Down syndrome and acute lymphoblastic leukemia. *J Clin Oncol.* 1993;11(7):1361–1367.

3.  Ribera JM, Oriol A, González M, et al.; Programa Español de Tratamiento en Hematología; Grupo Español de Trasplante Hemopoyético Groups. Concurrent intensive chemotherapy and imatinib before and after stem cell transplantation in newly diagnosed Philadelphia chromosome-positive acute lymphoblastic leukemia. Final results of the CSTIBES02 trial. *Haematologica.* 2010;95(1):87–95.

4.  Harvey RC, Mullighan CG, Chen IM, et al. Rearrangement of CRLF2 is associated with mutation of JAK kinases, alteration of IKZF1, Hispanic/Latino ethnicity, and a poor outcome in pediatric B-progenitor acute lymphoblastic leukemia. *Blood.* 2010;115(26):5312–5321.

5.  van der Veer A, Waanders E, Pieters R, et al. Independent prognostic value of BCR-ABL1-like signature and IKZF1 deletion, but not high CRLF2 expression, in children with B-cell precursor ALL. *Blood.* 2013;122(15):2622–2629.

6.  Asnafi V, Buzyn A, Le Noir S, et al. NOTCH1/FBXW7 mutation identifies a large subgroup with favorable outcome in adult T-cell acute lymphoblastic leukemia (T-ALL): a Group for Research on Adult Acute Lymphoblastic Leukemia (GRAALL) study. *Blood.* 2009;113(17):3918–3924.

7.  Kantarjian HM, O'Brien S, Smith TL, et al. Results of treatment with hyper-CVAD, a dose-intensive regimen, in adult acute lymphocytic leukemia. *J Clin Oncol.* 2000;18(3):547–561.

8.  Larson RA, Dodge RK, Burns CP, et al. A five-drug remission induction regimen with intensive consolidation for adults with acute lymphoblastic leukemia: cancer and leukemia group B study 8811. *Blood.* 1995;85(8):2025–2037.

9.  Mani S, Ghalib M, Chaudhary I, Goel S. Alterations of chemotherapeutic pharmacokinetic profiles by drug-drug interactions. *Expert Opin Drug Metab Toxicol.* 2009;5(2):109–130.

10. Relling MV, Hancock ML, Boyett JM, et al. Prognostic importance of 6-mercaptopurine dose intensity in acute lymphoblastic leukemia. *Blood.* 1999;93(9):2817–2823.

11. Stock W, La M, Sanford B, et al.; Children's Cancer Group; Cancer and Leukemia Group B studies. What determines the outcomes for adolescents and young adults with acute lymphoblastic leukemia treated on cooperative group protocols? A comparison of Children's Cancer Group and Cancer and Leukemia Group B studies. *Blood.* 2008;112(5):1646–1654.

12. Ribera JM, Oriol A, Sanz MA, et al. Comparison of the results of the treatment of adolescents and young adults with standard-risk acute lymphoblastic leukemia with the Programa Español de Tratamiento en Hematología pediatric-based protocol ALL-96. *J Clin Oncol.* 2008;26(11):1843–1849.

13. Rytting ME. Role of L-asparaginase in acute lymphoblastic leukemia: focus on adult patients. *Blood Lymphat Cancer.* 2012;2:117–124.

14. Thomas DA, O'Brien S, Faderl S, et al. Chemoimmunotherapy with a modified hyper-CVAD and rituximab regimen improves outcome in de novo Philadelphia chromosome-negative precursor B-lineage acute lymphoblastic leukemia. *J Clin Oncol.* 2010;28(24):3880–3889.

15. Kantarjian H, Thomas D, Jorgensen J, et al. Results of inotuzumab ozogamicin, a CD22 monoclonal antibody, in refractory and relapsed acute lymphocytic leukemia. *Cancer.* 2013;119(15):2728–2736.

16. Topp MS, Gökbuget N, Zugmaier G, et al. Long-term follow-up of hematologic relapse-free survival in a phase 2 study of blinatumomab in patients with MRD in B-lineage ALL. *Blood.* 2012;120(26):5185–5187.

17. Gökbuget N, Kneba M, Raff T, et al.; German Multicenter Study Group for Adult Acute Lymphoblastic Leukemia. Adult patients with acute lymphoblastic leukemia and molecular failure display a poor prognosis and are candidates for stem cell transplantation and targeted therapies. *Blood.* 2012;120(9):1868–1876.

18. Neale GA, Coustan-Smith E, Stow P, et al. Comparative analysis of flow cytometry and polymerase chain reaction for the detection of minimal residual disease in childhood acute lymphoblastic leukemia. *Leukemia.* 2004;18(5):934–938.

19. Hahn T, Wall D, Camitta B, et al. The role of cytotoxic therapy with hematopoietic stem cell transplantation in the therapy of acute lymphoblastic leukemia in adults: an evidence-based review. *Biol Blood Marrow Transplant.* 2006;12(1):1–30.

20. Goldstone AH, Richards SM, Lazarus HM, et al. In adults with standard-risk acute lymphoblastic leukemia, the greatest benefit is achieved from a matched sibling allogeneic transplantation in first complete remission, and an autologous transplantation is less effective than conventional consolidation/maintenance chemotherapy in all patients: final results of the International ALL Trial (MRC UKALL XII/ECOG E2993). *Blood.* 2008;111(4):1827–1833.

21. Faderl S, Thomas DA, O'Brien S, et al. Augmented hyper-CVAD based on dose-intensified vincristine, dexamethasone, and asparaginase in adult acute lymphoblastic leukemia salvage therapy. *Clin Lymphoma Myeloma Leuk.* 2011;11(1):54–59.

22. Thomas DA, Kantarjian HM, Stock W, et al. Phase 1 multicenter study of vincristine sulfate liposomes injection and dexamethasone in adults with relapsed or refractory acute lymphoblastic leukemia. *Cancer.* 2009;115(23):5490–5498.

23. Ravandi F, O'Brien S, Thomas D, et al. First report of phase 2 study of dasatinib with hyper-CVAD for the frontline treatment of patients with Philadelphia chromosome-positive (Ph+) acute lymphoblastic leukemia. *Blood.* 2010;116(12):2070–2077.

24. Cortes JE, Kim DW, Pinilla-Ibarz J, et al.; PACE Investigators. A phase 2 trial of ponatinib in Philadelphia chromosome-positive leukemias. *N Engl J Med.* 2013;369(19):1783–1796.

25. Fielding AK, Rowe JM, Buck G, et al. UKALLXII/ECOG2993: addition of imatinib to a standard treatment regimen enhances long-term outcomes in Philadelphia positive acute lymphoblastic leukemia. *Blood.* 2014;123(6):843–850.

26. Jain P, Kantarjian H, Ravandi F, et al. The combination of hyper-CVAD plus nelarabine as frontline therapy in adult T-cell acute lymphoblastic leukemia and T-lymphoblastic lymphoma: MD Anderson Cancer Center experience. *Leukemia.* 2014;28(4):973–975.

# 29

# Acute Myelogenous Leukemia

KAVITHA BEEDUPALLI AND GUSTAVO RIVERO

## EPIDEMIOLOGY, RISK FACTORS, NATURAL HISTORY, AND PATHOLOGY

Acute leukemias are heterogeneous malignant disorders resulting from molecular and genetic alterations in normal hematopoietic stem cells. These changes limit normal differentiation and lead to proliferation of abnormal leukemic cells or blasts. Acute myelogenous leukemia (AML) is the most common acute leukemia, accounting for about 80% of acute leukemia in adults. Approximately 18,860 people will be diagnosed with AML in 2014, and around 10,460 will die of the disease (1). In general, the risk for developing AML increases with age with a 10-fold increase from age 30 years (1 case per 100,000) to 65 years (1 case per 10,000), and a median age at diagnosis of 65–70 years. A notable exception to this escalating incidence with age is a rare (600–800 cases/yr in the United States) subtype of AML called acute promyelocytic leukemia (APL) or M3 (see the following). APL is very uncommon in children, but its incidence increases steadily during the teen years, reaches a plateau during early adulthood, and remains constant until it increases after age 60 years. Higher incidence of APL has been reported in Latin America and northwestern Italy. Obesity might also be a risk factor for developing APL, but this has not been reported in other forms of AML. AML is slightly more common in males than females.

AML presents de novo or can develop following another disorder (secondary AML). AML can evolve from a variety of bone marrow disorders including myelodysplastic syndrome (MDS), aplastic anemia, and inherited bone marrow failure syndromes including Fanconi anemia, dyskeratosis congenita, Diamond–Blackfan anemia, and amegakaryocytic thrombocytopenia. Down syndrome and Bloom syndrome also predispose affected persons to develop AML. Exposure to benzene, pesticides, petroleum products, and radiation increases the risk of developing leukemia. Chemotherapeutic drugs, particularly alkylating agents and topoisomerase inhibitors, can increase the risk of developing AML later in life ("therapy-related AML"). Acute leukemia resulting from exposure to alkylating agents usually has a latency period of 7–10 years, and it is frequently associated with MDS, monosomies or deletion of 5q and/or 7q, and complex cytogenetics (2). AML following exposure to topoisomerase II inhibitors has a shorter latency period of 2–3 years, is not typically preceded by MDS, and usually shows monocytic differentiation with chromosomal translocations involving the MLL locus at 11q23. Outcomes for these patients are historically poor compared to de novo AML.

Patients with AML present with fever and symptoms related to bone marrow failure including fatigue, infection, bruising, and bleeding. Some patients present with pain related to rapidly expanding disease in the marrow whereas those with elevated circulating blast count can have central nervous system (CNS) symptoms, retinal hemorrhage, or cardiopulmonary complications due to leukostasis. Patients with monocytic AML subtypes can present with infiltration of the gingiva or other tissues (chloroma). Disseminated intravascular coagulation (DIC) with abnormal clotting or bleeding is a common presentation in patients with APL due to the release of procoagulants from the abnormal granules; DIC can also be seen in other forms of AML. Physical examination might reveal hepatosplenomegaly or lymphadenopathy.

In recent years, considerable progress has been made in deciphering the molecular, genetic, and epigenetic basis of AML and in defining new diagnostic and prognostic markers. De novo AML must be distinguished from acute lymphoblastic leukemia (ALL), MDS, or AML arising in the setting of MDS because therapeutic strategies and prognosis vary considerably for these diseases. AML can be distinguished from ALL by demonstrating definitive commitment to the myeloid lineage through judicious use of morphological (e.g., presence of Auer rods), immuno-histochemical, and immunological methods. Diagnosis of AML requires identification of 20% leukemic blasts in the blood or bone marrow with a notable exception for AML with the recurrent genetic abnormalities t(8;21), inv(16), or t(16;16), t(15;17), and some cases of erythroleukemia, which are treated as AML regardless of blast counts. In order to make a diagnosis of AML, at least 200 leuko-cytes on blood smears and 500 nucleated cells in mar-row smears should be counted, with the latter containing spicules. Myeloblasts, monoblasts, and megakaryoblasts are included in the blast count. In AML with monocytic or myelomonocytic differentiation, monoblasts, and promonocytes, but not abnormal monocytes, are counted as blast equivalents. Erythroblasts are not counted as blasts except in the rare instance of pure erythroid leuke-mia. Once a clinical diagnosis of AML is made, the mor-phological and genetic subtype must be identified. AML is a heterogeneous disease caused by a variety of pathogenic mechanisms. At a morphological level, this heterogeneity is manifested by variability in the degree of commitment and differentiation of the cell lineage. This variability has been used to define specific morphological subgroups.

Immunophenotyping by flow cytometry is used to determine lineage involvement of a newly diagnosed acute leukemia. Quantifying expression of several surface and cytoplasmic antigens is necessary for lineage assignment, to diagnose mixed phenotype acute leukemia (MPAL), and to detect aberrant immunophenotypes allowing for measurement of minimal residual disease (MRD). Flow cytometric determination of blast count should not be used as a substitute for morphological evaluation. Acute leukemias of ambiguous lineage are rare leukemias and comprise those cases that demonstrate no evidence of lin-eage differentiation (i.e., acute undifferentiated leukemia [AUL]) or those with blasts that express markers of >1 lin-eage (i.e., MPAL). AULs often express HLA-DR, CD34, and/or CD38, but lack lineage-associated markers.

Conventional cytogenetic analysis is a mandatory com-ponent in the diagnostic evaluation of a patient with sus-pected acute leukemia. Chromosome abnormalities are detected in approximately 55% of adult AML. A mini-mum of 20 metaphase cells analyzed from bone marrow is considered mandatory to establish the diagnosis of a normal karyotype, and recommended to define an abnor-mal karyotype. In 2008, the World Health Organization (WHO) revised the classification for AML to include addi-tional recurrent genetic abnormalities created by reciprocal translocations/inversions and some of the molecular mark-ers that have been found to have prognostic impact (Table 29.1) (3). Furthermore, novel therapies are being developed

**Table 29.1** AML and Related Precursor Neoplasms, and Acute Leukemia of Ambiguous Lineage

**AML and Related Neoplasms**

**AML with recurrent genetic abnormalities**
  AML with t(8;21)(q22;q22);RUNX1-RUNX1T1
  AML with inv(16)(p13.1q22) or t(16;16)(p13.1;q22);CBFC-MYH11
  APL with t(15;17)(q22;q12);PML-RARA
  AML with t(9;11)(p22;23);MLLT3-MLL
  *AML with t(6;9)(p23;q34);DEK-NUP214*
  *AML with inv(3)(q21q26.2)or t(3;3)(q21;q26.2);RPN1-EVI1*
  *AML (megakaryoblastic) with t(1;22)(p13;q13);RBM15-MKL1*
  *Provisional entity: AML with mutated NPM1*
  *Provisional entity: AML with mutated CEBPA*

**AML With Myelodysplasia Related Changes**
**Therapy-related myeloid neoplasms**
**AML, not otherwise specified**
  AML with minimal differentiation
  AML without maturation
  AML with maturation
  Acute myelomonocytic leukemia
  Acute monoblastic/monocytic leukemia
  Acute erythroid leukemia
  Pure erythroid leukemia
  Acute megakaryoblastic leukemia
  Acute basophilic leukemia
  Acute panmyelosis with myelofibrosis

**Myeloid sarcoma**
**Myeloid proliferations related to Down syndrome**
  Transient abnormal myelopoiesis
  Myeloid leukemia associated with Down syndrome
  Blastic plasmacytoid dendritic cell neoplasm

**Acute leukemia of ambiguous lineage**
  Acute undifferentiated leukemia
  Mixed phenotypic acute leukemia with t(9;22)(q34;q11.2); BCR-ABL1
  Mixed phenotype acute leukemia with t(11q23); MLL rearranged
  Mixed phenotype acute leukemia, B-myeloid, NOS
  Mixed phenotype acute leukemia, T-myeloid, NOS
  Provisional entity: natural killer (NK) cell lymphoblastic leukemia/lymphoma

AML, acute myelogenous leukemia; APL, acute promyelocytic leukemia; MLL, mixed-lineage leukemia gene; NOS, not otherwise specified. *Source*: Adapted from Ref. (3). Vardiman JW, Thiele J, Arber DA, et al. The 2008 revision of the World Health Organization (WHO) classification of myeloid neoplasms and acute leukemia: rationale and important changes. *Blood*. 2009;114(5):937–951.

that target some of the genetic lesions. At presentation with the suspected diagnosis of acute leukemia, a marrow speci-men should routinely be obtained for molecular diagnostics. However, if this results in a "dry tap," the peripheral blood may be obtained for cytogenetic and molecular diagnostics.

Unfavorable prognostic factors include white blood cell (WBC) count >20,000/μL, prior MDS, previous cytotoxic

**Table 29.2**  Standardized Reporting of Cytogenetics, Incidence, and Treatment Outcome in AML

| Genetic Group | Subsets | Incidence (%) | CR Rate (%) | 5-Yr Survival (%) |
|---|---|---|---|---|
| Favorable | | 20 | 85 | 60 |
| | t(15;17); PML-RARα | | | |
| | t(8;21)(q22;q22); *RUNX1-RUNX1T1* | | | |
| | inv(16)(p13.1q22) or t(16;16)(p13.1;q22); *CBFB-MYH11* | | | |
| | Normal karyotype with mutated *NPM1* without *FLT3*-ITD | | | |
| | Normal karyotype with mutated *CEBPA* | | | |
| Intermediate | | 45 | 76 | 38 |
| | Normal karyotype with mutated *NPM1* and *FLT3*-ITD | | | |
| | Normal karyotype with wild-type *NPM1* and *FLT3*-ITD | | | |
| | Normal karyotype with wild-type *NPM1* without *FLT3*-ITD | | | |
| | t(9;11)(p22;q23); *MLLT3-MLL* | | | |
| Adverse | | 30 | 55 | 12 |
| | Complex karyotype, −5 or del(5q); −7; abnormal(17p); | | | |
| | inv(3)(q21q26.2) or t(3;3)(q21;q26.2); *RPN1-EVI1* | | | |
| | t(6;9), t(v;11)(v;q23); *MLL* rearrangement | | | |

AML, acute myelogenous leukemia; CR, complete remission; FLT3-ITD, FMS-like tyrosine kinase 3 internal tandem duplication; MLL, mixed-lineage leukemia gene; NPM, nucleophosmin.

therapy, and certain specific cytogenetic and molecular genetic changes in the leukemic cells at diagnosis. The cytogenetics represent the strongest prognostic factor for response to induction therapy and for survival. Recurrent genetic abnormalities, such as t(8;21), inv(16) or t(16;16), t(15;17), generally carry a favorable prognosis and are more commonly seen in younger adult patients. Monosomy 5 or 7, chromosome 3 abnormalities such as inv 3(q21q26.2), 11q23 abnormalities other than t(9;11)(p22;q23), and complex karyotype, which occurs in 10–12% of patients, have consistently been associated with very poor outcomes. Complex karyotype has been defined as the presence of 3 or more chromosome abnormalities in the absence of t(8;21), inv(16) or t(16;16), or t(15;17). Complex karyotypes include a paucity of balanced rearrangements, and a predominance of chromosomal imbalances. Chromosomal losses most frequently affect 5q, 17p, and 7q, and gains affect 8q, 11q, and 21q. Normal cytogenetics, trisomy 8, and t(9;11)(p22;q23) indicate intermediate risk (Table 29.2).

Recent work by The Cancer Genomic Atlas (TCGA) underscores the impact of mutations in 8 functionally relevant gene categories on disease pathogenesis and prognosis (Figure 29.1). These mutations are especially useful for risk stratification within the large and heterogeneous group of patients with cytogenetically normal (CN) AML (4). In general, 2 classes of molecular mutations have been identified in AML. Class I mutations

activate signal-transduction pathways and increase proliferation and/or survival of progenitors. Mutations that activate the receptor tyrosine kinase FMS-like tyrosine kinase 3 *(FLT3)*, particularly the internal tandem duplication *(FLT3*-ITD) or *N-RAS* (neuroblastoma RAS viral oncogene homolog) are good examples. Class II mutations affect transcription factors or components of the transcriptional coactivation complex and cause impaired differentiation. Mutations of this type include those in the *C/EBPα* (CCAAT/enhancer-binding protein a) referred to as *CEBPA*, *MLL* (myeloid/lymphoid or mixed-lineage leukemia), and *NPM1* (nucleophosmin) genes. More recently, mutations in genes encoding tumor suppressor proteins that participate in regulation of gene expression, such as *TET2*, *DNMT3 A* and *B*, and *IDH 1* and *2* (Figure 29.2) have been identified in AML. One consequence of *TET2* mutation is inhibition of passive demethylation, which is required for gene expression. *TET2* facilitates *DNMT3A/B* exclusion by converting 5-MC to 5-HMC. Despite the fact that *TET2* and *IDH 1/2* mutations are mutually exclusive, *IDH 1* and *2* gain of function mutations result in accumulation of 2-hydroglutarate (2-HG), which impairs *TET2* biological function. Epigenetic (DNA and chromatin) modifications are generally reversible, thus providing the potential for pharmacological intervention in gene expression during differentiation, cell division, and DNA repair.

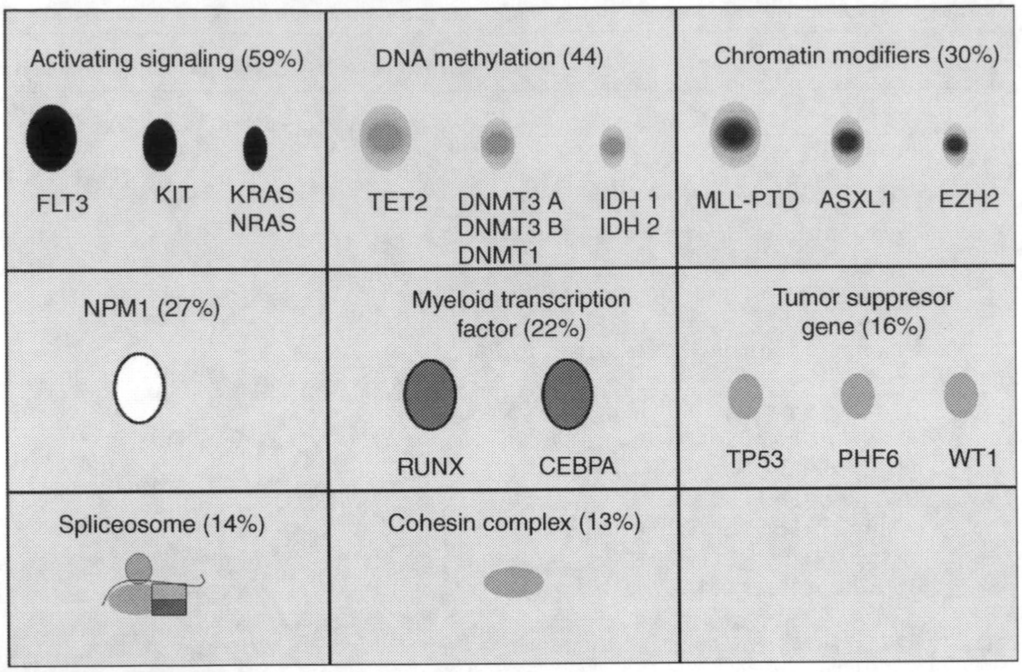

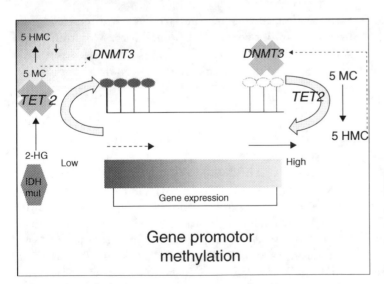

**Figure 29.1**

Representation of commonly mutated genes in AML. Epigenetic modifier mutations (*TET2, DNMT3 A/B, IDH1/2*) are actively investigated as potential disease initiating events. Activating signaling mutations provide proliferative advantage to leukemia clones. Myeloid specification genes, such as RUNX and CEBPA, are important participants in lineage specification, and once mutated, they can cooperate with leukemogenesis. AML, acute myelogenous leukemia.

**Figure 29.2**

Mechanism of promoter methylation induced by *TET2* mutation. Cells harboring *TET2* mutation would allow 5-MC to be readily available for DNMT3A/B enzymes. Incorporation of 5-MC into the gene promoter would facilitate methylation and repression of gene expression.

Prognostic significance within younger adults with CN-AML has consistently been shown for mutations in the *NPM1*, *CEBPA*, and *FLT3* genes. CN-AML patients harboring internal tandem duplication (ITD) of the *FLT3* gene have an inferior outcome. The *NPM1* mutation in CN-AML has been associated with higher complete remission (CR) rates and better relapse-free survival (RFS) and event-free survival especially if it occurs in the absence of *FLT3*-ITD. This observation also seems to hold among older patients. CN-AML with mutations in *CEBPA* is another AML subset associated with favorable prognosis (5) and survival, similar to AML patients with mutated NPM1 without *FLT3*-ITD. Although *FLT3* mutations are observed in APL and are associated with a higher WBC count at presentation, they do not add to the specific diagnosis of APL, influence management, or provide independent prognostic information. In the cytogenetically favorable core-binding factor (CBF) AMLs—that is, AML

**Table 29.3** Standardized Reporting of Correlation of Cytogenetic and Molecular Genetic Data in Acute Myeloid Leukemia With Clinical Data According to the ELN Guidelines

| ELN Genetic Risk Group | Subsets |
| --- | --- |
| Favorable | t(8;21)(q22;q22); RUNX1-RUNX1T1inv(16)(p13.1q22) or t(16;16)(p13.1;q22); CBFB-MYH11 |
| | Mutated NPM1 without FLT3-ITD (normal karyotype) |
| | Mutated CEBPα (normal karyotype) |
| Intermediate-I | Mutated NPM1 and FLT3-ITD (normal karyotype) |
| | Wild-type NPM1 and FLT3-ITD (normal karyotype) |
| | Wild-type NPM1 without FLT3-ITD (normal karyotype) |
| Intermediate-II | t(9;11)(p22;q23); MLLT3-MLL cytogenetic abnormalities not classified as favorable or adverse |
| Adverse | inv(3)(q21q26.2) or t(3;3)(q21;q26.2); RPN1-EVI1t(6;9)(p23;q34); DEK-NUP214t(v;11)(v;q23); MLL rearranged–5 or del(5q); –7; abnl(17p); complex karyotype |

CEBP, CCAAT enhancer-binding protein alpha; ELN, European Leukemia Network; FLT3-ITD, FMS-like tyrosine kinase-3-internal tandem duplication; MLL, mixed-lineage leukemia gene; NPM1, nucleophosmin 1.

with t(8;21) or inv(16)/t(16;16)—retrospective studies have demonstrated that several mutations in the *KIT* gene have an unfavorable influence on outcome (6). To date, the prognostic relevance of epigenetic modifier mutations in TET2 and IDH1/2 is not well established. However, data derived from a phase III AML trial including patients younger than 60 years demonstrated unfavorable overall survival (OS) impact in intermediate-risk patients independent of the FLT3 status (7,8). In the same study, high-dose daunorubicin (90 mg/m$^2$) significantly improved OS in patients with *DNMT3A* mutation compared to a standard dose of 45 mg/m$^2$. A growing list of genetic abnormalities in genes such as *WT1, RUNX1, MLL, KIT, RAS, TP53*, spliceosome, and cohesin complexes are being investigated for prognostic value in AML. Beyond mutational analysis, the impact of noncoding RNAs (ncRNA) on posttranscriptional gene regulation and distinctive epigenetic modification in gene expression are expected to facilitate risk stratification and provide potential therapeutic targets that could be evaluated in clinical trials.

Monitoring for MRD by reverse transcription-polymerase chain reaction (RT-PCR) detecting leukemia-specific targets or by flow cytometry identifying leukemia-associated aberrant phenotypes remains an active field of investigation. Except for APL, there is a paucity of prospective trial data regarding the timing, monitoring technique, and indications for MRD monitoring. Mutations in the *NPM1* gene are common (25–30%) in AML and likely provide one of the most promising new targets for MRD monitoring in AML. In a German–Austrian AML group study, *NPM1* mutation-based MRD monitoring during and after therapy revealed a subset of patients at high risk for relapse (9). However, the instability of *NPM1* mutations may result in false negatives. WT1 is a zinc finger transcription factor overexpressed at the mRNA level in 80–90% of AML cases at diagnosis. WT1 is detectable in the blood and bone marrow of normal donors. A promising observation that

poor leukemia-free survival is associated with higher transcript levels makes WT1 an attractive tool for postremission MRD monitoring (10,11).

AML with mutations in *NPM1* or *CEBPA* have been incorporated in the WHO classification as provisional entities in an effort to standardize the reporting system for molecular abnormalities. Screening for these 2 markers as well as for *FLT3* mutations should be done in clinical trials and is also recommended for patients undergoing intensive therapy for AML in routine practice. Table 29.2 provides a summary of cytogenetic features that are associated with a favorable, intermediate, or poor prognosis. Most recently, the European Leukemia Network (ELN) proposed a new classification integrating relevant molecular and cytogenetic predictors that result in improved risk stratification. The ELN classification incorporates 2 intermediate-risk subcategories (intermediate-I and intermediate-II) that are expected to enhance risk adaptive therapies (Table 29.3).

Response assessment is commonly performed between days 14 and 28 after the start of induction therapy. Definitions of response criteria are based primarily on those reported by Cheson et al. (12). A CR is defined as bone marrow blasts <5%; absence of blasts with Auer rods; absence of extramedullary disease; absolute neutrophil count >1.0 × 10$^9$/L (1000/μL); platelet count >100 × 10$^9$/L (100,000/μL), and independence from red cell transfusions. All criteria need to be fulfilled. Just as in initial diagnosis, marrow evaluation should be based on a count of 500 nucleated cells in an aspirate with spicules; if ambiguous, a repeat examination should be done in 5–7 days. A marrow biopsy should be performed in cases of dry tap, or if no spicules are obtained. No minimum duration of response is required. In cases with low blast percentages (5–10%), a repeat marrow should be performed to confirm relapse. Cytogenetics should be tested to distinguish true relapse from therapy-related MDS/AML.

## CASE SUMMARIES

### Management of APL

Y.A., a 28-year-old woman with no significant past medical history, was brought to the emergency department by her sister with reports of generalized weakness, excessive bruising, and continuous vaginal bleeding for 1 week. Her physical examination did not reveal lymphadenopathy or hepatosplenomegaly. She had ecchymoses on her thighs, arms, and upper torso that were not associated with trauma. There was oozing from IV line sites and some vaginal bleeding observed on a gynecological examination. A complete blood count (CBC) showed a WBC count of 1800/μL, hemoglobin level of 8.7 g/dL, and platelet count of 13,000/μL. Examination of the peripheral smear showed promyelocytes with a large nuclear:cytoplasmic ratio, prominent nucleoli, and several Auer rods. Coagulation parameters showed a prothrombin time (PT) of 18 s, partial thromboplastin time (PTT) of 38 s, and fibrinogen of 80 mg/dL.

### Evidence-Based Case Discussion

A presumptive diagnosis of APL should be made by review of the peripheral blood smear alone or with the bone marrow aspirate and core biopsy in the presence of the characteristic clinical findings. Immediate treatment must begin when the disease is suspected. As in the case of Y.A., the peripheral blood smear often shows leukopenia with circulating promyelocytes that usually have abundant, often irregular-appearing, primary azurophilic granules. Leukemic promyelocytes with multiple Auer rods may be found and are a distinctive feature of APL. Although often obscured by the granules, the nuclear contour is bilobed or reniform in appearance. The latter feature is important because patients with the microgranular variant (M3V) may not have easily visible granules, but have the same predisposition toward catastrophic bleeding and the same excellent outcome with appropriate treatment.

APL may be classified into 3 risk groups based on prognosis: (a) the low-risk group includes patients with WBC ≤10,000/μL and platelet count ≥40,000/μL with RFS of 98%; (b) the intermediate-risk group includes patients with WBC ≤10,000/μL and platelets ≤40,000/μL with RFS of about 90%; and (c) the high-risk group includes patients with WBC >10,000/μL and an RFS of 70%.

### Induction Therapy

Based on examination of the peripheral smear and laboratory parameters, APL was suspected and risk stratification placed Y.A. in the intermediate group. After a negative pregnancy test, Y.A. was started on all-*trans* retinoic acid (ATRA) and transfused with fresh frozen plasma, cryoprecipitate, and platelets. She was initiated on daunorubicin at 50 mg/m$^2$ for 4 days, 24 hours after ATRA initiation.

PCR for the *PML-RARα* transcript (performed on the peripheral blood) came back positive the following day. Subsequently, an analysis of the bone marrow aspirate and biopsy confirmed AML M3 (APL) and t(15;17).

The introduction of ATRA (tretinoin) and arsenic trioxide (ATO) into APL therapy has revolutionized the management and outcome of this disease. Treatment strategies using ATRA in combination with chemotherapy or ATO, have provided excellent results with survival rates exceeding 70%. Cure of patients with APL depends not only on the effective use of combination therapy, but also on supportive care measures that take into account the biology of the disease and the complications associated with molecularly targeted therapies. Once a diagnosis of APL is suspected, the disease should be managed as a medical emergency. Treatment with ATRA at 45 mg/m$^2$/d in divided doses should be initiated without waiting for genetic confirmation of the diagnosis, preferably the same day the diagnosis is suspected. ATRA is unlikely to have deleterious effects should genetic assessment fail to confirm the diagnosis of APL. Diagnosis should be further confirmed by molecular detection of *PML-RARα* fusion (or rare molecular variants). In addition to conventional karyotyping, fluorescent in-situ hybridization (FISH) and RT-PCR can be used for rapid diagnosis of APL. Intracranial and pulmonary hemorrhages are relatively common life-threatening complications of APL coagulopathy. Central venous catheterization, lumbar puncture, and other invasive procedures (e.g., bronchoscopy) should be avoided before and during induction therapy due to high risk of hemorrhagic complications, but patients with APL may also have a higher incidence of thrombosis. Aggressive supportive care should include liberal transfusion with fresh frozen plasma, cryoprecipitate, and platelet transfusions to maintain the fibrinogen concentration above 100–150 mg/dL, platelet count >30,000–50,000/μL and international normalized ratio (INR) <1.5. Heparin, tranexamic acid, and other anticoagulant or antifibrinolytic therapy should not be used routinely outside the context of a clinical trial.

For low- or intermediate-risk patients, initial induction with ATRA + ATO or ATRA + idarubicin alone or ATRA + daunorubicin with or without cytarabine is recommended. Choice of regimen is made based on risk stratification, age, and cardiovascular risk. Recently, APL 0406, an intergroup study conducted by Gruppo Italiano Malattie EMatologiche dell'Adulto (GIMEMA), showed that the combination of ATO + ATRA is noninferior to ATRA + chemotherapy with a 2-year event-free survival (EFS) of 97% in ATRA + ATO group versus 87.6% in ATRA + cytotoxic chemotherapy (13). Exclusion of anthracyclines may minimize the risk of long-term hematological malignancies in this group of patients. ATO regimens require monitoring of QTc interval with electrocardiogram and electrolytes. High-risk patients should begin chemotherapy without delay, *even if the molecular results are pending.* Leukapheresis should be avoided due to risk of precipitating fatal hemorrhage. Early institution of anthracycline-based chemotherapy (idarubicin or daunorubicin with or without cytarabine [Ara-C]) in combination with ATRA is the standard treatment approach in this life-threatening situation. Chemotherapy is generally started on day 1 within a few hours of the first dose of ATRA, aiming to control the coagulopathy and reduce the risk of APL differentiation syndrome (DS), formerly retinoic acid syndrome, which is particularly high in these patients. The role of cytarabine in combination with the anthracycline is a topic of debate. Patients who are not candidates for anthracycline may be treated upfront with a combination of ATRA and ATO.

APL DS, associated with the administration of ATRA or ATO, should be suspected clinically in the presence of dyspnea, unexplained fever, weight gain, peripheral edema, unexplained hypotension, acute renal failure, congestive heart failure, or a chest radiograph demonstrating pulmonary infiltrates, or pleural/pericardial effusion. Severe manifestations of the syndrome are characterized by systemic inflammatory response syndrome, disseminated endothelial damage, and capillary leak. ATRA induces upregulation of adhesion molecules that promote aggregation of promyelocytes and enhanced tissue trafficking. Prophylactic corticosteroids should be strongly considered at a dose of 10 mg IV twice daily and should be started in patients with WBC count >10,000/ μL or at the earliest symptoms or signs to prevent DS. However, recent recommendations from the Program Espanol de Tratamiento en Hematologia (PETHEMA) propose prophylactic dexamethasone initiation in patients with WBC >5000 × 10⁹/L or early evidence of renal impairment (creatinine >1.4 mg/dL). This intervention resulted in an overall DS-associated mortality of 1.0%. Discontinuation of ATRA or ATO is indicated in severe APL DS (i.e., patients developing renal failure or requiring admission to the ICU due to respiratory distress). If a favorable response is obtained, dexamethasone should be maintained until complete disappearance of symptoms, and then ATRA or ATO should be resumed.

Virtually all *PML-RARα*-positive APLs are sensitive to ATRA and anthracycline-based chemotherapy or to the combination of ATRA + ATO leading to CR in 90–95% of patients with excellent long-term outcomes. Inclusion of cytarabine is somewhat more controversial, but data from the European Group suggest that there may be a benefit of adding standard-dose cytarabine both during induction and consolidation. So long as the patient is tolerating therapy, ATRA is continued until CR is achieved (PCR negative for *PML-RARα* in the peripheral blood and bone marrow). No therapeutic modifications should be made on the basis of incomplete blast maturation (differentiation) detected up to 50 days or more after the start of treatment by morphology, cytogenetics, or molecular assessment.

Y.A. achieved complete hematological and morphological remission based on a bone marrow examination

performed 4 weeks after treatment with ATRA and idarubicin. An important aspect of bone marrow assessment after induction is that it should not be done too early as the terminal differentiation of blasts may be delayed. Molecular remission need not be achieved at the end of induction and no change in therapy course should be made if PCR testing for PML-RARα is still positive at this stage.

Y.A. experienced no major complications during induction therapy. She used contraception throughout the duration of her treatment. Acute leukemia during pregnancy is a special challenge that should be managed jointly by the hematologist, obstetrician, and neonatologist in a tertiary care center. In a pregnant woman with APL, treatment should be started immediately because delays may compromise maternal outcome. The risk of teratogenicity is highest in the first trimester, therefore, the crucial decision during this period is whether to continue with the pregnancy and receive chemotherapy or commit to terminate the pregnancy. Daunorubicin is the preferred anthracycline in pregnancy as idarubicin has a higher DNA affinity and is more lipophilic favoring an increased placental transfer. Chemotherapy delivered during the second and third trimester of pregnancy is safer for the fetus; however, delivery while the patient and fetus are cytopenic should be avoided. In APL, administration of ATRA is controversial in the second and third trimesters and should not be used in the first. ATO cannot be used in any stage of pregnancy.

## Consolidation Therapy

Consolidation strategies depend on the risk classification for relapse at diagnosis and the initial induction regimen. However, this is still an area of controversy and data continue to evolve on how to use the risk strata to help tailor consolidation. Three cycles of anthracycline-based chemotherapy are administered for low- and intermediate-risk patients in first CR (CR1). Many consolidation regimens incorporate ATRA in combination with chemotherapy or ATO whereas a few regimens do not incorporate ATRA. Although there is no consensus, there may be a benefit of adding cytarabine to the anthracycline in patients <60 years old who are in the high-risk group. Molecular remission should be assessed at the end of consolidation therapy.

Y.A. received consolidation therapy with first cycle of ATRA and idarubicin followed by ATRA with mitoxantrone and a third cycle of ATRA and idarubicin. At the end of consolidation therapy, she attained a molecular remission.

## Maintenance Therapy

Following consolidation, the decision for maintenance therapy is tailored based on individual patient disease characteristics. Despite historical recommendation that maintenance therapy might reduce relapse rates (14), previous maintenance study by GIMEMA group found no difference in relapses among maintenance arms. This highlights the fact that consideration for maintenance should include a careful evaluation of initial disease risk (low vs. intermediate vs. high risk); type, intensity, and duration of previous induction/consolidation; and MRD status given by $PMR\text{-}RAR\alpha$ positivity. For low- and intermediate-risk patients who are MRD negative after intensive induction/consolidation with chemotherapy and ATO, the long-term benefit appeared less important pointing to a need for individualized patient risk assessment. In high-risk patients, 1–2 years of consolidation with daily 6-mercaptopurine (6MP) and weekly methotrexate (with careful monitoring of cytopenias) given with a 2-week course of ATRA every 3 months is recommended. PCR monitoring should be performed every 3 months. Early treatment intervention in patients with evidence of MRD affords a better outcome than treatment in full-blown relapse. MRD monitoring of bone marrow or blood by PCR for $PML\text{-}RAR\alpha$ every 3 months should be offered to all patients for up to 3 years after completion of consolidation therapy. For patients testing PCR-positive at any stage after completion of consolidation, a bone marrow is repeated for MRD assessment within 2–4 weeks and samples are sent for confirmation. For patients with confirmed molecular relapse (defined as 2 successive PCR-positive assays with stable or rising $PML\text{-}RAR\alpha$ transcript levels), preemptive therapy should be started promptly to prevent frank relapse. Although ATRA in combination with chemotherapy can be used as salvage therapy, ATO-based regimens are presently regarded as the first option for treatment of relapsed APL. The role of ATO in patients who relapse following ATO containing induction and/or consolidation regimens remains unknown. Autologous hematopoietic stem cell transplant (HSCT) is considered the best option for patients without detectable MRD in the marrow (in second CR) and with an adequate PCR-negative harvest. Allogeneic HSCT is recommended for patients failing to achieve a second molecular remission. For patients in whom HSCT is not feasible, the available options include repeated cycles of ATO with or without ATRA and with or without chemotherapy. The CNS is the most common site of extramedullary disease in APL and at least 10% of hematological relapses are accompanied by CNS involvement. Because the majority of CNS relapses occur in patients presenting with hyperleukocytosis, some strategies include CNS prophylaxis for patients in this particular high-risk setting after the achievement of CR (lumbar puncture at presentation and during induction is extremely hazardous). Y.A. finished her consolidation therapy as outlined above. She declined maintenance therapy, but has continued PCR testing and has remained disease free for 3 years postconsolidation treatment.

## AML in Younger Adults (18–60 Years Old) With Favorable Risk Factors

A.M., a 48-year-old man with a history of hypertension, presented to his primary physician with a 1-month history of generalized weakness, fatigue, easy bruising, and intermittent epistaxis. He also reported a 1-week history of exertional dyspnea and chest pain. Physical examination revealed pallor with no hepatosplenomegaly or lymphadenopathy. There was no evidence of bruising, but some petechiae were visible on his lower extremities. WBC count was 46,000/μL with a hemoglobin level of 6.8 g/dL and a platelet count of 18,000/μL. A peripheral blood smear showed a large number of monocytoid appearing blasts and an increased number of eosinophils. A bone marrow aspirate and biopsy confirmed AML with cytogenetic showing inv(16). A baseline EKG and chest x-ray were normal. He was transfused with packed red cells for symptomatic anemia and aggressively hydrated in preparation for treatment. An echocardiogram demonstrated a normal ejection fraction (EF) with no wall motion abnormalities.

### Evidence-Based Case Discussion

Supportive care is an important part of induction therapy, including tumor lysis prophylaxis and management of hyperleukocytosis. A.M. has a WBC count <50,000/μL with no symptoms of hyperleukocytosis. Patients presenting with a WBC count of >100,000/μL have increased induction mortality mainly due to hemorrhagic events, tumor lysis syndrome, and end-organ damage caused by leukostasis. Increased blood viscosity due to hyperleukocytosis and leukostasis can lead to respiratory distress from sludging in the pulmonary circulation or lead to retinal or cerebral hemorrhages that require immediate medical attention. This is considered a medical emergency. Measures to rapidly reduce the white count to <50,000/ μL include leukapheresis or initiation of hydroxyurea. Leukapheresis has been shown to reduce blast counts quickly and may improve early outcomes of induction therapy in AML; however, it has not been clearly shown to improve survival. There are no randomized trials comparing use of hydroxyurea alone versus the combination of hydroxyurea and leukapheresis in patients presenting with elevated white counts. Excessive red blood cell (RBC) transfusions can lead to increased blood viscosity when white cell counts are elevated and should be avoided.

### Induction Therapy

A.M. was started on allopurinol for tumor lysis prophylaxis and hydroxyurea for 2 days to reduce his WBC count while waiting to obtain bone marrow biopsy results, cardiac workup, and central line placement. Induction therapy was begun with 3 days of an anthracycline (e.g., daunorubicin, at least 60 mg/m²;

idarubicin, 10–12 mg/m²; or mitoxantrone, 10–12 mg/m²) and 7 days of cytarabine (100–200 mg/m² continuous IV infusion). This regimen, commonly known as "3 + 7," remains the standard for induction therapy in AML. With such regimens, CR is achieved in 70–80% of younger adults. No other intervention has been shown to be superior. However, in a phase III Eastern Cooperative Oncology Group (ECOG) study of young adults with AML, induction therapy with daunorubicin dose escalation at 90 mg/m² for 3 days improved the rate of CR and the duration of remission duration as compared with the standard dose of 45 mg/m² (15). Induction chemotherapy should be started only after the diagnostic workup has been completed, preferably within 5 days of diagnosis. Randomized studies comparing high-dose versus low-dose cytarabine have demonstrated higher toxicity with higher doses, but no improvement in remission rates or disease-free survival (DFS). Thus, higher doses of cytarabine are not recommended outside of clinical trials. Attempts to increase response rates by the use of additional cytotoxic agents (thioguanine, etoposide, fludarabine, and topotecan) or modulators of multidrug resistance (MDR) in general have failed (16,17), and variable results have been obtained when attempting to sensitize leukemic cells with hematopoietic growth factors.

## Consolidation Therapy

Various consolidation strategies have been evaluated including intensive conventional chemotherapy, and high-dose therapy followed by autologous or allogeneic HSCT. Patients with CBF AMLs (expressing the cytogenetic abnormalities t[8;21], inv[16], or t[16;16]) have a relatively good prognosis when consolidated with high-dose cytarabine without HSCT in first remission. A landmark study performed by Cancer and Leukemia Group B (CALGB) showed that 4 cycles of high-dose cytarabine (3 g/m² per q12h on days 1, 3, and 5) are superior to 4 courses of intermediate-dose (400 mg/m² continuous IV on days 1–5) or standard-dose (100 mg/m² continuous IV on days 1–5) cytarabine. The beneficial effect of cytarabine dose intensification was restricted to patients with good-risk AML and, to a lesser extent, to patients with CN-AML. The outcome of patients with other cytogenetic abnormalities was not affected by cytarabine dose.

Allogeneic HSCT as a postremission strategy is associated with the lowest rates of relapse. This benefit is attributable to both the high-dose therapy of standard conditioning regimens and potent graft versus leukemia (GVL) effect. However, benefits of allogeneic HSCT have been limited by the high treatment-related mortality (TRM). Single-arm prospective trials have not shown a definitive survival advantage for allogeneic HSCT in patients with AML in first CR (CR1). A meta-analysis of clinical trials that prospectively assigned patients to allogeneic HSCT versus alternative consolidation therapies for AML in CR1 on an intent-to-treat donor versus no-donor basis showed that allogeneic HSCT

offers significant OS benefit for patients with intermediate- and high-risk AML. For individual patients, disease risk as assessed by the cytogenetic and molecular profile of the leukemia and the risks associated with the transplant itself including comorbidities and other transplant-related risk indices must be weighed. In patients with favorable risk AML (Table 29.2) consolidation therapy with repetitive cycles of high dose Ara-C (HiDAC; 3 g/m² per q12h on days 1, 3, and 5) is considered a reasonable choice for younger adults especially those with CBF AML and for AML with mutated NPM1 and wild-type FLT3 or with mutated CEBPA. For CBF AML, retrospective studies by CALGB suggest that 3 or more cycles of high-dose cytarabine (cumulative dose: 54–72 g/m²) are superior to 1 cycle (18 g/m²). No advantage has been shown for autologous or allogeneic HSCT for CBF AML in CR1. Nonetheless, there are subsets of patients with CBF AML who do not fare well (e.g., t[8;21] with high WBCs, CBF AML with KIT mutations, or molecular disease persistence); allogeneic HSCT may be considered in these patients, especially for those with a low transplant risk.

A.M. achieved a CR with induction chemotherapy consisting of idarubicin, 12 mg/m², and 7 days of cytarabine (100 mg/m² continuous IV). He had a complicated course with prolonged cytopenias requiring frequent transfusion. He developed transfusion-related acute lung injury (TRALI) and acute coronary syndrome that were medically managed. Subsequently, a bone marrow aspiration and biopsy showed that he was in cytogenetic and morphological remission. A cardiac evaluation was repeated to ensure his EF was still normal and his cardiac status was optimized. Based on his favorable risk AML, induction was followed by 4 courses of consolidation with HiDAC (high-dose cytarabine at dose 3 g/m² q12h on days 1, 3, and 5). He has remained disease free for 3 years.

## AML in Younger Adults (18–60 Years) With Unfavorable Risk Factors

T.R., a 57-year-old businessman with a history of hypercholesterolemia and hypertension, was brought to the hospital with an acute febrile illness and lethargy. On examination, he was found to have mild hepatosplenomegaly with no lymphadenopathy. Oral examination was significant for gingival hyperplasia and gum bleeding. Labs demonstrated a WBC of 60,000/μL with >50% blasts, a hemoglobin level of 9 g/dL, and a platelet count of 44,000/μL. A bone marrow biopsy confirmed AML and cytogenetic evaluation showed the following: 46XY, –7, +8, 21q-, and 11q- in all 20 of the analyzed cells.

## Evidence-Based Case Discussion

### Induction Therapy

T.R.'s AML displayed complex cytogenetics defined as >3 cytogenetic abnormalities in the absence of CBF mutations falls into the high-risk category with a poor prognosis. In choosing an induction strategy, several issues need to be considered including comorbid illnesses, performance status, ability to tolerate induction therapy, and existence of antecedent hematological disease. The standard induction regimen has continued to be 3 days of anthracycline with 7 days of infusional cytarabine commonly referred to as "3 + 7" (Figure 29.2). Moreover, there does not seem to be a clear benefit of adding additional chemotherapy agents such as etoposide to this regimen. Although a clear benefit of high-dose cytarabine in this high-risk population has not been established, multiple guidelines list HiDAC induction as an option. Patients who fall into the WHO adverse risk category typically have poor outcome with standard induction and consolidation. Hence, a clinical trial is also always appropriate in this setting. In the case of antecedent hematological disease or treatment-related AML, there is accumulating evidence that induction therapy with an allogeneic HSCT is an attractive option for poor-risk patients with a donor. For those with no donor, either a clinical trial may be offered or standard chemotherapy regimens may be given.

At the end of induction therapy, risk stratification is once again performed by obtaining a bone marrow biopsy. Unlike APL where bone marrow biopsy assessment is not recommended until count recovery, it is reasonable to perform a bone marrow assessment 7–14 days after induction is completed. At this juncture if the bone marrow is hypoplastic, it is recommended that bone marrow be reassessed at count recovery. If the bone marrow examination shows significant reduction in blasts, consolidation can be pursued or delayed until count recovery has occurred. If there is significant residual disease, reinduction would be a reasonable course of action.

The most challenging patients are those with refractory disease. Several studies have shown that lack of early blast clearance or no response to the first induction cycle are major predictors of poor outcome, and conventional chemotherapy offers almost no chance of cure for these patients. In these patients, the only chance of cure is allogeneic HSCT with a dismal success rate of about 10%. Clinical trials should be considered for all patients with primary refractory disease. In patients with relapsed disease, that is, patients who achieved a CR with initial induction therapy, the rate of response will depend on duration of CR. Patients with a relapse of >12 months in CR have about a 50% chance of responding to cytarabine containing induction regimens. This should be followed with allogeneic HSCT. Patients with shorter duration of CR will not fare as well and are best treated in clinical trials.

## Consolidation Therapy

Initial risk stratification can be useful in guiding consolidation therapy (Figure 29.2). For patients with intermediate- or poor-risk cytogenetics, a beneficial effect of allogeneic HSCT as consolidation therapy has been shown in CR1. This includes patients with unfavorable cytogenetics as well as CN-AML and unfavorable molecular markers, that is, those who lack the favorable genotypes of mutated NPM1 without FLT3-ITD mutation and biallelic CEBPA mutation. In particular, allogeneic HSCT should be considered in patients whose leukemic cells have FLT3-ITD. An allogeneic HSCT from a matched related donor is currently considered the treatment of choice for patients with unfavorable cytogenetics in CR1. The outcome after allogeneic HSCT from fully matched and unrelated donor appears to be similar when compared to allogeneic HSCT from matched related donors. The Center for International Blood and Marrow Transplant Research (CIBMTR) reported a long-term survival probability of 30% for AML patients with adverse cytogenetics transplanted in CR1 from matched unrelated donors.

In general, there is no indication for intrathecal prophylaxis in AML patients without CNS symptoms although it may be considered in special situations (e.g., hyperleukocytosis). In patients with CNS involvement, intrathecal chemotherapy with cytarabine, liposomal cytarabine, or methotrexate should be administered. Intrathecal therapy is administered twice a week until 2 consecutive negative CSF cytologies are obtained and then weekly for 4–6 weeks. Liposomal cytarabine is typically administered every 2 weeks. Longer duration of intrathecal treatment (particularly >6 months) can cause CNS complications with no benefit and is discouraged. For prevention of arachnoiditis, oral dexamethasone (4-mg TID) may be considered on the days of intrathecal treatment. In patients with a CNS recurrence, craniospinal irradiation has also been shown to be effective; however, its impact on long-term outcome is unknown.

T.R. had 7 siblings and a younger brother was an HLA identical match. After 3 + 7 standard induction, he attained a CR. Within 1 month, he proceeded to allogeneic stem cell transplant. Unfortunately, he had a prolonged period of neutropenia during which he developed a perirectal abscess and he succumbed to gram-negative sepsis despite antibiotic therapy.

## AML in the Older Adult (Age >60 Years)

H.T., a 72-year-old man with excellent performance status and hypertension, presented to the emergency department with fatigue. His physical examination revealed pallor and petechiae on his lower extremities. He had no hepatosplenomegaly, no lymphadenopathy, and no other evidence of bleeding. Routine labs showed a WBC count of 500/µL, a hemoglobin level of 6 g/dL, and a platelet count of 9,000/µL. Consultation with his primary physician revealed that his blood counts had been normal 2 months earlier. A peripheral smear showed normal red cell morphology, rare platelets, decreased WBC count, and a few circulating blasts with high nuclear:cytoplasmic ratio and several nucleoli. No Auer rods were observed in the blasts. The patient was admitted to the hospital and a platelet transfusion was begun followed by packed red cells. A bone marrow aspirate and biopsy was consistent with acute leukemia with 60% cellularity. The blasts constituted 50% of the bone marrow, and flow cytometry showed that they were positive for CD34, CD117, CD13, and CD33 consistent with myeloid blasts. Marrow cytogenetics was normal. FLT3-ITD was negative and NPM mutation was positive. Cardiac evaluation showed a normal ejection fraction.

## Evidence-Based Case Discussion

### Induction Therapy

Patients older than 60 years with AML form a distinct subgroup, and "AML in the older adult" is an active area of research. Adults older than 70 years tend to have increased comorbidities and less tolerance to therapy. These older patients have a worse prognosis that is thought to be due to biological differences including an increased frequency of secondary AML that is more resistant to therapy, adverse cytogenetic features, and overexpression of multidrug-resistant phenotypes. The decision to treat with intensive induction regimens versus less intensive treatments or supportive care alone needs to be individualized. Advanced age alone should not prohibit induction therapy. Recent studies have shown that older patients with good performance status can tolerate induction therapy reasonably well, and treatment with higher doses of daunorubicin at 90 mg/m² had a better outcome than a reduced dose of anthracycline at 45 mg/m². On the other hand, investigators at MD Anderson Cancer Center published data showing that the majority of patients older than 70 years at their institution did not benefit from intensive chemotherapy (18). A multivariate analysis of >900 elderly AML patients established that karyotype, age, NPM1 mutation status, WBC count, lactate dehydrogenase (LDH), and CD34 expression were independent predictors of prognosis. Patients were scored based on these variables and grouped into 4 prognostic risk groups: (a) favorable, (b) good intermediate risk, (c) adverse intermediate risk, and (d) high risk, and the corresponding 3-year OS rates were 39.5%, 30%, 10.6%, and 3.3% (19). Hence, induction regimens must be chosen keeping the patient's performance status and comorbidities in mind as well as the overall prognosis. In summary, the decision to give standard induction regimen has to be individualized. In fit patients with a favorable risk profile there is no benefit to reducing the dose of daunorubicin. Given his good performance status and relative lack of comorbidities, T.R. elected treatment with a standard induction regimen containing daunorubicin and cytarabine.

For patients with disease refractory to induction therapy, but suitable for intense intervention including reduced intensity conditioning and allogeneic transplantation, achievement of CR is critical. Several chemotherapy protocols are available as depicted in Table 29.4. Clinical trials should be considered for all patients with primary refractory disease. Concurrent with treatment, an evaluation for a suitable transplant donor should be performed.

Treatment strategies for fit elderly patients with high-risk AML, defined as evidence of complex cytogenetics, secondary AML and evidence of FLT3 mutation without availability of compatible donor is undefined and an area of active research. An ECOG-led phase III trial comparing induction therapy with single-agent clofarabine versus standard induction with cytarabine plus daunorubicin in patients older than 60 years followed by consolidation with either clofarabine or cytarabine is underway. Several agents, such as newer generation nucleoside analogs, liposomal

**Table 29.4** Chemotherapy Regimens Commonly Used in Primary Refractory/Relapsed AML

| Agents | Study Population | Outcome | Reference |
|---|---|---|---|
| Cladrabine + Cytarabine (Ara-C) + Mitoxantrone and G-CSF (CLAG-M) | "Polish initiative" Median age = 45 yr Relapse-refractory | CR = 58% | Wierzbowska et al., 2008 |
| Mitoxantrone + Etoposide + Ara-C (MEC) | Median age = 52 yr Relapse-refractory | CR = 59% | Trifilo et al., 2012 |
| Fludarabine + Ara-C + G-CSF and Idarubicin (FLAG-IDA) | Median age = 42 yr Relapse-refractory | CR = 51% | Pastore et al., 2003 |
| Clofarabine + Ara-C | Median age = 67 yr Relapse-refractory | CR= 32.5% TRM = 15% | Faderl et al., 2012 |
| Sorafenib | Phase II | CR/CRi[a] | Ravandi et al., 2010 |

CR, complete remission; CRi, complete remission with incomplete count recovery; G-CSF, granulocyte-colony stimulating factor; TRM, treatment-related mortality.
[a] Remission outcome improved when combined with induction chemotherapy.

**Table 29.5** Novel Therapeutic Agents in the Treatment of AML

| Agent | Mechanistic Target | Type of Study | Type of Response | Reference |
|---|---|---|---|---|
| Elacytabine | Nucleoside analog | Phase II | CR/CRi = 45% when combined with idarubicin | O Brien et al., 2012 |
| Flavopiridol | Inhibition of multiple serine-threonine kinases | Phase II Randomized FLAM vs. 7 + 3 | CR; FLAM vs. 7 + 3 68% vs. 48 % | Karp et al., 2010 |
| CPX351 | Liposomal cytarabine and daunorubicine | Phase II Randomized CPX351 vs. 7 + 3 | CR + CRi; CPX351 vs. 7 + 3 Patients >60 yrs = 57.6% vs. 31.6% | Lancet et al., ASH 2012 |
| Sapacitabine | Cytosine nucleoside analog | Phase II | ORR = 45% in patients >70 yr old | Kantarjian et al., 2012 |

AML, acute myelogenous leukemia; CR, complete remission; CRi, complete remission with incomplete count recovery; FLAM, flavopiridol, Ara-C, and mitoxantrone; ORR, overall response rate.

anthracycline, and cytarabine formulations have shown promising results (Table 29.5). For patients who may not tolerate standard induction, low-intensity therapy with a hypomethylating agent such as azacytidine (5-AC) or decitabine (DAC) or low-dose cytarabine is also an option. In elderly patients with low-marrow blast count (20–30%), azacitidine significantly prolongs OS and improves quality of life compared with conventional care regimens (20). Other agents such as single-agent clofarabine have also been used in this group with modest results.

## Consolidation Therapy

Postremission therapy in older adults is also a topic of debate. The tolerability of high-dose cytarabine is poor, and CBF mutations, which traditionally are thought to have higher response rates with HIDAC, are less common in older adults. Postremission therapy with agents such as gemtuzumab has not been shown to be effective in a randomized phase III trial (21). Some studies have examined allogeneic HSCT with reduced intensity conditioning with varying response. These data point to the heterogeneity of the disease and the patient population and highlight again that age alone should not preclude consideration of HSCT. There is a paucity of randomized clinical trials addressing the question of HSCT in the older adult.

T.R. went into remission after receiving standard 3 + 7 induction with idarubicin and cytarabine therapy. Other options included low-intensity therapy with agents such as azacytidine. However, given his good performance status and his personal preference, he was induced with standard induction therapy that he tolerated well. For consolidation therapy, he was given the option of 2 + 5 or reduced intensity conditioning and allogeneic transplant. Molecular studies revealed the leukemia to be *NPM1* positive and *FLT3*-ITD negative, which placed him in a relatively favorable risk group and he was not referred for transplant. He received 2 cycles of consolidation therapy with 2 + 5 (idarubicin at 12 mg/m² × 2 days and cytarabine at

100 mg/m² × 5 days). Both cycles were complicated by neutropenic fever and requirement for multiple transfusions of blood products. After the second cycle, the patient declined further chemotherapy. He relapsed 6 months after completing therapy. At that point, his performance status had declined considerably and he opted for supportive care alone with transfusion support. He succumbed to his disease 10 months after initial diagnosis.

## REVIEW QUESTIONS

1. A 75-year-old man presented to emergency department complaining of shortness of breath and fatigue. He has a history of congestive heart failure with an ejection fraction (EF) of 30%, osteoarthritis, and dyslipidemia. His complete blood cell count revealed a white blood cell count of 30,000 /μL, hemoglobin level of 9 g/dL, and platelet count of 75,000/μL. A review of his peripheral blood showed about 30% peripheral blasts. Bone marrow aspirate and flow cytometry confirmed the diagnosis of acute myelogenous leukemia. Standard G-band karyotyping revealed 45XY, –5, –7, and +8 in 14 of 20 metaphases analyzed. His performance status is 2.

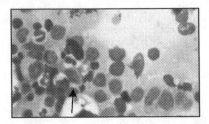

Bone marrow aspirate. Leukemia cells are noted (arrows) (hematoxylin and eosin stain, original magnification ×100).

Which of the following treatment options would most favorably impact his outcome?

(A) Decitabine
(B) Standard-dose daunorubicin plus cytarabine (3 + 7)

(C) Escalated-dose daunorubicin plus cytarabine

(D) Low-dose cytarabine

2. A 52-year-old woman presents to the emergency department with fatigue and easy bruising. Laboratory data revealed a leukocyte count of 50,000/µL, and a platelet count of 20,000/µL. Bone marrow aspirate showed a monocytic blast-like population staining positive for CD13, CD33, CD34, and CD117 (see figure [*arrow*]). Fluorescent in-situ hybridization analysis showed a fusion signal of *CBFB* and *MYH11* in 89 of 200 nuclei. Next-generation sequencing of DNA extracted from bone marrow cells identifies a *KIT* D816V mutation.

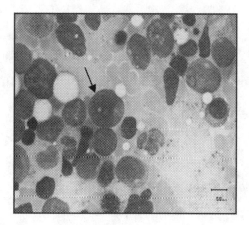

Bone marrow aspirate. Leukemia cells are noted (*arrows;* hematoxylin and eosin stain, original magnification ×100).

What would be the best consolidation strategy based on the mutational analysis provided?

(A) Standard induction with 7 + 3 followed by high-dose Ara-C consolidation

(B) Escalated-dose danorubicin + cytarabine

(C) Use of C-KIT inhibitor kinase inhibitor

(D) Standard induction/consolidation followed by allogeneic stem cell transplant

3. A 63-year-old man diagnosed with *FLT3-ITD* mutated, *NPM1* wild-type acute myelogenous leukemia achieved complete remission (CR) following 1 cycle of standard induction therapy (cytarabine plus daunorubicin). Four cycles of high-dose Ara-cytarabine (HiDAC) were administered under close medical monitoring. Two months after completion of his fourth cycle of HiDAC, a bone marrow biopsy shows 25% myeloblasts. His performance status is 0. Echocardiography is within normal limits. What treatment option would most likely be associated with more durable second remission in this patient?

(A) Reinduction with escalated-dose daunorubicin plus cytarabine followed by allogeneic stem cell transplantation

(B) Decitabine at 20 mg/m² for 4 cycles followed by allogeneic stem cell transplantation

(C) Clofarabine single agent at 40 mg/m² for 4 cycles followed by allogeneic stem cell transplantation

(D) Clofarabine plus cytarabine-containing regimen followed by allogeneic stem cell transplantation

4. A 25-year-old obese woman presents with 2 weeks of dyspnea and fatigability. Laboratory evaluation shows white blood cell count of 9,800/µL, hemoglobin level of 8.5 g/dL, and a platelet count of 70,000/µL. Flow cytometry showed myeloblasts positive for CD13, CD33, and CD117. Blasts were negative for CD34 and HLA-DR.

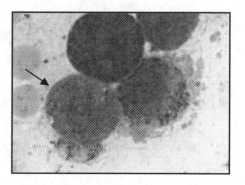

Which of the following induction regimens would yield the most favorable outcome in this patient?

(A) Arsenic trioxide (ATO) plus All-*trans* retinoic acid (ATRA)

(B) Cytarabine plus daunorubicin at 90 mg/m²

(C) Cytarabine plus daunorubicin at 45 mg/m²

(D) ATRA in combination with daunorubicin at 45 mg/m²

5. A 55-year-old woman presents to the ear–nose–throat clinic with decreased hearing and progressive nasal congestion. Sinonasal endoscopy shows mass prompting biopsy with immunostain analysis revealing tumor cells positive for CD117, CD34, myeloperoxidase and CD43; CD20, CD3, CD5, CD10, and CD23 were all negative. A diagnosis of granulocytic sarcoma was made. Complete blood count showed a white blood cell count of 3.9 K/µL, hemoglobin level of 12 g/dL, and platelets of 300 K/µL. A peripheral blood smear showed normal neutrophils. Her bone marrow aspiration showed normal cellularity with trilineage differentiation. Blast counts were not increased. Which treatment intervention would most likely improve clinical outcome in this patient?

(A) Standard induction with 7 + 3 (cytarabine plus danorubicin)

    (B) Radiation therapy followed by 4 cycles of high-dose cytarabine

    (C) Surgical resection followed by radiation

    (D) Neoadjuvant chemotherapy followed by radical surgery

6. A 33-year-old woman presents for treatment evaluation of normal cytogenetic *FLT3* wild type, *NPM1* mutated acute myelogenous leukemia. She receives standard induction with a combination of daunarubicin at 90 mg/m$^2$ IV for 3 days plus cytarabine at 200 mg/m$^2$ IV continuous infusion for 7 days. Her bone marrow 28 days after induction showed complete remission (CR). As part of her consolidation, she is initiated on high-dose Ara-cytarabine (HiDAC) at 3 g/m$^2$ IV twice daily on days 1, 3, and 5. On day 3 of treatment, she notes gait disturbances. Her physical examination reveals ataxia and nystagmus. Which of the following interventions would most likely favorably impact outcome on this patient?

    (A) Lumbar puncture plus empiric antibiotics for meningitis

    (B) High-dose steroids with prednisone at 1 mg/kg orally daily

    (C) Proceed with discontinuation of HiDAC

    (D) MRI of brain for investigation of potential central nervous system chloroma

7. A 35-year-old woman presents with a white blood cell count of 300,000/ µL with 70% circulating blasts. Her hemoglobin level is 9 g/dL and platelet count 30,000/µL. Her bone marrow showed a distinct monomorphic myeloblast population representing 80% of marrow cellularity. Three hours after admission, she complains of headache and becomes confused. Her physical examination reveals no focal neurological deficits. However, progressive shortness of breath develops with oxygen saturation of 85%. Chest radiograph reveals bilateral pulmonary infiltrates. Additional vital signs show a heart rate of 130 beats/min and temperature of 98°F. Broad-spectrum antibiotics are initiated. In addition to antibiotics, what important treatment intervention would most favorably impact outcome in this patient?

    (A) Addition of antifungal therapy

    (B) Initiation of low-molecular weight heparin

    (C) Leukapheresis

    (D) Addition of acyclovir

8. A 52-year-old woman diagnosed with acute myelogenous leukemia with normal karyotype receives 1 cycle of standard induction with 3 + 7 (daunorubicin intravenously at 60 mg/m$^2$ for 3 days plus cytarabine IV at 100 mg/m$^2$ for 7 days). Day 14 bone marrow examination showed persistent blasts of 70%.

Immunophenotyping shows a distinct blast population highlighting CD117, CD33, and CD13 positive cells. Which of the following is the most reasonable course of action?

    (A) Initiate FLAG plus IDA followed by allogeneic stem cell transplantation

    (B) Wait until day 28 and repeat the marrow examination

    (C) Begin decitabine at 20 mg/m$^2$ for 5 days every 28 days cycle (total 4 cycles) followed by allogeneic stem cell transplantation

    (D) Begin gemtuzumab ozogamicin at 9 mg/m$^2$ on days 1 and 15 followed by allogeneic stem cell transplantation

## REFERENCES

1. Siegel R, Ma J, Zou Z, Jemal A. Cancer statistics, 2014. *CA Cancer J Clin.* 2014;64(1):9–29.

2. Leone G, Pagano L, Ben-Yehuda D, Voso MT. Therapy-related leukemia and myelodysplasia: susceptibility and incidence. *Haematologica.* 2007;92(10):1389–1398.

3. Vardiman JW, Thiele J, Arber DA, et al. The 2008 revision of the World Health Organization (WHO) classification of myeloid neoplasms and acute leukemia: rationale and important changes. *Blood.* 2009;114(5):937–951.

4. Döhner H, Estey EH, Amadori S, et al.; European LeukemiaNet. Diagnosis and management of acute myeloid leukemia in adults: recommendations from an international expert panel, on behalf of the European LeukemiaNet. *Blood.* 2010;115(3):453–474.

5. Fröhling S, Schlenk RF, Stolze I, et al. CEBPA mutations in younger adults with acute myeloid leukemia and normal cytogenetics: prognostic relevance and analysis of cooperating mutations. *J Clin Oncol.* 2004;22(4):624–633.

6. Paschka P, Marcucci G, Ruppert AS, et al.; Cancer and Leukemia Group B. Adverse prognostic significance of KIT mutations in adult acute myeloid leukemia with inv(16) and t(8;21): a Cancer and Leukemia Group B Study. *J Clin Oncol.* 2006;24(24): 3904–3911.

7. Chou WC, Chou SC, Liu CY, et al. TET2 mutation is an unfavorable prognostic factor in acute myeloid leukemia patients with intermediate-risk cytogenetics. *Blood.* 2011;118(14): 3803–3810.

8. Metzeler KH, Maharry K, Radmacher MD, et al. TET2 mutations improve the new European LeukemiaNet risk classification of acute myeloid leukemia: a Cancer and Leukemia Group B study. *J Clin Oncol.* 2011;29(10):1373–1381.

9. Krönke J, Schlenk RF, Jensen KO, et al. Monitoring of minimal residual disease in NPM1-mutated acute myeloid leukemia: a study from the German-Austrian acute myeloid leukemia study group. *J Clin Oncol.* 2011;29(19):2709–2716.

10. Cilloni D, Renneville A, Hermitte F, et al. Real-time quantitative polymerase chain reaction detection of minimal residual disease by standardized WT1 assay to enhance risk stratification in acute myeloid leukemia: a European LeukemiaNet study. *J Clin Oncol.* 2009;27(31):5195–5201.

11. Polak J, Hajkova H, Haskovec C, et al. Quantitative monitoring of WT1 expression in peripheral blood before and after allogeneic stem cell transplantation for acute myeloid leukemia—a useful tool for early detection of minimal residual disease. *Neoplasma.* 2013;60(1):74–82.

12. Cheson BD, Bennett JM, Kopecky KJ, et al.; Revised recommendations of the International Working Group for Diagnosis, Standardization of Response Criteria, Treatment Outcomes, and

Reporting Standards for Therapeutic Trials in Acute Myeloid Leukemia. *J Clin Oncol.* 2003;21(24):4642–4649.

13. Lo-Coco F, Avvisati G, Vignetti M, et al.; Gruppo Italiano Malattie Ematologiche dell'Adulto; German-Austrian Acute Myeloid Leukemia Study Group; Study Alliance Leukemia. Retinoic acid and arsenic trioxide for acute promyelocytic leukemia. *N Engl J Med.* 2013;369(2):111–121.

14. Adès L, Guerci A, Raffoux E, et al.; European APL Group. Very long-term outcome of acute promyelocytic leukemia after treatment with all-trans retinoic acid and chemotherapy: the European APL Group experience. *Blood.* 2010;115(9):1690–1696.

15. Fernandez HF, Sun Z, Yao X, et al. Anthracycline dose intensification in acute myeloid leukemia. *N Engl J Med.* 2009;361(13):1249–1259.

16. Estey EH, Thall PF, Cortes JE, et al. Comparison of idarubicin + ara-C-, fludarabine + ara-C-, and topotecan + ara-C-based regimens in treatment of newly diagnosed acute myeloid leukemia, refractory anemia with excess blasts in transformation, or refractory anemia with excess blasts. *Blood.* 2001;98(13):3575–3583.

17. Ossenkoppele GJ, Graveland WJ, Sonneveld P, et al.; Dutch-Belgian Hemato-Oncology Cooperative Group (HOVON). The value of fludarabine in addition to ARA-C and G-CSF in the treatment of patients with high-risk myelodysplastic syndromes and AML in elderly patients. *Blood.* 2004;103(8):2908–2913.

18. Kantarjian H, Ravandi F, O'Brien S, et al. Intensive chemotherapy does not benefit most older patients (age 70 years or older) with acute myeloid leukemia. *Blood.* 2010;116(22): 4422–4429.

19. Röllig C, Thiede C, Gramatzki M, et al.; Study Alliance Leukemia. A novel prognostic model in elderly patients with acute myeloid leukemia: results of 909 patients entered into the prospective AML96 trial. *Blood.* 2010;116(6):971–978.

20. Fenaux P, Mufti GJ, Hellström-Lindberg E, et al. Azacitidine prolongs overall survival compared with conventional care regimens in elderly patients with low bone marrow blast count acute myeloid leukemia. *J Clin Oncol.* 2010;28(4):562–569.

21. Löwenberg B, Beck J, Graux C, et al.; Dutch-Belgian Hemato-Oncology Cooperative Group (HOVON); German Austrian AML Study Group (AMLSG); Swiss Group for Clinical Cancer Research Collaborative Group (SAKK). Gemtuzumab ozogamicin as postremission treatment in AML at 60 years of age or more: results of a multicenter phase 3 study. *Blood.* 2010;115(13):2586–2591.

# 30

# *Chronic Myeloid Leukemia*

ALISSA A. WEBER, RAMI N. KHORIATY, AND MOSHE TALPAZ

## EPIDEMIOLOGY, RISK FACTORS, NATURAL HISTORY, AND PATHOLOGY

Chronic myeloid leukemia (CML) accounts for about 15% of all adult leukemias. The annual incidence rate of CML is about 1.5/100,000, and the lifetime risk of developing CML is 0.16%. In the United States, an estimated 5430 new cases of CML were diagnosed in 2012, and approximately 610 deaths occurred from the disease. CML can occur at any age, but it is essentially a disease of adulthood, with a median age at diagnosis of 66 years. With the use of imatinib and second-generation tyrosine kinase inhibitors (TKIs), the annual mortality rate has been substantially reduced. This has resulted in an increase in the prevalence of CML from approximately 70,000 patients in the United States in 2010, to a projected 144,000 patients in 2030 (1).

Established CML risk factors include older age, high-dose radiation exposure or high-dose radiation therapy used to treat other cancers, and male sex (male-to-female preponderance is about 1.5:1). Although high-dose radiation is a risk factor for CML, most patients with CML do not have a history of radiation exposure, and most patients exposed to radiation do not develop CML. There are no known genetic factors associated with susceptibility to developing CML. A positive family history of CML is not a risk factor for the disease. There are no clear social or geographic risk factors for CML.

Without treatment, CML progresses from a chronic phase (CP) to an advanced phase (AP) and then to a blast phase (BP). In about 25% of cases, patients progress directly from CP to BP. The pace of the CP is highly variable; some patients stay in CP for more than a decade, whereas others progress to AP or BP within months. The median durations of the CP and AP in untreated patients are 3–5 years and 3–9 months, respectively. Prior to the development of TKIs, CML patients who did not undergo allogeneic stem cell transplantation (ASCT) had a median survival of about 5–7 years.

Patients with CML can be classified into low-, intermediate-, and high-risk groups according to the Sokal formulation that is based on age, spleen size, platelet count, and percentage of circulating blasts (2). Although the Sokal risk stratification scheme was conceived prior to the advent of TKIs, it continues to be useful to stratify patients treated with imatinib. The 5-year rates of complete cytogenetic response (CcyR) in patients in the low-, intermediate-, and high-risk Sokal groups treated with imatinib are 89%, 82%, and 69%, respectively ($P < .001$), and the 5-year rates of disease progression in those patients are 3%, 8%, and 17%, respectively ($P = .002$) (3).

CML is thought to develop when a hematopoietic stem cell becomes transformed by the breakpoint cluster region (BCR) and Abelson kinase *(ABL)* fusion gene. This transformation confers a proliferative advantage over normal hematopoietic stem cells. The t(9;22)(q34;q11.2) results in the fusion of *ABL* located on chromosome 9q34 and BCR located on chromosome 22q11.2. The *BCR–ABL* fusion gene, located on the shortened chromosome 22 (called the Philadelphia chromosome), encodes the *BCR–ABL* oncoprotein that constitutively activates tyrosine kinase activity and is sufficient to cause CML. This kinase regulates downstream targets, including c-Myc, Akt, and Jun, all of which are important in cell proliferation and survival. In addition, the fusion gene results in decreased DNA binding activity of *ABL* and increased binding of *ABL* to actin microfilaments, which affects differentiation and results in increased proliferation and decreased apoptosis. The fact that the t(9,22) is found in cells of myeloid, B-lymphoid, erythroid, and megakaryocytic lineages confirms that CML is a hematopoietic stem cell disease.

Depending on the specific location of the breakpoint in the *BCR* gene, the resulting fusion oncogene can have varying lengths. In CML, the *BCR* gene is typically disrupted at the e13 or e14 loci, and the resulting hybrid transcripts e13a2 and e14a2, respectively, both encode the p210 *BCR–ABL* oncoprotein. Less commonly, the breakpoint in the *BCR* gene occurs either more upstream near the e1 locus or downstream near the e19 locus, resulting in the e1a2 or e19a2 transcript variants, which correspond to oncoproteins p190 and p230, respectively. The p190 oncoprotein is more common in Philadelphia-positive acute lymphoblastic leukemia. The p230 oncoprotein is very rare in CML, but can be found in atypical CML and chronic neutrophilic leukemia cases. Other fusion proteins are less common.

## STAGING

There are multiple staging systems for CML, the most commonly used ones being the World Health Organization (WHO) and the MD Anderson staging systems.

### Chronic Myeloid Leukemia

| Phases of CML | WHO Criteria | MD Anderson Criteria |
|---|---|---|
| Chronic phase | CML diagnosis without features of accelerated or blastic phase | |
| Accelerated phase | PB or BM blasts 10–19%, PB basophils ≥20%, platelets <100 × 10⁹/L unrelated to therapy, or platelets >1000 × 10⁹/L unresponsive to therapy, cytogenetic evidence of clonal evolution, increasing spleen size, and WBC count unresponsive to therapy | PB blasts ≥15%, PB blasts + promyelocytes ≥30%, PB basophils ≥20%, platelets ≤100 × 10⁹/L unrelated to therapy, cytogenetic clonal evolution |
| Blastic phase | PB or BM blasts ≥20%, extramedullary blasts, large foci or clusters of blasts in BM | PB or BM blasts ≥30%, extramedullary disease |

BM, bone marrow; CML, chronic myeloid leukemia; PB, peripheral blood; WBC, white blood cell; WHO, World Health Organization.

## CASE SUMMARIES

### Diagnosis of CP CML

S.L. is a 61-year-old man who presented with generalized fatigue. His physical examination demonstrated palpable splenomegaly (about 5 cm below the left costal margin), and his complete blood count (CBC) revealed leukocytosis with a white blood cell (WBC) count of 52,000/µL. The WBC differential showed a left shift: 52% neutrophils, 20% band forms, 10% myelocytes, 6% metamyelocytes, 1% blasts, 6% lymphocytes, 2% basophils, and 3% eosinophils. His hemoglobin level was 15 g/dL, and his platelet count was 355,000/µL. A bone marrow biopsy was performed and showed a hypercellular marrow with an increased myeloid to erythroid ratio and no significant dysplasia. Maturation was preserved in the myeloid series, but there was a left shift; reticulin stain was negative for fibrosis, and cytogenetics showed t(9;22) (q34;q11.2) in all 20 cells examined. Peripheral blood polymerase chain reaction (PCR) for *BCR–ABL* revealed the p210 BCR–ABL transcript.

### Evidence-Based Case Discussion

S.L. has leukocytosis with a left shift, splenomegaly, t(9;22) (q34;q11.2) on metaphase cytogenetics, and the p210 *BCR–ABL* transcript. All myeloproliferative disorders (MPDs) share some common features; however, the patient presented here fits the diagnostic criteria for CML. CML should be suspected in patients with persistent leukocytosis, especially in the presence of basophilia, after infectious etiologies have been ruled out. The absence of polycythemia, thrombocytosis, marrow reticulin fibrosis, and dysplastic features in the bone marrow rule out the following diagnoses in respective order: polycythemia vera, essential thrombocytosis, myelofibrosis, and myeloproliferative disease/myelodysplastic syndrome-overlap disorders. Nevertheless, the clinical and laboratory tests overlap significantly among these syndromes (e.g., about 30% of patients with CML have thrombocytosis). Consequently, patients with similar blood count profiles require a bone marrow aspirate and biopsy, as well as cytogenetics and molecular testing to assign a specific diagnosis.

The diagnosis of CML requires presence of the Philadelphia chromosome t(9;22) identified by 1 of the following methods: metaphase karyotyping, fluorescent in situ hybridization (FISH), or PCR for BCR–ABL, either in bone marrow or peripheral blood. Peripheral blood PCR for *BCR–ABL* detects the p210 and p190 fusion transcripts, but not the p230 transcript. A bone marrow biopsy is necessary, not only for diagnostic purposes but also for staging the disease as well as providing a baseline for follow-up monitoring. Moreover, performing metaphase karyotyping on the bone marrow aspirate may identify unusual *BCR–ABL* translocations as well as additional cytogenetic abnormalities, which would otherwise not be detected by PCR. Approximately 90–95% of patients with CML have t(9;22) (q34;q11.2) detected by metaphase cytogenetics, which means that the absence of the Philadelphia chromosome does not completely rule out CML in the right clinical context. Of the remaining 5–10% of patients, 30–40% will have the translocation discovered by FISH or PCR. Patients without evidence of the Philadelphia chromosome may have "atypical CML," which is an entity with distinct clinical features and course. The absence of the Philadelphia chromosome and negative PCR testing for *BCR–ABL* should trigger an evaluation for diseases other than CML.

If bone marrow metaphase cytogenetics analysis cannot be performed (due to inability to collect marrow or technical difficulties with the test), FISH should be performed on the peripheral blood using probes for *BCR* and *ABL*. FISH should also be performed when the Philadelphia chromosome is not identified by conventional cytogenetics, in order to rule out a falsely positive PCR for *BCR–ABL*, and thus to confirm or refute the diagnosis of CML. There is no role for screening for *BCR–ABL* mutations at baseline.

In our patient, metaphase karyotyping performed on the bone marrow aspirate showed t(9;22) (q34;q11.2), and peripheral blood PCR for *BCR–ABL* revealed 1 of the typical transcript variants in CML encoding the p210

fusion protein, thus establishing the diagnosis of CML. On the basis of both the WHO and MD Anderson criteria, the stage of the patient's CML is chronic phase (CML-CP).

## Frontline Treatment of CP CML

T.S. is a 52-year-old man who presented with leukocytosis and splenomegaly and was diagnosed with CML-CP. He is otherwise healthy with no comorbidities and has a good performance status.

### Evidence-Based Case Discussion

Frontline treatment of CP-CML has evolved tremendously over the last 15 years. ASCT and interferon alpha were important strategies prior to the introduction of TKIs, but are now viewed as salvage therapeutic options. Currently, TKIs stand as preferred first-line treatment in this subset of CML (see Figure 30.1). TKIs block the adenosine

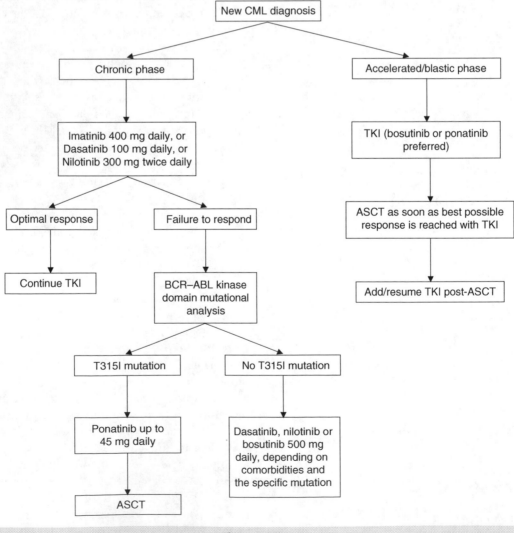

## Figure 30.1

Treatment algorithm for chronic myeloid leukemia. ABL, Abelson kinase; ASCT, allogeneic stem cell transplantation; BCR, breakpoint cluster region; CML, chronic myeloid leukemia; TKI, tyrosine kinase inhibitor.

triphosphate (ATP) binding site of *BCR–ABL*, suppressing downstream signaling associated with cellular proliferation. Imatinib, dasatinib, and nilotinib are TKIs approved by the Food and Drug Administration (FDA) for frontline CML-CP therapy. The response definitions are summarized in Table 30.1 (4).

## Imatinib as First-Line Therapy

Based on the promising results with imatinib in a phase II trial in patients with CML-CP who were resistant–refractory–intolerant to interferon alpha (96% complete hematologic response [CHR], 67% major cytogenetic response [McyR], 57% CcyR), a randomized phase III trial known as IRIS (International Randomized interferon [IFN] vs. STI571) was conducted comparing first-line imatinib 400-mg daily with the standard of care then, interferon alfa plus low-dose cytarabine, in patients with CML-CP. Patients receiving imatinib had impressive outcomes with rates of CHR, McyR, and CCyR of 96%, 85%, and 69%, respectively, at 12 months, and 98%, 92%, and 87%, respectively, at 60 months (3). The rate of major molecular response (MMR) increased from 24% at 6 months to 39% at 12 months, and to a best of 86% with 8 years

of follow-up. The response to imatinib was fairly durable, and the majority of patients who had an event or who progressed to AP CML did so in the first 2 years of therapy. The annual rates of transformation to AP or BP from years 1–8 were 1.5%, 2.8%, 1.8%, 0.9%, 0.5%, 0%, 0%, and 0.4% (5,6). This translates to a remarkable 92% rate of freedom from progression to AP or BP after 8 years of imatinib. After 8 years of follow-up on the IRIS trial, patients who were randomized to imatinib had estimated event-free survival (EFS) and overall survival (OS) of 81% and 86%, respectively. If only CML-related deaths and deaths prior to stem cell transplant were considered, the 8-year OS would be 93% (6). As discussed in detail earlier, CCyR and MMR are important milestones in patients with CML-CP. Among patients who achieved CCyR, only 3% progressed to AP or BP, the vast majority of whom progressed within 2 years of reaching CCyR. None of the 39% of patients who reached MMR at 12 months progressed to AP or BP. Despite these impressive results, an OS advantage of imatinib over interferon could not be established in the IRIS trial due to the high rate of crossover from the interferon alpha arm to the imatinib arm (about 90%). Nevertheless, a comparison between patients treated with imatinib and historical patients treated with interferon alfa with or without ara-c showed the anticipated survival advantage with imatinib (7,8).

It is important to note that in the IRIS trial, only patients who continued to receive imatinib were evaluated, and patients who stopped imatinib were censored. A single-center study examined a cohort of consecutively treated patients with CML-CP receiving first-line imatinib 400 mg/d, and estimated the outcomes by intention-to-treat analysis. In this study, CHR, MCyR, CcyR, and MMR were 97.1%, 71.1%, 57.4%, and 12.3% at 12 months and 98.5%, 85.1%, 82.7%, and 50.1% at 60 months, respectively. These numbers are slightly inferior (although fairly comparable) to those in the IRIS trial. Conversely, the 5-year EFS by intention-to-treat analysis was 62.7%, which is considerably lower than the 5-year EFS of 83% in the IRIS trial. However, the 5-year EFS was 81% in this trial when calculated using the IRIS trial definition. The 5-year progression-free survival (PFS) and OS by intention-to-treat analysis were 82.7% and 83.2%, respectively (9). The majority of patients on the imatinib arm of the IRIS study have remained on the drug long term.

Imatinib is generally well tolerated; common side effects are neutropenia, thrombocytopenia, gastrointestinal symptoms, rash, edema, musculoskeletal symptoms, hypophosphatemia, and possibly congestive heart failure (CHF) (the rate of CHF is 1.7% in patients receiving imatinib, which is comparable to the rate of CHF in the general population). An increased rate of peripheral arterial or atherosclerotic disease has not been demonstrated in imatinib-treated patients (10,11).

**Table 30.1** Response Definition in CML

**Hematologic Response**

| | |
|---|---|
| Complete hematologic response (CHR) | Platelets <450 × 10⁹/L, WBC <10 × 10⁹/L, basophils <5%, no circulating immature granulocytes, no palpable spleen |

**Cytogenetic Response**

| | |
|---|---|
| Major cytogenetic response (MCyR) | Ph positive metaphases: 0% |
| Complete cytogenetic response (CCyR) | Ph positive metaphases: 1–35% |
| Partial cytogenetic response (PCyR) | |
| Minor cytogenetic response (mCyR) | Ph positive metaphases: 36–65% |
| Minimal cytogenetic response (minCyR) | Ph positive metaphases: 66–95% |
| No cytogenetic response | Ph positive metaphases >95% |

**Molecular Response**

| | |
|---|---|
| Complete molecular response (CMR) | No detectable *BCR–ABL* transcripts by 2 PCR analyses of sensitivity >10⁻⁴ |
| Major molecular response (MMR) | Ratio of *BCR–ABL/ABL* (or other housekeeping genes) transcripts ≤0.1% on the international scale |

CML, chronic myeloid leukemia; WBC, white blood cell.

High-dose imatinib (either given continuously or using an induction strategy) has not proven superior to standard-dose imatinib in the first-line setting in patients with CML-CP (12,13). This unexpected result could be secondary to dose interruptions–reductions that occurred in a significant proportion of patients randomized to high-dose imatinib. Nevertheless, the recommended dose of imatinib in the first-line setting in patients with CML-CP is 400 mg/d.

## Frontline Second-Generation TKIs

After dasatinib and nilotinib were approved as second-line therapies for patients with imatinib resistance or intolerance, these agents were examined in the first-line setting with the hope of improving outcomes. Phase II studies testing dasatinib or nilotinib in the frontline setting for CML-CP showed promising results and led to randomized phase III trials comparing these agents to imatinib.

The ENESTnd (Evaluating Nilotinib Efficacy and Safety in Clinical Trials of Newly Diagnosed Ph⁺ CML Patients) phase III trial randomized newly diagnosed CML-CP patients to nilotinib 300-mg twice daily, nilotinib 400-mg twice daily, or imatinib 400-mg daily (14). MMR at 12 months, the primary end point of the study, was 44% in the nilotinib 300-mg arm, 43% in the nilotinib 400-mg arm, and 22% in the imatinib arm ($P < .0001$ for each nilotinib group compared to imatinib). The rates of MMR at 3, 6, and 9 months were also higher in patients receiving either dose of nilotinib compared to imatinib. Cytogenetic responses were superior for nilotinib both at 6 and 12 months, further indicating faster responses with nilotinib. Perhaps, the most important finding of the study is that progression to AP or BP occurred less commonly in patients receiving nilotinib 300-mg twice daily (0.7%, $P = .0095$ compared to imatinib), and in patients receiving nilotinib 400-mg twice daily (0.4%, $P = .0037$ compared to imatinib) compared to patients receiving imatinib (3.9%). If sustained, this finding would suggest that nilotinib is a better first treatment option than imatinib. Both drugs were fairly well tolerated, and no patient developed $QT_C > 500$ ms or a decrease in the left ventricular ejection fraction. Muscle spasm, nausea, diarrhea, vomiting, and fluid overload were more common in patients receiving imatinib, whereas rash, alopecia, headache, elevations in transaminases, bilirubin, and lipase were more common in patients receiving nilotinib. Grade 3 or 4 neutropenia and anemia were more common with imatinib, whereas grade 3 or 4 thrombocytopenia was more common with nilotinib.

DASISION (Dasatinib vs. Imatinib Study in Treatment-Naive CML Patients), a phase III clinical trial, randomized newly diagnosed CML-CP patients to dasatinib 100-mg daily or imatinib 400-mg daily (15). The rate of confirmed CCyR by 12 months, the primary end point of the study, was 77% in patients receiving dasatinib compared to 66% in patients receiving imatinib ($P = .007$). Cytogenetic responses were attained more rapidly with dasatinib. Molecular responses were also improved with dasatinib at 3, 6, 9, and 12 months (12-month MMR of 46% and 28%, respectively). Progression to AP or BP occurred in 1.9% of patients receiving dasatinib compared to 3.5% of patients receiving imatinib. Both drugs were well tolerated and the majority of the adverse events were grade 1 or 2 in both arms. The rates of grade 3 or 4 neutropenia were comparable in both arms, but grade 3 or 4 thrombocytopenia and anemia were more common in patients receiving dasatinib. Nausea, vomiting, myalgias, muscle inflammation, rash, fluid retention, superficial edema, and grade 3 or 4 hypophosphatemia were more common in patients receiving imatinib. Pleural effusion (grade 1 or 2) occurred exclusively in patients receiving dasatinib at a frequency of about 10%. Only 3 patients (1.2%) required thoracentesis, and the rest of the patients with pleural effusions were treated with dasatinib dose modifications or medically (steroids and/or diuretics). The rates of discontinuation secondary to drug-related side effects were similar in both arms.

The choice of initial therapy should take into account a series of issues, including administration, side effect profiles, and the aforementioned response rates. Nilotinib requires twice-daily dosage, whereas imatinib and dasatinib are given once daily. Nilotinib is the only TKI that must be taken on an empty stomach; patients cannot eat 2 hr before or 1 hr after taking it (food significantly increases the absorption of nilotinib). Proton pump inhibitors cannot be used with nilotinib because an acidic milieu is required for adequate absorption. Recent evidence suggests a risk of accelerated atherosclerosis in patients treated with nilotinib. In a prospective study, 129 CML patients were prospectively screened for pathological peripheral artery occlusive disease (PAOD), defined by <0.9 ankle-brachial index (ABI). Pathological PAOD was found in 6.3% of patients receiving imatinib, 26% receiving nilotinib as first-line therapy, and 35.7% receiving nilotinib as second-line therapy ($P < .05$), and clinically overt PAOD was seen in 5 patients who were exposed to nilotinib therapy (10). Additionally, 27 cases of overt PAOD from several centers were reviewed, and all but 1 of these patients were exposed to nilotinib therapy, with events severe enough to require percutaneous angioplasty in 33% of cases, stent placement in 22%, amputation in 22%, and surgery in 18.5% (11). Nilotinib has greater risk for causing QTc prolongation; thus caution is required in prescribing other medications that might increase QTc in patients receiving nilotinib. Dasatinib should not be used in patients with a history of pleural or pericardial effusions. Dasatinib should also be avoided in patients with bleeding tendencies and in patients receiving antiplatelet agents or anticoagulants because it can cause bleeding due to platelet dysfunction. Nilotinib should be avoided in patients with a history of pancreatitis. All 3 agents are substrates for CYP3A4; therefore, CYP3A4 inhibitors (macrolides, azoles, grapefruit juice, etc.) should be avoided in patients taking any 1 of the TKIs (particularly nilotinib) because they result in increased serum concentration of TKIs and accentuated side effects, the most worrisome of which is QTc prolongation. CYP3A4 inducers (e.g., dexamethasone, phenytoin, St. John's wort, etc.) result in lower area under the curve of the TKIs; thus, higher doses are required to attain the desired benefits. Patients on a CYP3A4 substrate (e.g. simvastatin) may need a reduction in the dose of this medication if a TKI is started.

To date, imatinib at 400-mg daily, nilotinib 300-mg twice daily, and dasatinib 100-mg daily are all acceptable first-line treatment options in CML-CP. Initial treatment of choice should take into account side-effect profiles as well as patient compliance and comorbidities.

T.S. was started on imatinib 400-mg daily.

## CML-CP Follow-Up and Response Evaluation

M.P. is a 59-year-old man who was diagnosed with CML-CP 4 months ago when he presented with asymptomatic leukocytosis (WBC = 46,000/µL) with a left shift (49% neutrophils, 17% band forms, 11% myelocytes, 8% metamyelocytes, 2% blasts, 8% lymphocytes, 2% basophils, and 3% eosinophils) and splenomegaly. His hemoglobin level was 13 g/dL, and his platelet count was 200,000/µL. His bone marrow biopsy at diagnosis showed t(9,22) in all 20 cells examined. He was started on imatinib 400-mg daily and was given a CBC every 2 weeks. His blood counts completely normalized 6 weeks after starting imatinib, as did his splenomegaly. A bone marrow aspirate and biopsy performed after 3 months of treatment showed no morphologic evidence of CML, and cytogenetic analysis demonstrated 8 out of 20 cells examined with the t(9;22).

## Evidence-Based Case Discussion

Several technical difficulties are associated with metaphase cytogenetics, including the need for a bone marrow biopsy, the necessity of timely processing of the bone marrow sample, the use of different marrow culture protocols in various labs, and the low sensitivity of this test (in the order of 5–10%); however, it remains the gold standard to document CCyR, given that it has been validated in large TKI clinical trials. Additional advantages of metaphase cytogenetics include the ability to detect cytogenetic abnormalities other than the Philadelphia chromosome, as well as the ability to detect clonal evolution that occurs in 5–10% of patients. Unlike metaphase cytogenetics, FISH analysis and qRT-PCR can be done on the bone marrow aspirate or peripheral blood with equivalent sensitivity. Modern FISH probes have improved sensitivity for

detecting BCR–ABL transcripts as low as 0.3–0.6%, and also allow for detection of der(9) deletions. FISH has not been adequately validated in large trials; thus, its use in monitoring CML is limited to the following circumstances: a bone marrow aspirate and biopsy cannot be performed; technical difficulties prevent performance of conventional cytogenetic analysis (as a supplement to metaphase karyotyping if qRT-PCR for BCR–ABL is not available); and cytogenetic and molecular results are incongruent. The most sensitive test for monitoring response to a TKI in CML-CP is qRT-PCR; the sensitivity of this test is on the order of $10^{-5}$ to $10^{-6}$. PCR for BCR–ABL has been standardized by a National Institutes of Health Consensus Group, which set the baseline BCR–ABL (defined by the IRIS trial) at 100%, and the 3-log reduction at 0.1% representing MMR (16).

The important response milestones are summarized in Table 30.2 (4). It is critical to adequately monitor patients receiving treatment for CML-CP (as summarized subsequently) and to initiate therapeutic changes immediately in patients who fail to respond, lose their responses, or achieve suboptimal responses (although this is still somewhat debatable). When a therapeutic change is necessary, immediate implementation results in better outcomes. For example, after switching to dasatinib, CCyR was achieved in 72% of patients who lost MCyR to imatinib compared to 42% in patients who lost both MCyR and CHR to imatinib. The 24-month EFS was 89% after loss of MCyR only, compared to 29% after loss of both MCyR and CHR on imatinib (17).

Response to imatinib should be monitored by performing a CBC twice a month until CHR is documented and confirmed. Subsequently, a CBC should be obtained at least every 3 months or as required. Cytogenetic monitoring should be performed at diagnosis (as mentioned earlier), at month 6, and then every 6 months until CCyR is attained and confirmed. The European Leukemia Net group recommends obtaining a bone marrow biopsy at 3 months after starting therapy; however, this is not absolutely necessary because the results will not necessarily alter the treatment. Subsequently, cytogenetic monitoring should be performed every 12 months if regular molecular monitoring cannot be obtained, if unexplained cytopenia/cytopenias are present, if treatment failure (primary or secondary resistance) occurs, and if myelodysplastic features are present. Molecular monitoring (qRT-PCR) should be done every 3 months until MMR is obtained and confirmed, and at least every 6 months afterward. BCR–ABL mutational analysis should be performed in patients who fail to respond or have a suboptimal response, and always before changing to second-generation TKIs or other therapies (4). Patients on second-generation TKIs should be monitored similarly; however, earlier and more frequent testing may be warranted as responses occur typically earlier with second-generation TKIs.

**Table 30.2** Response Milestones in CP-CML Warnings[a]

| Response | Optimal Response | Suboptimal Response | Failure to Respond |
|---|---|---|---|
| **CHR** | CHR at 3 mos | CHR at 3 mos | No CHR at 3 mos |
| CyR | At least mCyR at 3 mos | No mCyR at 3 mos | No CyR at 6 mos |
|  | At least PCyR at 6 mos | No PCyR at 6 mos | No PCyR at 12 mos |
|  | CCyR at 12 mos | PCyR at 12 mos | No CCyR at 18 mos |
| MR | MMR at 18 mos | Less than MMR at 18 mos |  |
|  |  | Loss of MMR; mutation | Loss of CHR or CCyR; clonal chromosomal abnormality |

CHR, complete hematologic response; CP-CML, chronic phase chronic myeloid leukemia; CyR, cytogenetic response; mos, months; MR, molecular response; mCyR, major cytogenetic response; MMR, major molecular response; PCyR, partial cytogenetic response.
[a]These include high-risk disease; clonal chromosomal abnormalities at diagnosis; less than MMR at 12 mos; increase in PCR transcript levels; or clonal chromosomal abnormalities in Ph-cells at any time during treatment.

The most important and best validated response end point in CML is CCyR; however, the importance of achieving early CCyR is under debate. The IRIS study showed no correlation between the time to achieving CCyR and outcome, as long as CCyR was reached (18). This analysis has been criticized because patients who received <12 months of imatinib were excluded from the analysis. Although not statistically significant, the duration of cytogenetic response was superior for patients who achieved CCyR at earlier time points. A recent study from MD Anderson Cancer Center showed that the likelihood of reaching CCyR decreases over time, whereas the risk of having an event increases (19). In this study, if CCyR was not reached at 12 months, the chance of achieving CCyR was 42%, whereas the chance of having an event was 38%. This highlights the importance of achieving early CCyR, especially within 12 months of therapy.

Monitoring the molecular responses may provide additional prognostic information for patients receiving imatinib therapy. Rapid achievement of MMR seems to correlate with a more durable response (20). Patients who achieve MMR by 6 months have fewer events (defined as loss of MMR or acquisition of *BCR–ABL* mutation), than patients who achieve MMR between 6 and 12 months or between 12 and 18 months (0%, 12%, and 19%, respectively). In addition, the probability of achieving complete molecular response (CMR) is higher in patients who achieve MMR earlier rather than later (93%, 69%, and 37% in patients who achieve MMR by 6 months, 6–12 months, and 12–18 months, respectively). However, faster MMR may reflect better disease biology, rather than a true representation of a particular drug's efficacy. Response at 3 months can predict risk of progression and indicate change of therapy, including addition of IFNα to frontline TKI treatments. Patients who achieve a cytogenetic remission (CCyR or MCyR) or reach a *BCR–ABL* level of <10% by PCR after 3 months have significantly better OS after 5 years (95% vs. 87%) (21–24). Thus, this prognostic

marker may be a key for optimizing treatment protocols early on and will likely replace the current definition of optimal response to imatinib at 3 months, which requires CHR and <95% Ph+ metaphases (25).

M.P. achieved a CHR and MCyR by 3 months after frontline imatinib therapy was started. His response is optimal and he should be continued on current therapy and monitored according to the above guidelines.

## CML After Imatinib or Other Frontline Treatment Failure

F.G. is a 72-year-old man who was diagnosed with CML-CP 18 months ago and started on imatinib 400-mg daily. He achieved a CHR at 3 months, but at 18 months had only achieved a partial cytogenetic response (PCyR).

### Evidence-Based Case Discussion

F.G. failed to respond to first-line imatinib for CML-CP. The treatment strategy for patients who fail first-line standard-dose imatinib depends on 2 factors: the stage of the disease at the time of imatinib failure and the identification of mutation in the *BCR–ABL* kinase domain. The threonine-to-isoleucine mutation at position 315 (T315I) accounts for up to 20% of patients who exhibit TKI resistance and portends a poor response to higher doses of imatinib or to second-generation TKIs. Until 2012, the preferred treatment option in cases of T315I mutation was ASCT. Yet, in December 2012, ponatinib, a potent multikinase inhibitor with activity against the T315I mutation was approved for second-line treatment of CML. The drug was approved on the basis of the pivotal Ponatinib in Philadelphia Chromosome-Positive Acute Lymphocytic Leukemia and Chronic Myeloid Leukemia Evaluation (PACE) trial, a phase II study of 449 heavily pretreated patients with CML or Ph+ acute lymphoblastic leukemia (ALL) (26). In this study, 56% of patients with CP-CML, including 70% of patients with the T315I mutation, achieved an (mCyR) after 12 months of treatment. Furthermore, 55% of AP patients (50% with T315I) achieved a CHR, and nearly 40% achieved an mCyR after 12 months. Of the 62 patients with BP-CML, 34% met the CHR end point, whereas nearly 25% achieved mCyR. Adverse events reported in this study included thrombocytopenia, rash, dry skin, and abdominal pain. Serious arterial thrombotic events were observed in 9% of patients, but only 3% were considered treatment related.

By November 2013, the FDA halted commercial sales and marketing of ponatinib because an increasing number of serious arterial events were reported after longer-term follow-up in all 3 phases of the drug's clinical trial development. In December 2012, when the drug was approved, 14% of ponatinib-exposed patients had experienced serious arterial events; however, by November 2013, these events had occurred in 24% of patients in the phase 2 trial and 48% of patients in the phase 1 trial after mean treatment durations of 1.3 years and 2.7 years, respectively (27). Serious arterial events included heart attack, stroke, loss of blood flow to extremities resulting in tissue death, and severe narrowing of blood vessels in the extremities, heart, and brain, requiring surgical procedures to restore blood flow. These events were seen in patients of all ages, including those in their 20s. Due to safety concerns, a phase 3 trial comparing ponatinib to imatinib in the frontline setting was stopped indefinitely. Shortly thereafter, following more investigation, ponatinib was reapproved with revised U.S. prescribing information alerting to the risk for vascular occlusive events and heart failure. The revised indication is for patients with CP-, AP-, or BP- T315I-positive CML; T315I-positive Ph+ ALL; or CP-, AP-, or BP-CML or Ph+ ALL for whom no other TKI therapy is indicated. Ponatinib remains a valuable treatment option for this group of patients with few second-line options, yet requires important risk–benefit discussions between patients and providers.

Alternative options for those patients with intolerance or contraindications to ponatinib include ASCT, omacetaxine (semisynthetic homoharringtonine) given subcutaneously, or standard cytoreductive agents (interferon alpha ± ara-c or hydrea). Treatment of patients with CML-CP who carry the T315I mutation with omacetaxine resulted in CHR of 80%, overall cytogenetic response of 20%, and CCyR of 13%. The BCR–ABL T315I clone was reduced to below detectable level in 60% of evaluable patients (28). The 2-year PFS with omacetaxine in patients with T315I mutation is 70%.

In patients without the T315I mutation, the treatment options include switching to an FDA-approved second-generation TKI (as discussed subsequently), enrolling on clinical trials, or undergoing stem cell transplantation. Given that these patients invariably respond well to other second-generation TKIs, stem cell transplantation should be reserved for a later stage; for example, when patients

fail or are intolerant to multiple second-generation TKIs. Some mutations have been shown to be more sensitive to a particular second-generation TKI; thus, the results of the mutational analysis should guide choice of therapy (4).

Dasatinib, nilotinib, and bosutinib are all second-generation TKIs approved for treatment of patients refractory/intolerant to imatinib. Bosutinib, like dasatinib, inhibits both BCR–ABL and Src kinases. Several phase 2 studies demonstrated its efficacy in treating advanced CML (29–31), and the FDA approved this TKI in September 2012, on the basis of a single-arm, open-label, multicenter trial of 546 patients with CP-CML (406 patients) AP-CML, or BP-CML (140 for both AP- and BP-CML). These patients were previously treated with at least 1 other TKI and all had received prior imatinib therapy. CCyR was achieved in 23–46% of CP-CML patients, including those resistant to imatinib, dasatinib, and/or nilotinib. Bosutinib also showed activity in patients with AP-CML and BP-CML. In the Bosutinib Efficacy and Safely in Chronic Myeloid Leukemia (BELA) trial, a multinational open-label trial comparing bosutinib with imatinib for first-line treatment of CP-CML, CCyR at 12 months was similar (P = .601) between bosutinib (70%) and imatinib (68%). Although cytogenetic and molecular responses were achieved more quickly with bosutinib, no survival difference was observed. Because the study did not achieve its primary efficacy end point of CCyR at 12 months, bosutinib's indication at this time is limited to second-line therapy (32). Responses with bosutinib appear to be durable; at 36 month follow-up in a phase 2 study (28), 42% of patients were still receiving therapy. Bosutinib is active against most baseline mutations, but has no activity against T315I. The FDA-approved starting dose is 500 mg daily. Its distinct safety profile includes a high incidence of diarrhea, liver function test abnormalities, abdominal pain, and hyperlipasemia. Overall, bosutinib has not yet demonstrated an advantage over other second-generation TKIs, though it remains an important option for patients with CP-CML who are resistant or intolerant to imatinib, nilotinib, or dasatinib.

The phase II START (SRC/ABL Tyrosine Kinase Inhibition Activity Research Trials of Dasatinib)–C study of dasatinib 70-mg twice daily in patients with resistance–intolerance to imatinib demonstrated a 2-year CCyR of 53%, PFS of 80%, and OS of 94%. This study was followed by the START-R trial, which randomized CML-CP patients with imatinib resistance to dasatinib 70-mg twice daily (BID) versus high-dose imatinib (800 mg/d) (33). The rate of MCyR at 12 weeks was not statistically different between the 2 groups (36% for dasatanib patients and 29% for high-dose imatinib patients; P = .402). The CCyR rate at 12 weeks was higher in patients on dasatinib than patients on imatinib (22% and 8%, respectively; P = .041). At the 2-year follow-up, the rates of MCyR, CCyR, and MMR were significantly higher in patients receiving dasatinib than in patients receiving imatinib. It is important to mention that 80% of patients receiving imatinib and 20% of patients receiving dasatinib crossed over to the other treatment arm. Among patients who crossed over, MCyR was enhanced with dasatinib in comparison to high-dose imatinib (49% and 15%, respectively). The 24-month PFS was 86% in patients receiving dasatinib compared to 65% in patients receiving imatinib (*P* = .0012). Grade 3 or 4 thrombocytopenia and neutropenia occurred in more patients in the dasatinib arm. Pleural effusions were exclusively reported in patients on dasatinib (grade 3 or 4 pleural effusion in 5%). These results provide support for switching imatinib-resistant patients to dasatinib instead of further intensifying the dose of imatinib, with the caveat of a worse side-effect profile.

The dose of dasatinib used in the START-R trial is not the currently recommended dose. A dose-optimization study of dasatinib in patients with CML-CP demonstrated that a dose of 100-mg daily induced comparable MCyR and CCyR rates, as well as PFS and OS and an improved side-effect profile compared to multiple other doses tested. In particular, pleural effusions occurred in 14% of patients receiving 100 mg of dasatinib (2% grade 3 or 4) compared to 23–25% in patients receiving the other doses (4–5% grade 3 or 4) (*P* = .049). The risk of neutropenia, thrombocytopenia, and severe thrombocytopenia was also statistically lower with 100 mg of dasatanib daily, and fewer drug interruptions and discontinuations resulted at that dose. Thus, the preferred dasatinib dose is now 100-mg daily (34).

Nilotinib's activity in the setting of imatinib resistance or intolerance in CML-CP was demonstrated in a pivotal open-label phase II trial where patients received nilotinib at a dose of 400-mg twice daily. At 24 months, CCyR was achieved in 46% of patients, of whom 84% maintained this response at 24 months. The overall MMR was 28% with a median time to MMR of 5.6 months. The rates of PFS and OS at 24 months were 64% and 87%, respectively. For F.G., BCR–ABL kinase domain mutational analysis was performed and found to be negative. The treatment options and side effect profiles were discussed with him, and he expressed interest in switching therapy to dasatinib.

## Advanced-Phase CML

S.N. is a 57-year-old otherwise healthy man who presented with fatigue occurring over several months. His CBC showed a WBC count of 120,000/μL, hemoglobin level of 11 g/dL, and platelet count of 88,000/μL. The WBC differential was as follows: 15% blasts, 15% promyelocytes, 11% myelocytes, 8% metamyelocytes, 20% neutrophils, 6% band forms, 3% lymphocytes, 20% basophils, and 2% eosinophils). Physical examination showed splenomegaly (spleen palpated 8 cm below the left costal margin). Cytogenetic analysis of the bone marrow sample showed t(9,22) in all 20 examined cells. Peripheral blood PCR for *BCR–ABL* was positive for the p210 *BCR–ABL* transcript.

## Evidence-Based Case Discussion

S.N. was diagnosed with AP-CML. The treatment of AP and BP CML is disparate from the treatment of CML-CP and is discussed subsequently. Traditional cytotoxic therapies are not very effective in patients with myeloid and undifferentiated blast crises; responses are infrequent, and when they occur, they tend to be short lived. The median OS of patients with myeloid BP-CML who received cytotoxic chemotherapy ranged between 1.3 and 12 months. In lymphoid blast crisis, responses are somewhat more common, but are short lived as well. Decitabine has been studied in AP-CML, but has not shown superiority over cytotoxic chemotherapy (median OS of 4–13 months). The second-generation TKIs, including bosutinib, and third-generation TKI, ponatinib, have activity in AP-CML, and should be utilized prior to or in combination with cytotoxic chemotherapy, unless previously exposed. Rational clinical trials should be strongly considered.

In CML-AP patients who are imatinib resistant/intolerant, dasatinib results in CHR and CCyR in 45% and 18% of patients, respectively. In myeloid BP, dasatinib induces CHR in 24–35% and CCyR in 26–27% of patients. Similarly, for CML-AP patients treated with nilotinib, CHR is achieved in 26–46% and CCyR in 13–19% of patients. Nilotinib results in CHR in 8% and CCyR in 4% of patients in myeloid BP. Combining cytotoxic chemotherapy agents or decitabine with imatinib in patients with AP-CML does not improve outcomes compared to treatment with single-agent dasatinib. In patients with lymphoid BP CML who are imatinib resistant/intolerant, dasatinib results in CHR and CCyR in about 70% and 30%, respectively, whereas nilotinib results in even poorer responses (11% rate of CCyR). Thus, the long-term outcome of patients with advanced CML treated with second-generation TKIs is poor.

Unlike the majority of patients with CML-CP, patients with AP- or BP-CML require ASCT because TKIs do not provide long-lasting responses in this setting (Figure 30.1). The outcomes of patients with CML who undergo ASCT depend on the stage of the disease at the time of ASCT. The incidence of hematologic relapse at 3 years post-ASCT is 5.7% in patients who are transplanted in CP-CML, compared to 25.3% in patients transplanted at AP-CML, 27% in patients transplanted in second CP-CML, and 26% in patients transplanted in BP-CML (*P* = .0001). Imatinib pre-SCT does not result in unfavorable outcomes or increased transplant-related mortality. Imatinib can be safely given post-ASCT as well, and in fact, it may delay early relapses following reduced-intensity ASCT. The newer TKIs are also being utilized in the posttransplant setting, although data, especially efficacy data, are limited (35). Patients treated with imatinib pre-SCT have inferior outcomes if they had a suboptimal response or loss of response at the time of transplant, further confirming the importance of achieving cytogenetic responses at the time of transplantation.

For our patient S.N., we recommend starting a TKI immediately in an attempt to control his disease. Even the patients with advanced CML who achieve an excellent response to a TKI relapse early, so we also recommend HLA typing for the patient and his siblings and initiation of an immediate donor search through the national registry if none of his siblings is a good match. The patient should undergo an ASCT as soon as he has achieved an optimal response with the TKI. We recommend adding/resuming a TKI post-ASCT.

## Duration of Therapy

The current standard of care in the management of CML is lifelong TKI therapy as long as response is maintained and treatment is tolerated. The only known curative therapy for CML is ASCT. However, in patients who achieve a durable CMR, there has been recent interest in whether TKI therapy can be safely discontinued. The largest trial to evaluate this was the Stop Imatinib (STIM) Trial, a prospective, non-randomized trial of 100 patients with CML on imatinib who had achieved a CMR for at least 2 years (36). Of 69 patients with at least 12 months of follow-up, 41% maintained a CMR. Of the nearly 60% of patients who demonstrated molecular relapse, all responded to reintroduction of imatinib, with either reduction in BCR–ABL1 transcripts by PCR or restoration of durable CMR (26 patients). This was after a median 24 months' follow-up. After longer-term follow-up at 60 months, the cumulative incidence of molecular relapse was 61%. Of these 61 patients who relapsed, 40 sustained treatment with a TKI, all achieving MMR or CMR, and 10 stopped treatment without molecular relapse. No deaths attributable to CML have been reported. In this study, having a low Sokal score plus being treated with imatinib for >5 years predicted a higher rate of survival without molecular relapse (0.68 [95% CI (45–83)] vs. 0.33 [95% CI (22–42)], $P = 0.007$) compared to all groups.

## REVIEW QUESTIONS

1.  A 56-year-old man presents with a 3-month history of fatigue. On examination, he is noted to have splenomegaly, and the remainder of his examination is unremarkable. Laboratory evaluation reveals a white blood cell count of 26,000 × 10⁶/L (70% neutrophils, 6% myelocytes, 3% metamyelocytes, 9% basophils, 10% lymphocytes, and % eosinophils), hemoglobin level of 12.6 g/dL, and platelet count of 230,000 × 10⁶/L. Which of the following is needed to confirm the diagnosis?

    (A) Bone marrow aspirate and biopsy, including conventional cytogenetics
    (B) Fluorescent in situ hybridization for the BCR–ABL fusion
    (C) RT-polymerase chain reaction (PCR) for BCR–ABL transcripts

    (D) Flow cytometry of peripheral blood
    (E) JAK2V617F mutational analysis
    (F) B or C
    (G) A, B, or C

2.  A 26-year-old woman is recently diagnosed with chronic myeloid leukemia. Her initial white blood cell count is 170,000 × 10⁶/L (65% neutrophils, 5% myelocytes, 4% metamyelocytes, 12% basophils, 17% lymphocytes, 5% eosinophils, and 2% blasts), hemoglobin level is 11.7 g/dL, and platelet count is 140,000 × 10⁶/L. The bone marrow aspirate shows 6% blasts. Which of the following is the best initial treatment for this patient?

    (A) High-dose interferon
    (B) Tyrosine kinase inhibitor (TKI) until major molecular response is achieved followed by allogeneic stem cell transplantation
    (C) TKI indefinitely
    (D) Cytarabine-based chemotherapy plus TKI
    (E) Observation

3.  A 64-year-old man is referred to you for a recent diagnosis of chronic phase chronic myeloid leukemia. He has no significant past medical history other than 1 episode of acute pancreatitis following acute alcohol intoxication 3 years ago. Which of the following tyrosine kinase inhibitors should be avoided in his treatment course?

    (A) Imatinib
    (B) Dasatinib
    (C) Nilotinib
    (D) Ponatinib

4.  A 73-year-old woman was recently diagnosed with chronic phase chronic myeloid leukemia. She has a history of coronary artery disease and mild ischemic cardiomyopathy. She was started on imatinib as initial tyrosine kinase inhibitor therapy. You are now seeing her in follow-up, 3 months after initiating imatinib. Laboratory evaluation from today reveals normal complete blood counts; fluorescent in situ hybridization for BCR–ABL fusion is positive in 5/200 cells (2.5% of cells) and polymerase chain reaction for BCR–ABL1 transcripts is positive at 7.5% by international scale. What do you recommend?

    (A) Continue imatinib at current dose
    (B) Switch to dasatinib
    (C) Switch to bosutinib
    (D) Switch to ponatinib
    (E) Obtain a mutation analysis

5.  What advantage has been demonstrated by the second-generation tyrosine kinase inhibitors nilotinib and dasatinib over imatinib in phase III clinical trials?

(A) Decreased rates of progression to AP-CML or BP-CML

(B) Improved rates of major molecular response

(C) Improved rates of complete cytogenic response

(D) Improved side effect profiles

(E) Better overall survival

(F) A, B, C

(G) All of the above

6. A 55-year-old woman has been treated with imatinib 400-mg daily for the past 2 years. At her most recent visit, her BCR–ABL polymerase chain reaction was found to be 1.5% on the international scale (IS), an increase from 0.05% on the IS 3 months ago. You order an ABL kinase mutation analysis, which reveals a Y253H mutation in the ATP-binding loop. What is the best next treatment option?

(A) Dasatinib

(B) Interferon

(C) Increase imatinib to 800-mg daily

(D) Ponatinib

7. A 75-year-old man has been treated with dasatinib for frontline therapy of his chronic myeloid leukemia (CML). His polymerase chain reaction for BCR–ABL transcripts begins to rise, and an ABL kinase mutation analysis is obtained, which reveals a T315I mutation. The CML is in chronic phase currently. Which of the following is the best next treatment?

(A) Nilotinib

(B) Ponatinib

(C) Bosutinib

(D) Referral for allogeneic transplant

8. A 40-year-old man with a 2-year history of chronic phase chronic myeloid leukemia, treated with imatinib, with intermittent compliance, is admitted to the hospital with fatigue, night sweats, and bone pain. His polymerase chain reaction for BCR–ABL 6 months into therapy was positive at 26% by international scale. Now, his white blood cell count is elevated to $200,000 \times 10^6$/L, hemoglobin level is 9.8 g/dL, and platelet count is $600,000 \times 10^6$/L. A bone marrow aspirate and biopsy are obtained, showing increased blasts estimated at 35%, immunophenotypically consistent with a lymphoid blast population. Conventional cytogenetics return as +8, t(9;22) [20/20]. An ABL kinase mutation analysis is negative. Which of the following is the best treatment strategy for this patient?

(A) Induction chemotherapy

(B) Increase Imatininb dose to 600-mg daily

(C) Any tyrosine kinase inhibitor plus chemotherapy followed by allogeneic stem cell transplantation (ASCT)

(D) Immediate ASCT

## REFERENCES

1. Cortes JE, Silver RT, Khoury J, et al. Chronic myeloid leukemia. *Cancer Manag J Oncol.* 2013: 1–4.

2. Sokal JE, Cox EB, Baccarani M, et al. Prognostic discrimination in "good-risk" chronic granulocytic leukemia. *Blood.* 1984;63(4):789–799.

3. Druker BJ, Guilhot F, O'Brien SG, et al.; IRIS Investigators. Five-year follow-up of patients receiving imatinib for chronic myeloid leukemia. *N Engl J Med.* 2006;355(23):2408–2417.

4. Baccarani M, Cortes J, Pane F, et al.; European LeukemiaNet. Chronic myeloid leukemia: an update of concepts and management recommendations of European LeukemiaNet. *J Clin Oncol.* 2009;27(35):6041–6051.

5. O'Brien SG, Guilhot F, Goldman JM, et al. International Randomized Study of Interferon versus STI571 (IRIS) 7-year follow-up: sustained survival, low rate of transformation and increased rate of major molecular response (MMR) in patients (pts) with newly diagnosed chronic myeloid leukemia in chronic phase (CML-CP) treated with Imatinib (Im). *Blood (ASH Annual Meeting Abstracts).* 2008(Abstract 186).

6. Deininger M, O'Brien SG, Guilhot F, et al. International Randomized Study of Interferon versus STI571 (IRIS) 8-year follow-up: sustained survival and low risk for progression or events in patients with newly diagnosed chronic myeloid leukemia in chronic phase (CML-CP) treated with imatinib. *Blood (ASH Annual Meeting Abstracts).* 2009(Abstract 1126).

7. Kantarjian HM, Talpaz M, O'Brien S, et al. Survival benefit with imatinib mesylate versus interferon-alpha-based regimens in newly diagnosed chronic-phase chronic myelogenous leukemia. *Blood.* 2006;108(6):1835–1840.

8. Roy L, Guilhot J, Krahnke T, et al. Survival advantage from imatinib compared with the combination interferon-alpha plus cytarabine in chronic-phase chronic myelogenous leukemia: historical comparison between two phase 3 trials. *Blood.* 2006;108(5):1478–1484.

9. de Lavallade H, Apperley JF, Khorashad JS, et al. Imatinib for newly diagnosed patients with chronic myeloid leukemia: incidence of sustained responses in an intention-to-treat analysis. *J Clin Oncol.* 2008;26(20):3358–3363.

10. Kim TD, Rea D, Schwarz M, et al. Peripheral artery occlusive disease in chronic phase chronic myeloid leukemia patients treated with nilotinib or imatinib. *Leukemia.* 2013;27(6):1316–1321.

11. Giles FJ, Mauro MJ, Hong F, et al. Rates of peripheral arterial occlusive disease in patients with chronic myeloid leukemia in the chronic phase treated with imatinib, nilotinib, or non-tyrosine kinase therapy: a retrospective cohort analysis. *Leukemia.* 2013;27(6):1310–1315.

12. Cortes JE, Baccarani M, Guilhot F, et al. Phase III, randomized, open-label study of daily imatinib mesylate 400 mg versus 800 mg in patients with newly diagnosed, previously untreated chronic myeloid leukemia in chronic phase using molecular end points: tyrosine kinase inhibitor optimization and selectivity study. *J Clin Oncol.* 2010;28(3):424–430.

13. Baccarani M, Rosti G, Castagnetti F, et al. Comparison of imatinib 400 mg and 800 mg daily in the front-line treatment of high-risk, Philadelphia-positive chronic myeloid leukemia: a European LeukemiaNet Study. *Blood.* 2009;113(19):4497–4504.

14. Saglio G, Kim DW, Issaragrisil S, et al.; ENESTnd Investigators. Nilotinib versus imatinib for newly diagnosed chronic myeloid leukemia. *N Engl J Med.* 2010;362(24):2251–2259.

15. Kantarjian H, Shah NP, Hochhaus A, et al. Dasatinib versus imatinib in newly diagnosed chronic-phase chronic myeloid leukemia. *N Engl J Med.* 2010;362(24):2260–2270.

16. Hughes T, Deininger M, Hochhaus A, et al. Monitoring CML patients responding to treatment with tyrosine kinase inhibitors: review and recommendations for harmonizing current methodology for detecting BCR-ABL transcripts and kinase domain mutations and for expressing results. *Blood.* 2006;108(1):28–37.

17. Quintás-Cardama A, Cortes JE, O'Brien S, et al. Dasatinib early intervention after cytogenetic or hematologic resistance to imatinib in patients with chronic myeloid leukemia. *Cancer.* 2009;115(13):2912–2921.

18. Guilhot F, Larson RA, O'Brien SG, et al. Time to complete cytogenetic response (CCyR) does not affect long-term outcomes for patients on imatinib therapy. *Blood (ASH Annual Meeting Abstracts).* 2007;110(Abstract 27).

19. Quintás-Cardama A, Kantarjian H, Jones D, et al. Delayed achievement of cytogenetic and molecular response is associated with increased risk of progression among patients with chronic myeloid leukemia in early chronic phase receiving high-dose or standard-dose imatinib therapy. *Blood.* 2009;113(25):6315–6321.

20. Branford S, Fletcher L, Cross NC, et al. Desirable performance characteristics for BCR-ABL measurement on an international reporting scale to allow consistent interpretation of individual patient response and comparison of response rates between clinical trials. *Blood.* 2008;112(8):3330–3338.

21. Jabbour E, Kantarjian H, O'Brien S, et al. The achievement of an early complete cytogenetic response is a major determinant for outcome in patients with early chronic phase chronic myeloid leukemia treated with tyrosine kinase inhibitors. *Blood.* 2011;118(17):4541–6; quiz 4759.

22. Hanfstein B, Müller MC, Hehlmann R, et al.; SAKK; German CML Study Group. Early molecular and cytogenetic response is predictive for long-term progression-free and overall survival in chronic myeloid leukemia (CML). *Leukemia.* 2012;26(9):2096–2102.

23. Marin D, Ibrahim AR, Lucas C, et al. Assessment of BCR-ABL1 transcript levels at 3 months is the only requirement for predicting outcome for patients with chronic myeloid leukemia treated with tyrosine kinase inhibitors. *J Clin Oncol.* 2012;30(3):232–238.

24. Mahon FX, Fabères C, Pueyo S, et al. Response at three months is a good predictive factor for newly diagnosed chronic myeloid leukemia patients treated by recombinant interferon-alpha. *Blood.* 1998;92(11):4059–4065.

25. Baccarani M, Cortes J, Pane F, et al.; European LeukemiaNet. Chronic myeloid leukemia: an update of concepts and management recommendations of European LeukemiaNet. *J Clin Oncol.* 2009;27(35):6041–6051.

26. Cortes JE, Kim DW, Pinilla-Ibarz J, et al.; PACE Investigators. A phase 2 trial of ponatinib in Philadelphia chromosome-positive leukemias. *N Engl J Med.* 2013;369(19):1783–1796.

27. Suspension of Marketing and Sales: Iclusig (ponatinib). US Food and Drug Administration website. http://www.fda.gov.proxy. lib.umich.edu/Drugs/InformationOnDrugs/ApprovedDrugs/ucm373072.htm. Accessed October 31, 2013.

28. Cortes J, Khoury HJ, Corm S, et al. Safety and efficacy of subcutaneous (SC) omacetaxine mepesuccinate in imatinib (Im)-resistant chronic myeloid leukemia (CML) patients (pts) with the T315I mutation—results of an ongoing multicenter phase II study. *Blood (ASH Annual Meeting Abstracts).* 2008;112:Abst 3239.

29. Cortes JE, Kantarjian HM, Brümmendorf TH, et al. Safety and efficacy of bosutinib (SKI-606) in chronic phase Philadelphia chromosome-positive chronic myeloid leukemia patients with resistance or intolerance to imatinib. *Blood.* 2011;118(17):4567–4576.

30. Khoury HJ, Cortes JE, Kantarjian HM, et al. Bosutinib is active in chronic phase chronic myeloid leukemia after imatinib and dasatinib and/or nilotinib therapy failure. *Blood.* 2012;119(15):3403–3412.

31. Gambacorti-Passerini C, Cortes JE, Khoury HJ, et al. Safety and efficacy of bosutinib in patients with AP and BP CML and Ph+ ALL following resistance/intolerance to imatinib and other TKIs: update from study SKI-200. *J Clin Oncol.* 2010;28(suppl):6509.

32. Cortes JE, Kim DW, Kantarjian HM, et al. Bosutinib versus imatinib in newly diagnosed chronic-phase chronic myeloid leukemia: results from the BELA trial. *J Clin Oncol.* 2012;30(28):3486–3492.

33. Kantarjian H, Pasquini R, Lévy V, et al. Dasatinib or high-dose imatinib for chronic-phase chronic myeloid leukemia resistant to imatinib at a dose of 400 to 600 milligrams daily: two-year follow-up of a randomized phase 2 study (START R). *Cancer.* 2009;115(18):4136–4147.

34. Shah NP, Kim DW, Kantarjian H, et al. Potent, transient inhibition of BCR-ABL with dasatinib 100 mg daily achieves rapid and durable cytogenetic responses and high transformation-free survival rates in chronic phase chronic myeloid leukemia patients with resistance, suboptimal response or intolerance to imatinib. *Haematologica.* 2010;95(2):232–240.

35. Klyuchnikov E, Schafhausen P, Kröger N, et al. Second-generation tyrosine kinase inhibitors in the post-transplant period in patients with chronic myeloid leukemia or Philadelphia-positive acute lymphoblastic leukemia. *Acta Haematol.* 2009;122(1):6–10.

36. Mahon FX, Réa D, Guilhot J, et al.; Intergroupe Français des Leucémies Myéloïdes Chroniques. Discontinuation of imatinib in patients with chronic myeloid leukaemia who have maintained complete molecular remission for at least 2 years: the prospective, multicentre Stop Imatinib (STIM) trial. *Lancet Oncol.* 2010;11(11):1029–1035.

# 31

# Chronic Lymphocytic Leukemia

RAMI N. KHORIATY AND SAMI N. MALEK

## EPIDEMIOLOGY, NATURAL HISTORY, AND RISK FACTORS

In the Western world, chronic lymphocytic leukemia (CLL) is the most common hematologic malignancy (about 30% of all leukemias), whereas in Asia, CLL has a lower incidence (about 5% of all leukemias). In 2014, an estimated 15,720 new CLL cases will be diagnosed in the United States and about 4600 patients will die of the disease. CLL is mainly a disease of the elderly, with a median age at diagnosis of 72 years. The life expectancy of patients with CLL is significantly lower than that of matched controls, but it is also highly variable and influenced by multiple clinical and biological factors. Patients with Rai stage 0, for example, have a life expectancy of about 130 months, whereas patients with Rai stage III or IV have a life expectancy of about 60–70 months. Patients within the same Rai stage may display diverse clinical behavior. To address the limitation of the clinical CLL staging system (in particular Rai stages 0–II), multiple laboratory variables have been developed as prognostic markers for CLL (discussed in detail in the first case and reviewed by Malek) (1).

Traditionally, CLL has been regarded as an accumulative disease with defects in apoptosis. Recent evidence indicates that CLL has a proliferative fraction that is primarily located in the lymph nodes (LNs) and the bone marrow. Stimulation of the B-cell receptor by antigens is 1 factor driving CLL proliferation, but the exact etiology of CLL remains uncertain and no gene has been found to be mutated at a high frequency in this disease. In untreated CLL, *SF3B1*, *NOTCH1*, and *TP53* are the most frequently mutated genes, with mutation frequencies of approximately 6–10% each. In relapsed CLL, *TP53* mutation frequency is higher. The 13q14 chromosomal deletion is involved early in CLL pathogenesis and mice with engineered 13q14 deletions develop CLL-like illnesses

after variable latency periods. Although CLL is typically an acquired disorder, a family history of CLL is found in 10% of cases and multiple (>20) gene loci and alleles have been identified that confer incremental risk to CLL development. A positive family history of CLL or other lymphoid malignancy is one of the strongest risk factors for developing the disease. Additional risk factors for development of CLL include older age, male sex (male-to-female ratio of approximately 2:1), and ethnicity. CLL is more common in whites than in African Americans, and is rare in Hispanics, Native Americans, and Asians. CLL is not associated with radiation exposure.

## STAGING

There are 2 major staging systems in CLL; the Rai staging system and the Binet staging system. The original Rai staging system was modified to a simpler classification scheme. Both the Rai and Binet staging systems are easily

| Chronic Lymphocytic Leukemia | | |
| --- | --- | --- |
| Rai Stage | Modified Rai Stage | Definition |
| 0 | Low risk | Lymphocytosis only |
| I | Intermediate risk | Lymphocytosis and lymphadenopathy |
| II | Intermediate risk | Lymphocytosis with hepatomegaly or splenomegaly |
| III | High risk | Lymphocytosis and anemia[a] (Hb <11 g/dL) |
| IV | High risk | Lymphocytosis and thrombocytopenia[a] (platelets <100,000/μL) |

[a]Cytopenias must not be immune mediated.

implemented because they rely only on physical examination and a complete blood count (CBC). The Rai system is the most commonly used of these 2 staging systems in the United States.

| Binet Stage | Definition |
|---|---|
| A | <3 nodal sites[a] |
| B | Three or more nodal sites[a] |
| C | Anemia (Hb <10 g/dL) and/or thrombocytopenia (platelets <100,000/µL) |

[a]The sites for Binet staging are cervical (including Waldeyer's ring), axillary (both axillae count as 1 area), inguinal (involvement of both groins is considered as 1 area), spleen, and liver.

From a clinical perspective, the diagnosis of Rai stage III or IV and/or Binet stage C CLL requires that the bone marrow be packed with CLL cells. Otherwise, alternative causes of anemia–thrombocytopenia need to be investigated (discussed further in the last case summary).

## CASE SUMMARIES

### Early-Stage CLL

D.S. is a 73-year-old man referred to the hematology clinic because of incidental lymphocytosis. The patient is asymptomatic; his energy level is good, and he has no fevers, night sweats, or weight loss. His physical examination is normal without palpable lymphadenopathy or hepatosplenomegaly. His CBC shows a white blood cell (WBC) count of 25,000/µL, hemoglobin level of 15 g/dL, and a platelet count of 250,000/µL. The WBC differential is as follows: 90% lymphocytes, 7% neutrophils, and 3% monocytes. A peripheral blood smear shows small mature lymphocytes with a narrow border of cytoplasm and dense nuclei, as well as scattered smudge cells. Flow cytometry shows the following pattern: CD5+, CD10–, CD19+, CD20 (dim), CD23+, and surface immunoglobulin (sIg) dim. The lymphocytes are lambda restricted. Fluorescent in-situ hybridization (FISH) testing shows del 13q14 as the sole abnormality in 68% of the nuclei. Zeta-associated protein of 70-kDa (ZAP-70) expression by flow cytometry in the CD5+/CD19+ cells is negative (<20%), immunoglobulin variable region heavy chain (IGVH) gene mutation analysis discloses a mutated genotype (94.5% homology to germ line), and CD38 expression by flow cytometry is negative (<30%).

### Evidence-Based Case Discussion

D.S. is an elderly patient with asymptomatic lymphocytosis. The most common presentation of CLL is incidental lymphocytosis or asymptomatic lymphadenopathy. Signs and symptoms related to CLL may include fatigue and malaise (most common); early satiety or abdominal discomfort secondary to splenomegaly; B symptoms: fevers, night sweats, and weight loss (<10% incidence); recurrent infections (rare); and autoimmune cytopenias (approximately 15% incidence).

The differential diagnosis of CLL includes various lymphomas (mantle cell lymphoma, marginal zone lymphoma (MZL), lymphoplasmacytic lymphoma, and follicular lymphoma); leukemias (prolymphocytic leukemia [PLL], hairy cell leukemia, and large granular lymphocytic leukemia); reactive lymphocytosis, and monoclonal B-cell lymphocytosis (MBL). The diagnosis of CLL must be confirmed before making any therapeutic plans. All of the following criteria should be met: (a) the peripheral blood monoclonal B-lymphocytes count must be ≥5000/µL; (b) the immunophenotype of the peripheral blood lymphocytes should be characteristic of CLL; and (c) prolymphocytes should not comprise >55% of the lymphocytes. Flow cytometry provides indirect evidence for clonality of the B cells by demonstrating uniform expression of either kappa or lambda immunoglobulin light chains and confirms the characteristic immunophenotype of the CLL cells. CLL cells typically coexpress the T-cell antigen CD5, the B-cell markers CD19 and CD23, and have characteristically dim expression of CD20, CD79b, and sIgs (dimmer in the CLL cells compared to normal B cells). CLL can be distinguished from other lymphomas by a distinct immunophenotypic pattern (Table 31.1). Positive expression of CD5, CD19, and CD20 is shared only by CLL and mantle cell lymphoma (rarely observed in the leukemic phase of diffuse large B-cell lymphoma [DLBCL] or MZL). Unlike CLL, mantle cell lymphoma cells typically do not express CD23, and have the characteristic translocation t(11;14) resulting in aberrant expression of cyclin D1 (this translocation should be tested in the CLL FISH panel test). In rare cases, the mantle cell lymphoma cells may express CD23 or lack t(11;14) or cyclin D1 expression, and the CLL cells may lack CD23 expression (atypical CLL). In those situations, the degree of expression of CD20 and sIg is helpful in making the distinction between these 2 diseases. CD20 and sIg are characteristically dimly expressed in CLL.

Small lymphocytic lymphoma (SLL), PLL, and MBL may all have the same immunophenotype as CLL. The criteria in distinguishing CLL from these other diseases are summarized in Table 31.2. For clinical purposes, CLL and SLL are the same disease. The progression risk from MBL to CLL is approximately 1%/yr.

Our patient fulfills the diagnostic criteria of CLL. In addition, his peripheral blood smear is classic for CLL and shows small mature lymphocytes, with a narrow border of cytoplasm, and clumped nuclear chromatin. Smudge cells are characteristic of CLL. Our patient's CLL stage is Rai stage 0.

After the diagnosis of CLL is confirmed, the next step in management is to determine whether or not therapy is

**Table 31.1** CLL Can be Differentiated From Other Lymphomas Through Immunophenotyping by Flow Cytometry

| Malignancy | CD5 | CD10 | CD19 | CD23 | sIg | cIg | Cyclin D1 |
|---|---|---|---|---|---|---|---|
| CLL | + | – | + | + | + dim | +/– | – |
| MCL | + | – | + | – | + | – | + |
| FL | – | + | + | – | + | – | – |
| Splenic MZL | – | – | + | – | + | +/– | – |
| MZL | +/– | – | + | +/– | + | +/– | – |
| LPL | – | – | + | – | + | + | – |

– Indicates >90% negative; + indicates >90% positive. cIg, cytoplasmic immunoglobulin; CLL, chronic lymphocytic leukemia; FL, follicular lymphoma; LPL, lymphoplasmacytic lymphoma; MCL, mantle cell lymphoma; MZL, marginal zone lymphoma; sIg, surface immunoglobulin.

**Table 31.2** Comparison of CLL and Other Diseases That Have a Similar Immunophenotypic Pattern

| | Clonal B Cells of CLL Phenotype | Monoclonal Peripheral B Cells ≥5000 / μL | LN Enlarge- ment or HSM | Prolym- phocytes ≥55% |
|---|---|---|---|---|
| CLL | + | + | +/– | – |
| SLL | + | – | + | – |
| MBL[a] | + | – | – | – |
| PLL | +/–[b] | + | +/– | + |

CLL, chronic lymphocytic leukemia; HSM, hepatosplenomegaly; LN, lymph node; MBL, monoclonal B-cell lymphocytosis; PLL, prolymphocytic leukemia; SLL, small lymphocytic lymphoma.

[a]In order for a diagnosis of MBL to be made, patients should not have cytopenias or disease-related symptoms. MBL without CD5 expression exists.

[b]It is important to mention that about one half of patients with PLL are CD5⁻.

required. The initiation of treatment in early-stage asymptomatic CLL does not impact survival, although published clinical trials employed low potency drugs. Therefore, asymptomatic CLL patients with Rai stage 0 should be monitored closely without starting therapy. One of the following consensus criteria defined by the International Workshop on CLL (IWCLL) should be met in order to justify starting therapy in patients with CLL (2): (a) new or worsening anemia or thrombocytopenia from marrow failure; (b) symptomatic, progressive, or massive lymphoid tissue enlargement (massive is defined as spleen >6 cm below the left costal margin, or LN >10 cm in longest diameter); (c) autoimmune hemolytic anemia (AIHA) or autoimmune thrombocytopenia that is poorly responsive to steroids or other standard therapy; (d) lymphocyte doubling time of <6 months or >50% increase in absolute lymphocyte count (ALC) over a period of 2 months (this criterion should not be used in patients with ALC <30,000; additionally infections as a cause of worsening lymphocytosis need to be ruled out); and (e) fevers (>100.5°F or >38.0°C for >2 weeks with no proof of infection), night sweats (for >1 month with no evidence of infection), unintentional weight loss (≥10% over a 6-month period), and fatigue (Eastern Cooperative Oncology Group [ECOG] performance status of ≥2). An elevated WBC count alone, is not a reason to treat patients with CLL. The same is true for hypogammaglobulinemia and paraproteinemia. In the author's clinic, >90% of patients are treated based on the first 2 listed criteria.

Our patient has asymptomatic Rai stage 0 CLL and does not have any criteria for treatment. Therefore, the patient should be monitored closely.

The median overall survival (OS) of patients with Rai stages 0, I, II, III, and IV CLL are 130, 106, 88, 58, and 69 months, respectively, but prognostication based on Rai stage alone should be done with caution. Multiple biological variables have been found to predict outcome of CLL patients (1). One of the most important and robust prognostic tests is the clinically available CLL FISH panel. FISH can identify abnormalities in >80% of patients with CLL. Del 13q (found in approximately 50% of the cases), del 11q (15%), trisomy 12 (20%), del 17p (approximately 7–10%), and complex FISH (≥2 FISH findings found in approximately 10% of CLL) are the most common of these abnormalities and are prognostic for both OS and treatment-free survival. Compared to patients with normal karyotypes (median OS > 10 years), del 17p and del 11q portend a poorer prognosis (median OS of approximately 3–5 years and 7 years, respectively), trisomy 12 predicts an intermediate prognosis (median OS of approximately 10 years), and isolated del 13q portends a "favorable" prognosis (median OS >10 years). Complex FISH karyotype also predicts a poor prognosis (OS of approximately 3–8 years). However, with changes in CLL therapies, the value of a FISH-based CLL prognostic system needs reassessment. Importantly, >90% of all cases of del 17p CLL show mutation of the second copy of *TP53*. CLL patients with mutated *TP53* have been found to have a poor prognosis regardless of the presence or absence of del 17p (rare isolated mono-allelic *TP53* mutations). Other molecular–biological factors that predict outcome in CLL are IGVH mutation status, high CD49 expression, *SF3B1* mutations, high ZAP-70 expression, and high CD38 protein expression.

About 60% of all CLL patients have mutated *IGVH* (*M-IGVH*), defined as <98% homology with the germline sequences. *M-IGVH* generally portends an excellent OS; however, patients expressing the *VH3–21* gene usually belong to the *M-IGVH* group; but their survival is as poor as that of patients with unmutated *IGVH* (*U-IGVH*). Positive ZAP-70 expression was initially thought to be a surrogate of *U-IGVH* CLL, but proved to be an independent predictor of short time to treatment (TTT). ZAP-70 is a flow cytometric test and should be measured in $CD19^+/CD5^+$ cells. ZAP-70 expression >20% is considered positive; nonetheless, lower expression may also be associated with a short TTT. Regarding CD38, the optimal cutoff of positive expression is controversial (>30% is considered positive by most investigators). Bimodal expression of CD38 could be seen in some patients. High CD38 expression predicts short TTT. Mounting evidence suggests that *SF3B1* mutations and high CD49 expression by flow cytometry independently confer a poor prognosis in CLL, with shorter TTT and worsened survival.

In clinical practice, a combination of molecular factors including FISH testing appears to provide the most accurate prognostic classification. The CLL Research Consortium assessed the relative impacts of *IGVH*, ZAP-70, and CD38 in predicting TTT in CLL, and showed that patients can be grouped into 3 risk groups: low-, intermediate-, and high-risk groups (3). Patients who are ZAP-70 positive are at high risk for short TTT, while patients with ZAP-70 negative CLL can be classified into intermediate risk if *IGVH* is unmutated, and low risk if *IGVH* is mutated. CD38 has no added prognostic significance to ZAP-70 and IGVH. However, given persistent difficulties in measuring ZAP-70 accurately in the routine clinical setting, testing is not advised.

Our patient has good prognostic features including del 13q as a sole abnormality on FISH, negative ZAP-70, *M-IGVH*, and negative CD38. We predict that the patient will not require therapy for his CLL for many years.

## First-Line Therapy in Advanced CLL

D.S. is a 61-year-old gentleman diagnosed with CLL 3 years ago. FISH testing at diagnosis showed del 11q as the sole abnormality. He was observed closely with physical examinations and serial CBCs. On his most recent follow-up, he is asymptomatic and his ECOG performance status is 0. He has 3 palpable cervical LNs (all <3 cm in size), and his spleen is palpable 8 cm below the left costal margin. His ALC, which was 9000/µL at diagnosis, has reached 160,000/µL. The patient's hemoglobin level is 9.5 g/dL, and his platelet count is 90,000/µL. Lactate dehydrogenase (LDH) is 160 IU/L (normal 120–240 IU/L), and reticulocyte percentage is 0.5%. A bone marrow aspirate and biopsy show that the majority of the marrow space is occupied by CLL cells.

## Evidence-Based Case Discussion

D.S. now has Rai stage IV CLL. He has multiple indications for therapy including massive splenomegaly, and anemia and thrombocytopenia resulting from marrow failure.

Monotherapy with alkylating agents has long been used for frontline treatment of CLL. Chlorambucil (Clb) has been regarded as the "gold standard" first-line therapeutic option in CLL for many decades. More recently, fludarabine (F), bendamustine (B), and alemtuzumab (A) were each compared head to head to Clb in first-line CLL in phase III randomized control trials (reviewed in Refs. 4,5). These trials showed superiority of single-agent F, single-agent B, and single-agent A over Clb in terms of improved response rates and progression-free survival (PFS). F was also compared with other alkylator combination regimens, CAP (cyclophosphamide, doxorubicin, and prednisone) and CHOP (cyclophosphamide, doxorubicin, vincristine, and prednisone) and the results were in favor of F. Other purine analogs, cladribine (Cla) and pentostatin, are active in CLL as well.

Fludarabine and cyclophosphamide (FC) were found to have synergistic cytotoxicity in CLL cells. Three randomized control trials compared FC with F in first-line CLL and showed superiority of FC, with improved complete response (CR and PFS) (4,5). FC did not result in an increased rate of severe infections compared to F. Another purine analog, Cla was also combined with cyclophosphamide (C) in clinical trials. One trial compared Cla alone versus Cla and cyclophosphamide (C) versus Cla, C, and mitoxantrone (M), and showed superior CR with the 3-drug combination, and a trend toward superior CR with the 2-drug combination compared to Cla alone; however, the PFS was fairly similar among the 3 groups. The combination Cla and C was equally effective and safe as FC in first-line CLL.

Fludarabine and rituximab (FR) also showed synergistic activity in preclinical studies in CLL. The Cancer and Leukemia Group B (CALGB) 9712 phase II randomized control trial compared concurrent FR followed by 4 weekly doses of R to single-agent F followed by 4 weekly R infusions (6). The response rates (CR and overall response rate [ORR]) were higher in the concurrent group. When these patients were compared retrospectively to patients enrolled in the previous CALGB trial (CALGB 9011) where therapy was with F only, patients receiving FR had a better PFS and OS than patients receiving F only (7).

The combination FCR, pioneered by Dr. Keating, showed very promising results in a large phase II study conducted at the MD Anderson Cancer Center (8). This led the German CLL Study Group (GCLLSG) to conduct a phase III randomized trial (CLL 8 trial) comparing FCR with FC in frontline CLL (9). This trial showed superiority of FCR in terms of response rates (ORR and CR), PFS, as well as OS (although the OS benefit was modest). The benefit of FCR was at a cost of increased grade 3 or 4 neutropenia (34% vs. 21%), but there was no increase in treatment-related mortality (2% with FCR and 1.5% with FC). All cytogenetic prognostic subgroups benefited from FCR with the exception of patients with del 17p (see the third case #for treatment of CLL patients with del 17p). Specifically, in the subgroup of patients with del 11q (as in the case of our patient), the addition of R to FC resulted in a 3-fold increase in the rate of CR from 15.5% to 53.2%, and marked statistically significant improvement in PFS and OS. The results of this study suggest that FCR may overcome the negative prognostic impact of del 11q, and that del 11q is likely a predictive marker for increased benefit from FCR therapy. It is important to note that 8 patients out of 300 enrolled in the MD Anderson phase II FCR study developed treatment-related myelodysplastic syndrome (MDS) (8), a life-threatening complication and that patients older than 70 years did not benefit from FCR.

Multiple modifications have been made to the FCR regimen in an attempt to reduce its toxicity. The FCR-Lite regimen using reduced doses of F and C, and an intensified R schedule followed by R maintenance demonstrated promising results with a lower rate of grade 3 or 4 neutropenia (13%) than that observed in FCR (10). Another variation in FCR was the substitution of pentostatin (P) for F with the hope of reducing the myelotoxicity of FCR. A phase II trial of PCR in untreated CLL patients showed promising results with a fairly low toxicity profile; grade 3 or 4 neutropenia only occurred in 16% of the cycles (41% of the patients). Patients older than 70 years had a similar benefit without excess morbidity or adverse outcomes compared to patients younger than 70 years (11). PCR was then compared to FCR in a phase III community-based randomized trial in untreated or minimally treated CLL patients. There was no difference in the ORR and OS between PCR and FCR. The infection rate—the primary end point of the trial—was not different between both arms of the study (12). However, it is important to note that the P dose was higher in this phase III trial (4 mg/m$^2$) compared to the P dose in the phase II PCR trial (2 mg/m$^2$) mentioned previously, and that the FCR schedule and dose were different from the traditional FCR regimen, making it difficult to make comparisons between the more traditional PCR and FCR regimens. Another promising chemoimmunotherapy (CIT) regimen in CLL is B + R (BR). BR showed encouraging results in a phase II CLL trial, which led to a phase III GCLLSG trial comparing BR to FCR in previously untreated CLL patients. Planned interim analysis of this trial demonstrated that FCR-treated patients had higher CR rates than BR-treated patients (47% vs. 38%, respectively) as well as higher rates of PFS at 2 years

(85% and 78%, respectively). This benefit was offset by an increased rate of severe adverse events in patients treated with FCR, including a higher risk of severe infections as compared to BR-treated patients (39% and 25.4%, respectively). An OS difference was not apparent between patients treated with FCR compared to BR in the interim analysis (13).

Attempts have been made to eliminate chemotherapy altogether from first-line CLL therapy, particularly because some patients have many comorbidities and a poor performance status. A phase II trial of high-dose methylprednisolone and weekly R (R-HDMP) in previously untreated CLL patients showed encouraging results (even in patients with del 17p), but long-term follow-up data are not available (14). This regimen was fairly well tolerated and non-myelotoxic, but was associated with frequent infections despite prophylaxis. R-HDMP is a reasonable consideration in patients with baseline cytopenias, elderly patients with poor performance status, and patients with del 17p. Early-phase clinical trials incorporating new agents (such as the PI3 kinase delta inhibitor idelalisib or the Bruton tyrosine kinase inhibitor ibrutinib) in frontline CLL therapy are promising. Phase III clinical trials with these agents in the frontline setting are currently planned/underway, the results of which may transform the approach to CLL therapy.

In summary, current evidence supports the use of CIT in frontline CLL therapy. The 4 best-studied CIT regimens in this setting are FR, FCR, PCR, and BR. There is growing evidence that FCR abrogates the poor prognostic impact of del 11q; thus, we favor FCR in young and medically fit patients. In all other circumstances, awaiting the results of the CALGB phase III randomized clinical trial comparing FR and FCR, and the final results of the GCLLSG trial comparing FCR and BR in frontline CLL therapy, we favor using FR or BR, given their lower toxicity profiles.

Our patient is young (<65 years of age) with a good performance status, and has del 11q only. We recommend treating him with FCR. Physicians should be vigilant when administering R with the first cycle of therapy in patients who have an elevated WBC count because of the reported risk of severe tumor lysis syndrome and rarely death, likely secondary to a cytokine storm. We recommend splitting the R dose in the first cycle of therapy, and giving 100 mg on day 1 and the remaining of the R dose on day 2 (high-risk R protocol). Allopurinol should also be given to patients who have a high tumor burden and thus a high risk of tumor lysis syndrome. F is a lymphotoxic agent, and it decreases predominantly the CD4+ cells. Anti-pneumocystis prophylaxis with bactrim should be initiated during therapy, and continued until the CD4 count increases to >200, or alternatively for 1 year after completion of therapy. Herpes simplex virus prophylaxis is also recommended.

## First-Line Therapy in Patients With Deletion 17p

B.P. is a 59-year-old man with CLL diagnosed 1 month ago. He presented with low-grade fevers and night sweats for which he had an extensive negative infectious workup. He has palpable lymphadenopathy (up to 3 cm in diameter) and modest splenomegaly. His CBC shows a WBC count of 75,000/µL (ALC 69,000/µL), a hemoglobin level of 9 g/dL, and a platelet count of 80,000/µL. LDH, haptoglobin, and indirect bilirubin are normal. Bone marrow biopsy shows that the majority of the marrow space is occupied by CLL cells. CLL FISH panel shows del 17p together with del 13q.

## Evidence-Based Case Discussion

B.P. is a relatively young patient with symptomatic Rai stage IV CLL characterized by del 17p and lack of bulky lymphadenopathy.

Symptomatic CLL patients with del 17p or *TP53* mutation have a poor prognosis. There is no widely accepted standard of care in this setting. The response rate of these patients to F or FC is poor. The ORR to FCR is higher (68%), with a 5% rate of CR; however, the duration of response remains fairly short (11.3 months). The 3-year OS of patients with del 17p treated with FR is 33%, compared to 53% in patients with del 11q and 86% in patients with normal cytogenetics. In the GCLLSG randomized trial of first-line FC versus FCR, the 3-year survival of patients with del 17p was not improved with CIT (37% with FC vs. 38% with FCR) (9).

Agents that act independently of the DNA damage pathway and/or p53 have been studied in frontline treatment of del 17p CLL. Single-agent A, for example, results in an ORR of 64% and a PFS of only 10.7 months in this setting (15). In an attempt to improve outcomes, a phase II clinical trial combined A with methylprednisolone in CLL patients with *TP53* deletion. In this study, previously untreated patients exhibited ORR = 88%, CR = 65%, PFS = 18 months, and OS = 39 months (a subset of patients in this study underwent allogeneic stem cell transplantation [ASCT]) (16). In another trial, del 17p CLL patients receiving frontline therapy with A combined with dexamethasone also exhibited encouraging outcomes: ORR 98%, CR 19%, PFS 38 months, and median OS not reached at 36 months. About two thirds of patients enrolled in the latter trial received maintenance A for upto 2 years or underwent ASCT. There was a trend for improved outcomes with ASCT compared to maintenance A, though more follow-up time and a multivariate analysis are needed to confirm this trend (17).

ASCT is currently the only treatment that may provide prolonged survival in this CLL group. There is mounting evidence that ASCT may partially mitigate the unfavorable prognostic impact of del 17p (18). The treatment strategy for patients with del 17p is therefore distinct from other CLL patients (Figure 31.1). In the absence of a clinical trial, CLL patients with del 17p or *TP53* mutation should be treated with an A-containing regimen (A, AR, A + methylprednisolonene/dexamethasone) or with FCR, followed by reduced-intensity ASCT (RI-ASCT) in first remission, if transplant eligible. R-HDMP is another regimen that could be used prior to ASCT (see the previous case).

RI-ASCT rather than myeloablative ASCT represents the standard ASCT modality in CLL (15). However, in young patients with a good performance status and poorly controlled disease, myeloablative ASCT may be the preferred option. A matched sibling donor is preferred over a matched unrelated donor (MUD) whenever possible, but MUD is an acceptable alternative in the event that a matched sibling is not available.

B.P. could be treated with a regimen containing A or with FCR, followed by RI-ASCT. Patients with significantly enlarged LNs (particularly when >3 cm) do not respond well to single-agent A, and a combination of HDMP and A is preferred. In patients with >3 cm LNs, FCR followed by ASCT is another option. B.P. and his siblings should have HLA-typing performed; if no siblings match, an unrelated donor search should be initiated. In the near future, frontline treatment of patients with del 17p will likely shift to targeted agents including BTK inhibitors, PI3K inhibitors and BH3 mimetics.

## First-Line Therapy in Elderly CLL Patients

T.L. is a 79-year-old man with a recent diagnosis of CLL. He has early satiety resulting in decreased oral intake and weight loss. The patient's ECOG performance status is 2. On physical examination, he has palpable lymphadenopathy and splenomegaly (spleen palpated about 8 cm below the left costal margin). The patient's CBC shows a WBC count of 80,000/µL (ALC = 71,000/µL), hemoglobin level of 10.5 g/dL, and platelet count of 140,000/µL. His ALC was 30,000/µL 6 months ago. A CLL FISH panel was negative for all the chromosomal abnormalities tested.

## Evidence-Based Case Discussion

T.L. has symptomatic Rai stage III CLL with a rapidly doubling ALC (<6 months' doubling time), and requires therapy. He is elderly with a poor performance status that has important implications for the choice of therapy. The majority of patients with CLL are elderly. The performance status of many of these elderly patients is poor enough that aggressive therapy, like FCR, could not be safely administered. In a single center cohort of 125 elderly patients (including untreated and relapsed patients) who received FC or FCR, the response rates were favorable; however, the toxicity profile was unacceptable (grade 3 or 4 myelotoxicity of 65–82%), resulting in high rates of treatment discontinuation.

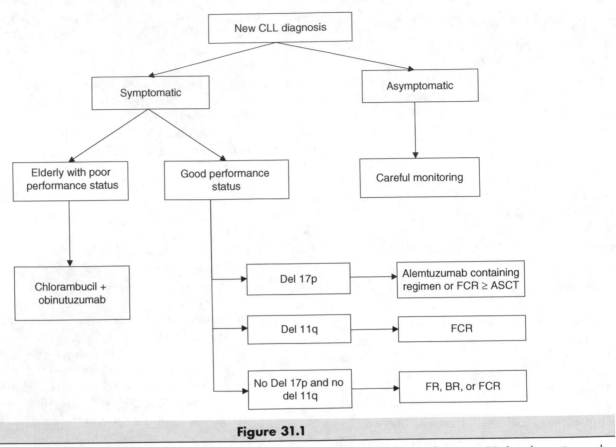

**Figure 31.1**

First-line treatment algorithm for chronic lymphocytic leukemia. ASCT, allogeneic stem cell transplantation; BR, bendamustine and rituximab; CLL, chronic lymphocytic leukemia; FCR, fludarabine, cyclophosphamide, and rituximab; FR, fludarabine and rituximab.

The majority of the CLL trials have enrolled younger patients than the typical CLL population. Therefore, the results of these trials cannot be generalized to the elderly CLL patients. For example, the median age of patients enrolled on the CALGB 9011 trial, which showed superiority of F over Clb, was 62–64 years (19). A similar GCLLSG randomized trial targeting only patients older than 65 showed equivalence of F and Clb in terms of PFS and OS (despite the higher response rates with F), suggesting that Clb is still a valid first-line treatment option in elderly CLL patients who are not candidates for more intensive combination regimens (20). Other agents–regimens that may be considered in elderly CLL patients include the single agents: B, A (for patients with del 17p), and Cla; and the combination BR. Recently, a phase III clinical trial randomized CLL patients with preexisting comorbid conditions (median age = 73 years) to receive Clb alone; Clb + obinutuzumab (a humanized and glycoengineered anti-CD20 monoclonal antibody); or Clb + R as first-line therapy (21). This study demonstrated improved outcomes (ORR, CR, and PFS) with the addition of an anti-CD20 monoclonal antibody to Clb, suggesting that elderly patients (or patients with comorbidities) may benefit from this approach. Physically fit elderly patients without significant comorbidities may tolerate more intensive

regimens; thus FR and PCR (with a P dose of 2 mg/m$^2$ and not 4 mg/m$^2$) are valid treatment options for these more fit patients (11).

T.L. was treated with Clb plus obinutuzumab.

## Second-Line Therapy in CLL

S.C. is a 64-year-old man, who was diagnosed with CLL 10 years ago. He was treated with FCR 4 years ago. A CLL FISH panel performed before FCR was administered showed trisomy 12 as the sole abnormality. The patient achieved CR after FCR treatment. Nine months ago he showed signs of disease recurrence that manifested as an increase in the ALC to 12,000/µL and palpable lymphadenopathy in the cervical area. His ALC steadily increased reaching 100,000/µL a week ago, and his cervical lymphadenopathy became uncomfortable. Repeat CLL FISH showed trisomy 12 with no other abnormalities. The patient is physically fit with no significant comorbidities, and an ECOG performance status of 0.

## Evidence-Based Case Discussion

S.C. has symptomatic relapsed CLL 3.5 years after FCR, and no del 17p and thus likely has a chemoresponsive disease.

Despite major improvements in first-line therapy in CLL, the vast majority of the patients will relapse (median PFS is approximately 3.5–4 years after FCR). Patients asymptomatic at relapse should be monitored closely, and therapy should be instituted when 1 of the IWCLL criteria (described in the first-line treatment section) develops. Treatment of relapsed CLL is not standardized, and depends on the duration of the first remission, the performance status of the patient, and the presence or absence of del 17p or del 11q or complex FISH findings. In general, if the duration of first remission is >24 months, it is reasonable to repeat the first-line treatment. In patients who are refractory to nucleoside analogs, defined as no response or response lasting <2 years, the outlook is poor and therapy is individualized; enrollment into a well-designed clinical trial is highly recommended. Physically fit patients with del 17p should be treated with an A-containing regimen or novel oral agents, followed by ASCT. Physically fit patients who lack del 17p have a variety of treatment options if a clinical trial is not available, but survival times are short. Treatment options include CIT (if prior therapy only comprised F); A, AR, or A + dexamethasone (if LN <3 cm); BR; or ofatumumab, and should be followed by ASCT.

New therapeutic agents have demonstrated promising results in relapsed CLL, including del 17p CLL. A phase III clinical trial comparing idelalasib + R to placebo + R, demonstrated improved ORR, PFS, and OS in patients randomized to the idelalisib arm (22). A phase I/II clinical trial of ibrutinib in relapsed CLL showed promising results at 26 months of follow-up with ORR = 71%, OS = 83%, and PFS = 75% (23). Bcl-2 inhibitors are currently under evaluation in relapsed CLL. Ongoing and future studies with these agents should provide further insight into their use in relapsed CLL.

S.C. had recurrence of CLL > 2 years after FCR and lacks del 17p. He could be retreated with dose-reduced FCR; other CIT regimens (like FR, BR) may be used as well and may be less toxic.

## AIHA in CLL

D.A. is a 63-year-old man diagnosed with CLL more than a year ago. He has been monitored closely, but has not yet received treatment. His hemoglobin level has fallen from 14 g/dL at diagnosis to 8 g/dL. His WBC count is 17,000/µL and his platelet count is 255,000/µL. LDH is elevated at 650 IU/L (normal = 120–240 IU/L); haptoglobin is undetectable (normal = 22–239 mg/dL); unconjugated bilirubin is 2.5 mg/dL (normal = 0–1 mg/dL); and the absolute reticulocyte count is 150,000/µL. The direct antiglobulin test (DAT) is positive (IgG). A bone marrow aspirate and biopsy show 45% involvement of the marrow space with CLL cells, and an expanded erythroid compartment. The patient is asymptomatic from the CLL standpoint, and his physical examination shows no enlarged lymphadenopathy or splenomegaly.

## Evidence-Based Case Discussion

D.A. has CLL and anemia. His anemia is secondary to autoimmune hemolysis. It is essential to identify the cause of anemia or thrombocytopenia in CLL patients; if the cause is progressive marrow failure from CLL, then treatment of CLL should be instituted. On the other hand, if the anemia or thrombocytopenia is from an autoimmune process, then treatment should be directed toward the autoimmune process. Another rare cause of anemia in CLL is pure red cell aplasia. This diagnosis should be suspected in anemia with no reticulocyte response, and is confirmed by the absence of erythroid precursors in the bone marrow. Viral infections including Epstein–Barr virus, cytomegalovirus, and parvovirus should be ruled out before assuming that pure red cell aplasia is due to an autoimmune process (Figure 31.2).

About 15% of CLL patients develop autoimmune cytopenias (AIHA, idiopathic thrombocytopenic purpura [ITP], and Evans syndrome) in the course of the disease with AIHA being most the most common. Half of autoimmune cytopenias develop during or after therapy. The diagnosis of AIHA relies on a fall in hemoglobin in the absence of bleeding, a positive DAT and laboratory values suggesting hemolysis including elevated LDH, low or undetectable haptoglobin, increased reticulocyte count, and elevated unconjugated bilirubin. Elevation in the mean corpuscular volume (MCV) may be an early diagnostic clue. It is important to note that about 14% of CLL patients with AIHA have a negative DAT, thus a positive DAT is not needed for the diagnosis of AIHA. Conversely, about one third of patients with CLL have a positive DAT during the course of their disease, and most of them do not develop clinically evident AIHA.

There are no randomized controlled trials defining treatment of AIHA in CLL. We follow the algorithm presented in Figure 31.2. Patients who have an indication for CLL treatment should have directed CLL therapy. In patients who do not have an indication for CLL therapy, the first-line treatment of AIHA is prednisone 1 mg/kg/d (capped usually at 80 mg) for 4 weeks together with folic acid and pneumocystis pneumonia prophylaxis, followed by a slow taper (fast tapers are a common cause of relapse). In patients who do not respond to steroids or who relapse during the steroid taper or after steroids withdrawal, the treatment options include rituximab, intravenous immunoglobulins, cyclosporine A, mycophenolate mofetil, azathioprine, daily low-dose oral cyclophosphamide, and rarely alemtuzumab, and splenectomy. We generally recommend a trial of 1 immunosuppressive agent and rituximab before consideration of splenectomy. Treatment-refractory AIHA is an indication for CIT directed at CLL.

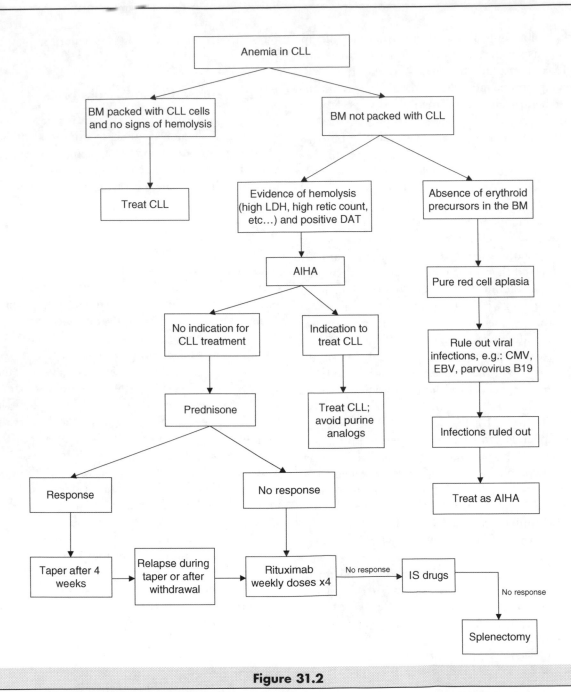

**Figure 31.2**

Treatment algorithm for anemia in chronic lymphocytic leukemia. AIHA, autoimmune hemolytic anemia; BM, bone marrow; CLL, chronic lymphocytic leukemia; CMV, cytomegalovirus; DAT, direct antiglobulin test; EBV, Epstein–Barr virus; LDH, lactate dehydrogenase; IS drugs, immunosuppressive drugs.

In the early 1990s, multiple reports made the observation of severe (and sometimes fatal) AIHA in patients treated with purine analogs (mostly fludarabine). Even though the majority of these cases occurred in heavily pretreated patients and in the setting of active immune cytopenias, it is prudent to avoid fludarabine in patients with active AIHA, and in patients with a history of AIHA (particularly if purine analog induced). Otherwise, among patients who lack a history of AIHA, the latter does not develop more commonly in patients treated with F-containing regimens (4%) compared to patients treated with Clb (5%) (24). Furthermore, the incidence of AIHA may be reduced with the addition of C to F (5%), compared to patients receiving F (12%) and patients receiving Clb (12%) (25). In the GCLLSG trial, the incidence of AIHA was 1% with FC and <1% with FCR.

D.A. has AIHA and lacks any indication for CLL therapy. Prednisone is the first-line treatment of choice for his AIHA. If the patient's CLL progresses to the point where it needs to be treated, fludarabine should probably be avoided.

## REVIEW QUESTIONS

1. A 62-year-old gentleman is found to have multiple bilateral enlarged cervical lymphadenopathy on routine physical examination. A core biopsy of an enlarged cervical lymph node demonstrated kappa restricted lymphocytes that are CD5+, CD10−, CD19+, CD20, Dim, CD23+, sIg Dim, and cyclin D1 negative. What is the most likely diagnosis?

   (A) Reactive lymphadenopathy
   (B) Follicular lymphoma
   (C) Small lymphocytic leukemia
   (D) Mantle cell lymphoma
   (E) Diffuse large B-cell lymphoma

2. A 50-year-old woman has a complete blood count (CBC) performed during a routine physical examination that demonstrates a white blood cell (WBC) count of 38,000, hemoglobin level of 15, and platelet count of 320,000. WBC differential shows 88% lymphocytes, 10% neutrophils, 1% monocytes, and 1% eosinophils. Flow cytometry demonstrates lambda-restricted lymphocytes with a characteristic chronic lymphocytic leukemia (CLL) immunophenotype. CLL fluorescent in situ hybridization panel shows del 11q as the sole abnormality. The patient is asymptomatic. A CBC 1 year ago demonstrated a WBC count of 19,000 (85% lymphocytes). Which is the best current treatment option for this patient?

   (A) Fludarabine
   (B) Fludarabine, cyclophosphamide, and rituximab
   (C) Bendamustine and rituximab
   (D) Alemtuzumab
   (E) Observation

3. A 61-year-old woman was diagnosed with chronic lymphocytic leukemia 3 years ago, but has not required therapy thus far. Over the last 2 months, the patient has had significant fatigue on minimal exertion, but no fevers, night sweats, or weight loss. Complete blood count (CBC) demonstrates a white blood cell (WBC) count of 35,000 with 90% lymphocytes, hemoglobin level of 8 (mean corpuscular volume = 85), and platelet count of 300,000. CBC from 3 months ago demonstrated WBC count of 30,000 with 89% lymphocytes, hemoglobin level of 14, and platelet count of 310,000. The patient denies any blood loss. Iron studies, B12, and folic acid levels are normal. Direct antiglobulin test (DAT) is negative. Lactate dehydrogenase is 170 and haptoglobin is 85. Retic count is 0.2%. Which is the next step in the management of the patient?

   (A) Chemoimmunotherapy
   (B) Bone marrow biopsy, polymerase chain reaction for parvovirus B19, Epstein–Barr virus, and cytomegalovirus

   (C) Initiate single-agent rituximab
   (D) Start Prednisone and observe for response
   (E) Observe closely with no therapy

4. A 57-year-old man diagnosed with chronic lymphocytic leukemia (CLL) 5 years ago has not received any CLL therapy. Complete blood count (CBC) from 6 months ago demonstrated a white blood cell (WBC) count of 60,000 (91% lymphocytes), a hemoglobin level of 13, and a platelet count of 185,000. Over the last 3 months, the patient has developed fatigue and drenching night sweats, but no fevers. An extensive infectious workup was negative. There is no lymphadenopathy, but spleen is palpable 8 cm below the left costal margin. CBC showed a WBC count of 86,000 (89% lymphocytes), a hemoglobin level of 11.5, and a platelet count of 125,000. CLL fluorescent in situ hybridization panel demonstrates del 11q as the sole abnormality. The patient's current Eastern Cooperative Oncology Group performance status is 1. Which is the best treatment option for the patient?

   (A) Fludarabine, cyclophosphamide, and rituximab
   (B) Alemtuzumab
   (C) Fludarabine and rituximab
   (D) Broad spectrum antibiotics and continued observation of CLL
   (E) Chlorambucil plus obinutuzumab

5. The patient is a 76-year-old lady recently diagnosed with chronic lymphocytic leukemia. Her physical examination is normal with no palpable lymphadenopathy or splenomegaly. Her most recent complete blood count demonstrates a white blood cell count of 66,000 (87% lymphocytes), a hemoglobin level of 9, and a platelet count of 82,000. A bone marrow biopsy demonstrated that the marrow space is packed with lambda restricted CD5+, CD19+, CD23+, and cyclin D1 negative lymphocytes. The Eastern Cooperative Oncology Group performance status is 2. Which of the following is the best treatment option?

   (A) Fludarabine and rituximab
   (B) Fludarabine, cyclophosphamide, and rituximab
   (C) Chlorambucil plus obinutuzumab
   (D) Chlorambucil
   (E) Observation

6. A 64-year-old man with untreated chronic lymphocytic leukemia (CLL) presents with an absolute lymphocyte count (ALC) of 135,000. Five years ago at diagnosis his ALC was 13,000 and 6 months ago his ALC was 40,000. Physical examination demonstrates scattered palpable lymphadenopathy (2–3 cm in size) and splenomegaly (spleen palpated 7 cm below the left costal margin). His hemoglobin level is 11 and his platelet

count is 110,000. CLL fluorescent in situ hybridization panel demonstrated del 17p. Performance status is excellent. Which of the following is not an appropriate treatment option?

(A) Fludarabine, cyclophosphamide, and rituximab followed by reduced intensity allogeneic stem cell transplantation (ASCT)
(B) Chlorambucil followed by reduced intensity ASCT
(C) High-dose methylprednisolone plus rituximab followed by reduced intensity ASCT
(D) Fludarabine and rituximab followed by reduced intensity ASCT
(E) Alemtuzumab plus high-dose methylprednisolone followed by reduced intensity ASCT

7. A 62-year-old man was diagnosed with chronic lymphocytic leukemia 5 years ago. He was observed initially, and 2 years ago he received fludarabine, cyclophosphamide, and rituximab (FCR). Over the last 6 months, his disease has progressed and currently needs to be treated. The patient has no comorbidities and his Eastern Cooperative Oncology Group performance status is 0–1. Which of the following is the best treatment option?

(A) Chemoimmunotherapy followed by reduced intensity allogeneic stem cell transplantation
(B) FCR
(C) Alemtuzumab
(D) Lenalidomide and rituximab
(E) Chemoimmunotherapy followed by autologous stem cell transplantation

8. Prophylaxis against which infectious pathogen/ pathogens is recommended for patients receiving fludarabine-based therapy for chronic lymphocytic leukemia?

(A) Bacteria
(B) Herpes simplex virus
(C) Bacteria, herpes simplex virus, and pneumocystis pneumonia
(D) Herpes simplex virus and pneumocystis pneumonia

9. All the following laboratory tests have prognostic value in chronic lymphocytic leukemia (CLL) except:

(A) CLL fluorescent in situ hybridization test
(B) Albumin
(C) Immunoglobulin heavy chain variable region gene mutation status
(D) p53 mutation
(E) Complex karyotypes

10. A 73-year-old woman with chronic obstructive pulmonary disease and coronary artery disease was diagnosed with chronic lymphocytic leukemia 4 years ago. She underwent therapy with reduced dose bendamustine plus rituximab and achieved a partial response. Recently, her disease progressed and therapy is indicated. Her Eastern Cooperative Oncology Group performance status is currently 2. Which of the following is the best treatment option for the patient?

(A) Fludarabine and rituximab
(B) Fludarabine, cyclophosphamide, and rituximab
(C) Ibrutinib
(D) Chemoimmunotherapy followed by reduced intensity allogeneic stem cell transplantation
(E) Single-agent rituximab

## REFERENCES

1. Malek SN. Clinical utility of prognostic markers in chronic lymphocytic leukemia. In: *The American Society of Clinical Oncology Education Book*; 2010:263–267.
2. Hallek M, Cheson BD, Catovsky D, et al.; International Workshop on Chronic Lymphocytic Leukemia. Guidelines for the diagnosis and treatment of chronic lymphocytic leukemia: a report from the International Workshop on Chronic Lymphocytic Leukemia updating the National Cancer Institute-Working Group 1996 guidelines. *Blood*. 2008;111(12):5446–5456.
3. Rassenti LZ, Jain S, Keating MJ, et al. Relative value of ZAP-70, CD38, and immunoglobulin mutation status in predicting aggressive disease in chronic lymphocytic leukemia. *Blood*. 2008;112(5):1923–1930.
4. Foon KA, Hallek MJ. Changing paradigms in the treatment of chronic lymphocytic leukemia. *Leukemia*. 2010;24(3):500–511.
5. Hallek M. State-of-the-art treatment of chronic lymphocytic leukemia. *Hematology Am Soc Hematol Educ Program*. 2009: 440–449.
6. Byrd JC, Peterson BL, Morrison VA, et al. Randomized phase 2 study of fludarabine with concurrent versus sequential treatment with rituximab in symptomatic, untreated patients with B-cell chronic lymphocytic leukemia: results from Cancer and Leukemia Group B 9712 (CALGB 9712). *Blood*. 2003;101(1):6–14.
7. Byrd JC, Rai K, Peterson BL, et al. Addition of rituximab to fludarabine may prolong progression-free survival and overall survival in patients with previously untreated chronic lymphocytic leukemia: an updated retrospective comparative analysis of CALGB 9712 and CALGB 9011. *Blood*. 2005;105(1): 49–53.
8. Tam CS, O'Brien S, Wierda W, et al. Long-term results of the fludarabine, cyclophosphamide, and rituximab regimen as initial therapy of chronic lymphocytic leukemia. *Blood*. 2008;112(4):975–980.
9. Hallek M, Fischer K, Fingerle-Rowson G, et al.; International Group of Investigators; German Chronic Lymphocytic Leukaemia Study Group. Addition of rituximab to fludarabine and cyclophosphamide in patients with chronic lymphocytic leukaemia: a randomised, open-label, phase 3 trial. *Lancet*. 2010;376(9747):1164–1174.
10. Foon KA, Boyiadzis M, Land SR, et al. Chemoimmunotherapy with low-dose fludarabine and cyclophosphamide and high dose rituximab in previously untreated patients with chronic lymphocytic leukemia. *J Clin Oncol*. 2009;27(4):498–503.
11. Kay NE, Geyer SM, Call TG, et al. Combination chemoimmunotherapy with pentostatin, cyclophosphamide, and rituximab shows significant clinical activity with low accompanying toxicity in previously untreated B chronic lymphocytic leukemia. *Blood*. 2007;109(2):405–411.
12. Reynolds C, DiBella N, Lyons RM, et al. Phase III trial of fludarabine, cyclophosphamide, and rituximab vs.

pentostatin, cyclophosphamide and rituximab in B-cell chronic lymphocytic leukemia. *Blood (ASH Annual Meeting Abstracts)*. 2008;112:abstract 327.

13. Eichhorst B, Fink AM, Busch R, et al. Chemoimmunotherapy with fludarabine, cyclophosphamide, and rituximab versus bendamustine and rituximab in previously untreated and physically fit patients with advanced chronic lymphocytic leukemia: results of a planned interim analysis of the CLL10 trial, and international, randomized study of the German CLL study group (GCLLSG). *Am Soc Hemat*. 2013(abstract 526).

14. Castro JE, James DF, Sandoval-Sus JD, et al. Rituximab in combination with high-dose methylprednisolone for the treatment of chronic lymphocytic leukemia. *Leukemia*. 2009;23(10): 1779–1789.

15. Hillmen P, Skotnicki AB, Robak T, et al. Alemtuzumab compared with chlorambucil as first-line therapy for chronic lymphocytic leukemia. *J Clin Oncol*. 2007;25(35):5616–5623.

16. Pettitt AR, Jackson R, Carruthers S, et al. Alemtuzumab in combination with methylprednisolone is a highly effective induction regimen for patients with chronic lymphocytic leukemia and deletion of TP53: final results of the national cancer research institute CLL206 trial. *J Clin Oncol*. 2012;30(14):1647–1655.

17. Stilgenbauer S, Cymbalista F, Leblond V, et al. Alemtuzumab plus dexamethasone followed by alemtuzumab maintenance or allogeneic transplantation in ultra high-risk CLL: updated results from a phase II study of the GCLLSG and FCGCLL/MW. *Am Soc Hematol*. 2012:abstract 716.

18. Dreger P. Allotransplantation for chronic lymphocytic leukemia. *Hematol Am Soc Hematol Educ Prog*. 2009:602–609.

19. Rai KR, Peterson BL, Appelbaum FR, et al. Fludarabine compared with chlorambucil as primary therapy for chronic lymphocytic leukemia. *N Engl J Med*. 2000;343(24):1750–1757.

20. Eichhorst BF, Busch R, Stilgenbauer S, et al.; German CLL Study Group (GCLLSG). First-line therapy with fludarabine compared with chlorambucil does not result in a major benefit for elderly patients with advanced chronic lymphocytic leukemia. *Blood*. 2009;114(16):3382–3391.

21. Goede V, Fischer K, Busch R, et al. Obinutuzumab plus chlorambucil in patients with CLL and coexisting conditions. *N Engl J Med*. 2014;370(12):1101–1110.

22. Furman RR, Sharman JP, Coutre SE, et al. Idelalisib and rituximab in relapsed chronic lymphocytic leukemia. *N Engl J Med*. 2014;370(11):997–1007.

23. Byrd JC, Furman RR, Coutre SE, et al. Targeting BTK with ibrutinib in relapsed chronic lymphocytic leukemia. *N Engl J Med*. 2013;369(1):32–42.

24. Moreno C, Hodgson K, Ferrer G, et al. Autoimmune cytopenia in chronic lymphocytic leukemia: prevalence, clinical associations, and prognostic significance. *Blood*. 2010 (e-pub ahead of print).

25. Dearden C, Wade R, Else M, et al.; UK National Cancer Research Institute (NCRI); Haematological Oncology Clinical Studies Group; NCRI CLL Working Group. The prognostic significance of a positive direct antiglobulin test in chronic lymphocytic leukemia: a beneficial effect of the combination of fludarabine and cyclophosphamide on the incidence of hemolytic anemia. *Blood*. 2008;111(4):1820–1826.

# 32

# Myelodysplastic Syndrome

SUMANA DEVATA, JOHN MAGENAU, AND DALE BIXBY

## EPIDEMIOLOGY, RISK FACTORS, NATURAL HISTORY, AND PATHOLOGY

Myelodysplastic syndrome (MDS) represents a compilation of clonal myeloid neoplasms resulting in various degrees of ineffective hematopoiesis leading to neutropenia, anemia, and/or thrombocytopenia, with anemia being the most common presenting symptom. Because of the asymptomatic nature of early-stage disease that can smolder for years, the reported incidence of approximately 10,000–15,000 cases per year in the United States likely underrepresents the true frequency of the disease. There is a slight male predominance, and the incidence rises exponentially with age, with a median age of 68 years and a peak occurring in the ninth decade of life (1). Nearly all cases of MDS are sporadic rather than familial. However, 5 genes have been linked to a genetically inherited predisposition for the development of MDS or acute myeloid leukemia (AML), including *RUNX1, CEBPA, TERC, TERT,* and *GATA2.* Most of these mutations are somatic rather than congenital (2). A number of rare congenital disorders can also predispose younger patients to the development of MDS, including Down syndrome, neurofibromatosis 1, congenital neutropenia disorders, Fanconi's anemia, and dyskeratosis congenita. Risk factors for development of acquired MDS include exposure to chemotherapeutic agents including alkylators and topoisomerase II inhibitors, high doses of radiation, and solvents such as benzene and carbon tetrachloride. A prior diagnosis of bone marrow (BM) failure disorders, including aplastic anemia or paroxysmal nocturnal hemoglobinuria (PNH), also increases an individual's risk for MDS. However, >95% of patients have no identifiable risk factor other than advanced age.

The term MDS incorporates distinct pathological processes that carry a variable risk for disease progression, including worsening cytopenias and transformation into AML. The diagnosis and classification of MDS is challenging, and the molecular pathogenesis and evolution of the disease is not well understood.

Establishing the diagnosis of MDS includes evaluation of the peripheral blood, a BM aspirate and core biopsy, and cytogenetics to assess for the following (3,4):

(a) Cytopenias: Defined by the World Health Organization (WHO) as hemoglobin <10 g/dL, absolute neutrophil count (ANC) <1.8 × 10$^9$/L, and platelets <100 × 10$^9$/L. If cytopenias do not meet these criteria, but there is a morphological conformation of dysplasia, a diagnosis of MDS can still be established.

(b) Morphological dysplasia: Seen in >10% of at least 1 BM cell line, which includes erythroid, granulocytic, and megakaryocytic lineages. The preferred method of evaluation is via BM aspirate. Secondary causes of dysplasia should be excluded. If a patient presents with cytopenias consistent with MDS but has inconclusive morphological changes, a presumptive diagnosis of MDS can be made if certain specific clonal chromosomal abnormalities are identified (3). Asynchronous expression of maturation-associated antigens on myeloid cells detected by flow cytometry is not considered diagnostic of MDS when morphological features are inconclusive.

(c) Myeloid blast count: An increase in the number of myeloid blasts, but <20% of total cells in the BM or peripheral blood, is evidence of dysplasia.

(d) Cytogenetics: According to the WHO 2008 criteria, 14 recurrent karyotypic abnormalities are recognized as presumptive evidence of MDS, even in the absence of other definitive features. These cases are now included in the "MDS unclassified" subtype. Fluorescent in-situ hybridization (FISH) for specific chromosomal changes can complement standard cytogenetics, but should not replace this testing. Developments in microarray technologies have prompted the application of single-nucleotide polymorphisms (SNPs) for high-resolution genome-wide genotyping in hematological disorders, including MDS. According to the European leukemia net (ELN), the use of routine SNP array testing cannot currently be recommended. In the future, molecular testing may be used to confirm the diagnosis in patients with suspected but morphologically occult MDS.

## TREATMENT CONSIDERATIONS

The Food and Drug Administration (FDA) has approved 3 chemotherapeutic agents, azacitidine (Vidaza; Celgene), decitabine (Dacogen; Eisai), and lenalidomide (Revlimid; Celgene) for the treatment of MDS. Understanding the pathogenesis and prognosis of this clinically heterogeneous disease is increasingly important. Due to an incomplete understanding of the predictive variables for treatment response to individual therapies, a lack of understanding as to the true mechanism of action of these medications, and the dearth of prospective randomized clinical trials, there is a continued challenge in optimally caring for patients with MDS.

## CASE SUMMARIES

### Low-Risk Disease

L.S. is a 68-year-old woman with a prior history of hypertension and hyperlipidemia who presented to her physician for a health maintenance examination. She described some increasing fatigue and mild dyspnea on exertion. A complete blood count (CBC) with differential was performed that demonstrated a white blood cell (WBC) count of $3.3 \, K/mm^3$ (ANC of $1.9 \, K/mm^3$), a hemoglobin of $8.1 \, g/dL$, and a platelet count of $111 \, K/mm^3$. After receiving a red blood cell (RBC) transfusion, a BM biopsy demonstrated an overall cellularity of 80% with trilineage dysplasia in >20% of the myeloid, erythroid, and megakaryocytic progenitor cells. A 500-cell differential of the aspirate smear contained 1.6% blasts. Cytogenetics demonstrated a normal female karyotype in all 20 cells examined: 46, XX [20]. The erythropoietin (EPO) level was 89 mU/mL.

### Evidence-Based Case Discussion

The diagnosis of MDS is established by demonstrating cytologic dysplasia in 1 or more cell lineages together with cytopenias and/or an increase in myeloblasts. Two major classification systems have been developed for MDS, including the French American British (FAB) system and the WHO scheme. The WHO system additionally recognized unilineage versus multilineage dysplasia, delineated sideroblastic anemias into those with and without multilineage dysplasia, incorporated cytogenetic information into subtyping (5q-syndrome), further divided the distinction of refractory anemia with excess blasts based on blast percentage, and lowered the threshold for transformation into AML to the presence of 20% blasts in the peripheral blood or BM (Table 32.1) (5).

Although both the FAB and WHO diagnostic categories stratify prognosis, they were not originally designed to aid in therapeutic decision making. The International MDS Risk Analysis Workshop collected data from 7 prior studies on 816 patients and built a prognostic model based on the BM blast percentage, BM karyotype, and number of cytopenias—termed the International Prognostic Scoring System (IPSS) (Table 32.2) (6). Since the advent of the IPSS in 1997, it has been the standard prognostic tool for stratification of MDS risk. However, the more recently developed revised IPSS score (IPSS-R), was released to address gaps in the predictive utility of the IPSS (7,8). The revised IPSS prognostic score was created by analyzing the outcomes of 7012 MDS cases. It incorporates several additional factors to the IPSS, including additional cytogenetic abnormalities, additional stratification of BM blast percentage, and assigns a prognostic score to the individual cytopenias (Table 32.2). The WHO Prognostic Scoring System (WPSS) has been validated as a system that could be used throughout the disease course. It considers the WHO disease subtype rather than blast percentage and takes into account the number of transfusions received rather than just the number of cytopenias (9). However, few pathology centers report the WHO subtype of the biopsy, limiting the applicability of the system. Moreover, there appears to be a large variability in outcomes in patients designated "low-risk" by the WPSS. The MD Anderson Comprehensive Scoring System (MDS-CSS) was developed after analysis of 1915 patients. This risk model further refines outcomes, segregating patients with traditionally low-risk disease into lower- and higher-risk populations, and includes groups of patients that were excluded in prior models, such as those with previously treated disease, secondary MDS, and chronic myelomonocytic leukemia (CMML) (10).

The IPSS-R stratifies patients into 1 of 5 categories: very low, low, intermediate, high, and very high risk. Patients identified as having very low-risk MDS by the IPSS-R have a median survival of 8.8 years, while patients with low risk according to the IPSS model have a median survival of 5.5 years. Both groups have a low rate of progression to AML, with a 25% rate at 9.4 years in the low-risk IPSS group. At >10 years of follow-up, AML progression in the very low IPSS-R group was under 25%.

The focus of therapy in this patient (IPSS score of 0, low risk; IPSS-R score of 2, low risk) should be symptom control, including correction of transfusion-dependent anemia (Figure 32.1). EPO-stimulating agents (ESAs)—including epoetin alfa (Epogen; Amgen and Procrit; Ortho Biotech) and darbepoetin (Aranesp; Amgen)—can reduce RBC transfusion dependency, especially in patients with low-transfusion needs and a low-endogenous EPO level of <500 mU/mL (Hellström–Lindberg Score—Figure 32.2) (11). Indeed, the Eastern Cooperative Oncology Group (ECOG) published a randomized phase III trial of ESAs with or without myeloid growth factor support compared to best supportive care (BSC) with transfusions alone

**Table 32.1** WHO and FAB Classification Scheme of Myelodysplastic Syndrome

| WHO Classification (15) | | FAB Classification (6) | |
|---|---|---|---|
| Classification | PB and BM Findings | Classification | PB and BM Findings |
| Refractory anemia (RA) | Anemia, <5% blasts, <15% ringed sideroblasts | Refractory anemia (RA) | Anemia, <5% blasts, <15% ringed sideroblasts |
| Refractory anemia with ringed sideroblasts (RARS) | Anemia, <5% blasts, >15% ringed sideroblasts | Refractory anemia with ringed sideroblasts (RARS) | Anemia, <5% blasts, >15% ringed sideroblasts |
| Refractory cytopenia with multilineage dysplasia (RCMD) | Multiple cytopenias and multilineage dysplasia, <5% blasts, >15% ringed sideroblasts | | |
| Refractory cytopenia with multilineage dysplasia and ringed sideroblasts (RCMD-RS) | Multiple cytopenias and multilineage dysplasia, <5% blasts, >15% ringed sideroblasts | | |
| Refractory anemia with excess blasts—type 1 (RAEB-I) | Multiple cytopenias and 5–9% blasts in the BM | Refractory anemia with excess blasts (RAEB) | Multiple cytopenias and 5–20% blasts in the BM |
| Refractory anemia with excess blasts—type 2 (RAEB-II) | Multiple cytopenias and 10–19% blasts in the BM | | |
| Acute myeloid leukemia (AML) | ≥20% blasts in the PB or BM | Refractory anemia with excess blasts in transformation (RAEB-t) | Multiple cytopenias with 21–30% blasts |
| MDS—unclassified (MDS-U) | Multiple cytopenias, but with findings not classifiable in other categories | | |
| MDS associated with isolated del(5q) | Anemia, <5% blasts, normal to elevated platelet count, increased megakaryocytes with hypolobated nuclei, isolated del(5q) on karyotype | | |

BM, bone marrow; FAB; French American British; MDS, myelodysplastic syndrome; PB, peripheral blood; WHO, World Health Organization.

**Table 32.2** Prognostic Scoring Systems in Myelodysplastic Syndrome (MDS)

**International Prognostic Scoring System (IPSS)**

| Entity | Score | | | | |
|---|---|---|---|---|---|
| | 0 | 0.5 | 1.0 | 1.5 | 2 |
| Percentage of bone marrow blasts | <5 | 5–10 | — | 11–20 | >20 |
| Number of cytopenias | 0 or 1 | 2 or 3 | | | |
| Karyotypic risk | Good | Intermediate | Poor | | |

Cytopenias: Hemoglobin <10 g/dL, absolute neutrophil count <1,800/μL, and/or platelet count <100,000/μL.
Karyotype risk: Good: Normal, –Y, del (5q), or del (20q)/Intermediate: all others/Poor: complex karyotype (≥3 abnormalities) or abnormal chromosome 7.
Risk groups: Low—0 points; Intermediate-1 (Int-1)—0.5 to 1 points; Intermediate-2 (Int-2)—1.5 to 2 points; High—2.5 to 3.5 points.
*Source:* From Ref. (6). Greenberg P, Cox C, LeBeau MM, et al. International scoring system for evaluating prognosis in myelodysplastic syndromes. *Blood.* 1997;89(6):2079–2088.

*(continued)*

**Table 32.2** Prognostic Scoring Systems in Myelodysplastic Syndrome (MDS) (continued)

Revised International Prognostic Scoring System (IPSS-R)

| Entity | Score | | | | | | |
|---|---|---|---|---|---|---|---|
| | 0 | 0.5 | 1 | 1.5 | 2 | 3 | 4 |
| Cytogenetics | Very good | | Good | | Intermediate | Poor | Very poor |
| BM blasts (%) | ≤2 | | >2–<5 | | 5–10 | >10 | |
| Hemoglobin, g/dL | ≥10 | | 8–<10 | <8 | | | |
| Platelets, × 10⁹/L | ≥100 | 50–<100 | <50 | | | | |
| ANC, 10⁹/L | ≥0.8 | <0.8 | | | | | |

Cytogenetics: Very good: –Y, del(11q); Good: del (5q), del(12p), del(20q), del(5q) +1 additional; Intermediate: del(7q), +8, +19, i(17q), other abnormalities not in other groups; Poor: –7, inv(3)/t(3q)/del(3q), –7/del(7q) + 1 additional, complex (3 abnormalities); Very poor: complex (>3 abnormalities).
Risk groups: Very low – ≤1.5; low – >1.5–3; intermediate – >3–4.5; high – >4.5–6; very high – >6
ANC, absolute neutrophil count; BM, bone marrow; IPSS, International Prognostic Scoring System.
*Source*: From Ref. (8). Greenberg PL, Tuechler H, Schanz J, et al. Revised international prognostic scoring system for myelodysplastic syndromes. *Blood*. 2012;120(12):2454–2465.

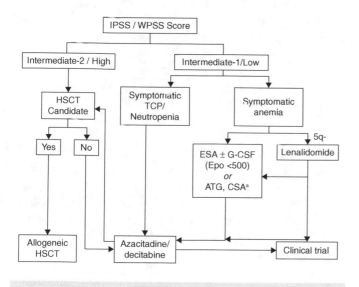

**Figure 32.1**

Treatment algorithm for myelodysplastic syndromes.
ATG, antithymocyte globulin; CSA, cyclosporin A; ESA, erythropoiesis-stimulating agent; G-CSF, granulocyte colony-stimulating factor; HSCT, hematopoietic stem cell transplant; IPSS, international prognostic scoring system; PNH, paroxysmal nocturnal hemoglobinuria; TCP, thrombocytopenia; WPSS, WHO prognostic scoring system.

ᵃConsider for patients ≤60 years, hypocellular marrow, HLA-DR 15, and/or demonstrating a PNH-positive clone.

(12). While there was no difference in progression-free survival (PFS) or overall survival (OS) on an intention-to-treat analysis, the erythroid response rates were higher in the patients receiving ESA support, and survival was longer in those patients responding to ESAs versus non-responders (median, 5.5 vs. 2.3 years). Although ESAs are currently not FDA indicated for use in MDS, they are frequently employed off-label given the benefits noted previously, and are currently recommended by the National Comprehensive Cancer Network (NCCN) guidelines as well as the ELN guidelines. Iron overload may be associated

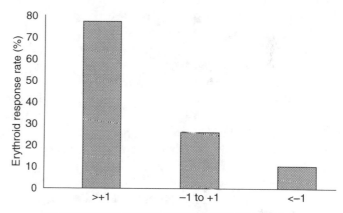

Total Hellström–Lindberg Score

| Factor | Level | Score |
|---|---|---|
| Erythropoietin level (mU/mL) | <100 | +2 |
| | 100–500 | +1 |
| | >500 | –3 |
| RBC transfusions per month | <2 | +2 |
| | ≥2 | –2 |

RBC, red blood cells.

**Figure 32.2**

Hellström–Lindberg predictive model. The graph represents the percentage of transfusion-dependent MDS patients responding to erythropoietin with or without granulocyte colony-stimulating factor (G-CSF). A predictive model was developed based upon a score for the patients' endogenous erythropoietin level (measured in mU/mL) added to the score for the number of red blood cell transfusions received per month. MDS, myelodysplastic syndrome.
*Source*: From Ref. (11). Hellström-Lindberg E, Negrin R, Stein R, et al. Erythroid response to treatment with G-CSF plus erythropoietin for the anaemia of patients with myelodysplastic syndromes: proposal for a predictive model. Br J Haematol. 1997;99(2):344–351.

with poorer survival in lower-risk MDS patients receiving significant RBC transfusion support. However, only retrospective analyses are available describing improved OS in MDS patients receiving iron-chelation therapy (13). Nonetheless, chelation therapy is also recommended by the NCCN, especially in those patients receiving >20 RBC transfusions and having elevated ferritin levels. ELN guidelines also note the limited prospective data and lack of evidence that it impacts OS. Therefore, they advise that iron chelation could be considered in transfusion-dependent patients with RA, refractory anemia with ringed sideroblasts (RARS), or MDS with isolated 5q deletion and a serum ferritin level >1000 ng/mL after approximately 25 units of red cells, but note that this is based upon level 3 and 4 evidence.

In summary, patients with MDS should have a prognosis calculated based on either the IPSS or IPSS-R. Those patients with lower-risk disease (very low-, low- or intermediate-1 [Int-1] risk) should be counseled about average survival and rates of transformation to AML, while understanding that each case is unique and medical observation is continuously required. In the lower-risk population, symptom control with transfusion support and/or the use of growth factors (ESAs) is common, but ESAs should be employed in the appropriate clinical setting (those with a low Hellström–Lindberg score) (11). In this case, L.S. required a transfusion and had an inappropriately normal endogenous EPO level. She had an IPSS score of 0 (low risk) and an IPSS-R score of 2 (low risk). Given that her age is >60 years, a median survival of 2.7 years is predicted based upon the IPSS score. With a Hellström–Lindberg score of +4, she would be predicted to have a 74% chance of an erythroid response to ESAs and can be counseled on their potential use to decrease transfusion needs, with the understanding that there would likely be no OS advantage. In addition, an evaluation of her iron status (ferritin) would be appropriate, and iron chelation may be required if her transfusion needs continue despite ESAs.

## 5q-Syndrome

E.L. is a 78-year-old woman with osteoarthritis and hyperlipidemia who presented with complaints of increasing fatigue and dyspnea on minimal exertion. A CBC with differential was performed and demonstrated a WBC of 5.2 K/mm$^3$ (ANC of 3.1 K/mm$^3$), a hemoglobin of 7.6 g/dL with mean corpuscular volume (MCV) of 102, and a platelet count of 525 K/mm$^3$. She was transfused, and an evaluation demonstrated no evidence of vitamin or mineral deficiency. Endoscopy failed to identify a source of gastrointestinal (GI) blood loss. BM biopsy demonstrated an overall cellularity of 30%, with normal erythroid and granulocytic maturation. Increased numbers of small, unilobate megakaryocytes were seen. A 500-cell

differential of the aspirate smear demonstrated 1.1% blasts. Cytogenetics revealed an abnormal female karyotype: 46,XX,del(5)(q13q33)[16]/46,XX[4]. The EPO level was 510 mU/mL.

### Evidence-Based Case Discussion

In 2000, the WHO began to recognize the central importance of cytogenetic abnormalities in the pathogenesis as well as the prognosis of patients with MDS. Therefore, a unique subgroup of MDS was defined, using the term 5q-syndrome. This syndrome is characterized by an older female predominance (median age, 65–70 years), with blood counts demonstrating an isolated macrocytic anemia along with a normal or elevated platelet count (14,15). The BM typically displays micromegakaryocytes with monolobated and bilobated nuclei together with a low myeloid blast count. Cytogenetics demonstrate an isolated interstitial deletion of variable length on the long arm of chromosome 5, most often del(5)(q13q33), with nearly all cases lacking a 1.5-Mb segment extending from bands 5q31 to 5q32.3. Thus, the diagnosis is based on a compilation of morphological and cytogenetic information. Because of the normal neutrophil and platelet counts seen in most patients, there is a low incidence of infection and bleeding, but RBC transfusions are frequently needed. The disease typically has an indolent course, with few cases of progression to AML and a reported median survival of 63 months. Subsequent work identified *RPS14*, a protein required for the function of the 40S ribosomal complex, as a critical player in the pathogenesis of this syndrome, but haploinsufficiency of 2 microRNAs (miRNAs), miR-145 and miR-146a, may also be involved (16).

During an early phase clinical trial with lenalidomide (Revlimid; Celgene) in patients with MDS who did not respond to ESAs, clinicians observed that 10 of 12 patients with the 5q deletion no longer needed red cell transfusions and had a complete or partial cytogenetic response. A subsequent phase II study (MDS-003) involving 148 low- or Int-1 risk transfusion-dependent patients, demonstrating a chromosome 5q31 deletion that was either isolated or accompanied by additional cytogenetic abnormalities, showed that 67% became transfusion independent and 62% had a complete cytogenetic response (17). Moreover, the median time to transfusion independence was only 4.6 weeks, and the median duration of transfusion independence was not reached. Based on these data, the FDA-approved lenalidomide for IPSS low- or Int-1 risk transfusion-dependent MDS patients with a deletion 5q in isolation or accompanied by additional cytogenetic abnormalities (Figure 32.1). Additional trials in patients with MDS without del(5q) demonstrated an overall response rate of 26%, indicating lower response rates than compared with studies utilizing hypomethylating agents, and it has limited use in patients without del(5q). To date, no studies have demonstrated a survival advantage for patients receiving lenalidomide versus other supportive measures, including patients with the 5q-syndrome.

In summary, E.L. is a prototypical 5q-syndrome patient having an isolated macrocytic anemia, elevated platelet count, low blast percentage, and a karyotype displaying an isolated loss of the distal portion of the long arm of chromosome 5. Although this cytogenetic change is not a perfect predictive marker, therapy using lenalidomide may be optimal in this patient population. However, the goal would be to provide transfusion independence, with no evidence currently indicating an OS advantage.

## High-Risk MDS

B.H. is a 77-year-old man with a history of gout and coronary artery disease with a history of myocardial infarction 5 years ago, but without recurrent angina or heart failure symptoms. He presented to his primary care provider with increasing bruising and fatigue. A CBC with differential demonstrated a WBC of 1.2 K/mm$^3$ (ANC of 0.2 K/mm$^3$), hemoglobin of 7.2 g/dL (MCV 98), and platelet count of 25,000 K/mm$^3$. His EPO level was 922 mU/mL. He was transfused twice with RBCs and platelets over the next month. BM biopsy demonstrated an overall cellularity of 70%, with trilineage dysplasia in a substantial number of myeloid, erythroid, and megakaryocytic precursors. There were 14% myeloid blasts in the aspirate. Cytogenetics demonstrated a complex male karyotype: 46,XY,del(13)(q12q22)[14]/50,sl,+8,+9,+13,del(13)(q12q22),+14[6].

## Evidence-Based Case Discussion

Unlike their lower-risk counterparts, patients with higher-risk MDS (IPSS Int-2 and high-risk) have shorter latency periods for transformation to AML and a median survival measured in months. Therefore, the focus of therapy is not only in improving symptoms but also in prolonging survival. As previously discussed, BM transplantation remains the only curative option in MDS. Due to the increased risk of therapy-related morbidity and mortality with increased age, allogeneic hematopoietic stem cell transplantation (alloHSCT) use has been restricted to those patients with higher-risk MDS who are under the age of 70–75 years (Figure 32.1) (18). Because the average MDS patients are typically in their 70s, the majority of patients will not be transplant eligible due to age, underlying comorbidities, and limited sibling donor options. Thus, alternative therapy options are desperately needed.

Both azacitidine (Vidaza; Celgene) and decitabine (Dacogen; Eisai) are agents that are thought to alter gene expression through inhibition of DNA methylation, although they may also demonstrate cytotoxic capacity through incorporation into DNA and RNA, resulting in strand cessation. Azacitidine was recently compared with ...tional care options (transfusions alone, low-dose

cytarabine, or induction chemotherapy) in a randomized phase III clinical trial (19). Restricted to those with IPSS Int-2 or high-risk MDS and FAB-defined refractory anemia with excess blasts, refractory anemia with excess blasts in transformation (AML per WHO), or type II CMML, patients randomized to receive azacitidine had an improved median survival of 24.5 versus 15 months in the conventional care arms. The survival benefit held for most subgroups, including those with high-risk disease, age >75 years, poor-risk karyotype, as well as patients only achieving hematological improvement rather than a morphological remission. Notably, the median number of cycles of therapy received was 9 and there was no limit on the total number of treatment cycles, as long as the patient was tolerating the therapy. Prior studies had reported that a median of 4 cycles of azacitidine were needed for a response, and 80% of responses occur by the eighth cycle. Cytopenias are common during the initial cycles of treatment, and patients should be counseled that transfusion support is often required during this time. Decitabine has also been evaluated in a number of phase II as well as a registration phase III clinical trial, but demonstrated no evidence of improved survival compared with BSC (20). However, patients received on an average only 3 cycles of therapy in the pivotal trial. The European Organization for Research and Treatment of Cancer (EORTC) also compared the outcome of patients receiving decitabine versus BSC (21). Importantly, patients could only receive 2 cycles past a complete remission and the maximum number of cycles was 8, with patients receiving on average only 4 cycles of therapy. Again, there was no survival difference between the decitabine-treated patients and those receiving BSC.

Although alloHSCT remains the only curative option for patients with MDS, treatment-related toxicities make this approach challenging, particularly given the older age of MDS patients. Retrospective evaluation of allogeneic transplant in low-risk MDS patients (IPSS-low or Int-1) demonstrated a superior OS for those receiving BSC instead of transplant, likely secondary to the low rate of disease progression in those patients receiving supportive care alone (18). In 2010, the Centers for Medicare and Medicaid Services (CMS) stated that there was insufficient evidence that the use of alloHSCT improves health outcomes in Medicare beneficiaries with MDS. They are currently restricting its use through the act through coverage with evidence development (CED) to patients participating in an approved clinical study addressing the long-term effectiveness of transplant in MDS. However, most private insurers continue to cover allogeneic transplant for patients with advanced MDS. For the cohort of patients that are refractory to or relapse after ESA use, other treatment options to consider are hypomethylating agents, although there are no good data to demonstrate a survival benefit in low-risk MDS patients. Reduced-intensity conditioning (RIC) regimens may limit organ toxicities in older patients, but these benefits may be offset by higher relapse rates (22). There have been nonrandomized reports on the benefit of the use of the hypomethylating agents azacitidine or decitabine either prior to or after allogeneic transplant, and therefore, their associated use remains an active area of investigation (23). To date, no prospective trial has demonstrated a benefit of utilizing a hypomethylating agent to reduce the blast percentage prior to an alloHSCT.

Alternatively, immunosuppressive therapy may be considered for a subgroup of patients with specific characteristics of their MDS, including younger patients with hypocellular BMs (hypocellular MDS), low- or Int-1 risk disease (especially normal cytogenetics), a shorter duration of red cell transfusion dependence, presence of PNH-positive cells, and the presence of an HLA-DR15 (DR2) haplotype (Figure 32.1) (24). Prior therapies employing cyclosporine alone or in combination with antithymocyte globulin in these patients have demonstrated hematological improvement in 30–70% of patients, with relatively good durability in those responding to therapy (25).

In summary, B.H. presents with advanced MDS, with an IPSS score of 3—high risk (1.5 for blast percentage, 1 for karyotype, and 0.5 for cytopenias), and thus has an anticipated median survival of only 0.4 months in the absence of therapy. His advanced age precludes the current use of alloHSCT, and his age in combination with the hypercellular marrow and the complex karyotype makes immunosuppressive therapy a poor choice. His elevated EPO level and transfusion requirements would predict only a 7% chance of responding to an ESA. Options in this case should focus on supportive care, either alone or concurrent with the use of either azacitidine or decitabine, with the potential aim of decreasing transfusion dependency as well as delaying transformation to AML and improving OS. If he were younger without significant comorbidities, consideration for alloHSCT should be incorporated into his treatment plan as early as possible.

## REVIEW QUESTIONS

1. A 74-year-old gentleman presents with increasing fatigue and shortness of breath. A complete blood count showed a macrocytic anemia, with hemoglobin at 8.1 g/dL (mean corpuscular volume 105), normal white blood cell count and absolute neutrophil count, and platelet count of 550 K/mm³. Erythropoietin (EPO) level was 560 mU/mL. Vitamin B12 and folate levels were normal. There was no history of alcohol abuse and no evidence of gastrointestinal blood loss. A bone marrow biopsy showed overall cellularity of 80% with 2% blasts in the aspirate. Karyotypic analysis demonstrated the following male karyotype: 46, XY, del(5q)(q13q33) in all 20 cells. What is the most appropriate step in his initial management?

   (A) Start treatment with EPO
   (B) Initiate treatment with lenalidomide
   (C) Observation
   (D) Intermittent transfusion therapy

2. A 45-year-old gentleman was treated for Hodgkin lymphoma with 6 cycles of adriamycin, bleomycin, vinblastine, dacarbazine 2 years ago and now presents with anemia. Myelodysplastic syndrome has been most strongly associated with prior exposure to which of the following type of chemotherapy agents?

   (A) Antimetabolites, vinca alkaloids
   (B) Taxanes, anthracyclines
   (C) Alkylators, topoisomerase II inhibitors
   (D) Platinum agents, hypomethylating agents 3

3. A 79-year-old woman with a history of hypertension, diabetes, and gastroesophageal reflux disease presented after developing shortness of breath when walking up stairs. Physical examination revealed pallor and scattered ecchymosis. Complete blood count showed hemoglobin 6.6 g/dL, mean corpuscular volume 103 fL, white blood cell count 1.9 K/mm³ with 10% neutrophils, 1% circulating blasts, and a platelet count of 27 K/mm³. The reticulocyte count was 0.5%. Vitamin B12 and folate levels were normal. Erythropoietin level was 570 mU/mL. Her bone marrow aspirate and biopsy demonstrated an overall cellularity of 35% with trilineage dysplasia. Nine percent blasts were seen on the aspirate smear. An abnormal female karyotype revealed the following changes: 47,XX,+11[10]/48,sl,+8[5]/46, sl, −7[3]/46,XX[2]. She was given 2 units of red blood cells for her symptomatic anemia. What is the most appropriate initial treatment for this patient?

   (A) Azacitidine
   (B) Lenalidomide
   (C) Referral for hematopoietic stem cell transplant
   (D) Low-dose cytarabine

4. A 64-year-old gentleman presented with increased fatigue. A complete blood count showed a hemoglobin of 7.1 g/dL, white blood cell count of 4 K/mm³ with normal differential, and platelet count of 115 K/mm³. A bone marrow aspiration and biopsy showed a 70% overall cellularity with trilineage dysplasia in >20% of the erythroid and megakaryocytic progenitor cells. The aspirate smear revealed 4% myeloid blasts. Cytogenetics showed a normal karyotype. Folate, vitamin B12, and iron levels were within normal limits. An erythropoietin (EPO) level was 28 mU/mL. A blood transfusion was given for symptomatic anemia and an EPO-stimulating agent (ESA) was ordered. According to the Hellström–Lindberg score, this patient would have which of the following estimated response rate to an ESA?

(A) 50%

(B) 74%

(C) 33%

(D) 25%

5. A 54-year-old woman presents after a routine complete blood count performed at her primary care physician's office demonstrated a hemoglobin of 11.1 g/dL, white blood cell count of 3.6 K/mm³ with normal differential, and platelet count of 155 K/mm³. Folate, vitamin B12, and iron levels were within normal limits. Bone marrow aspiration and biopsy showed 50% overall cellularity and no evidence of dysplasia. The aspirate smear revealed 1.2% myeloid blasts. Which of the following tests, if abnormal, would establish a diagnosis of myelodysplastic syndrome despite the normal morphology and blast percentage?

(A) *JAK2* V617F mutation

(B) −5 or del(5q) seen on a karyotype

(C) *ASXL1* mutation

(D) +8 seen on a karyotype

6. Which of the following has been identified as a predictive factor for hematological response in patients receiving a hypomethylating agent for intermediate II risk myelodysplastic syndrome?

(A) del (5q) seen on a karyotype

(B) +8 seen on a karyotype

(C) A *TET2* mutation combined with an MLL partial tandem duplication (PTD)

(D) None of the above

## REFERENCES

1. Ma X, Does M, Raza A, Mayne ST. Myelodysplastic syndromes: incidence and survival in the United States. *Cancer.* 2007;109(8):1536–1542.

2. Holme H, Hossain U, Kirwan M, et al. Marked genetic heterogeneity in familial myelodysplasia/acute myeloid leukaemia. *Br J Haematol.* 2012;158(2):242–248.

3. Vardiman JW, Thiele J, Arber DA, et al. The 2008 revision of the World Health Organization (WHO) classification of myeloid neoplasms and acute leukemia: rationale and important changes. *Blood.* 2009;114(5):937–951.

4. Malcovati L, Hellström-Lindberg E, Bowen D, et al.; European Leukemia Net. Diagnosis and treatment of primary myelodysplastic syndromes in adults: recommendations from the European LeukemiaNet. *Blood.* 2013;122(17):2943–2964.

5. Vardiman JW, Harris NL, Brunning RD. The World Health Organization (WHO) classification of the myeloid neoplasms. *Blood.* 2002;100(7):2292–2302.

6. Greenberg P, Cox C, LeBeau MM, et al. International scoring system for evaluating prognosis in myelodysplastic syndromes. *Blood.* 1997;89(6):2079–2088.

7. Bejar R. Prognostic models in myelodysplastic syndromes. *Hematology Am Soc Hematol Educ Program.* 2013;2013:504–510.

8. Greenberg PL, Tuechler H, Schanz J, et al. Revised international prognostic scoring system for myelodysplastic syndromes. *Blood.* 2012;120(12):2454–2465.

9. Malcovati L, Germing U, Kuendgen A, et al. Time-dependent prognostic scoring system for predicting survival and leukemic evolution in myelodysplastic syndromes. *J Clin Oncol.* 2007;25(23):3503–3510.

10. Kantarjian H, O'Brien S, Ravandi F, et al. Proposal for a new risk model in myelodysplastic syndrome that accounts for events not considered in the original International Prognostic Scoring System. *Cancer.* 2008;113(6):1351–1361.

11. Hellström-Lindberg E, Negrin R, Stein R, et al. Erythroid response to treatment with G-CSF plus erythropoietin for the anaemia of patients with myelodysplastic syndromes: proposal for a predictive model. *Br J Haematol.* 1997;99(2):344–351.

12. Greenberg PL, Sun Z, Miller KB, et al. Treatment of myelodysplastic syndrome patients with erythropoietin with or without granulocyte colony-stimulating factor: results of a prospective randomized phase 3 trial by the Eastern Cooperative Oncology Group (E1996). *Blood.* 2009;114(12):2393–2400.

13. Leitch HA. Controversies surrounding iron chelation therapy for MDS. *Blood Rev.* 2011;25(1):17–31.

14. Boultwood J, Lewis S, Wainscoat JS. The 5q-syndrome. *Blood.* 1994;84(10):3253–3260.

15. Bennett JM. World Health Organization classification of the acute leukemias and myelodysplastic syndrome. *Int J Hematol.* 2000;72(2):131–133.

16. Ebert BL, Pretz J, Bosco J, et al. Identification of RPS14 as a 5q- syndrome gene by RNA interference screen. *Nature.* 2008;451(7176):335–339.

17. List A, Dewald G, Bennett J, et al.; Myelodysplastic Syndrome-003 Study Investigators. Lenalidomide in the myelodysplastic syndrome with chromosome 5q deletion. *N Engl J Med.* 2006;355(14):1456–1465.

18. Cutler CS, Lee SJ, Greenberg P, et al. A decision analysis of allogeneic bone marrow transplantation for the myelodysplastic syndromes: delayed transplantation for low-risk myelodysplasia is associated with improved outcome. *Blood.* 2004;104(2):579–585.

19. Fenaux P, Mufti GJ, Hellstrom-Lindberg E, et al.; International Vidaza High-Risk MDS Survival Study Group. Efficacy of azacitidine compared with that of conventional care regimens in the treatment of higher-risk myelodysplastic syndromes: a randomised, open-label, phase III study. *Lancet Oncol.* 2009;10(3):223–232.

20. Kantarjian H, Issa JP, Rosenfeld CS, et al. Decitabine improves patient outcomes in myelodysplastic syndromes: results of a phase III randomized study. *Cancer.* 2006;106(8):1794–1803.

21. WijerMans P, Suciu S, Baila L, et al. Low dose decitabine versus best supportive care in elderly patients with intermediate or high risk MDS not eligible for intensive chemotherapy: final results of the randomized phase III study (06011) of the EORTC leukemia and German MDS study groups. *ASH Annual Meeting Abstracts.* 2008;112(11):226.

22. Martino R, Iacobelli S, Brand R, et al.; Myelodysplastic Syndrome subcommittee of the Chronic Leukemia Working Party of the European Blood and Marrow Transplantation Group. Retrospective comparison of reduced-intensity conditioning and conventional high-dose conditioning for allogeneic hematopoietic stem cell transplantation using HLA-identical sibling donors in myelodysplastic syndromes. *Blood.* 2006;108(3):836–846.

23. de Lima M, Giralt S, Thall PF, et al. Maintenance therapy with low-dose azacitidine after allogeneic hematopoietic stem cell transplantation for recurrent acute myelogenous leukemia or myelodysplastic syndrome: a dose and schedule finding study. *Cancer.* 2010;116(23):5420–5431.

24. Sloand EM, Wu CO, Greenberg P, et al. Factors affecting response and survival in patients with myelodysplasia treated with immunosuppressive therapy. *J Clin Oncol.* 2008;26(15):2505–2511.

25. Molldrem JJ, Leifer E, Bahceci E, et al. Antithymocyte globulin for treatment of the bone marrow failure associated with myelodysplastic syndromes. *Ann Intern Med.* 2002;137(3):156–163.

# Answers

## CHAPTER 1: HEAD AND NECK CANCER

1. **(A)** Primary surgical approach with adjuvant radiation with/without chemotherapy
2. **(C)** Adjuvant chemoradiation
3. **(D)** Cetuximab
4. **(D)** Concurrent chemoradiation
5. **(B)** Human papillomavirus (HPV)
6. **(C)** Carboplatin/5-fluorouracil (5-FU) plus cetuximab
7. **(A)** Chemoradiation with/without adjuvant chemotherapy

## CHAPTER 2: THYROID CANCER

1. **(A)** Nuclear thyroid scan
2. **(E)** C and D
3. **(C)** Offer sorafanib
4. **(B)** *RET*
5. **(D)** Age
6. **(D)** Offer cabozantinib
7. **(A)** Offer hospice

## CHAPTER 3: NON-SMALL-CELL LUNG CANCER

1. **(D)** None of the above
2. **(D)** Concurrent chemotherapy plus radiation therapy
3. **(B)** Erlotinib
4. **(A)** Secondary T790M mutations in EGFR
5. **(D)** Stop afatinib and start carboplatin/paclitaxel
6. **(C)** Stop crizotinib indefinitely
7. **(D)** Start cisplatin/paclitaxel
8. **(A)** Start carboplatin/pemetrexed/bevacizumab for 4–6 cycles and if stable or responding disease, switch to maintenance pemetrexed
9. **(B)** Start erlotinib and refer to palliative care

## CHAPTER 4: SMALL CELL LUNG CANCER

1. **(A)** Two-thirds of patients have hematogenous metastases at time of diagnosis
2. **(B)** Cisplatin plus etoposide for 4 cycles
3. **(C)** Cisplatin plus etoposide for 4 cycles with concurrent thoracic radiotherapy delivered twice daily to a total dose of 45 Gy
4. **(D)** Prophylactic cranial irradiation
5. **(C)** Carboplatin plus etoposide
6. **(E)** Prophylactic cranial irradiation
7. **(B)** Topotecan

## CHAPTER 5: BREAST CANCER

1. **(E)** B plus C
2. **(B)** Adjuvant aromatase inhibitor therapy, with or without radiotherapy
3. **(C)** Adjuvant aromatase inhibitor hormonal therapy
4. **(C)** Neoadjuvant "dose dense" chemotherapy consisting of doxorubicin, cyclophosphamide, and paclitaxel
5. **(A)** Neoadjuvant anastrozole for 4–6 months
6. **(B)** Administer doxorubicin and cyclophosphamide for 4 cycles, followed by weekly paclitaxel for 12 weeks, followed by breast radiotherapy, followed by 5 years of anastrozole
7. **(A)** Systemic hormonal therapy with letrozole
8. **(C)** Cycles of cyclophosphamide, doxorubicin, and 5-fluorouracil; alternating with cycles of docetaxel
9. **(E)** A or B
10. **(B)** Resection of the brain lesion followed by whole-brain radiotherapy
11. **(B)** She should have a mammogram, breast ultrasound, axillary lymph node fine needle aspiration, chest x-ray, labwork, and an abdominal ultrasound

## CHAPTER 6: ESOPHAGEAL CANCER

1. (A) Hypertension
2. (B) HER2 immunohistochemistry
3. (C) Smoking and alcohol use
4. (D) Capecitabine and oxaliplatin
5. (B) Radiation plus cisplatin and fluorouracil
6. (C) Referral for surgical resection with perioperative chemotherapy
7. (D) Radiation plus concurrent fluoropyrimidine-based chemotherapy

## CHAPTER 7: GASTRIC CANCER

1. (C) The incidence of gastric cancer is far greater in Japan, China, and Korea than in North America
2. (D) Vitamin C exposure
3. (B) *E cadherin*
4. (D) Total gastrectomy and lymph node dissection followed by observation
5. (B) Immunohistochemical (IHC) staining for HER2-neu expression
6. (C) Docetaxel, cisplatin, and 5-FU
7. (D) All of the above statements are correct

## CHAPTER 8: PANCREATIC CANCER

1. (B) Combination therapy of 5-fluorouracil (5-FU)/leucovorin plus irinotecan and oxaliplatin (FOLFIRINOX)
2. (B) Clinical trial or gemcitabine/nab-paclitaxel chemotherapy
3. (C) Concurrent chemoradiation followed by systemic chemotherapy
4. (B) Gemcitabine
5. (C) Chemotherapy such as FOLFIRINOX or gemcitabine/nab-paclitaxel
6. (D) A and C
7. (D) Obtain a baseline chromogranin A level, then observe and repeat imaging in a few months
8. (A) Everolimus
9. (C) Cisplatin/etoposide

## CHAPTER 9: NEUROENDOCRINE CANCER

1. (C) Cisplatin and paclitaxel
2. (C) Insulin and glucose

3. (A) Everolimus
4. (D) Perform radical resection of tumor with regional lymphadenectomy
5. (C) Plasma metanephrine
6. (A) Re-exploration and right hemicolectomy
7. (D) Octreotide LAR
8. (D) B and C
9. (A) Cisplatin/etoposide
10. (C) Menin, 11q13

## CHAPTER 10: HEPATOBILIARY CANCERS

1. (D) Dynamic MRI
2. (D) Transarterial chemoembolization
3. (E) Supportive measures
4. (C) Sorafenib
5. (B) Surgical resection
6. (A) Liver transplantation
7. (B) Systemic chemotherapy with cisplatin and gemcitabine

## CHAPTER 11: COLORECTAL CANCER

1. (D) Start FOLFOX chemotherapy
2. (D) Chemotherapy for 3 months followed by consideration for resection of the liver metastasis, 3 more months of chemotherapy, then resection of the primary tumor
3. (D) FOLFIRI/cetuximab
4. (C) Omit the oxaliplatin for now, but consider adding back later if her disease progresses on i5-FU/leucovorin and her neuropathy has improved
5. (E) FOLFOX for 6 months
6. (A) Observation
7. (E) A and B
8. (D) Neoadjuvant radiation with concurrent capecitabine, followed by surgery and adjuvant chemotherapy
9. (C) Endoscopic placement of a rectal stent followed by chemotherapy
10. (D) APC
11. (E) A and B
12. (B) Colonoscopy now, then again in 3 years if no advanced adenoma or cancer, then every 5 years if no advanced adenoma or cancer

## CHAPTER 12: ANAL CANCER

1. **(E)** All of the above
2. **(C)** Concurrent chemoradiation therapy
3. **(B)** Begin surveillance with periodic DRE, anoscopy, and annual CT scans
4. **(D)** Surgical (abdominoperitoneal) resection
5. **(D)** Cisplatin plus 5-FU

## CHAPTER 13: PROSTATE CANCER

1. **(C)** *HOXB13* mutation
2. **(E)** Watchful waiting
3. **(B)** Adjuvant RT
4. **(A)** Testosterone level
5. **(B)** Enzalutamide
6. **(A)** The patient should have continuous ADT until disease progression
7. **(F)** All of the above

## CHAPTER 14: TESTICULAR CANCER

1. **(D)** Surveillance or RPLND is a reasonable option at this point
2. **(D)** BEP × 3 cycles or EP × 4 cycles and removal of undescended testicle
3. **(D)** EP × 2 cycles
4. **(B)** RPLND and resection of lung lesion
5. **(A)** FISH analysis frequently reveals an isochromosome i(12p)
6. **(C)** Obtain a second pathology consultation
7. **(D)** Adjuvant radiation
8. **(A)** BEP × 4 cycles
9. **(C)** Repeat tumor markers
10. **(C)** Etoposide, ifosfamide, cisplatin × 4 cycles
11. **(B)** Paclitaxel, ifosfamide, cisplatin
12. **(D)** Surveillance
13. **(B)** Because some of the chemotherapy agents in first-line regimens for testicular cancer have blood–brain barrier penetrance, it may be reasonable to manage brain metastases with systemic chemotherapy, particularly in chemotherapy-naïve-patients with limited CNS compromise

## CHAPTER 15: KIDNEY CANCER

1. **(D)** Continue sunitinib and evaluate thyroid function
2. **(E)** Initiate pazopanib, 800 mg by mouth every day
3. **(C)** Referral to urology for surgical resection of kidney mass
4. **(D)** Observation
5. **(C)** Smoking and obesity have been associated with an increased risk of kidney cancer
6. **(C)** Temsirolimus

## CHAPTER 16: BLADDER CANCER

1. **(E)** Female gender
2. **(B)** Schedule the patient to have repeat cystoscopy under anesthesia with transurethral resection of the bladder tumor and complete resection of the bladder mass
3. **(B)** Administration of adjuvant intravesical bacillus Calmette–Guerin in conjunction with surveillance cystoscopy every 3–6 months
4. **(D)** Cystectomy
5. False
6. **(B)** Administration of neoadjuvant chemotherapy followed by radical cystectomy or definitive radiotherapy
7. **(A)** Aggressive TUR of the tumor followed by administration of concurrent chemotherapy and radiation therapy

## CHAPTER 17: CERVICAL CANCER

1. **(A)** Starting an exercise and weight loss regimen
2. **(D)** Radical trachelectomy with pelvic lymph node dissection and possible para-aortic lymph node sampling
3. **(D)** Pelvic radiation therapy with or without concurrent cisplatin sensitization
4. **(B)** Carboplatin, paclitaxel, and bevacizumab
5. **(C)** Cancel surgery and refer her to radiation oncologist to proceed with concurrent pelvic radiation therapy with cisplatin sensitization
6. **(C)** Close surveillance with routine Pap smears

## CHAPTER 18: UTERINE CANCER

1. **(D)** Omentectomy
2. **(B)** Disease confined to the endometrial cavity
3. **(C)** Time interval between antecedent pregnancy and diagnosis of GTD
4. **(C)** African American race
5. **(A)** Endometrial biopsy
6. **(B)** TAH and BSO
7. **(D)** Vaginal brachytherapy
8. **(B)** Chemotherapy

## CHAPTER 19: OVARIAN CANCER

1. **(C)** Observation
2. **(C)** Three to six cycles Q3 weekly IV carboplatin/ paclitaxel
3. **(A)** Six cycles of IP cisplatin and IV/IP paclitaxel
4. **(D)** Six cycles of every 3 week IV carboplatin/ paclitaxel
5. **(B)** Ms. V. does meet criteria for genetic testing, given her personal history of ovarian cancer
6. **(A)** Start every 4 week IV pegylated liposomal doxorubicin
7. **(B)** Three to six cycles of every 3 week IV carboplatin/ paclitaxel

## CHAPTER 20: MELANOMA

1. **(C)** MRI of the brain
2. **(C)** Autoimmune lymphocytic hypophysitis
3. **(B)** Wide local excision with a 1-cm margin
4. **(D)** *BRAF*
5. **(A)** Improvement in disease-free survival at 7 years
6. **(C)** 20–25%

## CHAPTER 21: BONE SARCOMA

1. **(B)** Bone scan and CT chest
2. **(B)** Chemotherapy alternating vincristine, cyclophosphamide, and doxorubicin with ifosfamide and etoposide
3. **(C)** Absence of constitutional symptoms
4. **(C)** Methotrexate, cisplatin, and doxorubicin
5. **(A)** Osteosarcoma
6. **(C)** Denosumab
7. **(B)** Hypocalcemia

## CHAPTER 22: SOFT TISSUE SARCOMA

1. **(C)** Combination chemotherapy with doxorubicin and ifosfamide
2. **(A)** Hemorrhagic cystitis secondary to ifosfamide toxicity
3. **(D)** Resection of the primary mass and evaluation for wedge resection of the right upper lobe
4. **(C)** Increase dose of imatinib to 400-mg BID
5. **(B)** Imatinib starting at 400-mg daily
6. **(A)** Increased chance of postoperative infection

7. **(A)** Continue HAART therapy and continue to observe lesions
8. **(D)** Age of patient
9. **(C)** Studies have shown improved OS for the combination of doxorubicin and ifosfamide compared to single-agent therapy

## CHAPTER 23: PRIMARY BRAIN TUMORS

1. **(C)** After a 4-week break from end of chemoradiation, start temozolomide 150 mg/m² daily for 5 days per 28-day cycle
2. **(B)** 60 Gy radiation therapy followed by adjuvant procarbazine, CCNU, and vincristine (PCV) chemotherapy
3. **(C)** Start bevacizumab
4. **(B)** Patients with MGMT methylation have an improved survival but knowledge of its status will not change management for this patient
5. **(C)** Concurrent chemoradiation with temozolomide 75 mg/m² daily with radiation 60 Gy followed by temozolomide 150–200 mg/m² for 5 days every 28 days for at least 6 cycles
6. **(B)** Hypofractionated radiotherapy or temozolomide alone
7. **(C)** Reoperation to verify pathology, and reinitiate treatment with temozolomide
8. **(D)** Treatment with temozolomide, on the 5-day regimen every 28 days
9. **(A)** Radiation with concomitant temozolomide followed by adjuvant temozolomide (Stupp regimen)

## CHAPTER 24: CANCER OF UNKNOWN PRIMARY

1. **(B)** Colon carcinoma
2. **(D)** Extragonadal germ cell tumor
3. **(D)** Breast carcinoma
4. **(D)** Mucinous ovarian carcinoma
5. **(C)** Small cell carcinoma of the lung
6. **(B)** 55-year-old man with adenocarcinoma with multiple metastases involving liver, lung, and bone
7. **(C)** Surgery–radiotherapy
8. **(A)** Platinum-based chemotherapy
9. **(C)** A CT of the chest
10. **(C)** βhCG
11. **(C)** Breast MRI
12. **(C)** PSA

## CHAPTER 25: HODGKIN LYMPHOMA

1. (C) Its age incidence has a bimodal pattern of distribution
2. (A) Two cycles ABVD + 20-Gy ISRT
3. (B) Four to six cycles ABVD + 30-Gy ISRT
4. (D) Eight cycles of ABVD alone
5. (D) High-dose chemotherapy followed by ASCT
6. (B) It has a higher risk of transformation to non-Hodgkin lymphoma compared to CHL
7. (A) 30-Gy ISRT alone

## CHAPTER 26: NON-HODGKIN LYMPHOMA

1. (C) Entecavir prophylaxis
2. (B) *myc*
3. (A) Surveillance only
4. (D) Biopsy of the axillary mass
5. (A) Systemic treatment with high-dose methotrexate 3.5 g/m$^2$ body surface area backbone
6. (D) Two cycles of R-ICE chemotherapy, if in remission then proceed with high-dose chemotherapy with autologous stem cell rescue
7. (E) Bendamustine with rituximab therapy only followed by observation
8. (A) t(8;14)
9. (D) Urease breath test or stool antigen for *H. pylori*

## CHAPTER 27: MULTIPLE MYELOMA

1. (C) del17p
2. (B) MGUS
3. (B) Induction therapy with lenalidomide and dexamethasone, then proceed to repeat ASCT
4. (B) Thalidomide
5. (D) Bortezomib/cyclophosphamide/dexamethasone
6. (D) Start acyclovir for prevention of varicella zoster reactivation
7. (E) Risk of thalidomide neuropathy increases with the duration of maintenance therapy
8. (B) Bortezomib/dexamethasone

## CHAPTER 28: ACUTE LYMPHOBLASTIC LEUKEMIA

1. (D) Detection of *ETV6–RUNX1 (TEL–AML1)* fusion transcripts
2. (B) Pre-B ALL

3. (E) Peg-asparaginase associated pancreatitis
4. (C) Continue dasatinib
5. (B) TPMT
6. (C) Ponatinib

## CHAPTER 29: ACUTE MYELOGENOUS LEUKEMIA

1. (A) Decitabine
2. (D) Standard induction/consolidation followed by allogeneic stem cell transplant
3. (D) Clofarabine plus cytarabine-containing regimen followed by allogeneic stem cell transplantation
4. (A) ATO plus ATRA
5. (A) Standard induction with 7 + 3 (cytarabine plus danorubicin)
6. (C) Proceed with discontinuation of HiDAC
7. (C) Leukapheresis
8. (A) Initiate FLAG plus IDA followed by allogeneic stem cell transplantation

## CHAPTER 30: CHRONIC MYELOID LEUKEMIA

1. (G) A, B, or C
2. (C) TKI indefinitely
3. (C) Nilotinib
4. (A) Continue imatinib at current dose
5. (F) A, B, C
6. (A) Dasatinib
7. (B) Ponatinib
8. (C) Any tyrosine kinase inhibitor plus chemotherapy followed by allogeneic stem cell transplantation (ASCT)

## CHAPTER 31: CHRONIC LYMPHOCYTIC LEUKEMIA

1. (C) Small lymphocytic leukemia
2. (E) Observation
3. (B) Bone marrow biopsy, polymerase chain reaction for parvovirus B19, Epstein–Barr virus, and cytomegalovirus
4. (A) Fludarabine, cyclophosphamide, and rituximab
5. (C) Chlorambucil plus obinutuzumab
6. (B) Chlorambucil followed by reduced intensity ASCT
7. (A) Chemoimmunotherapy followed by reduced intensity allogeneic stem cell transplantation

8. **(D)** Herpes simplex virus and pneumocystis pneumonia

9. **(B)** Albumin

10. **(C)** Ibrutinib

2. **(C)** Alkylators, topoisomerase II inhibitors

3. **(A)** Azacitidine

4. **(B)** 74%

5. **(B)** −5 or del(5q) seen on a karyotype

6. **(D)** None of the above

## CHAPTER 32: MYELODYSPLASTIC SYNDROME

1. **(B)** Initiate treatment with lenalidomide

# Index

Note: Page numbers followed by "*f*" and "*t*" denote figures and tables, respectively.

Printed in the United States
By Bookmasters